Essential Revision Notes
in Paediatrics
for the MRCPCH

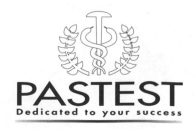

PASTEST
Dedicated to your success

Acknowledgements

The publisher wishes to thank the following publishers for their kind permission to reproduce or amend and reproduce various images in this book.

Page 6: LifeART, Lippincott Williams & Wilkins 2002. Pages 517 and 518: figures produced by Professor G Haycock, reproduced courtesy of The British Journal of Urology, Vol 81, supplement 2, p33-38, Blackwell Scientific, April 1998. Page 555: Pediatrics, Vol. 67, Page(s) 396, Figure 2, Copyright 1981. Page 522: Clinical Paediatric Physiology, Godfrey S and Baum JD, Blackwell Scientific, 1979. Page 538: Paediatric Nephrology third edition, Holliday, Barrett and Avner, Lippincott Williams and Wilkins, 1994. Page 626 top: Paediatric Ophthalmology second edition, Taylor D, Blackwell Scientific 1997. Pages 626 bottom and 661: Slide Atlas of Paediatric Physical Diagnosis, second edition, Eds: Zitelli, B and Davis, HW, Gower Medical Publishing, 1992. Page 637 Clinical Ophthalmology by Kanski. Reprinted by permission of Elsevier Science Limited.

Essential Revision Notes in Paediatrics for the MRCPCH

edited by

Mark Beattie BSc MBBS MRCP FRCPCH
Consultant Paediatric Gastroenterologist
Paediatric Medical Unit
Southampton General Hospital
Southampton

Mike Champion BSc MBBS MRCP MRCPCH
Consultant in Paediatric Metabolic Medicine
Department of Paediatric Metabolic Medicine
Guy's Hospital
London

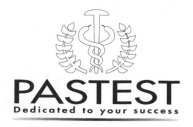

PASTEST
Dedicated to your success

© 2002 PasTest Ltd
Egerton Court
Parkgate Estate
Knutsford
Cheshire WA16 8DX

Telephone: 01565 752000

First edition 2002
Reprinted 2003

ISBN: 1 901198 64 2

A catalogue record for this book is available from the British Library.

The information contained within this book was obtained by the authors from reliable sources. However, while every effort has been made to ensure its accuracy, no responsibility for loss, damage or injury occasioned to any person acting or refraining from action as a result of information contained herein can be accepted by the publisher or the authors.

PasTest Revision Books and Intensive Courses

PasTest has been established in the field of postgraduate medical education since 1972, providing revision books and intensive study courses for doctors preparing for their professional examinations. Books and courses are available for the following specialties:

MRCGP, MRCP Part 1 and Part 2, MRCPCH Part 1 and Part 2, MRCOG, DRCOG, MRCS, MRCPsych, DCH, FRCA and PLAB.

For further details contact:

PasTest Ltd, Freepost, Knutsford, Cheshire, WA16 7BR

Tel: 01565 752000   **Fax: 01565 650264**
Email: enquiries@pastest.co.uk   **Web site:** www.pastest.co.uk

Typeset by Saxon Graphics Ltd
Printed and bound in Europe by the Alden Group

Contents

Contributors

Mark Beattie BSc MBBS MRCP FRCPCH
Consultant Paediatric Gastroenterologist
Paediatric Medical Unit
Southampton General Hospital
Southampton

Michael L Capra MBBCH DCH Dip.Obst MRCP MMedSci (Clinical education)
Clinical Fellow
Department of Haematology/Oncology
Hospital for Sick Children
Toronto
Canada

Mike Champion BSc MBBS MRCP MRCPCH
Consultant in Paediatric Metabolic Medicine
Department of Paediatric Metabolic Medicine
Guy's Hospital
London

Ruth M Charlton MBBS MRCP MRCPCH
Consultant Paediatrician
Paediatric Department
Epsom & St. Helier NHS Trust
Epsom
Surrey

Jane C Davies MBChB MRCP MD
Honorary Consultant
Dept of Paediatric Respiratory Medicine
Royal Brompton Hospital
London

Katy Fidler BSc MBBS MRCPCH
Clinical Research Fellow in Paediatric Infectious Diseases
Department of Infectious Diseases and Microbiology
Institute of Child Health
London

Grenville F Fox MBChB MRCP FRCPCH
Consultant Neonatologist
Department of Neonatology
Guy's and St. Thomas' Hospital
London

Bobby Gaspar BSc MBBS MRCP PhD MRCPCH
Senior Lecturer and Consultant in Paediatric Immunology
Molecular Immunology Unit
Institute of Child Health
University College London
London

Helen M Goodyear MBChB MRCP FRCPCH MD DipMedEd
Consultant Paediatrician and Associate Postgraduate Dean
Birmingham Heartlands and Solihull NHS Trust
Department of Child Health
Birmingham

Nathan Hasson MBChB FRCPCH
Honorary Consultant in Paediatric Rheumatology
Great Ormond Street Hospital for Sick Children
London

Majeed H Jawad MBChB FRCP FRCPCH DCH
Consultant Paediatrician
East Surrey Hospital
Redhill
Surrey

Nigel Klein BSc MBBS MRCP FRCPCH PhD
Reader/Honorary Consultant in Paediatric ID and Immunology
Department of Infectious Diseases and Microbiology
Institute of Child Health
London

Heather Mitchell BM.BCh MA MRCP MRCPCH MRCGP DCH DRCOG
SpR in Paediatric Endocrinology
Department of Paediatric Endocrinology
University College London Hospitals
London

Vasanta R Nanduri MBBS DCH MRCP MRCPCH
Consultant Paediatrician
Department of Paediatrics
Watford General Hospital
Watford
Hertfordshire

Joanne Philpot BA MBBS DCH MRCPCH
Consultant Paediatrician
Paediatric Department
Frimley Park Hospital
Frimley
Surrey

Waseem Qasim BMedSci MB BS MRCPCH
Clinical Research Fellow in Immunology
Molecular Immunology Unit
Institute of Child Health
University College London
London

Christopher J D Reid MB ChB MRCP(UK) FRCPCH
Consultant Paediatric Nephrologist
Department of Paediatric Nephrology and Urology
Guy's Hospital,
London

Neil H Thomas MA MB BChir FRCP FRCPCH DCH
Consultant Paediatric Neurologist
Department of Paediatric Neurology
Southampton University Hospitals NHS Trust
Southampton General Hospital
Southampton

Stephen R Tomlin MRPharmS
Principal Paediatric Pharmacist
Pharmacy Department
Guy's and St. Thomas' Hospitals NHS Trust
Guy's Hospital
London

Robert M R Tulloh BM BCh MA DM MRCP FRCPCH
Consultant Paediatric Cardiologist
Department of Congenital Heart Disease
Guy's and St Thomas' Hospital NHS Trust
London

Angie M Wade MSc PhD CSTAT ILTM
Senior Lecturer in Medical Statistics
Centre for Epidemiology and Biostatistics
Institute of Child Health
London

Louise C Wilson BSc MBChB FRCP
Consultant in Clinical Genetics
Clinical and Molecular Genetics Unit
Institute of Child Health
London

Robert A Wheeler MS FRCS FRCPCH
Consultant Paediatric and Neonatal Surgeon
Wessex Regional Centre for Paediatric Surgery
Southampton General Hospital
Southampton

Preface

There are numerous question books useful in the preparation for the paediatric membership. The feedback is that it is often the concise and focused summary notes that are the most helpful. This book attempts to bring all that together in one text. We hope prospective candidates will find it useful in the preparation for the exam and subsequently as a reference text.

We have tried to emphasise topics which are of particular relevance to the exam and therefore future practice.

We hope the book will also be useful for GP trainees studying for the DCH and to allied health care professionals who want to broaden their general paediatric knowledge base.

We are indebted to PasTest for their considerable expertise and support, our impressive list of contributors all of whom are experts in their fields and experienced teachers, and the candidates who on many MRCPCH courses by their commitment and enthusiasm for the speciality have provided the inspiration for the book.

Mark Beattie
Mike Champion

Chapter 1

Cardiology

Robert M R Tomlin

CONTENTS

Cardiology

1. DIAGNOSIS OF CONGENITAL HEART DISEASE

1.1 Fetal cardiology

Diagnosis

In South-East England, most children (>70%) who require surgery for congenital heart disease are diagnosed during pregnancy at 16–20 weeks' gestation. This gives significant advantage to the parents who are counselled by specialists. Some undergo termination of pregnancy (depending on the diagnosis). Those who continue with the pregnancy can be offered delivery within the cardiac centre if there could be neonatal complications or if treatment is likely to be needed within the first 2 days of life.

Screening (by a fetal cardiologist) is offered to those with:

- Abnormal 4-chamber view on routine-booking, antenatal-anomaly ultrasound scan
- Increased nuchal translucency (thickness at back of the neck), which also increases the risk of Down's syndrome
- Previous child with or other family history of congenital heart disease (CHD)
- Maternal risk factors, such as phenylketonuria or diabetes
- Suspected Down's or other syndrome

Surgical intervention during fetal life is not yet available.

Important normal findings on fetal echocardiography include echodensities:

- Used to be called 'Golf-balls'
- Found on anterior mitral valve papillary muscle
- Thought to be calcification during development
- No importance for congenital heart disease
- Positive association with Down's syndrome
- Do not need echocardiogram after delivery

Arrhythmias

- Diagnosed at any time during pregnancy: an echocardiogram is required to confirm normal anatomy and to confirm type of arrhythmia. Fetal ECG is not yet a routine investigation.
- Multiple ectopics are usually not treated
- Supraventricular tachycardia is treated with maternal digoxin or flecainide
- Heart block may be treated with maternal isoprenaline or salbutamol
- Presence of hydrops is a poor prognostic sign

1.2 Epidemiology

8:1,000 live births have congenital heart disease of which the commonest are:

- Ventricular septal defect   30%
- Persistent arterial duct   12%
- Atrial septal defect   7%
- Pulmonary stenosis   7%
- Aortic stenosis   5%
- Coarctation of the aorta   5%
- Tetralogy of Fallot   5%
- Transposition of the great arteries   5%
- Atrioventricular septal defect   2%

Incidence increased by a positive family history:

- Previous sibling with CHD   2%
- Two siblings with CHD   4%
- Father with CHD   3%
- Mother with CHD   6%

Incidence increased by presence of other anomaly or syndrome.

1.3 Cardiac anatomy

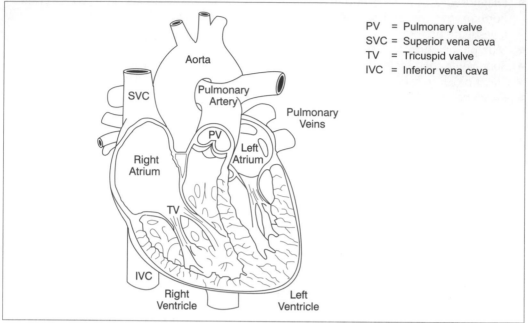

PV = Pulmonary valve
SVC = Superior vena cava
TV = Tricuspid valve
IVC = Inferior vena cava

Normal heart

1.4 Nomenclature for sequential segmental arrangement

The European (as opposed to American) system for complete heart diagnosis is referred to as 'sequential segmental arrangement'. The advantage is that it is no longer necessary to remember the pattern of an eponymous syndrome. The disadvantage is that it is quite long-winded. The idea is that each component is described in turn:

Atrial arrangement (atrial situs)

Usual (solitus)
Mirror image (inversus)
Right isomerism (Asplenia syndrome)
Left isomerism (Polysplenia syndrome)

Atrioventricular (AV) connection

Type of atrioventricular connection
Biventricular	Concordant
	Discordant
	Ambiguous (with atrial isomerism)
Univentricular	Absent left AV connection
	Absent right AV connection
	Double inlet AV connection

Mode of atrioventricular connection

- Two AV valves
- Common AV valve
- Straddling right or left AV valve
- Imperforate right or left AV valve
- Overriding right or left AV valve

Ventricular topology

- Right-hand (normal) or left-hand topology

Ventriculoarterial connection

Type of ventriculoarterial connection

- Concordant
- Discordant
- Double outlet
- Single outlet:
  - Common arterial trunk
  - Solitary arterial trunk
  - With pulmonary atresia
  - With aortic atresia

Mode of ventriculoarterial connection

- Two perforate valves
- Left or right imperforate valve

Infundibular morphology

Arterial relationships

Associated malformations

- Position of heart in the chest — left, right or middle
- Systemic and pulmonary veins
- Atrial septum
- Atrioventricular valves
- Ventricular septum
- Semilunar valves
- Anomalies of great arteries (e.g. double aortic arch)

Surgical or interventional procedures

Acquired or iatrogenic lesions

1.5 Examination Technique

To many candidates the diagnosis of congenital heart disease is daunting. Certainly, if the candidate examines the child, listens to the heart and then tries to make a diagnosis, this will prove difficult. The following system should be used instead.

History

The history-taking is short and to the point. The candidate needs to know:

- Was the child born preterm?
- Are there any cardiac symptoms of:
  - heart failure (breathlessness, poor feeding, failure to thrive, cold hands and feet)
  - cyanosis
  - neonatal collapse
- Is it an asymptomatic heart murmur found on routine examination?
- Is there a syndrome such as Down's?
- Is there any family history of congenital heart disease?
- Did the mother have any illnesses or take any medication during pregnancy?

Examination

- Introduce yourself to mother and patient. Ask if you can examine the child.
- Position child according to age:
  - For a 6-year-old — at an angle of 45 degrees
  - For a toddler — upright on mother's knee
  - For a baby — flat on the bed
- Remove clothes from chest
- Stand back and look for:
  - Dysmorphism
  - Intravenous infusion cannula
  - Obvious cyanosis or scars

Examine for:

Heart failure

'The delivery of oxygen to the peripheral vascular bed is insufficient to meet the metabolic demands of the child.' Usually due to left to right shunt with good heart pump function.

- Breathlessness +/– subcostal or intercostal recession
- Poor peripheral perfusion with cold hands and feet
- A large liver
- A thin, malnourished child (failure to thrive)
- Excessive sweating around the forehead
- Tachycardia
- Never found with ventricular septal defect (VSD) or other left to right shunt in first week of life

- An emergency if found up to 7 days of age implies a duct dependent lesion, e.g. HLMS

Cyanosis

- Mild cyanosis is not visible — use the pulse oximeter

Clubbing

- Visible >6 months old
- First apparent in the thumbs or toes
- Best demonstrated by holding thumbs together, back to back to demonstrate loss of normal nail-bed curvature
- Disappears a few years after corrective surgery

Pulses

- Rate (count for 6 seconds × 10)
- Rhythm (only 'regular' or 'irregular', need ECG for 'sinus rhythm')
- Character at the antecubital fossa with the elbows straight, using the thumbs — on both arms together

Head and neck

- Anaemia — for older children only — ask the patient to look up and examine the conjunctiva (not appropriate in a baby).
- Cyanosis — the tongue should be examined for central cyanosis. If in doubt ask the child to stick out their tongue and ask the mother to do the same. This will detect oxygen saturations of <85%.
- Jugular venous pressure (JVP) — the head is turned towards the candidate so that the other side of the neck (the left side) can be seen with the JVP visible, outlined against the pillows. In a child who is under 4 years, the JVP should not be assessed.
- Carotid thrill — essential part of the examination, midway up the left side of the neck, felt with the thumb, proof of the presence of aortic stenosis.

Precordium

Inspection
- Respiratory rate
- Median sternotomy scar (= open heart surgery — see section 8)
- Lateral thoracotomy scar (Blalock–Taussig (BT) shunt, patent ductus arteriosus (PDA) ligation, pulmonary artery (PA) band, coarctation repair)
- Additional scars, e.g. on the abdomen

Palpation

- Apex beat 'the most inferior and lateral position where the index finger is lifted by the impulse of the heart'. Place fingers along 5th intercostal space of both sides of chest (for dextrocardia) and count down apex position only if patient is lying at 45 degrees.
- Left ventricular heave

9

- Right ventricular heave at the left parasternal border
- Thrills at upper or lower left sternal edge

Auscultation

- Heart sounds and their character
- Additional sounds
- Murmurs, their character, intensity and where they are best heard

Heart sounds

First heart sound is created by closure of the mitral and then tricuspid valves. It is not important for the candidate to comment on the nature of the first heart sound.

Second heart sound, however, is more important, created by closure of first the aortic and then the pulmonary valves.

- Loud pulmonary sound — pulmonary hypertension
- Fixed splitting of second sound. (Usually with inspiration the sounds separate and then come together during expiration.) Listen when sitting up, at the mid-left sternal edge in expiration
  - Atrial septal defect
  - Right bundle-branch block
- Single second sound in transposition of great arteries (TGA) or pulmonary atresia, or hypoplastic left heart syndrome
- Quiet second sound may occur in pulmonary valve stenosis or pulmonary artery band

Additional sounds

Added sounds present may be a normal 3rd or 4th heart sound heard in the neonate or these sounds can be pathological, for example in a 4-year-old with a dilated cardiomyopathy and heart failure. An ejection click is heard at aortic valve opening, after the first heart sound, and is due to a bicuspid aortic valve in most cases.

Murmurs

Before listening for any murmurs, the candidate should have a good idea of the type of congenital heart disease, which is being dealt with. The candidate should know whether the child is blue (and therefore likely to have Fallot's Tetralogy) or is breathless (likely to have a left to right shunt) or has no positive physical findings before auscultation of the murmurs (and therefore more likely to either be normal, have a small left to right shunt or mild obstruction). By the time the murmurs are auscultated, there should only be two or three diseases to choose between, with the stethoscope being used to perform the fine tuning. It is best to start at the apex with the bell, and move to the lower left sternal edge with the diaphragm. Then on to the upper left sternal edge and upper right sternal edge both with the diaphragm. Additional areas can be auscultated, but provide little additional information. Murmurs are graded out of 6 for systolic, 2 = soft, 3 = moderate, 4 = loud with a thrill. Murmurs are graded out of 4 for diastolic, again 2, 3 and 4.

Ejection systolic murmur

Upper sternal edge — implies outflow tract obstruction. Right or left ventricular outflow tract obstruction can occur at valvar (+ ejection click), subvalvar or supravalvar level.

- Upper right sternal edge (carotid thrill) = Aortic stenosis
- Upper left sternal edge (no carotid thrill) = Pulmonary stenosis or atrial septal defect (ASD)
- Mid/lower left sternal edge = Innocent murmur (see below)
- Long harsh systolic murmur + cyanosis = Fallot's tetralogy

Pansystolic murmur

- Left lower sternal edge (+/– thrill) = Ventricular septal defect
- Apex (much less common) = Mitral regurgitation
- Rare at left lower sternal edge (+/– cyanosis) = Tricuspid regurg. (Ebstein)

Continuous murmur

- Left infraclavicular (+/– collapsing pulse) = Persistent arterial duct
- Infraclavicular (+ cyanosis + lateral thoracotomy) = Blalock–Taussig shunt
- Any site (lungs, shoulder, head, hind-quarter) = Arterio venous fistula

Diastolic murmurs

- Unusual in childhood
- Left sternal edge/apex (+/– carotid thrill or ventricular septal defect (VSD)) = Aortic regurgitation
- Median sternotomy (+/– PS murmur) = Fallot's Tetralogy repaired
- Apical (+/– VSD) = Mitral flow/(rarely stenosis)

Listening to the back gives no useful information, but is useful thinking time.

Presentation

Few candidates pay enough attention to the case presentation. This should be done after the examination is complete. The candidate should stand, look the examiner in the eye, put hands behind his/her back and present. The important positives and negatives should be stated quickly and succinctly with no 'umms' or 'errrs'. It is important to judge the mood of the examiner, if he/she is looking bored, then go faster. Practise with a tape recorder or video-recording.

To complete the examination you would:

- Measure the blood pressure
- Measure the oxygen saturation
- Feel the femoral pulses
- Feel the liver edge

The presentation should be rounded off with the phrase 'the findings are consistent with the diagnosis of …'.

Algorithm for clinical examination

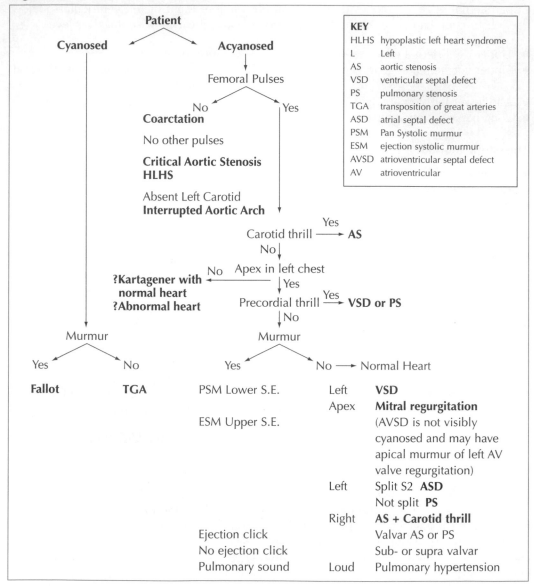

The patient with surgical scars:

Left lateral thoracotomy	PA band	Thrill + ESM at upper left sternal edge
	Coarctation	+/– left brachial pulse
	Shunt	Blue + continuous murmur
	PDA	No signs
Right lateral thoracotomy	Shunt	Blue + continuous murmur
Median sternotomy	Any intracardiac operation	

1.6 Innocent murmurs

The commonest murmur heard in children is the functional, innocent or physiological heart murmur (40% of all children). They are often discovered in children with an intercurrent infection or with anaemia. These all relate to a structurally normal heart but can cause great concern within the family. There are several different types depending on the possible site of their origin. It is clearly important to make a positive diagnosis of a normal heart. The murmur should be:

- **S**oft (no thrill)
- **S**ystolic and short, never pansystolic
- **A**symptomatic
- Left **s**ternal edge

May change with posture.

Innocent murmurs do not require antibiotic prophylaxis.

Diastolic murmurs are not innocent.

An innocent murmur is not associated with abnormal or added heart sounds. Types of innocent murmur include:

- Increased flow across branch pulmonary artery — this is frequently seen in preterm neonates, is a physiological finding and resolves as the pulmonary arteries grow. The murmur disappears after a few weeks of age, and never causes symptoms.
- Still's murmur — this is vibratory in nature and is found at the mid-left sternal edge. It may be caused by turbulence around a muscle band in the left ventricle.
- Venous hum — it may be easy to hear the venous blood flow returning to the heart, especially at the upper sternal edge. This characteristically occurs in both systole and diastole and disappears on lying the child flat.

2. LEFT TO RIGHT SHUNT

(Pink +/– breathless)

General principles

No signs or symptoms on first day of life due to high pulmonary vascular resistance. Later, at 1 week, can develop symptoms of heart failure:

- Tachypnoea
- Poor feeding, failure to thrive
- Cold hands and feet

- Sweating
- Vomiting

Signs of heart failure

- Thin
- Tachypnoea
- Displaced apex
- Dynamic precordium
- Apical diastolic murmur
- Hepatomegaly

2.1 Atrial septal defect (ASD)

Types of defect

- Secundum ASD
- Primum ASD (partial atrioventricular septal defect)
- Sinus venosus ASD
- Other

Secundum ASD

Defect in centre of atrial septum involving fossa ovalis

Clinical features

- Asymptomatic
- 80% of ASDs
- Soft systolic murmur at upper left sternal edge
- Fixed split S2 (difficult to hear)

ECG

- Partial right bundle-branch block (90%)
- Right ventricle hypertrophy

CXR

- Increased pulmonary vascular markings

Management

- Closure at 3–5 years (ideally)
- 70% surgical closure
- 30% device closure in catheter laboratory

Primum ASD (partial atrioventricular septal defect)

Defect in lower atrial septum, involving the left atrioventricular valve which has three leaflets and tends to leak.

Clinical features

- Asymptomatic
- 10% of ASDs
- Soft systolic murmur at upper left sternal edge
- Apical pansystolic murmur (atrioventricular valve regurgitation)
- Fixed split S2 (difficult to hear)

ECG

- Partial right bundle-branch block (90%)
- Right ventricle hypertrophy
- Superior axis

CXR

- Increased pulmonary vascular markings

Management

- Closure at 3–5 years
- 100% surgical closure (due to need to repair valve)

Sinus venosus ASD

Defect at upper end of atrial septum, such that superior vena cava (SVC) overrides the atrial septum. The right pulmonary veins are usually anomalous and drain directly into the SVC or right atrium adding to the left to right shunt.

Clinical features

- Asymptomatic or heart failure
- 5% of ASDs
- Soft systolic murmur at upper left sternal edge
- Fixed split S2 (easily heard)

ECG

- Partial right bundle-branch block
- Right ventricle hypertrophy

CXR

- Increased pulmonary vascular markings
- Cardiomegaly

Management

- Closure at 1–5 years
- 100% surgical closure and repair to anomalous pulmonary veins

There are other rare types of ASD, which are similarly treated.

2.2 Ventricular septal defect

Small defect

Defect anywhere in the ventricular septum (perimembranous or muscular, can be inlet or outlet). Restrictive defects are smaller than the aortic valve. There is no pulmonary hypertension.

Clinical features

- Asymptomatic (80–90%)
- May have a thrill at left lower sternal edge
- Loud pansystolic murmur at lower left sternal edge (the louder the murmur, the smaller the hole)
- Quiet P2

ECG

- Normal

CXR

- Normal

Management

- Review with echocardiography
- Spontaneous closure, but may persist to adult life

Large defect

Defects anywhere in septum. Large defects tend to be the same size or larger than the aortic valve. There is always pulmonary hypertension.

Clinical features

- Symptomatic with heart failure after age 1 week
- 10–20% of VSDs
- Soft or no systolic murmur
- Apical mid-diastolic heart murmur
- Loud P2

ECG

- Biventricular hypertrophy at 2 months (see *ECG*, section 13)

CXR

- Increased pulmonary vascular markings
- Cardiomegaly

Management

- Initial medical therapy, diuretics +/– captopril + added calories

- Surgical closure at 3–5 months

2.3 Persistent ductus arteriosus (PDA)

There is persistence of the duct beyond 1 month after the date the baby should have been born.

Clinical features

- Asymptomatic usually, rarely have heart failure
- Continuous or systolic murmur at left infraclavicular area

ECG

- Usually normal
- If large, have left ventricle volume loading (see *ECG*, section 13)

CXR

- Usually normal
- If large, have increased pulmonary vascular markings

Management

- Closure in cardiac catheter laboratory with coil at 1 year
- If large, surgical ligation age 1–3 months

NB. The presence of an arterial duct in a preterm baby is not congenital heart disease. If a clinical problem, with difficulty getting off the ventilator, or signs of heart failure with bounding pulses, it is usually treated with indomethacin or ibuprofen (<34 weeks). If medical management fails, surgical ligation is undertaken.

2.4 Aortopulmonary window

Defect in the wall between the aorta and pulmonary artery.

Clinical features

- Rare
- Usually develop heart failure
- Continuous murmur as for PDA

ECG

- If large, have left ventricle volume loading (see *ECG*, section 13)

CXR

- If large, have increased pulmonary vascular markings

Management

- If large, surgical ligation age 1–3 months

2.5 Others

There are other rare causes of significant left to right shunt, such as arteriovenous malformation. These are all individually rare. Medical and surgical treatment is similar to large ducts or VSDs.

Summary

Disease	Symptoms	Treatment
ASD	Minimal	Surgery/catheter device at 3–5 years
VSD	None	None (in 80–90% of cases)
	Moderate	Diuretics/captopril/ added calories then review early
	Severe	Surgery at 3–5 months (10–20% cases)
PDA	None	Coil occlusion at cardiac catheter (at 1 yr old)
	Mod/severe	Surgery especially in preterm babies
Others rare (A-P window, etc.)		Surgery at 3–4 months

3. RIGHT TO LEFT SHUNT

(Cyanosed)

General principles

Cyanosis in a newborn can be caused by:

- Cardiac (cyanotic heart disease)
- Respiratory (diaphragmatic hernia, etc.)
- Metabolic (lactic acidosis, etc.)
- Infective (pneumonia, etc.)

Cardiac cases which present on day 1–3 are usually duct-dependent:

- Transposition of great arteries (common)
- Fallot with pulmonary atresia (less common)

- Pulmonary atresia with intact ventricular septum (PA/IVS) (rare)
- Tricuspid atresia or other complex hearts (rare)
- Ebstein's (rare)

Investigations

- CXR (to exclude lung pathology and large 'wall to wall' heart in Ebstein)
- Blood culture (to exclude infection)
- ECG (superior axis in tricuspid atresia)
- Hyperoxia test, 10 min in 100% O_2 + blood gas from right radial arterial line. If PaO_2 >20kPa then it is not cyanotic heart disease — **you must not use a saturation monitor, since this is notoriously inaccurate in the presence of acidosis.**
  (Echo not first line if you are in a hospital without this facility, but should be thought of early on.)

Management

- Resuscitate first
- Ventilate early
- Prostaglandin E_1 or E_2 infusion (5–20 ng/kg per min) (may cause apnoeas)
- Transfer to cardiac centre
- Treat as for specific condition

3.1 Tetralogy of Fallot

Ventricular septal defect + subpulmonary stenosis + overriding aorta + right ventricular hypertrophy (RVH)

Clinical features

- Asymptomatic usually, rarely have severe cyanosis
- Loud, harsh murmur at upper sternal edge day 1
- Do not usually develop heart failure

ECG

- Normal at birth
- RVH when older

CXR

- Usually normal
- If older have upturned apex (boot shaped) + reduced vascular markings

Management

- Blalock–Taussig shunt in newborn if severely cyanosed
- Most have elective repair at 6–9 months

3.2 Transposition of the great arteries

Aorta is connected to the right ventricle, and pulmonary artery is connected to the left ventricle. The blue blood is therefore returned to the body and the pink blood is returned to the lungs. These children have high pulmonary blood flow and are severely cyanosed, unless there is an ASD, PDA or VSD to allow mixing.

Clinical features

- Cyanosed when duct closes
- No murmur usually
- Can be very sick, unless diagnosed antenatally
- May be associated with VSD, coarctation or PS

ECG

- Normal

CXR

- Normal (unusual to detect 'egg-on-side' appearance)
- May have increased pulmonary vascular markings

Management

- Resuscitate as above
- Balloon atrial septostomy at cardiac centre in 20% (via umbilical vein — see *Cardiac Catheterization*, section 15)
- Arterial switch operation before 2 weeks

3.3 Pulmonary atresia

Duct-dependent pulmonary atresia

Clinical features

- Cyanosed when duct closes
- No murmur usually
- Can be very sick, unless diagnosed antenatally
- May have IVS or VSD

ECG

- Normal

CXR

- Normal at birth (unusual to diagnose 'boot-shaped' heart, until much older)
- Decreased pulmonary vascular markings

Management

- Resuscitate as above
- BT shunt inserted surgically
- Radiofrequency perforation of atretic valve — if appropriate

Pulmonary atresia with VSD and collaterals

Collaterals are abnormal arterial connections direct from the aorta to the lung substance.

Clinical features

- Not usually duct-dependent
- No murmur usually
- Usually present with heart failure at 1 month, but may present with cyanosis at any age if collaterals are small

ECG

- Bi-ventricular hypertrophy

CXR

- Boot-shaped heart
- Cardiomegaly
- Increased pulmonary vascular markings if in heart failure, or reduced vascular marking if severely cyanosed

Management

- Diuretics, if in failure
- Further imaging with cardiac catheter or magnetic resonance imaging (MRI)
- Staged surgical repair

3.4 Ebstein anomaly

The tricuspid valve is malformed such that it leaks, and is set further into the right ventricle than normal.

Clinical features

- Cyanosed at birth
- Loud murmur of tricuspid regurgitation
- Can be very sick
- May be associated with maternal lithium ingestion

ECG

- May have a superior axis

CXR

- Massive cardiomegaly (wall to wall heart)
- Reduced pulmonary vascular markings

Management

- Resuscitate as above
- Pulmonary vasodilator therapy (ventilation, oxygen, etc., see section 10)
- Try to avoid surgical shunt insertion, in which case prognosis is poor

3.5 Eisenmenger

This is secondary to a large left to right shunt (usually VSD or AVSD (atrioventricular septal defect) where the pulmonary hypertension leads to pulmonary vascular disease (increased resistance) over many years. Eventually the flow through the defect is reversed (right to left) so the child becomes blue, typically at 15–20 years of age.

Clinical features

- Cyanosed in teenage life
- Uncommon
- Usually secondary to untreated VSD or AVSD
- No murmur usually
- Develop right heart failure eventually

ECG

- Severe RVH + strain

CXR

- Decreased pulmonary vascular markings

Management

- Supportive
- May need diuretic and anticoagulant therapy
- Oxygen at night, consider other therapy (see *Pulmonary hypertension*, section 10)
- Consider heart/lung transplantation

Summary of right to left shunts

Disease	Symptoms	Treatment
Fallot	Loud murmur Minimal cyanosis	Surgery at 6–9 months
TGA (transposition of great arteries)	No murmur Neonatal cyanosis	Septostomy at diagnosis (20%) Arterial switch at <2 weeks
Pulmonary atresia (duct-dependent)	No murmur Neonatal cyanosis	BT shunt or radiofrequency perforation
Pulmonary atresia (VSD + collaterals)	No murmur Heart failure/cyanosis	Staged surgical repair
Ebstein	Loud murmur of tricuspid regurgitation Cardiomegaly	Pulmonary vasodilation (O_2, NO, etc.)
Eisenmenger	Severe cyanosis No murmur, loud P2	Pulmonary vasodilators Diuretics Transplantation

4. MIXED SHUNT

(Blue and breathless)

General principles

- Tend to present either antenatally (most often) or at 2–3 weeks. Symptoms are that of mild cyanosis and heart failure
- Includes most of the complex congenital heart diseases

4.1 Complete atrioventricular septal defects

There is an atrial and ventricular component to the defect, so there is pulmonary hypertension as with a large VSD. There is a common atrioventricular valve with five leaflets, not a separate mitral and tricuspid valve.

Clinical features

- May be cyanosed at birth
- No murmur usually at birth, may develop in first few weeks
- Often present on routine echo screening (neonatal Down's)
- May present with heart failure at 1–2 months

ECG

- Superior axis
- Bi-ventricular hypertrophy at 2 months old

CXR

- Normal at birth
- Increased pulmonary vascular markings and cardiomegaly after 1 month

Management

- Treat increased pulmonary vascular resistance at birth if blue
- Treat as for large VSD if in failure (diuretics, captopril, added calories)
- Surgical repair at 3–5 months

4.2 Tricuspid atresia

There is no tricuspid valve and usually the right ventricle is very small.

Clinical features

- Cyanosed when duct closes if duct-dependent
- No murmur usually
- Can be very well at birth

ECG

- Superior axis
- Absent right ventricular voltages
- Large P wave

CXR

- May have decreased or increased pulmonary vascular markings

Management

- BT shunt inserted surgically if very blue
- PA band if in heart failure
- Hemi-Fontan after 6 months old (see Section 8.2)
- Fontan at 3–5 years old

4.3 Others

There are many other types of complex congenital heart disease.

- Common arterial trunk

- Double inlet left ventricle
- Total or partial anomalous pulmonary venous connection (unobstructed)
- Right or left atrial isomerism +/– dextrocardia

Individually, these are quite rare and their management is variable, depending on the pulmonary blood flow, the sizes of the two ventricles, etc. For further information a larger textbook of congenital heart disease should be consulted.

5. OBSTRUCTION IN THE WELL CHILD

(Neither blue nor breathless)

General principles

- Often present to GP with murmur
- Asymptomatic

5.1 Aortic stenosis

The aortic valve leaflets are fused together, giving a restrictive exit from the left ventricle. There may be two or three aortic leaflets.

Clinical features

- Asymptomatic
- Always have a carotid thrill
- Ejection systolic murmur at upper sternal edge
- May be supravalvar, valvar, (and ejection click) or subvalvar
- Quiet A2 (second heart sound aortic component)

ECG

- Left ventricular hypertrophy

CXR

- Normal

Management

- Review with echocardiography
- Balloon-dilate when gradient reaches 64 mmHg across the valve

5.2 Pulmonary stenosis

The pulmonary valve leaflets are fused together, giving a restrictive exit from the right ventricle.

Clinical features

- Asymptomatic (not cyanosed)
- May have a thrill at upper left sternal edge
- Ejection systolic murmur at upper sternal edge from day 1
- May be supravalvar, valvar, (ejection click) or subvalvar
- Quiet P2

ECG

- Right ventricular hypertrophy

CXR

- Normal

Management

- Review with echocardiography
- Balloon-dilate when gradient reaches 64 mmHg across the valve

5.3 Adult-type coarctation of the aorta

Not duct-dependent, this gradually becomes more severe over many years.

Clinical features

- Rare
- Asymptomatic
- Always have systemic hypertension in the right arm
- Ejection systolic murmur at upper sternal edge
- Collaterals at the back
- Radiofemoral delay

ECG

- Left ventricular hypertrophy

CXR

- Rib-notching
- '3' sign, with a visible notch on the chest X-ray in the descending aorta, where the coarctation is.

Management

- Review with echocardiography
- Stent insertion at cardiac catheter when gradient reaches 64 mmHg, or surgery via a lateral thoracotomy

5.4 Vascular rings and slings

Embryological remnant of aortic arch and pulmonary artery development.

Clinical features

- Often present with stridor
- May have no cardiac signs or symptoms

ECG

- Normal

CXR

- May have lobar emphysema due to bronchial compression

Management

- Diagnose with barium/gastrograffin swallow
- Review with echocardiography
- Additional imaging often required (CT (computed tomography), MRI, angiogram)
- Surgical treatment

6. OBSTRUCTION IN THE SICK NEWBORN

General principles

- Present when duct closes or antenatally
- Often have normal ECG and CXR when first present
- Must feel pulses!!

6.1 Coarctation of the aorta

Duct-dependent narrowing, the ductal tissue encircles the aorta and causes an obstruction when the duct closes.

Clinical features

- Very common diagnosis
- Often diagnosed antenatally

- Should be born in a cardiac centre
- If not detected antenatally, presents sick with absent femoral pulses
- No murmur, usually
- Signs of right heart failure (large liver, low cardiac output)
- May be breathless and severely acidotic
- Associated with VSD and bicuspid aortic valve

ECG

- Normal

CXR

- Normal, or cardiomegaly with heart failure

Management

- Resuscitate
- Commence prostaglandin E_1 or E_2 (5–20 ng/kg per min)
- Ventilate early (prior to transfer to cardiac centre)
- Surgery 24 hours later, usually through a left lateral thoracotomy, to resect the narrow segment, unless the whole aortic arch is small, when the surgery is then performed via a median sternotomy on bypass.

6.2 Hypoplastic left heart syndrome

A spectrum of disorders where the mitral valve, left ventricle and/or the aortic valve are too small to sustain the systemic output.

Clinical features

- Common diagnosis (200–400 born annually in UK)
- Usually diagnosed antenatally
- Should be born in a cardiac centre
- If sick, presents with absent femoral + brachial pulses
- No murmur
- Signs of right heart failure (large liver, low cardiac output)
- May be breathless and severely acidotic
- Anatomy varies from mitral stenosis to mitral and aortic atresia

ECG

- Absent left ventricular forces

CXR

- Normal, or cardiomegaly with heart failure

Management

- Resuscitate
- Commence prostaglandin E_1 or E_2 (5–20 ng/kg per min)
- Ventilate early (prior to transfer to cardiac centre)
- Surgery (*Norwood*, see section 8.3) 3–5 days later

6.3 Critical aortic stenosis

Critical means duct-dependent, i.e. there is not enough flow across the stenotic valve to sustain the cardiac output.

Clinical features

- Rare diagnosis
- Usually diagnosed antenatally
- Should be born in a cardiac centre
- If sick, presents with absent femoral + brachial pulses
- No murmur
- Signs of right heart failure (large liver, low cardiac output)
- May be breathless and severely acidotic
- Poor prognosis

ECG

- Left ventricular hypertrophy

CXR

- Normal, or cardiomegaly with heart failure

Management

- Resuscitate
- Commence prostaglandin E_1 or E_2 (5–20 ng/kg per min)
- Ventilate early (prior to transfer to cardiac centre)
- Balloon dilation 24 hours later, may require cardiac surgery

6.4 Interruption of the aortic arch

A gap in the aortic arch, which may occur at any site from the innominate artery around to the left subclavian artery. It is always duct-dependent.

Clinical features

- Rare diagnosis
- Presents with absent left brachial + femoral pulses
- No murmur
- Heart failure (large liver, low cardiac output)

- Breathless and severely acidotic
- Associated with VSD and bicuspid aortic valve
- Associated with 22q11.2 deletion and Di George syndrome (see section 9.5)

ECG

- Normal

CXR

- Normal, or cardiomegaly with heart failure

Management

- Resuscitate
- Commence Prostaglandin E_1 or E_2 (5–20 ng/kg per min)
- Ventilate early (prior to transfer to cardiac centre)
- Surgery 24 hours later

6.5 Total anomalous pulmonary venous connection

The pulmonary veins have not made the normal connection to the left atrium. Can drain up to innominate vein (supracardiac) drain to the liver (infracardiac) or to the coronary sinus (intracardiac).

Clinical features
- Uncommon diagnosis
- Not a duct-dependent lesion
- If obstructed, presents day 1–7 with cyanosis and collapse
- No murmur
- Signs of right heart failure (large liver, low cardiac output)
- May be breathless and severely acidotic
- May, however present later up to 6 months of age if unobstructed, with murmur or heart failure

ECG
- Normal in neonate
- RVH in older child

CXR

- Normal, or small heart
- 'Snowman in a snowstorm' or 'cottage loaf' due to visible ascending vein and pulmonary venous congestion. Appearance usually develops over a few months.

Management
- Resuscitate
- Ventilate early (prior to transfer to cardiac centre)
- Prostaglandin not effective if obstructed
- Emergency surgery if obstructed

Summary of obstructed hearts

Disease	Symptoms	Treatment
Coarctation	Absent femoral pulses	Surgery at 24 hours
Hypoplastic left heart	+Absent brachial pulses	Norwood 3–5 days
Interrupted aortic arch	+Absent left brachial	Surgery >24 hours
Critical aortic stenosis	+Absent brachial pulses	Balloon >24 hours
Total anomalous pulmonary venous connection	Cyanosed sick if obstructed	Emergency surgery

Overview

Left to right shunt	Right to left shunt	Mixed	Well obstructions	Sick obstructions
VSD	Fallot's	AVSD	AS	TAPVC
ASD			PS	HLHS
PDA	TGA			AS
				CoA
	Eisenmenger			Int Ao Arch

There are other causes in each column, but these are less common and are unlikely to appear in exams.

VSD	=	Pansystolic murmur at LLSE
ASD	=	Ejection systolic murmur at ULSE + fixed split S2
Partial AVSD	=	ASD + apical pansystolic murmur of mitral regurgitation.
PDA	=	Continuous murmur under left clavicle +/– collapsing pulses
Fallot	=	Blue + harsh long systolic murmur at ULSE
TGA	=	No murmur $^2/_3$ have no other abnormality, never in exams
Eisenmenger	=	10-years-old +/– Down's, often no murmurs, loud P2
Complete AVSD	=	Never in exams
AS	=	Ejection systolic murmur at URSE + carotid thrill
PS	=	Ejection systolic murmur at ULSE +/– thrill at ULSE

TAPVC/HLHS/AS/CoA/Interrupted aortic arch

Never in clinical exam, but common in vivas, grey cases, data; present in first few days of life. May see postoperative cases

Key:

AVSD	=	Atrioventricular septal defect
CoA	=	Coarctation
UL/RSE	=	Upper left/right sternal edge
TAPVC	=	Total anomalous pulmonary venous connection
HLHS	=	Hypoplastic left heart syndrome
Int Ao Arch	=	Interrupted aortic arch

7. NON-BYPASS SURGERY FOR CONGENITAL HEART DISEASE

Non-bypass surgery is performed by means of a lateral thoractomy, right or left. The scar is found underneath the right or left arm, the anterior border of the scar tends to end under the axilla and may not be seen from the front of the chest. It is imperative that the arms are lifted and the back inspected as a routine during clinical examination otherwise the scars will be missed.

7.1 Shunt operation

- Right or left modified Blalock–Taussig shunt (RMBTS, LMBTS)
- Modified shunts will mean an intact brachial pulse on that side
- Most likely to be for Tetralogy of Fallot with pulmonary atresia
- If there is no median sternotomy, will still be cyanosed
- Definitive repair will be performed usually by age 18 months

7.2 Coarctation of the aorta repair

- May have absent left brachial pulse (subclavian flap technique) or a normal left brachial pulse
- May have no murmur and normal femoral pulses

7.3 Pulmonary artery band

- Uncommon operation these days
- Usually for complex anatomy which may be palliated in the neonatal period
- The band is often removed at 1–2-years-old
- When present, the child is cyanosed
- There may be a thrill at the upper left sternal edge

7.4 Arterial duct ligation

- Rare except for the ex-preterm neonate
- No murmurs and no abnormal pulses
- Usually not associated with other defects

8. BYPASS SURGERY FOR CONGENITAL HEART DISEASE

Any child who undergoes open cardiac surgery, cardiopulmonary bypass, placement of a central shunt or repair of the proximal aortic arch will need a median sternotomy. Therefore any repair of intracardiac pathology will need to be done via a midline incision.

8.1 Switch operation

- Performed for transposition of the great arteries
- Undertaken before 2-weeks-old (if no VSD present)
- Involves cutting aorta and pulmonary artery and changing them round
- Have to relocate coronary arteries as well
- Mortality is low now, around 5%
- Outcome affected by presence of associated defects, such as VSD, coarctation, abnormal coronary artery patterns

8.2 Fontan

- Any child with a complex heart arrangement which is not suitable for a repair with two separate ventricles will end up with a Fontan operation. If the pulmonary blood flow is too low at birth (cyanosis), they will have a BT shunt. If the pulmonary blood is too high (heart failure) they will have a PA band. If balanced physiology, then conservative treatment will be undertaken until the hemi-Fontan is performed.
- At about 6–8 months, the venous return from the head and neck is routed directly to the lungs. A connection is therefore made between the superior vena cava and the right pulmonary artery. Nowadays, it is halfway to the Fontan circuit.
- Hemi-Fontan (also known as Glenn or Cavopulmonary shunt) is performed on bypass, via a median sternotomy. Following the operation, the oxygen saturations will typically be 80–85%.
- At 3–5 years, there will be insufficient blood returning from the head to keep the child well. Hence a Fontan operation will be performed, where a channel is inserted to drain blood from the inferior vena cava up to the right pulmonary artery. This means that the child will be almost pink, saturations around 90–95%.
- When completely palliated, the ventricle pumps pink oxygenated blood to the body, whereas the blue deoxygenated blood flows direct to the lungs.

8.3 Norwood

- Used to palliate hypoplastic left heart syndrome
- Stage I at 3–5 days of age
  - Pulmonary artery disconnected + sewn to aorta so that RV pumps blood to body
  - Atrial septectomy so that pulmonary venous blood returns to RV
  - BT shunt from innominate artery to right pulmonary artery
- Stage II (Hemi-Fontan) at 6–8 months old
- Stage III (Fontan) at 3–5 years old
- Results of survival to 5 years are approximately 70–80%
- Unknown long-term results

8.4 Rastelli

- Used for TGA/VSD/PS

- Left ventricle is channelled through VSD to aorta
- VSD is closed with a patch of Gortex material
- Right ventricle is connected to pulmonary artery with a homograft (donor artery)
- Homograft is replaced every 20 years

8.5 Other operations

- A child with median sternotomy scar and lateral thoracotomy scar with a systolic and diastolic murmur at the left sternal edge

  This is typical of a child who has undergone insertion of a Blalock–Taussig shunt, and then complete repair for Tetralogy of Fallot.

- The child with Down's syndrome who has a murmur at the left lower sternal edge and a median sternotomy scar

  Atrioventricular septal defect or ventricular septal defect, who has undergone repair and who has a residual ventricular septal defect — the child may also have residual left atrioventricular valve (i.e mitral) regurgitation with systolic murmur at the apex

- Bikini incision — in girls, for cosmetic reasons who have undergone closure of atrial septal defect
- Groin puncture site — it may be worth inspecting the area of the right and left femoral vein to look for the small puncture scar of previous cardiac catheterization, for example for balloon dilation of pulmonary stenosis

For further information, consult a larger textbook (see further reading list).

9. SYNDROMES IN CONGENITAL HEART DISEASE

General principles
- Septal defects are the most common
- Anomalies of kidneys, vertebra or limbs are often connected with cardiac disorders
- Genetic causes of many syndromes now known

9.1 Isomerism

Right atrial isomerism

Heart defects
- Both atria are morphological right atria
- May have apex to right (dextrocardia)

- Must have anomalous pulmonary venous connection (no left atrium to connect to)
- May have complex anatomy, with AVSD, pulmonary atresia, etc.

Associated defects

- Asplenia (penicillin prophylaxis)
- Midline liver
- Malrotation of small bowel
- Two functional right lungs

Left atrial isomerism

Heart defects

- Both atria are morphological left atria
- May have anomalous pulmonary venous connection
- May have complex with AVSD, etc.

Associated defects

- Polysplenia (usually functional)
- Malrotation (less often than in right isomerism)
- Two functional left lungs

9.2 Trisomy

Down's syndrome (trisomy 21)

Heart defects

- 30% have CHD
- Usually VSD and AVSD
- All offered surgery with low risk

Associated defects

- Diagnosed antenatally — increased nuchal translucency

Edward's syndrome (trisomy 18)

Heart defects

- VSD
- Double outlet right ventricle

Associated defects

- Rocker bottom feet
- Crossed index finger
- Developmental delay

Patau's syndrome (trisomy 15 or 13)

Heart defects

- VSD
- Double outlet right ventricle

Associated defects

- Holoprosencephaly
- Midline facial cleft
- Renal anomalies

9.3 William's syndrome

Heart defects

- Supravalve aortic stenosis
- Peripheral pulmonary artery stenosis

Associated defects

- Gene abnormality on long arm of chromosome 7
- Hypercalcaemia
- Serrated teeth
- Carp-shaped mouth
- Hypertelorism
- Cocktail party chatter

9.4 Noonan's syndrome

Heart defects

- Hypertrophic cardiomyopathy
- Pulmonary valve stenosis
- ASD

Associated defects

- Almond-shaped eyes + shallow orbits
- Shield-shaped chest, widely spaced nipples
- Short
- Not 'male Turner', can be girls

9.5 Di George, 22q11.2 deletion

It is increasingly recognized that Di George syndrome may not always occur with the classical form of hypocalcaemia, absent thymus, lymphopenia, cardiac defect and characteristic facies (CATCH 22). Chromosomal abnormalities have been recognized in partial cases, or even in those with familial VSD or Fallot's Tetralogy (22q11.2 deletion). Deletions of the chromosome are detected using fluorescent *in situ* hybridization probes (FISH).

Heart defects

- Conotruncal anomalies
- Common arterial trunk
- Interrupted aortic arch
- Fallot
- Familial VSD

Associated defects

- 22q11.2 deletion
- Only have full Di George if deletion + heart + 2/3 of:
  - Cleft palate
  - Absent thymus (T cells low)
  - Absent parathyroids, hypocalcaemia
- Small jaw, small head, pinched nose, hypertelorism
- Small baby, slow development

Physical examination

Features to describe or exclude in this are as follows:

- Dysmorphic features of face, skull or pelvis
- Exclude cleft palate
- Check spine for scoliosis
- Check males for hypospadias

Investigations

- Full blood count and film (ask for haematologist's report)
- Calcium and magnesium levels
- Thyroid function tests
- Check total CD4 count
- Measure total IgE levels
- CXR
- Thymic ultrasound
- If abnormal: T-cell precursors and response to tetanus, Haemophilus influenzae type B (HIB) and pneumococcus vaccination

Medical treatment (If T-cell deficient)

- Maintenance co-trimoxazole (if lymphocyte count <1.5 × 10^9/l)
- Regular intravenous immunoglobulin infusions
- CMV-negative, irradiated blood until immunological status is known
- No live vaccines, but with component or fixed vaccines

9.6 Alagille

Heart defects

- Peripheral pulmonary artery stenosis

Associated defects

- Prominent forehead; wide-apart, deep-set eyes
- Small, pointed chin
- Butterfly vertebra
- Intrahepatic biliary hypoplasia – jaundice
- Embryotoxon (slit lamp for cornea)
- Kidney, growth, abnormalities of development, high-pitched voice

9.7 Turner

Heart defects

- Coarctation of the aorta

Associated defects

- Webbed neck
- Short stature
- Shield-shaped chest, wide-spaced nipples
- Infertility

9.8 VACTERL

Heart defects

- VSD
- Fallot
- Coarctation
- PDA

Associated defects

- Vertebral
- Anorectal
- Cardiac
- Tracheo-
- Esophageal fistula
- Renal/Retardation
- Limb

9.9 Holt Oram/TAR/Fanconi

Heart defects

- ASD

Associated defects

- Radial aplasia
- Limb abnormalities

9.10 CHARGE

Heart defects

- VSD
- Fallot

Associated defects

- Coloboma
- Heart
- Atresiae choanae
- Renal/retardation
- Genital/growth
- Ear

9.11 Pentalogy of Cantrell

Heart defects

- Fallot

Associated defects

- Absent sternum
- Absent pericardium
- Absent diaphragm
- Absent heart (ectopic, on the front of the chest)
- Absence of normal heart (Fallot)

9.12 Dextrocardia

- A clinical diagnosis with the apex beat in the right chest. It is not used in cardiology, as it gives no information about the connections or orientation of the heart. For example, if the right lung was collapsed and there was a tension pneumothorax on the left, it would be possible to find the apex beat in the right chest. However, the child would not suddenly have developed a cardiac anomaly. We use the term 'apex to right' to imply the orientation of the heart and then talk about the connections such as situs inversus (right atrium is on the left and left atrium is on the right) or other situs.

- In practice, most children with dextrocardia have a normal heart. This is most often the case when the liver is on the left. May be part of Kartagener's syndrome (ciliary dyskinesia) where the organs failed to rotate properly during embryological development. Easily diagnosed by performing nasal brushings to look at the dynein arms of the cilia on electron microscopy. Associated with bronchiectasis, sinus occlusion and infertility.
- If the child is blue with dextrocardia, there is almost always complex heart disease with right atrial isomerism (see above).

9.13 Other syndromes

- Cri du chat (5p-gene defect) = VSD, ASD
- Tuberous sclerosis   = Cardiac rhabdomyoma, get smaller in time

and many more. In general, cardiac defects may be associated with other defects. The commonest cardiac defect is a septal defect (ASD or VSD).

10. PULMONARY HYPERTENSION

For children, pulmonary hypertension is when the systolic pulmonary artery pressure is higher than 50% systemic systolic pressure. Needless to say this is normal in the 1-day-old baby, but is abnormal after that time.

10.1 Persistent pulmonary hypertension of the newborn

Aetiology

A relatively uncommon scenario, there are numerous causes, most commonly:

- Structural lung disease (e.g. congenital diaphragmatic hernia)
- Respiratory distress syndrome (hyaline membrane disease)
- Group B streptococcal infection
- Idiopathic

Diagnosis

- Persistent hypoxia
- Low cardiac output
- Loud P2 on examination
- Oligaemic lung fields
- Hepatomegaly
- Episodic desaturation, preceding a fall in blood pressure
- Echocardiographic appearance of pulmonary hypertension

- High-velocity tricuspid regurgitation jet
- Dilated right ventricle
- Right to left shunt via atrial septum
- Long right ventricle ejection time
- High-velocity pulmonary regurgitation jet
- Right to left shunt via arterial duct

Treatment

- Good ventilation (High O_2, low CO_2)
- Use oscillation ventilation if necessary
- Sedation with morphine or fentanyl
- Paralysis
- Good chest physiotherapy
- Restricted fluids
- Pharmacology
  - Nitric oxide (5–20 ppm, inhaled)
  - Prostacyclin (50 ng/kg, nebulized each 15 minutes)
  - Magnesium sulphate (200 mg/kg i.v.)
- Extracorporeal membrane oxygenation (ECMO) as last resort

10.2 Increased pulmonary blood flow

Post-tricuspid shunts

- Ventricular septal defect
- Arterial duct
- Common arterial trunk
- Aortopulmonary window

Treatment

- Repair defect by 3 months of age to avoid irreversible pulmonary vascular disease

10.3 Chronic hypoxia

Aetiology

- Bronchopulmonary dysplasia
- High altitude
- Cystic fibrosis
- Upper airway obstruction
- Chronic bronchiectasis

Investigation

- Sleep studies
- ECG (right ventricular hypertrophy)
- ENT opinion (upper airway obstruction)
- Chest X-ray
- Echocardiogram
- Cardiac catheterization with pulmonary vascular resistance study

Treatment

- Ensure good airway mechanics
- Treat underlying cardiac condition if appropriate
- Added O_2 to keep SaO_2 >94%
- Maintain low CO_2 (consider night-time ventilation)
- If responsive to vasodilators:
  - Nifedipine (0.1 mg/kg three times per day)
  - Dipyridamole (2.5 mg/kg/12 hourly)
  - Nebulized or intravenous prostacyclin
- Consider heart/lung transplantation if appropriate

10.4 Pulmonary venous hypertension

Aetiology

- Uncommon
- Mitral valve stenosis rare in children
- Total anomalous pulmonary venous connection
- Pulmonary vein stenosis
- Hypoplastic left heart syndrome

Investigation and treatment as per aetiology.

11. DRUG THERAPY FOR CONGENITAL HEART DISEASE

11.1 Heart failure

- Diuretics (furosemide (frusemide) and spironolactone or amiloride)
- Captopril
- Added calories

(NB. Digoxin not routinely used now in left to right shunts)

11.2 Anticoagulation

- Aspirin   for arterial platelet aggregation prevention orally (5 mg/kg per day)
- Heparin   for arterial anticoagulation, i.v.
- Warfarin   for venous or arterial thrombus prevention
- Streptokinase for thrombolysis
- tPA.   Tissue plasminogen activator for thrombolysis

11.3 Pulmonary hypertension

- Oxygen   Therapeutic vasodilation
- Low CO_2 Good ventilation
- Alkalosis   Bicarbonate if needed
- Dipyridamole   Increases cyclic guanosine monophosphate (cGMP) levels
- Nifedipine   Only if proven to tolerate it
- Nitric oxide   2–20 parts per million
- Prostacyclin   Nebulized (Iloprost) or i.v.
- Bosentan   Endothelin (ET_A) antagonist (experimental)
- Sildenafil   Increases cGMP levels (experimental)

11.4 Antiarrhythmia

- Supraventricular tachycardia (SVT)

  Vagal manoeuvres first
  Adenosine i.v. 50–250 µg/kg
  DC synchronized cardioversion 0.5–2 J/kg

- Ventricular tachycardia (VT)

  Cardioversion if pulse present — synchronized
       0.5–2 J/kg
  Defibrillation if no pulse   — 2–4 J/kg

Prophylaxis for arrhythmias

This tends to be very variable from unit to unit. Suggestions are:

- SVT   Flecainide, sotalol, digoxin or propranolol
- VT   Flecainide, sotalol, amiodarone (toxic side-effects on thyroid, skin and lungs)

12. ACQUIRED HEART DISEASE

12.1 Kawasaki disease

Clinical features
- Fever >5 days
- + 4/5 of:
  - Rash

- Lymphadenopathy
- Mucositis (sore mouth, strawberry tongue)
- Conjunctivitis
- Extremity involvement (red fingers/toes)
- +/–Coronary artery aneurysms (25% of untreated cases, 4.6% of treated cases)
- +/–Abdominal pain, diarrhoea, vomiting, irritable, mood change, hydrops of gallbladder, peeling extremities, thrombocytosis

Pathology

- Marked similarity to toxic shock syndrome
- Perhaps immune response to disease or toxin

Investigation

Erythrocyte sedimentation rate (ESR), C-reactive protein (CRP), white blood count (WBC), blood culture, antistreptolysin-O test (ASOT), viral, throat swab, ECG

Heart

- Pericardial effusion
- Myocardial disease (poor contractility)
- Endocardial disease (valve regurgitation)
- Coronary disease
  - Ectasia, dilatation
  - Small 3–5 mm aneurysms — resolve
  - Medium 5–8 mm aneurysms — usually resolve
  - Giant aneurysms >8 mm — ischaemia later

Greatest risk if male, <1 year, fever >16 days, ESR >100, WBC >30,000

Echo at 10–14 days, 6 weeks, 6 months or longer if abnormal.

Treatment

- Immunoglobulin 2 g/kg over 12 h
- Aspirin 30 mg/kg per day (four times per day dosage) reduce to 5 mg/kg per day when fever resolves
- Continue aspirin until 6 weeks or longer if abnormal echocardiogram

12.2 Dilated cardiomyopathy

History

- Multiple transfusions, recent viral illness, family history of myopathy or autoimmune diseases. Consider nutritional deficiencies (e.g. selenium, thiamine, etc.)

Examination

- Full cardiovascular examination
- Exclude myopathy

ECG

- Evidence of ischaemia
- Arrhythmias — unrecognized tachycardia

Echo (echocardiogram)

- Exclude anomalous coronary artery

X-ray

- Look for arterial calcification

Blood

- Metabolic
  - Carnitine (and acylcarnitine profile)
  - Amino acids, organic acids, lactate
  - Creatinine and electrolytes (incl. phosphate)
  - Liver function tests (LFTs) and lactate dehydrogenase (LDH), creatine kinase-membrane bound (CK-MB)
  - Selenium and thiamine
- Autoimmune
  - Antinuclear, anti-DNA antibodies; immune complexes
- Virology
  - FBC, ESR, CRP,
  - PCR for Epstein–Barr virus (EBV) coxsackie-, adeno-viruses, echoviruses
  - Stools for viral culture

Other investigations include abdominal ultrasound for arterial calcification, electromyography (EMG) and muscle biopsy if myopathy. Rare causes include endomyocardial fibrosis, tropical diseases, amyloid.

12.3 Hypertrophic cardiomyopathy

History
Family history of sudden unexplained death, cardiomyopathy, or myopathy. If neonate, check infant of diabetic mother, or if mother was given ritodrine. Hypertrophic more suggestive of metabolic cause compared to dilated. For example, consider inherited causes such as consanguineous or X-linked Barth syndrome with neutropenia.

Examination

- Exclude syndromes, Noonan's, Leopard, Friedreich's ataxia, neurofibromatosis, lipodystrophy

- Exclude endocrine disease, thyroid (hyper- and hypo-), acromegaly
- Exclude hypertension; check for gross hepatomegaly
- Check for cataracts, ophthalmoplegia, ataxia, deafness, myopathy
- Look for signs of mucopolysaccharidosis

ECH

- Exclude tumours, amyloid, endocardial infiltration

ECG

- Look for short PR + giant complexes (Pompe's)
- Look for QRS–T axis dissociation (Friedreich's)

Blood tests

- Carnitine (decreased) + acylcarnitine profile
- Creatine phosphokinase (CPK) (increased suggests Glycogen storage disease type III (GSD III))
- Blood film for vacuolated lymphocytes, if positive check white cell enzymes (suggesting storage disorders)
- Calcium (hyperparathyroidism)
- Thyroid function tests (TFTs), fasting blood sugar
- Lactate, amino acids

Urine

- Glycosaminoglycans (GAGs) (for mucopolysaccharidosis)
- Organic acids
- Vanillylmandelic acid (VMA)

If no cause found screen family for hypertrophic obstructive cardiomyopathy (HOCM) and consider gene probe for HOCM

12.4 Suspected bacterial endocarditis (SBE)

All children and adults with congenital and many with acquired heart disease need antibiotic prophylaxis prior to dental extraction and potentially septic procedures. Only those with secundum ASD do not. After surgery, prophylaxis is required for 1 year — if no residual defect or until the residual defect closes.

History

- If a child is admitted with an unexplained fever, has or might have congenital heart disease, has murmurs (? changing), think of SBE
- Ask for history of recent boils, sepsis, dental extraction, etc.
- SBE may be found postoperatively following insertion of prosthetic material such as homograft or prosthetic valve

Examination

- Full cardiovascular examination
- Hepatosplenomegaly, fever, heart sounds and signs of infected emboli: Osler's nodes, Roth's spots, septic arthritis, splinter haemorrhages, haematuria, nephrosis

Investigations

- Six blood cultures from different sites at different times over 2 days, using the most sterile technique possible, but do not clean blood culture bottles with alcohol (or else the organisms will be killed off)
- Full blood count, ESR, CRP, ASOT throat swab
- Echocardiogram and ECG
- Consider V/Q scan, white cell differential
- Urine test for blood
- Dental opinion

Treatment

- If proven, treatment is for 6 weeks, predominantly intravenous
- Blood antibiotic levels may be taken for back titration after stabilization on antibiotic regime — this will be used to assess that there is sufficient antibiotic present to cause bacteriocidal effect
- Antibiotics chosen should be those with a good record of deep-tissue penetration, e.g. fusidic acid, gentamicin

12.5 Rheumatic fever

- Uncommon in UK
- Increasing incidence with reduced use of antibiotics to treat sore throats
- Diagnosed by Modified Duckett-Jones criteria (2 major or 1 major + 2 minor):
  - Major   Carditis
              Polyarthritis
              Chorea
              Erythema marginatum
              Subcutaneous nodules
  - Minor   Fever
              Arthralgia
              Previous rheumatic fever or carditis
              Positive acute-phase reactants (ESR, CRP)
              Leucocytosis
              Prolonged P–R interval

Investigations

- ASOT
- Throat swab for streptococcus A
- ECG

- Echocardiogram (mitral regurgitation, myocarditis, pericarditis)

Treatment

- Penicillin or cefuroxime (if sensitive)
- Prophylactic penicillin V orally for 25 years

12.6 Pericarditis

Aetiology

- Coxsackieviruses
- Enteroviruses
- Staphylococcus
- TB
- Oncological
- Rheumatic fever

Presentation

- Chest pain (inspiratory)
- Acute collapse (effusion)
- Soft, muffled heart sounds

Examination

- Pericardial friction rub
- Fever

ECG

- ST elevation, convex upwards
- T-wave inversion

Treatment

- Anti-inflammatory drugs (ibuprofen)
- Drain large pericardial effusion

13. ECG

13.1 The ECG and how to read it

Before interpreting a paediatric ECG it is essential to know the following:

a) How old is the child?
b) Is it recorded at a normal rate (25 mm/s) and voltage (10 mm/mV)?

Rate

When measuring the heart rate on the ECG, the number of large squares is counted between the R waves. The rate is calculated as 300/number of squares.

Rhythm

Sinus rhythm can only be inferred if there is one P wave before each QRS and that the P wave axis is between 0–90°.

Axis

QRS axis

This is calculated by adding the total positive deflection (R wave) and subtracting the negative deflection (Q+S wave). The resulting vector is plotted for lead I and AVF:

Lead I = 0°

Lead AVF = +90°

The P-wave and T-wave axis should be plotted similarly. This is important. For example, if there is left atrial isomerism, there is no sinoatrial node (a right atrial structure). This means that the P-wave axis is abnormal (superior) and can lead to the diagnosis. Similarly in cardiomyopathies, such as Friedreich's, there is a difference in the axis between QRS and T of more than 75°. This can help to make the diagnosis (see below).

Normal QRS axis for   newborn   =   90–180°
2–5 years   =   45–135°
>5 years   =   -10–100°

Causes of a superior axis (>180°)

- Atrioventricular septal defect
- Tricuspid atresia
- Ebstein's anomaly
- Noonan's syndrome
- W–P–W (Wolff–Parkinson–White) syndrome
- <1% of normals

Note: AVSD will have RV hypertrophy, whereas tricuspid atresia usually has no RV forces. Either can have large P waves.

P wave

The axis should be from 0 to 90°. The normal size is 2×2 little squares (0.08 seconds, 0.2 mV). If there are not regular P waves before each QRS consider the following:

- Complete heart block — there is complete dissociation between the QRS and P waves i.e. with no fixed relationship; see below for list of causes
- Atrial flutter. Usually with 2:1 block, there is a typical sawtooth baseline

- Inverted P waves. These are typically seen with:
  - Left atrial isomerism (no RA → no sinus node)
  - Postoperatively
  - Occasionally in normals (coronary sinus rhythm).
- Peaked P waves — seen in right atrial hypertrophy:
  - Tricuspid regurgitation (e.g. Ebstein's anomaly)
  - Atrioventricular septal defect
  - Pulmonary hypertension
  - Cardiomyopathy

P–R interval

Normal in children is 2–4 little squares (0.08–0.16 seconds).

Causes of a long P–R interval

- Atrioventricular septal defects
- Myocarditis
- Digoxin toxicity
- Hyperkalaemia
- Duchenne's
- Hypothermia
- Diphtheria

Causes of a short P–R interval

- W–P–W (Wolff–Parkinson–White) syndrome
- Pompe's disease (Wide QRS)
- Lown–Ganong–Levine (Normal QRS)

Q wave

Not often seen in paediatrics. Rare to see signs of infarct. Normal Q waves are seen in V1, V2 in young children and are allowed in other leads if small <0.2 mV.

Causes of Q waves

- Dextrocardia
- Left ventricular volume overload V5, V6 (e.g. large PDA or VSD)
- Congenitally corrected transposition
- Ischaemia (Kawasaki, anomalous left coronary artery from pulmonary artery)
- Ischaemia postoperatively

QRS wave

Normal duration is 0.08 seconds. Prolonged in right bundle-branch block, e.g. after Fallot's repair.

- Delta (δ) wave — seen in W–P–W syndrome, the slurred upstroke to R wave, represents depolarization via the accessory pathway, with a short P–R interval. There will be a wide QRS and the QRS axis will be unusual, even superior. Likely to have supraventricular tachycardias (re-entry).
- R–S progression — The best way to assess ventricular hypertrophy. The following pattern should be seen:

	Lead V1		Lead V6	
Newborn (0–1 month)	Dominant R	∧	Dominant S	∨
Infant (1–18 months)	Dominant R	∧	Dominant R	∧
Adult (>18 months)	Dominant S	∨	Dominant R	∧

Therefore, if there is persistence of the newborn pattern in an infant then RV hypertrophy is suggested. Other features of hypertrophy are:

- RV hypertrophy   Upright T waves V1 (from 1 week to 16 years is abnormal)
  Q wave in V1
  R waves >20 mm in V1
- LV hypertrophy   Inverted T waves V6
  Q waves in V6
  Left axis deviation for age
  R waves >20 mm in V6
- Bi-ventricular hypertrophy
  Total voltage (R+S) in V3/V4 of >60 mm only sign of large VSD

Q–T interval

Measured from the start of the Q wave to the end of the T wave (U wave if present). This represents the total time taken for depolarization and repolarization. Normal is <0.44 seconds for a heart rate of 60/min. To correct for the heart rate use the formula (Bazett)   QTc=QT/√(RR)
QT (corrected) = QT measured/(square root of time from R to R).

for example: QT measured = 0.30 s at rate of 120
QTc = 0.3/√(0.5) = 0.4 (normal)

If Q–T interval is long, abnormal T waves and a slow heart rate may result. The cause of long Q–T is thought to be differential sympathetic drive to the two sides of the ventricle, allowing one side to repolarize before the other, hence prolonging the total time of repolarization. This also explains why the T waves are abnormal.

Causes of long Q–T interval

- Romano–Ward (autosomal dominant, non-lethal)

- Jervell–Lange–Nielsen (autosomal recessive, deaf. Lethal — causes VT/VF)
- Hypocalcaemia
- Hypokalaemia
- Hypomagnesaemia
- Head injury
- Hypothermia
- Drug administration such as cisapride or erythromycin

S–T segment

Unusual to get marked changes in S–T segments. May represent ischaemia in Kawasaki, anomalous left coronary artery from pulmonary artery and postoperative cardiac surgery.

T waves

Normally T waves are downward in V1 from 1 week to 16 years of age.
T-wave axis should be within 75° of QRS. If not think of:

- Friedreich's ataxia
- Dilated cardiomyopathy
- Noonan's syndrome
- Long Q–T syndrome

Peaked T waves seen in hypokalaemia and digoxin toxicity.

13.2 Tachycardias

SVT

- Likely if the heart rate is >240/min
- Tend to be faster rates ~300/min
- Tend to be narrow complex (<0.08 s, unless aberrant conduction)
- Often caused by W–P–W
- Respond to adenosine (i.v. rapid bolus) or vagal manoeuvres such as immersion in ice-cold water, carotid sinus massage or valsalva in older children

Can use flecainide, propranolol, sotalol, esmolol, amiodarone for treatment/prophylaxis.

Do NOT use eyeball pressure, or i.v. verapamil.

For atrial flutter, adenosine challenge brings out flutter waves. Standard treatment is then to use synchronized D.C. cardioversion (0.5 J /kg)

VT

- Tend to be slower rates ~200/min
- Tend to be wide complex (>0.08 s)

- There is P-wave dissociation
- Can have torsade de points, which can degenerate to VF
- Treatment is usually amiodarone (can use flecainide, etc.)

13.3 Bradycardias

Complete heart block

Often present at birth but may be diagnosed antenally. Baby is born (sometimes following emergency caesarean section) with heart rate ~70/min but is perfectly well. Usually needs no treatment for several years. Intervene if failure to thrive, collapses, heart failure, Stokes-Adams attacks or resting heart rate <40/min. These would be indications for pacemaker insertion.

Causes

- Maternal systemic lupus erythematosus (SLE)
- Congenitally corrected transposition of the great arteries
- Post-operative
- Myocarditis
- Rheumatic fever

Sick sinus syndrome

- Tachy/brady syndrome
- May be seen after heart surgery
- Caused by scar formation over sinus node
  (To be differentiated from sinus arrhythmia which is normal variation in heart rate caused by the effects of respiration)

If symptomatic needs pacemaker insertion

14. CHEST X-RAYS

14.1 Cardiac outlines

Neonatal

- 'Egg-on-Side'
  Transposition of great arteries
  Narrow vascular pedicle (aorta in front of pulmonary artery)
  Boot-shaped
  Fallot's with pulmonary atresia
  Pulmonary artery bay due to absent pulmonary artery
- 'Snowman in a snowstorm'
  Obstructed total anomalous pulmonary venous connection (TAPVC)
  Small heart with pulmonary venous congestion

- Wall-to-wall heart
  Ebstein's anomaly
  Massive cardiomegaly with right atrial dilation

Infantile

- Cottage loaf
  TAPVC
  Visible ascending vein on upper left border

The older child

- Cardiomegaly with increased pulmonary vascular markings
  Atrial septal defect
- Small heart with pulmonary oligaemia
  Eisenmenger's syndrome
  Probably secondary to VSD or AVSD

Globular heart
Usually associated with pericardial effusions, perhaps secondary to pericarditis or dilated cardiomyopathy.

Situs
Check the heart is on the left along with the stomach bubble, and that the liver is on the right. This may be helpful in diagnosing right atrial isomerism, etc., as above.

Oligaemic lung fields
Reduced pulmonary blood flow such as Fallot, Ebstein, persistent pulmonary hypertension.

Plethoric lung fields
Left to right shunts, especially VSD and AVSD. Useful in transposition of the great arteries.

Normal lung fields
Those lesions with no shunt, such as pulmonary stenosis and aortic stenosis.

15. CARDIAC CATHETERIZATION

15.1 Diagnostic cardiac catheterization

Normal

Right Atrium
SaO_2= 65%
Press = 4 mmHg

Left Atrium
SaO_2= 99%
Press = 6 mmHg

Right Ventricle
SaO_2= 65%
Press = 25/4

Left Ventricle
SaO_2= 98%
Press = 75/6 (age dependent)

PA
SaO_2 = 65%
Press = 25/15

Aorta
SaO_2 = 97%
Press = 75/50 (age dependent)

In order to analyse cardiac catheter data, it is important to start with the aortic saturations. Follow the algorithm below.

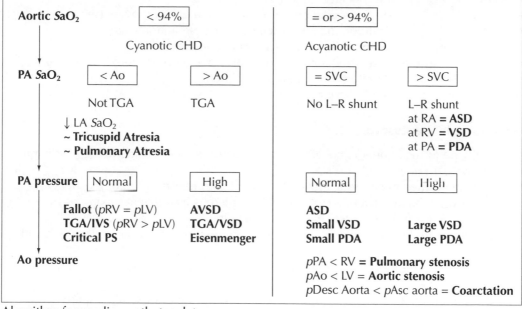

Algorithm for cardiac catheter data

- If pink (Ao SaO_2 ≥ 94%) check PA SaO_2. If this is > systemic venous SaO_2, then there is a left to right shunt. If same as venous then look for a pressure drop (AS/CoA).
- If blue (Ao SaO_2 < 94%) check PA SaO_2. If this is > $AoSaO_2$, then it is transposition of the great arteries. If PA SaO_2 < $AoSaO_2$ then not TGA. Check PA pressure. If less than RV pressure then there is RV outflow obstruction, probably Fallot's tetralogy.

- True diagnostic catheters rarely performed, use echocardiography instead
- Usually for assessment between staged surgical operations
- Pulmonary vascular resistance assessments for left to right shunts to determine operability
  - Measure pulmonary artery pressure and resistance (PVR) at baseline
  - Measure oxygen consumption for accurate determination
  - Repeat measurement in nitric oxide at two different doses
  - Repeat measurement in oxygen or prostacyclin
  - If PVR >7 Wood units $\times$ m^2, then inoperable
  - If PVR falls by more than 20% then is partly reversible

15.2 Interventional cardiac catheterization

Interventional cardiac catheters

75% of cardiac catheters are for interventional treatment

- ASD   Septal occlusion device in 30% of secundum ASD after 3 years old
- VSD   Not usually used, but may be appropriate in apical muscular VSDs
- PDA   Coil occlusion at 1 year
- AS   Balloon dilation is standard treatment at any age (see above)
- PS   Balloon dilation is standard treatment at any age
- Coarctation   Stent insertion in teenagers or adults
- Pulmonary atresia   Radiofrequency perforation as newborn or shunt insertion surgically
- Branch PS   Stent insertion in older children
- Arrhythmias   Radiofrequency ablation

Balloon atrial septostomy

- Usually performed under echocardiographic control at the bedside in the paediatric intensive care unit (PICU).
- Mostly performed in babies less than 2 days old with transposition of the great arteries (see above), who are severely cyanosed where there is insufficient mixing or where it is not possible to perform a neonatal switch operation.
- May be required in other conditions, such as pulmonary atresia with intact ventricular septum.
- Most are performed via the umbilical vein and the procedure only takes a few minutes.
- If the child is older than 3 days, the femoral vein approach is usually required.
- A catheter is passed via the vein into the right atrium and hence into the left atrium across the foramen ovale. The balloon on the end of the catheter is inflated and the balloon withdrawn rapidly into the right atrium. This tears a hole in the atrial septum allowing blood to pass freely from right to left and vice versa.

16. IMAGING

16.1 Echocardiography

- Mainstay of diagnostic tools
- Doppler to assess velocity (and hence pressure gradient) across valves or VSD
- Colour-flow to highlight small defects or turbulent blood flow
- Transoesophageal echo for posterior heart structures or during interventional cardiac catheterization, especially in adults with congenital heart disease
- Future uses for intravascular ultrasound, 3D ultrasound and contrast echocardiography

16.2 Magnetic resonance imaging (MRI)

- Standard diagnostic imaging for complex diseases where echocardiogram insufficient
- Spin-echo for routine imaging
- Contract-enhanced for blood flow
- 3D MRI reconstruction

16.3 Positron emission tomography (PET)

- Uses ammonium ion to give blood-pool images
- Best for myocardial perfusion imaging

16.4 Radionuclear angiography

- For quantifying left to right shunt (e.g. ASD)
- For determining right or left ventricle function and ejection fraction

17. FURTHER READING

How to read paediatric ECG's. Park MK, Gunteroth WG. 3rd Edition. Year Book Publishers Chicago.

Andrews RE, Tulloh RMR. Hypoplastic left heart syndrome: diagnosis and management. *Hosp Med.* Jan: **63** (1):24–7 2002.

Brogan PA, Bose A, Burgner D, Shingadia D, Tulloh R, Michie C, Klein N, Booy R, Levin M, Dillon MJ. Kawasaki disease: an evidence-based approach to diagnosis, treatment, and proposals for future research. *Arch Dis Child.* Apr: **86** (4):286–90 2002.

Andrews RE and Tulloh RMR. Management of Pulmonary Hypertension in Paediatrics. *Current opinion in Paediatrics.* July 2002.

Paediatric Cardiology. Anderson RH, Baker EJ, Macartney FJ, Rigby ML, Shinbourne EA, Tynan M (Eds). 2nd Edition. Churchill Livingstone London 2002.

Chapter 2

Child Development, Child Psychiatry and Community Paediatrics

Joanne Philpot and Ruth M Charlton

CONTENTS

Child Development

1. DEVELOPMENTAL ASSESSMENT

This is a key part of the assessment of any child. It is important to learn the common milestones.

1.1 Milestones

It is important to consider the four areas:

- Gross motor
- Fine motor and vision
- Speech and hearing (language)
- Social

Age	Gross motor	Fine motor and vision	Language	Social
6 weeks	Head lag still present on pulling from a supine to sitting position When held in ventral suspension, head can be held in the same plane as the body	Maintains fixation and follows an object through 90° in the horizontal plane	Makes throaty noises	Smiles in response to appropriate stimuli
3 months	Able to raise head and chest on forearms in the prone position No head lag on pulling to sit	Will fix and follow an object through 180° in the horizontal plane Hands beginning to be brought to the mid-line Attempts to make contact with offered object	Vowel sounds and noises uttered on social contact Turns head to sound, level to the ear	Social smile (infant has awareness that smile attracts attention) May show displeasure on interruption of social contact
6 months	Can roll over Sits briefly or with some support	Transfers Reaches out for objects Mouthing objects	Unintelligible babble Will turn when name is called	Plays with feet Holds onto bottle when fed
9 months	Sits steadily Pivots to reach objects Stands holding onto objects	Looks for toy fallen from view Pokes objects with index finger	Shouts to gain attention Understands 'no' Two-syllable babble	Finger feeds Resists when objects removed
12 months	Crawling Pulls to stand Cruising	Pincer grip Banging bricks together	Two words with meaning Responds to 'give it to me' Shows recognition of objects by using them, e.g. brush	Waves bye bye Claps hands Empties cupboards

continues

	Gross motor	Fine motor and vision	Language	Social
15 months i.e.	Walking well	Pincer grip refined, tiny objects can be picked up delicately Casting	Expression several words Understands words such as cup, names of brothers and sisters Jargon and jabbering Echolalia (repetition of words spoken to the child)	Drinks from a cup Indicates wants without crying, pointing, pulling, asking
18 months	Stoops and retrieves objects Carries toys while walking	Delicate pincer grasp Scribbles	Points to parts of body Understands up to 50 words Knows common objects by name, e.g. cat Follows one-step command, e.g. 'give me a doll' Expression 25 to 50 words	Holds spoon and gets food to mouth Into everything Takes shoes and socks off Indicates toilet needs
2 years to 2.5 years	Climbs and descends stairs one step at a time Kicks a ball Climbs furniture	Copies vertical line Tower of eight bricks	Uses plurals Follows two-step request, e.g. 'get the ball and put it in the box' Identifies objects from hearing their use Selects toy from others, i.e. 'Give me the sheep, brush'	Plays alone Eats with spoon and fork
3 years	Pedal tricycle Jumps well Momentarily balancing on one foot	Copies a circle Matches two colours	Knows some colours Three- to four-word sentences Name, age and sex on request Pronouns and plurals Knows more about time, today and not today Starts to tell stories	Out of nappies during the day Separates from mother easily (less apprehensive about you the candidate) Eats with knife and fork Dresses with supervision
4 years	Stands on one foot well Hops	Copies a cross and square Draws man with three parts	Count to 10 Identifies several colours 100s of questions Tells story Understands numbers Past tense Increasing concentration	Shares toys Out of nappies by night Brushes teeth Toilet alone

continues

	Gross motor	Fine motor and vision	Language	Social
5 years	Walks down stairs one foot per step Bounces and catches ball	Copies triangle Draws man with six parts Writes name Do up buttons	Comprehension: 'what do you do if you are hungry, cold, tired?' Comprehension of prepositions: 'put brick on, under, in front of' Opposites: hot, cold; if elephant is big, a mouse is small Definition of words, e.g. ball, banana	Chooses friends Comforts in distress Acts out role play

Primitive reflexes

- Sucking and rooting present from 0–6 months
- Palmar grasp present from 0–3 months
- Stepping present from 0–6 weeks
- Asymmetrical tonic neck reflex (ATNR) present from 1–6 months — with the child supine, the head is rotated to one side leading to extension of the arm and leg on the side towards which the head is turned and flexion of the arm and leg on the opposite side
- Moro present from 0–4 months
- Head-righting present from 6 months and persists
- Parachute reflex present from 9 months and persists

1.2 Developmental examination for the Short Case examination

It is important when assessing development to make comments under the four main headings (see above).

Inspect

- Look for clues. Remember the families will have come equipped for the day. Look for feeding equipment, nappy bag, the toys they have brought.
- Is the child well?
- Does the child look dysmorphic?
- Are there any obvious neurological abnormalities?

Assessment

- Pitch in at around the age you think the child is, i.e. if they look around 18 months do not start asking them to copy circles, etc.
- Assess each of the four developmental categories. Once you have demonstrated they can do one level push up to the next level until they are not able to perform the task. For example: if you have demonstrated the child can copy a square do not ask them to copy a circle as you have already demonstrated the child is past this level, instead see if they can copy a triangle.

- Keep control of the situation. If the child is playing already WATCH. You may be able to complete the whole assessment by observation alone.
- If the child is already sitting use the opportunity to assess language, social and fine-motor development. Do not disrupt the child to do gross-motor tests — you may well have difficulty settling him again and in the older child gross motor gives you the least additional information. Leave it to the end.
- Use the parents if the child is shy or apprehensive, e.g. ask the parents to draw a circle for the child to copy or test the child about colours, numbers, stories, etc.
- If the child does not co-operate do not panic. You can still get clues from observing. Remember stranger awareness and non-compliance are developmental milestones in themselves.

Presentation

- Summarize any relevant clinical findings, e.g. this girl looks ill, has a drip in, a Hickman line, etc. which may be affecting your assessment. If the child looks dysmorphic then say so.
- This child has a developmental age of X because:
  - Gross motor — I have demonstrated that they can do this but not that
  - Fine motor — I have demonstrated, etc.

'Demonstrated' is better than 'can' or 'cannot'. It means that the parents cannot correct you by saying 'yes he can'! Remember you are only assessing the child over a few minutes.

If you have a developmental discrepancy between the four areas then present this, e.g. this child has a developmental age of 4 in gross- and fine-motor skills but a developmental level of 2 years in speech and language and social skills. Follow this by saying what you would like to do next, e.g. I would like to formally test his hearing to exclude a hearing problem.

Children likely to be seen

- Normal
- Dysmorphic, e.g. Down's syndrome. Just keep to the same format and in each of the four sections demonstrate what they can and cannot do to determine their developmental level.
- Global developmental delay
- Gross-motor delay (cerebral palsy)

1.3 Management of the child with global developmental delay

Developmental delay can result from many causes:

- 40% have chromosomal abnormalities
- 5–10% have developmental malformations
- 4% have metabolic disorders

Causes of developmental delay

Static causes

Prenatal
Chromosomal abnormalities
Intrauterine infections
Teratogens
Congenital brain malformations, e.g. neuronal migration defects
Specific syndromes

Perinatal
Prematurity
Ischaemic hypoxic encephalopathy
Birth trauma
Meningitis

Postnatal
Trauma
Intracranial infections

Progressive causes

Metabolic
Hypothyroidism
Aminoacidurias
Galactosaemia
Mucopolysaccharidoses
Lesch–Nyhan
Degeneration of the cerebral grey matter
       Tay–Sachs disease
       Gaucher disease
       Niemann–Pick disease
       Batten disease
       Leigh disease
       Menkes disease
Degeneration of the cerebral white matter
       Krabbe disease
       Metachromatic leucodystrophy
       Canavan disease
Peroxisomal disorders
       Zellweger syndrome

Infection
Subacute sclerosing panencephalitis (SSPE)

History

A good history is essential to help determine the cause and appropriate investigations. Information is required on prenatal history, perinatal history and postnatal development. Are there any associated symptoms such as seizures? General health is important when considering metabolic disorders. Family history may give the strongest clue to a chromosomal disorder. Enquire about previous pregnancy losses.

Examination

Thorough examination is essential.

Neurodegenerative conditions affecting grey matter tend to present with dementia and seizures. Conditions affecting the white matter tend to present with spasticity, cortical deafness and blindness.

Inspect for

- Sex of child. X-linked conditions such as fragile X, Menkes, Hunter, Lesch–Nyhan syndromes.
- Age of the child:
  - First 6 months: Tay–Sachs disease, Leigh's disease, infantile spasms, tuberose sclerosis
  - Toddlers: infantile metachromatic leucodystrophy, mucopolysaccharidoses, infantile Gaucher, Krabbe's disease
  - Older children: juvenile Batten disease, SSPE, Wilson disease, Huntington chorea
- Dysmorphic features: Down's syndrome, mucopolysaccharidoses
- Neurocutaneous signs: ataxia telangiectasia, Sturge–Weber syndrome, incontinentia pigmenti, tuberose sclerosis
- Extrapyramidal movements: cerebral palsy, Wilson's, Huntington chorea
- Tremor: Wilson, Friedreich's ataxia, metachromatic leucodystrophy

Note growth of child

- Large head: Alexander, Canavan, Tay–Sachs, mucopolysaccharidoses
- Small head: cerebral palsy, autosomal recessive microcephaly, Rubinstein–Taybi, Smith–Lemli–Opitz, Cornelia de Lange
- Growth pattern (e.g. failure to thrive with metabolic disease, gigantism with Soto's)

Systematic examination

- Eyes: corneal clouding, cataract, cherry-red spot, optic atrophy
- Neurological examination including gait, scoliosis, tremor, extrapyramidal movements, tone, power and reflexes of limbs
- Associated system involvement (e.g. cardiac abnormalities, organomegaly in metabolic disease)
- Genitalia
- Hearing and vision should be checked

Further assessment often involves input from other professionals of the child development team, e.g. speech and language therapists and physiotherapist.

Investigations

A thorough history and examination may lead to targeted investigations, e.g. a specific genetic test or metabolic test. For approximately 40% of cases no cause is found. The two most useful investigations are genetic studies and brain imaging.

If no specific diagnosis is suggested then consider:

- **Blood tests**

  - Chromosomal analysis
  - Thyroid function tests
  - TORCH serology in infants (TORCH, **t**oxoplasmosis, **o**ther (congenital syphylis and viruses), **r**ubella, **c**ytomegalovirus and **h**erpes simplex virus)
  - Plasma amino acids
  - Ammonia
  - Lactate
  - White cell enzymes

- **Urine tests**

  - Urinary organic acids
  - Urinary amino acids
  - Urinary mucopolysaccharidoses

- **Brain imaging**

  This will identify congenital brain abnormalities and diagnose degenerative conditions such as the leucodystrophies and grey matter abnormalities.

- **EEG**

  Will identify SSPE, Batten

Management

This is multidisciplinary. The precise make-up of the team depends on local resources.

It can include:

- Community paediatrician
- Speech and language therapist
- Physiotherapist
- Occupational therapist
- Child psychologist/psychiatrist
- Play therapist
- Pre-school therapist, e.g. portage
- Nursery teachers
- Health visitors
- Social workers

2. VISION

Each year around 500 children are registered blind or partially sighted. Early diagnosis is important because:

- Appropriate treatment may reduce the severity of the disability or stop progression
- Other medical conditions associated with visual problems can be diagnosed
- Genetic counselling can be offered
- Pre-school learning support can be started

Causes of visual impairment in childhood

- Cataract
- Glaucoma
- Optic nerve
  Leber's optic atrophy
  Septo-optic dysplasia
  Raised intracranial pressure, e.g. hydrocephalus
- Retinal
  Retinopathy of prematurity
  Hereditary Leber's amaurosis
  Retinoblastoma
- Amblyopia due to squint, refractive error, ptosis

2.1 Assessment of visual acuity

There is no national policy on visual screening or who should do it (primary care or orthoptists). At present there are different screening policies in different health authorities. Visual screening is under review in conjunction with the results from trials on treatment of amblyopia.

Current recommendations are:

- Newborn screening inspecting the eyes for anomalies
- Repeat eye examination at the 6-week check
- Orthoptist's assessment of all children in the 4- to 5-age group. This is to assess acuity and to detect squints. The advantage of screening at this age is easier testing of visual acuity compared to younger children. Parents will usually recognize a squint but amblyopia due to refractive error will only be detected when the child's vision is assessed monocularly
- Screening very low birth-weight babies to detect retinopathy of prematurity
- Visual screening in children with other major disabilities

Between the age of 6 weeks and 4 years identification of visual defects will rely on concern being raised by the parents or other professionals.

Methods of testing visual acuity

1. **Newborn** inspection of the eye for cataract and other abnormalities — including red reflex.

2. **6 weeks'** inspection of the eye. The child should also be able to fix and follow an object held at arms' length through 90° in the horizontal plane.

3. **12 weeks** — the child should be able to fix and follow an object 180° in the horizontal and vertical planes.

4. **10 months** — an infant can pick up a raisin. By one year they can pick up individual '100 and 1000s' sweets. If possible try to test acuity of both eyes.

5. **2 to 3 years** — test each eye individually. Various tests for visual acuity are available. *Preferential looking test*: This can be used in a child too young to identify objects. Large cards with pictures on in different positions, i.e. top right-hand corner, bottom left-hand corner are shown to the child and the eye movements are observed as the child focuses on the picture as it moves around the card. *Picture cards*: Children asked to identify picture cards at a set distance. Picture size varies to determine the acuity.

6. **3 years** — visual acuity should be assessed in each eye. By this age the Sheridan–Gardner test can usually be used. The child has a card with five letters on, the Key card. The examiner stands 6 m away and holds up a letter which the child has to identify on his card.

7. **4 years and upwards** — by this age the child can usually verbally identify letters and therefore a Snellen chart can be used.

2.2 Squints

Squints are common, occurring in approximately 4% of all children. There is a strong familial incidence. A squint is usually noticed by the parents first and parental report of squint should be taken seriously.

A squint is:

- A misalignment of the visual axis of one eye

It is either:

- Latent, i.e. only there at certain times (such as fatigue, illness, stress)
- Manifest, i.e. present all the time

It is either:

- Alternating: the patient uses either eye for fixation while the other eye deviates. As each eye is being used in turn, vision develops more or less equally in both.
- Monocular: only one eye is used for fixation and the other eye consistently deviates. The child is more prone to develop amblyopia as the deviated eye is consistently not being used.

It is either:

- Convergent, i.e. turns in
- Divergent, i.e. turns out

It is either:

- Non-paralytic
- Paralytic

Non-paralytic squint

This is the more common type of squint and includes the following:

- Comprises the majority of the congenital and infantile convergent squints.

- The accommodative convergent squint. In some infants accommodation results in over-convergence or crossing of the eyes. This type of deviation most commonly occurs around 18 months to 2 years of age. The child is also usually long-sighted. In most cases the eye crossing can be controlled with glasses that correct for the long-sightedness.

- In a few cases a non-paralytic squint is due to an underlying ocular or visual defect, e.g. cataract, high refractive errors, retinopathy of prematurity, retinoblastoma.

Paralytic squints

These are due to weakness or paralysis of one or more of the extraocular muscles. They are less common.

- The deviation worsens on gaze into the direction of action of the affected muscle.

- Congenital paralytic squints are more commonly due to developmental defects of the cranial nerves, muscle disease, congenital infection.

- Acquired paralytic squints usually signify a serious pathological process, e.g. brain tumour, central nervous system infection, neurodegenerative disease.

Assessment of squint

- Ocular movements assessed to exclude paralytic squint.

- Corneal reflex examined, looking for symmetry of the light reflex.

- Cover/uncover test. The child sits comfortably on a parent's lap. Their attention is attracted and while they are looking at an object one of the eyes is covered. If the uncovered eye moves to fix on the object there is a squint present, a manifest squint. This may be a:

  Unilateral squint. The squinting eye takes up fixation of the object when the other eye is covered. When the cover is removed the squinting eye returns to its original squinting position

  Alternating squint. The squinting eye takes up fixation of the object when the other eye is covered. When the cover is removed the squinting eye maintains fixation and the previously fixing eye remains in a deviated position, i.e. the squint alternates from one eye to the other.

- Rapid cover/uncover test. Sometimes a squint is not present all the time but only when tired or stressed. In the rapid cover test the occluder is moved quickly between the eyes. If the eye that has been uncovered moves to take up fixation there is a latent squint.

Principles of treatment for a squint

- Develop best possible vision for each eye:
  - Correct any underlying defect, e.g. cataract
  - Correct refractive errors with glasses
  - Treat any amblyopia with occlusion therapy

- Achieve best ocular alignment:
  - In accommodative squints correction of long-sightedness by glasses usually controls the excessive convergence.
  - For other types of squints surgery is required. This is particularly important for congenital squints. The longer the defect persists untreated the less chance there is for development of good visual function.

2.3 Examination of the eyes for the Short Case

- Observe for obvious eye abnormalities, e.g. coloboma, ptosis, squint
- Assess visual acuity of both eyes separately
- Assess visual fields
- Test eye movements
- Cover test for squint
- Direct and consensual light reflex
- Examination of the fundi

Order of examination may be influenced by your findings along the way, e.g. if you find an abnormality such as a squint you may focus on the assessment of that.

3. HEARING

Some 1–2 children per 1,000 population have permanent childhood deafness, 84% congenital and 16% acquired. Early detection of hearing problems and treatment have permanent beneficial effects.

Possible interventions

- Hearing aids
- Cochlear implant — will allow more deaf children to develop spoken language
- Involvement of Speech and Language therapy services
- Pre-school/in school learning support, e.g. signing

Routine hearing screening programme

- **Neonatal screening**

Move towards universal neonatal screening to allow early detection of deafness. At present in many areas only high-risk infants are screened.

- Low birth weight
- Jaundice at the exchange level
- Anomalies of the ears, preauricular pits, tags
- Special Care Baby Unit (SCBU) admission for more than 72 hours
- Family history of deafness
- Gentamicin treatment

Screening test used: Otoacoustic emissions test or auditory brainstem response testing

- **At 8 months for all children** by health visitor
  Screening test used: hearing distraction test

- **At pre-school entry at 4–5 years for all children** by school nurse
  Screening test used: sweep audiogram

If the screening test is positive the child is referred to an audiologist for further assessment. Referrals to audiology can also be made at any time if concerns are raised about hearing or speech and language development, e.g. by the parents.

3.1 Assessment of auditory function

- **Babies**
  - Diagnostic auditory brainstem response testing
  - Otoacoustic emissions test

- **8 months**
  - Hearing distraction test
- **2 years**
  - Visual reinforcement audiometry
  - Performance games
  - Speech discrimination test
  - Free-field audiometry
- **3 years and over**
  - Pure-tone audiometry

It is important to consider both the developmental and the chronological age when deciding which test to use.

Otoacoustic emissions test

Otoacoustic emissions are thought to arise from the cochlear sensory mechanism and are only present if the cochlear is functioning. This test does not test the whole of the hearing pathway, but pure problems distal to the cochlear are very rare and this test detects most causes of deafness. For measuring emissions a soft tip probe is placed into the ear. The test is easy, quick with minimum preparation. This test is now widely used to screen infants in the neonatal period for sensorineural deafness.

Auditory brainstem response (ABR)

This test measures sound-induced electrical activity in the brain using scalp electrodes. It tests the whole hearing system but takes longer to perform, more equipment is needed and baby needs to stay calm. It is time-consuming, but it is very useful for babies and children who are difficult to test by behavioural means because they have developmental difficulties.

Distraction test

This test is performed routinely by health visitors on all infants at 8 months. The child sits on the mother's lap with a distracter sitting in front of them and the noise stimulus presenter remaining behind the child (out of sight). The test relies on the normal child's response to turn to locate the source of the sound and on the fact that they have not yet developed permanence of objects, so that once they have been distracted again by the person in the front they forget about the tester behind them. A series of sounds at different frequencies are presented at a level of about 40 dB at a set distance of 1 metre behind the child at ear level. There are standardized sounds and test materials — Manchester rattle, warbler, Nuffield rattle, voice.

Visual reinforced audiometry

Sounds are presented to the child via a loudspeaker arrangement that enables the sound to be presented precisely at different decibels for each frequency tested. If the head turns to the sound the child is rewarded by a visual stimulus, e.g. a toy lighting up in a box. Headphones can be used in a compliant child so allowing individual ears to be tested.

Performance test or Go games

These tests are useful for children aged 2 to 4 years actual or developmental level. They require some understanding and co-operation. The child is asked to perform a task when they hear a noise, i.e. put man in boat. It can be performed by health visitors.

Speech discrimination test

This test is useful for children 2.5 years plus actual or developmental level. An example is the McCormick Toy Test. Toys are laid out in front of the child on the table and the examiner asks the child to identify the toy called. The examiner must test voice against a sound meter level. The mouth is covered to prevent lip reading and the tester has to be careful not to give visual clues. The toys are in pairs to test for consonants, e.g. duck/cup.

Free-field testing

Suitable for children 2 years and over. It does not require understanding or co-operation so useful for children with developmental delay or behavioural problems. Sounds are produced within a free field at different frequencies. The child's reaction to sound is observed and assessed if satisfactory.

Pure-tone audiometry

By 4 years of age a child should be able to co-operate with this test. Both ears can be tested separately. The audiometer delivers sounds at different frequencies and intensity. It is possible to determine the child's threshold at each sound frequency. It takes at least 10 minutes to perform.

The audiogram

Key to symbols used:

X axis   = frequency (Hz)
Y axis = hearing level (dBHL)
O   = air conduction right ear
X   = air conduction left ear
△   = bone conduction unmasked — vibrator vibrates whole skull no matter which
           mastoid it is placed on. Assesses both cochleas unless one ear masked.
[= masked bone conduction right
]   = masked bone conduction left
↓   = off scale (no response)

Air conduction assesses whole auditory system, bone conduction assesses auditory pathway from the cochlea and beyond. A difference between the two suggests a conductive loss (middle or outer ear). Equal impairment suggests a sensorineural loss. Impairment greater in air than bone suggests a mixed loss.

Normal range	−10 –>+20 dBHL
Moderate hearing loss	20 –>40 dBHL
Profound hearing loss	90 –>120 dBHL

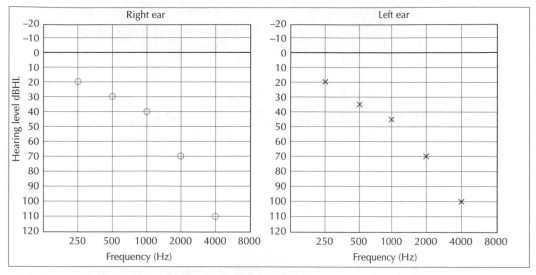

High-frequency hearing loss in a child with speech delay

Sweep audiometry

Same principle as above but quicker to perform as various sound frequencies tested at only one intensity (around 25 dB). It is used as a screening test at the pre-school entry. If the child fails at any frequency then full audiometry is performed.

Tympanometry

The compliance of the tympanic membrane and ear ossicles is assessed by a probe that fits snugly in the external auditory canal and which is able to generate positive and negative pressures whilst recording the sound reflected back from a small microphone within the probe. Suitable for any age child. Primarily used to check for 'glue ear'. In the normal ear, the peak is at 0 pressure, reflecting the equal pressures either side of the drum. The trace is flattened if a middle-ear effusion is present.

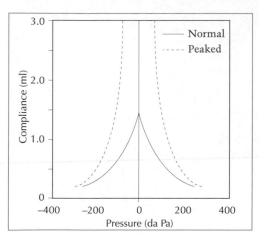

Normal trace
(If compliance much greater than normal (peaked) consider flaccid drum or disarticulation of the ossicles)

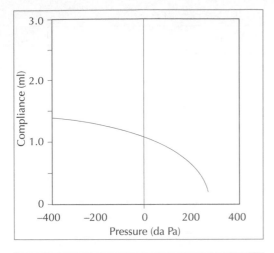

Flattened trace with no clear peak
– middle-ear effusion
– fixed ear ossicles

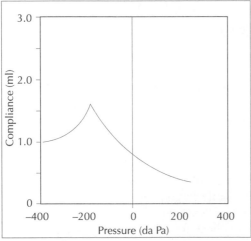

Peak at negative pressure (shift to left)
– eustachian tube dysfunction (retracted drum)

4. SPEECH AND LANGUAGE

4.1 Communication

Acquisition of communication involves:

- **Speech**
  - Expressive: production of speech
  - Comprehension: understanding what is being said
  - Comprehension development is ahead of expressive

- **Non-verbal communication**
  - Eye contact, pointing, body gestures

- **Social communication**
  - Reciprocity and sharing of communication, insight into what is socially acceptable, sharing communication, listening skills.

Problems in speech and language development are very common in pre-school children (5–10%). It is commoner in boys.

4.2 Differential diagnosis of speech and language problem

Problem with language input

- Hearing deficit
- Reduced exposure to spoken language, e.g. social circumstances, twins, poor parenting skills

Problems with language processing

- Specific speech and language delay
- Associated with general developmental delay
- Associated with reduced communicative intent and poor social skills, i.e. autistic spectrum disorder
- Associated with brain abnormalities, e.g. epilepsy, Llandau–Kleffner

Problems with language output

- Neurological or muscular problems, e.g. cerebral palsy

4.3 Specific speech and language delay

Problems in auditory/linguistic processing leading to difficulties with:

- Phonology: articulation and making the speech sounds
- Grammar: understanding the forms and structure of language

Problems in understanding the appropriate meaning and use of language

- Semantics: the meaning of words and sentences
- Pragmatics: the appropriate social use of language

Many children have a mixture of problems.

4.4 Clinical assessment

Clinical assessment determines:

- The nature of the speech and language problem
- If there are other problems such as general delay, autistic spectrum
- Any underlying cause, e.g. deafness

Investigations

- It is important to confirm that the hearing is normal (see earlier)
- EEG if clear history of loss of language skills to exclude epilepsy syndromes
- Chromosomal studies if other associated difficulties

Management of speech and language problem

- If speech and language delay is the only problem it is usually managed by speech and language therapists alone without continuing paediatric input.
- If other additional problems, multidisciplinary assessment is usually necessary involving some or all of the multidisciplinary team.
- It is also important that advice is given to education about the child's difficulties to enable them to access the national curriculum. Children with severe difficulties are sometimes placed in language units with access to on-site speech and language therapists. The majority, however, are managed in mainstream school with a speech and language programme incorporated into their individual education plans. Speech and language therapists then review the programme intermittently.

5. AUTISTIC SPECTRUM DISORDER

Recent studies suggest that autism is becoming more common and the prevalence in indus-trialized countries may be as high as 1 per 1,000, not including Asperger's syndrome. Boys tend to outnumber girls by 3:1.

There is a wide variation in clinical presentation (Autistic Spectrum Disorder). Three areas of development are affected:

Social skills

- Non-verbal behaviours, e.g. eye contact, body posture
- Failure to develop peer relationships
- Lack of social and emotional sharing

Verbal and non-verbal communication

- Delay in development of spoken language
- No attempt to communicate by other means
- Inability to initiate conversation
- Stereotyped and repetitive language, lack of imaginative play

Repetitive and stereotype patterns of behaviour

- Adherence to routines
- Lack of imaginative play and behaviour
- Restrictive patterns of interest
- Preoccupation with parts of objects
- Repetitive motor mannerisms, e.g. hand flapping, door closing

Other features

- The abnormal functioning is observed in one of these areas of development prior to age of 3 years.
- The behaviour is not accounted for by another diagnosis. A large number of children with syndromes and chromosomal abnormalities have autistic features.
- Over 50% also have associated intellectual impairment that can affect the behaviours observed.
- By middle age 30% have developed epilepsy
- Hearing and visual problems are common
- Dyspraxia is common

Asperger's syndrome is a condition at the mild end of the autistic spectrum. There is normal early language development and intellectual functioning. In early childhood it becomes apparent that the child has behavioural and social difficulties and some speech and language problems. The diagnosis can often be missed.

5.1 Assessment of children on the autistic spectrum

This is by multidisciplinary assessment. The format varies depending on local services but should include: a developmental paediatrician, a psychiatrist/psychologist and a speech and language therapy assessment.

- **History**: important to get thorough history including developmental milestones. Information about behaviour from other sources is helpful, e.g. nursery.
- **Examination**: to exclude any other diagnosis presenting with autistic features, e.g. fragile X syndrome. If possible, try to watch the child in different settings to observe the behavioural difficulties. A child in a one to one consultation situation may behave very differently when put into a group. Hearing and vision should also be checked.
- **Investigations**: there is no consensus regarding investigations. Some perform EEGs and chromosomal studies routinely. Others only perform the tests if there is a clinical indication, e.g. chromosomes if dysmorphic features are found, EEG if variation in symptoms or associated developmental regression.

Management: each child needs to be assessed as an individual to determine the degree of difficulty in social and communication skills, and an individual management plan decided upon.

Health: communication with parents about their concerns and difficulties with management of the child is essential. Access to more information should be provided, e.g. the National Autistic Society. Access to psychiatric/psychology services for the individual and the family are essential.

Education: liaison with education is essential. Pre-school intervention within the home and nursery is possible with early diagnosis. Local outreach services may be available to go into the home to give management advice. Formal pre-school notification by health to education allows the child's needs to be assessed prior to school placement. School placement can vary from mainstream with support through to a special unit depending on the individual child. They often require high teacher to pupil ratio in a highly structured environment to minimize disruptions. Speech and language input to help communication skills also important.

Social Services: living with a child on the autistic spectrum affects all members of the family. Families often need respite care and support in the home.

6. DYSPRAXIA

Dyspraxia is a common type of sensory processing problem that causes difficulty in performing co-ordinated actions. The child is often described as clumsy. There may be associated problems of language, perception and thought processing. Concern about dyspraxia is one of the commonest reasons for a referral to a paediatrician from education.

In the younger child symptoms include:

- Slow gross-motor development
- Poor motor skills, e.g. running, jumping, not able to catch a ball
- Difficulty dressing
- Poor pencil grip
- Difficulty with jigsaws
- Anxiety

In the older child symptoms include:

- Avoidance of physical education
- Slow school progress
- Reduced attention span
- Difficulty with maths, reading
- Trouble copying from blackboard
- Poor writing skills
- Inability to follow instructions
- Poor organizational skills

Differential diagnosis

- Learning disability
- Neuromuscular problem
- Attention-deficit hyperactivity disorder
- Specific speech and language delay
- Visual problem

Remember that a child can have more than one difficulty, e.g. dyspraxia and attention-deficit hyperactivity disorder.

Assessment

In the pre-school child initial assessment is usually by a paediatrician to exclude other pathologies, including general developmental delay. The school-age child is also often assessed by a paediatrician, but information should also be obtained from the school about the child's difficulties and overall progress. Often a speech and language assessment and occupational therapy assessment are also required.

The occupational therapist examines:

- Fine- and gross-motor developmental levels
- Visual motor integration (e.g. doing puzzles or copying shapes)
- Visual perception
- Balance and posture
- Responses to sensory stimulation
- Bilateral co-ordination
- Motor planning

Management

Dyspraxia is not curable but the child often improves in some areas with maturity. Liaison between education, health professionals and the child and parents is crucial to help the child within the classroom and the home environment. The school's special educational needs co-ordinator (SENCO) and school nurse can play an important role in the communication between health and education. Speech and language therapists and occupational therapists give advice to the school to help with difficulties in the classroom. Sometimes group and individual therapy can help, e.g. a phonology course for articulation difficulties. Advice for parents to help with home activities is also important.

7. SPECIAL EDUCATIONAL NEEDS AND THE EDUCATIONAL STATEMENT

Many children have special educational needs, but only a small percentage (approximately 2%) need statements because their difficulties are such that they require provision which is additional to or different from that normally available to children. In a statement the child's needs are clarified and a plan of how to meet these needs within the education setting is made. The statement is a legal contract and allows extra funding for the individual child to meet the special educational needs. Information from health is requested because:

- With the pre-school child it is often health that first becomes aware of the special educational needs, e.g. global developmental delay, Down's syndrome, cerebral palsy.

- Some medical conditions may have significant impact on the child's academic attainment and the ability to participate fully in the curriculum. Some of the commonest medical conditions are congenital heart disease, epilepsy, cystic fibrosis, haemophilia and childhood cancers.

Pre-school children

- Health are required by law to notify the local education authority (LEA) of children over the age of 2 years who may have special educational needs.
- The parents, nursery and social services are also able to notify education.
- The LEA then collects information about the child, which is passed onto the educational psychologist who decides if a formal assessment for statementing is appropriate.
- If formal assessment is requested health are asked to write a report on the child's needs, the 'E medical'. This report will give information about health, e.g. hearing, vision, epilepsy, physical problems and a summary of the developmental problems. It also informs education of other therapists involved such as physiotherapy, speech and language. It also describes the practical needs of the child, e.g. toileting, feeding, dressing, what to do if the child has a fit. Other professionals also submit reports including the parents.

Once the formal assessment is completed the local education authority decides whether to statement the child or not. (The majority of children are issued a statement after formal assessment.)

Schoolchildren

The process is the same, but the initial notification usually comes from the school or the parents rather than health, as the children are in school.

Child Psychiatry

8. ATTENTION-DEFICIT HYPERACTIVITY DISORDER (ADHD)

Estimated that 1% of school-age children meet the diagnostic criteria for ADHD. Commoner in boys.

Diagnosis

Characterized by exhibiting problems in three areas:
- Inattention
- Hyperactivity
- Impulsiveness

It is possible to have one of these features without the others, e.g. marked inattention without the hyperactivity and hyperactivity without inattention.

In addition:

- The behaviour should have persisted for at least 6 months
- The behaviour should be inconsistent with the child's developmental age
- There must be clinically significant impairment in social or academic development
- The symptoms should occur in more than one setting
- There should be no other explanation for the symptoms, e.g. psychiatric illness

Diagnosis requires detailed history and information gathering from parents, school and other professionals involved.

Children with ADHD develop emotional and social problems, poor school performance and problems within the home because of the difficult behaviour. Associated with unemployment, substance abuse and crime in adulthood.

Differential diagnosis

- Inappropriate expectations
- Language/communication disorder
- Social problem
- Specific learning difficulty
- Chronic illness, e.g. asthma
- Epilepsy
- Dyspraxia

Management

Management involves a comprehensive treatment programme. There needs to be multi-professional collaboration including the parents.

- **Psychological/behavioural interventions** — range of interventions from support groups through to psychotherapy
- **Educational support** — close communication with school is vital, development of individual education plan if necessary
- **Social services** — support if necessary
- **Drug treatment and dietary manipulation**

Dietary interventions are possibly useful. Some parents observe that certain foods aggravate the symptoms.

Methylphenidate (Ritalin) is used for the treatment of ADHD. It is a central nervous system stimulant and is usually given twice a day, morning and lunchtime. An evening dose is avoided because of difficulties with sleep. A drug holiday is recommended once a year. Side-effects include weight and growth retardation and hypertension. Treatment should be started by child psychiatrists or paediatricians with expertise in ADHD. Height, weight, pulse and BP should be monitored at least 6-monthly. Drug treatment does not cure ADHD. It improves the symptoms to allow the other interventions an opportunity to take effect.

The National Institute for Clinical Excellence (NICE) has recently issued guidance on the use of methylphenidate. It has recommended:

- Methylphenidate can be used as part of a comprehensive treatment programme for children with severe ADHD
- Not licensed for those under 6 years and diagnosis should be made by a psychiatrist or paediatrician with expertise in ADHD
- The clinical expert should supervise the medication
- Treatment should be stopped if there is no effect
- Treatment should also include advice and support to parents and teachers
- Children should be regularly monitored

NICE is part of the NHS. It provides guidance on medicines, medical equipment, diagnostic tests and clinical procedures and where they should be used.

9. SCHIZOPHRENIA WITH CHILDHOOD ONSET

Schizophrenia is rare in childhood and adolescence with an incidence of less than 3:10,000. A genetic component can be implicated in at least 10% of cases, but other factors including perinatal difficulties, psychosocial factors and difficulties with premorbid personality are also important. Boys outnumber girls by approximately 2:1.

Presentation

May be acute or insidious (gradual withdrawal and failing schoolwork).

Major symptoms include:
- Delusions
- Hallucinations
- Distortions of thinking (thought insertion and withdrawal)
- Movement disorders, commonly catatonia

Differential diagnosis

- May be difficult to distinguish from major mood disturbance, e.g. manic depressive psychosis or organic causes of psychosis e.g. neurodegenerative or drug-induced episode, SLE, epilepsy, Wilson disease, thyrotoxicosis and vasculitis. (Any child presenting with psychotic symptoms should have an EEG and brain MRI scan).

Treatment

- Drugs — antipsychotics, e.g. clozapine (few extrapyramidal side-effects but risk of agranulocytosis), chlorpromazine, haloperidol
- Individual and family therapy
- Adequate educational provision essential

Prognosis

- Chronic or relapsing course common
- Good prognostic factors include high intelligence, acute onset, precipitating factors, older age at onset and normal premorbid personality

10. DEPRESSION IN CHILDHOOD AND ADOLESCENCE

Depressive illness is rare in childhood with a frequency of less than 2% in primary school-aged children. This rises to around 5% in adolescents. There is an association with physical illness, including infectious mononucleosis (acute trigger) or chronic disease. There is also a strong association with neglect, anxiety and behavioural problems. A careful assessment of suicidal ideation must be made. Treatment is with antidepressants, and individual and family therapy are usually instituted. The prognosis is usually good.

Depression becomes more prevalent during adolescence. Whilst mild depressive episodes may be difficult to diagnose, moderate and severe episodes follow the same pattern as in adults. A family history of affective disorders is not uncommon. Appropriate practical support is essential and individual psychotherapy may be helpful.

First-line drug treatment usually comprises a trial of a selective serotonin-reuptake inhibitor (SSRI) such as fluoxetine. These drugs are safe with few side-effects. Although there is evidence that children commenced on fluoxetine have some improvement in their symptoms, in contrast to adults complete remission is uncommon. It is now widely accepted that the risks of tricyclic antidepressants outweigh any potential therapeutic benefits and there is evidence that tricyclics are no more effective than placebo for depression in children and adolescents. The true efficacy of pharmacotherapy is contentious and the long-term outcome of adolescent depression unpredictable.

11. SUICIDE AND SUICIDAL BEHAVIOUR

Suicide is rare before puberty, yet it is the third leading cause of death for adolescents with rates in young men continuing to rise. Methods include drug overdose, hanging, inhalation of car exhaust fumes and shooting. It is by far the minority of adolescents who make suicide attempts who have either an underlying psychiatric disorder or serious suicidal intent. All individuals who attempt suicide must undergo psychiatric assessment. The use of violent methods, attempts which take place in isolated places and the writing of a suicide note should ring particular alarm bells.

Risk factors for suicide in adolescents

- Male sex
- Broken home, disturbed relationships with parents
- Living alone
- Immigrant status
- Family history of affective disorder, suicide or alcohol abuse
- Recent loss or stress
- Previous suicide attempt
- Drug or alcohol addiction

Characteristics of deliberate self-harm in adolescents

Self-poisoning

- Much more common in females
- Accounts for over 90% of cases of deliberate self-harm
- Overdose often taken in environment where patient is likely to be found
- Drugs most commonly taken include paracetamol, aspirin, benzodiazepines and antidepressants
- Multiple drug ingestion common (often with alcohol)
- Under 20% need intensive medical management but all should be admitted until assessed by child psychiatrist/social services as appropriate
- Mortality well below 1%
- Blood and urine toxicology screen are useful as there is often a poor correlation between quantity of drugs taken and clinical effect
- Paracetamol and aspirin levels should be taken routinely

Self-mutilation

- Includes scratching, cutting, cigarette burns, tattooing, bruising, biting and inserting needles
- Typically seen in teenage girls with personality problems, e.g. aggressive/impulsive behaviour, eating disorders, poor self-esteem
- Also occurs in those with schizophrenia/learning disability

Difficult to treat — need to address underlying personality/emotional problems.

Over 10% of adolescents who attempt suicide will repeat within 1 year.

12. EATING DISORDERS IN CHILDHOOD AND ADOLESCENCE

The eating disorders anorexia nervosa and bulimia nervosa have become increasingly recognized in paediatric practice over the last two decades. Both are rare in pre-pubertal children. Anorexia nervosa increases in incidence through mid and late adolescence, bulimia nervosa most commonly presents in late teens or early 20s. Over 90% of those affected by eating disorders are female.

Many clinical features are common to both anorexia and bulimia nervosa and patients may satisfy criteria for anorexia or bulimia at different stages of their illness.

Diagnostic criteria for anorexia nervosa

- Self-induced weight loss of >15% body weight (avoidance of 'fattening' foods aggravated by self-induced vomiting, purging or exercise)
- Intense fear of gaining weight or becoming fat, even though underweight
- Abnormal perception of body image
- Amenorrhoea in post-menarchal female (absence of at least three menstrual cycles)

Diagnostic criteria for bulimia nervosa

- Recurrent episodes of binge eating, characterized by consuming an excessive amount of food within a short, defined time span, with lack of control of eating during the episode
- Recurrent inappropriate compensatory behaviour to prevent weight gain, e.g. laxative abuse or self-induced vomiting
- Binges and compensatory behaviour occur at least twice per week for 3 months
- Self-evaluation unduly influenced by body shape and weight
- Disturbance does not occur exclusively during periods of anorexia nervosa

Epidemiology of eating disorders
There is an overall incidence of between 1 and 5 cases per 100,000 population for anorexia nervosa. Prevalence studies suggest 'true' anorexia nervosa occurs in 0.5% of adolescent girls but partial forms may occur in up to 10% of young women. Occasional episodes of binge eating and purging have been reported in up to 40% of female college students, the true prevalence of bulimia is probably around 1.5%.

Aetiology

- **Familial factors:** concordance rate for anorexia nervosa in monozygotic twins is 50%, as compared to 10% for dizygotic twins. Other risk factors include family history of depression, alcoholism, obesity or eating disorder. Children with anorexia nervosa often come from overprotective and rigid families where there is a lack of conflict resolution.
- **Individual factors:** e.g. previous obesity, fear of losing control, self-esteem dependent on the opinion of others and previous or ongoing abuse

- **Sociocultural factors:** there is a higher prevalence in high social classes and certain occupations, e.g. ballet dancers
- **Neurohumoral factors:** controversy remains over the exact role of substances such as serotonin in the pathogenesis of eating disorders

Clinical features

Anorexia nervosa
Usually this begins as a 'typical' adolescent diet to reduce stigmatization from obesity. Once weight begins to reduce, weight goals are constantly reset and compulsive weighing becomes a feature. Often physical activity is increased and social contacts diminish. Disordered thinking and poor concentration develop as the disease process progresses.

Bulimia nervosa
Bulimia is even more common than anorexia in those with a past history of obesity. Self-loathing and disgust with the body are also greater than in anorexia. Patients are more likely to seek medical help for their symptoms. Coexisting substance abuse is not uncommon. Both bulimia and anorexia are frequently associated with major depressive and anxiety disorders.

Medical complications of anorexia nervosa and bulimia

CNS
- Reversible cortical atrophy
- Non-specific EEG abnormalities

Dental
- Caries
- Periodontitis

Pulmonary
- Aspiration pneumonia (rare)

Cardiovascular
- Bradycardia
- Hypotension
- Arrhythmias
- Cardiomyopathy (rare)

Gastrointestinal
- Parotitis
- Delayed gastric emptying
- Gastric dilation
- Constipation
- Raised amylase (bulimia)

Renal/electrolyte
- Hypokalaemia
- Hypochloraemic metabolic alkalosis
- Oedema
- Renal calculi (rare)

Neuroendocrine
- Amenorrhoea
- Oligomenorrhea (bulimia)

Musculoskeletal
- Myopathy
- Osteoporosis and pathological fractures

Haematological
- Anaemia
- Thrombocytopenia
- Hypercholesterolaemia
- Hypercarotenaemia

Dermatological
- Dry, cracking skin
- Lanugo
- Callous on dorsum of hand (from vomiting)
- Perioral dermatitis

Course and prognosis

Five to ten years after the diagnosis of anorexia nervosa around 50% will have recovered, 25% will have improved but still have some features of an eating disorder and the remainder will either not have improved or be dead. Mortality rates are around 5% but may rise further with longer term follow-up.

Good prognostic factors

- Younger age at onset
- Less denial
- Improved self-esteem

Poor prognostic factors

- Parental conflict
- Bulimia nervosa
- Coexisting behavioural disorders

The long-term outcome of bulimia nervosa is less clear.

Treatment

Most patients with anorexia can be treated as outpatients, with hospital admission only if adequate weight gain at home is not possible or there are complications such as depression.

A combined multidisciplinary approach with monitoring of eating and weight, biochemical monitoring and ongoing psychotherapy is required. At present the psychotherapy usually involves behavioural, cognitive and psychodynamic components. Rarely medication such as antipsychotics or antidepressants may be required. Appetite stimulants are used even less often. Prokinetics such as cisapride and domperidone may be useful in patients with delayed gastric emptying. Adequate provision for education is essential.

13. COMMON BEHAVIOURAL PROBLEMS IN PRE-SCHOOL CHILDREN

13.1 Sleep disorders

Reluctance to settle at night and persistent waking during the night are common problems in young children, with one in five 2-year-olds waking at least five times per week.

Factors contributing to sleep difficulties

- Adverse temperamental characteristics in child
- Perinatal problems
- Maternal anxiety
- Poor accommodation
- Physical illness

- Medication, e.g. theophyllines
- Timing of feeds
- Co-sleeping with parents

Medication is usually unhelpful in this situation. A behavioural strategy is usually successful but often needs to be combined with some respite for the parents.

Nightmares are most common between 3 and 5 years with an incidence of between 25% and 50%. The child who awakens during them is usually alert and can recall the dream and frightening images. They are usually self-limiting and may be related to obvious frightening or stressful events. In severe cases the involvement of a psychologist or psychiatrist may be needed.

13.2 Feeding problems in infancy and childhood

Most children at some point will be 'picky eaters' — a phase which will usually pass spontaneously. Infants and children may also, however, refuse to feed if they find the experience painful or frightening. Reasons contributing to this may include:

- Unpleasant physical experiences associated with eating, e.g. gastro-oesophageal reflux, oral candidiasis, stricture post-oesophageal atresia repair
- Oral motor dysfunction
- Children who have required early nasogastric tube feeds
- Maternal depression
- Being forced to eat by caregiver
- Developmental conflict with caregiver
- Emotional and social deprivation

Non-organic failure to thrive is a diagnosis of exclusion.

Evaluation of feeding disorders

- Complete history including detailed social history
- Complete physical examination — need to exclude physiological, anatomical and neurological abnormalities
- Assess emotional state and developmental level
- Observe feeding interaction
- Help parents understand infants and children may have different styles of eating and food preferences

Management of feeding disorders

- Eliminate and/or treat physical cause
- Multidisciplinary approach including paediatrician, GP, health visitor, speech therapist, dietician and/or psychologist
- Child's behaviour may need modification
- If failure to thrive also exclude medical disorders and maltreatment

Pica (the ingestion of inedible material such as dirt and rubbish) may be normal in toddlers but persistent ingestion is found in children with learning difficulties, psychotic and socially deprived children. Lead poisoning is a theoretical risk from pica.

13.3 Temper tantrums

These are common in the pre-school child and generally occur when the child is angry or has hurt themselves. Usually they are typified by screaming and/or crying, often in association with collapsing to the floor. It is rare for the child to injure themselves during such episodes. If necessary the child should be restrained from behind by folding one's arms around the child's body. It is important to minimize any additional attention to the child and to respond and praise only when behaviour is back to normal.

13.4 Breath-holding attacks

These episodes typically occur after a frustrating or painful experience. The child cries inconsolably, holds his breath and then becomes pale or cyanosed. In the most serious cases loss of consciousness may ensue and there may be stiffening of the limbs or brief clonic movements. Clearly it may be difficult to distinguish from a generalized seizure, however the fact that after a breath-holding attack the child will take a deep breath and immediately regain consciousness may facilitate differentiation. Typical onset is between 6 and 18 months. No specific treatment is needed and the episodes diminish with age.

14. COMMON PROBLEMS IN THE SCHOOL-AGED CHILD

14.1 School refusal

This problem refers to the child's irrational fear about school attendance and most commonly is seen at the beginning of schooling or in association with a change of school or move to secondary school. Typically the child is reluctant to leave home in the morning and they may develop headache or abdominal pain.

Factors contributing to school refusal include:

- Separation anxiety
- Specific phobia about an aspect of school attendance, e.g. travelling to school, mixing with other children, games lessons, etc.
- A more generalized psychiatric disturbance such as depression or low self-esteem
- Bullying

Characteristics of school refusers

- Good academic achievements
- Conformist at school
- Oppositional at home

Treatment

- Avoid unnecessary investigation of minor somatic symptoms
- Early, if necessary graded return to school
- Support for parents and child
- Close liaison with school

In chronic cases a gradual reintegration back into school is required, possibly with a concurrent specific behavioural programme and targeted family therapy.

Overall two-thirds of children will return to school regularly. Those who do badly are often adolescents from disturbed family backgrounds.

Truancy

In contrast to the above, truancy always reflects a lack of desire to go to school rather than anxiety re school attendance and as such may be part of a conduct disorder.

Bullying

Bullying may be defined as 'the intentional unprovoked abuse of power by one or more children to inflict pain or cause distress to another child on repeated occasions'. Estimates on the prevalence of bullying vary widely, but many studies report that between 20% and 50% of school-aged children have either participated in or been victims of bullying. Verbal harassment is the commonest form of bullying and is often not recognized as such.

Although it is important not to stereotype, certain characteristics are commonly exhibited by bullies:

- Poor psychosocial functioning
- Unhappiness in school
- Concurrent conduct disorders
- Emotional problems
- Social problems
- Alcohol and nicotine abuse

Children who suffer at the hands of bullies may consequently suffer from:

- Anxiety
- Insecurity
- Low self-esteem and self-worth
- Mental health problems
- Sleep difficulties
- Bed wetting
- Headaches
- Abdominal pain

Carefully planned programmes may reduce the incidence of bullying by 50% or more. Such strategies rely on teaching children who bully appropriate social skills, developing clear rules which they are expected to adhere to, providing an increased level of supervision, particularly within the school environment, and facilitating access to other services they may require, e.g. child psychiatry, social services, etc.

14.2 Non-organic abdominal pain/headache/limb pains

Over 10% of children experience such symptoms. It is important to exclude organic pathology promptly and to search for any underlying stresses. Most run a short course but if symptoms are persistent and involve several systems the term 'somatization disorder' is used.

14.3 Sleep problems in the school-aged child

In order to understand sleep disorders a basic knowledge of the sleep cycle is necessary:

Sleep stages

Sleep consists of several stages that cycle throughout the night. One complete cycle lasts 90–100 minutes.

Sleep stage	Features
1 Slow wave sleep (SWS) or non-rapid eye movement (NREM)	Transition state between sleep and wakefulness Eyes begin to roll slightly Mostly high-amplitude, low-frequency theta waves Brief periods of alpha waves — similar to those when awake Lasts only few minutes
2 SWS or NREM	Peak of brain waves higher and higher sleep spindles Lasts only few minutes
3 SWS or NREM	Also called delta sleep or deep sleep Very slow delta waves account for 20–50% of brain waves
4 SWS or NREM	Also called delta sleep or deep sleep Over 50% of brain waves are delta waves Last and deepest of sleep stages before REM sleep
5 REM	Frequent bursts of rapid eye movement and occasional muscular twitches Heart rate increases Rapid shallow respirations Most vivid dreaming during this phase

14.4 Night terrors

These are most commonly seen in children between the ages of 4 and 7 years. Typically the child wakes from deep or stage 4 sleep apparently terrified, hallucinating and unresponsive to those around them. Usually such episodes last less than 15 minutes and the child goes back to sleep, with no recollection of the events in the morning. It is unusual to find any underlying reason or stresses contributing to the problem.

14.5 Nightmares

These occur during REM sleep and the child remembers the dream either immediately or in the morning. Underlying anxieties should be sought.

14.6 Sleep walking

This occurs during stages 3 or 4 of sleep and is most often seen in those between 8 and 14 years.

14.7 Tics

These occur transiently in 10% of children and are much more commonly seen in boys. Onset is usually around the age of 7 years and, whilst simple tics are seen most commonly, Gilles de la Tourette syndrome may occur in childhood. This phenomenon is characterized by complex tics occurring in association with coprolalia (obscene words and swearing) and echolalia (repetition of sounds or words).

Factors predisposing to tics

- Positive family history
- Stress (including parental)
- Neurodevelopmental delay

Treatment

- Most resolve spontaneously
- Reassure accordingly
- Behavioural or family therapy if appropriate
- Medication: haloperidol, pimozide, clonidine (in very severe cases only)

Outcome

- Simple tics: complete remission
- Tourette's syndrome: 50% have symptoms into adult life

15. ENURESIS

This is defined as the involuntary passage of urine in the absence of physical abnormality after the age of 5 years. Nocturnal enuresis is much more common than diurnal enuresis, affecting at least 10% of 5-year-olds. Although most children with nocturnal enuresis are not psychiatrically ill, up to 25% will have signs of psychiatric disturbance. Diurnal enuresis is much more common among girls and those who are psychiatrically disturbed.

Aetiology

- Positive family history in 70%
- Developmental delay
- Psychiatric disturbance
- Small bladder capacity
- Recent stressful life events
- Large family size
- Social disadvantage

Treatment

- Exclude physical basis (history, examination, urine culture, +/– imaging)
- Look for underlying stresses
- Reassure child and parents of benign course
- Star chart
- Enuresis alarm (7 years and older)
- Drugs (short-term control only) desmopressin, tricyclic antidepressants

16. ENCOPRESIS AND SOILING

This is defined as the inappropriate passage of formed faeces, usually onto the underwear, after the age of 4 years. It is uncommon, with a prevalence of 1.8% amongst 8-year-old boys and 0.7% for girls. Psychiatric disturbance is common and enuresis often coexists. Broadly speaking, children with encopresis may be divided into those who retain faeces and develop subsequent overflow incontinence (retentive encopresis) and those who deposit faeces inappropriately on a regular basis (non-retentive).

Type of encopresis common family characteristics

- Retentive: obsessional toilet-training practices
- Non-retentive: continuous, disorganized, chaotic families

Other risk factors for encopresis

- Poor parent/child relationship
- Emotional stresses (including sexual abuse)
- Past history of constipation/anal fissure

Treatment

- Exclude physical problems, e.g. Hirschsprung's/hypothyroidism/hypercalcaemia
- Laxatives to clear bowel
- Education for parents and child
- Star chart
- Individual psychotherapy
- Family therapy

It is unusual for this problem to persist into adolescence

17. CONDUCT DISORDERS

Persistent antisocial or socially disapproved of behaviour often involving damage to property and unresponsive to normal sanctions.

Prevalence

- Approximately 4%
- Strong male predominance

Clinical features

- Temper tantrums
- Oppositional behaviour (defiance of authority, fighting)
- Overactivity
- Irritability
- Aggression
- Stealing
- Lying
- Truancy
- Bullying
- Delinquency, e.g. stealing, vandalism, arson in older children/teenagers

'Oppositional defiant disorder' is a type of conduct disorder characteristically seen in children under 10 years. It is characterized by markedly defiant, disobedient, provocative behaviour and by the absence of more severe dissocial or aggressive acts that violate the law or the rights of others.

Aetiology

- Family factors: lack of affection, marital disharmony, poor discipline, parental violence/aggression
- Constitutional factors: low IQ, learning difficulties, adverse temperamental features
- Oppositional peer group values
- Urban deprivation/poor schooling

Differential diagnosis

Young people with conduct disorders have an increased incidence of neurological signs and symptoms, psychomotor seizures, psychotic symptoms, mood disorders, ADHD and learning difficulties.

Treatment

- Family/behavioural therapy
- Practical social support, e.g. rehousing

Prognosis

Half have problems into adult life

Community Paediatrics

18. CHILD HEALTH SURVEILLANCE

The health authority is responsible for ensuring that an adequate surveillance programme is offered to all children and that it is monitored effectively. The programme should comprise:

- Oversight of health and physical growth of all children
- Monitoring developmental progress of all children
- Provision of adequate advice and support to parents
- Programme of infectious disease prophylaxis
- Participation in health education and training in parenthood
- Identification of 'children in need' in accordance with the Children Act
- Identification and notification of children with special educational needs in accordance with the 1981 Education Act

18.1 Pre-school children

At present in the UK, all children, at birth, are assigned a health visitor who has regular contact with the child and their family at home and at child health clinics. A parent-held child health record 'red book' is given at birth. All contact that professionals have with the child and family should be clearly documented. The current pre-school child health programme is:

- **Neonatal examination:** done by hospital doctor, nurse practitioner or GP. Full physical examination including weight, head circumference, heart, eyes, hips, eyes for red reflexes, genitalia. Screening for phenylketonuria (PKU), hypothyroidism +/– haemoglobinopathy done by midwife around day 5. In some regions in the UK screening is also performed for cystic fibrosis and Duchenne Muscular Dystrophy
- **6 week check:** physical examination by doctor and health visitor
- **7–9 month check:** physical examination, hearing distraction test, squint assessment, assessment of growth and development (doctor and health visitor)
- **18–24 months:** developmental assessment by health visitor (has been stopped in some areas)
- **36–54 months:** physical examination and identification of health problems that will either affect education or require medication in school

All these visits provide the opportunity for appropriate health promotion. The immunization schedule is discussed in detail below.

18.2 School-aged children

Programmes differ significantly between local authorities. A health questionnaire is completed on school entry and reviewed by the school nurse. Screening of hearing and vision is also undertaken. In most areas medical examination is carried out only on a selective basis.

Regular health interviews are subsequently carried out with intermittent screening of vision. Informal school nurse run 'drop in centres' provide valuable support to the child and their family. A full medical may be requested if parents, teachers or school nurse have concerns.

19. IMMUNIZATION IN CHILDHOOD

19.1 Immunization schedule

The current immunization schedule for infants and children in the UK is summarized below.

Age	Vaccine
Neonatal period	BCG if in high-risk category*
2 months	1st diphtheria, tetanus, pertussis, *haemophilus influenza* type b (Hib) — single vaccine + 1st meningococcal group C (men C) + 1st oral polio
3 months	2nd diphtheria, tetanus, pertussis, Hib + 2nd Men C + 2nd oral polio
4 months	3rd diphtheria, tetanus, pertussis, Hib + 3rd Men C + 3rd oral polio
12– 15 months	Measles, mumps, rubella (MMR)
3–5 years	Diphtheria and tetanus booster + Oral polio booster + Measles, mumps, rubella booster (MMR)
10–14 years	BCG (after skin test, if not given in infancy)
13–18 years	Diphtheria and tetanus booster + Oral polio booster

Notes on immunization schedule

*BCG vaccine
High-risk categories include:

- Infants born to immigrants from countries with high prevalence of TB
- Infants who are to travel abroad to high-prevalence areas
- Infants born in UK where high prevalence of TB

Meningitis C vaccine
Immunization as part of the primary vaccination schedule began in Autumn 1999 and a 'catch up' programme to immunize all other children commenced at the same time. The following groups are being immunized, in order, as vaccine becomes available.

- 15–17-year-olds — school and college-based programmes
- Infants (other than those who had Men C with primary immunizations) — with MMR vaccine
- Other children — special appointments as vaccine becomes available

Rubella vaccine
Any girl who missed the MMR should be immunized between the ages of 10 and 14 years.

Hepatitis B vaccine
At present the vaccine is recommended only for:

- Babies born to mothers who are chronic carriers of hepatitis B virus or to mothers who have had acute hepatitis B during pregnancy
- Families adopting children from countries such as SE Asia, in whom hepatitis status is unknown

19.2 Contraindications to immunization

General considerations

- **Acute illness**
  Immunization should be deferred if the individual is acutely unwell but not if they have a minor infection without fever or systemic upset.

- **Previous severe local or general reaction**
  If there is a definite history of severe local or general reaction to a preceding dose, then subsequent immunization with that particular vaccine should not be performed.

- **Local reactions**: extensive redness and swelling which becomes indurated and involves most of the anterolateral surface of the thigh or a major part of the circumference of the upper arm.

- **General reactions**: this is defined as: fever over 39.5 °C within 48 hours of vaccine; anaphylaxis; bronchospasm; laryngeal oedema; generalized collapse. In addition, prolonged unresponsiveness; prolonged inconsolable or high-pitched screaming for more than 4 hours; convulsions or encephalopathy within 72 hours.

Live vaccines (e.g. BCG, MMR, polio)

Contraindications to live vaccine administration include:

- Prednisolone (orally or rectally) at a daily dose of 2 mg/kg per day for at least a week or 1 mg/kg per day for a month; corticosteroid use via other routes (e.g. intra-articular or inhaled) does not contraindicate live vaccine administration
- Children on lower doses of steroid also on cytotoxic drugs or with immunosuppression secondary to an underlying disease process
- Those with impaired cell-mediated immunity, e.g. Di George syndrome
- Children being treated for malignant disease with chemotherapy and/or radiotherapy, or those who have completed such treatment within the last 6 months
- Children who have had a bone marrow transplant within 6 months
- Immunoglobulin administration within previous 3 months

Myths surrounding contraindications

The following are **NOT** contraindications to immunization:

- Family history of adverse immunization reaction
- Stable neurological condition, e.g. Down's syndrome or cerebral palsy
- Egg allergy: hypersensitivity to egg contraindicates influenza vaccine and yellow fever vaccine, but there is good evidence that MMR can be safely given to children who have had previous anaphylaxis after egg
- Personal or family history of inflammatory bowel disease does not contraindicate MMR immunization
- Family history of convulsions
- Mother is pregnant (often concerns raised that oral polio vaccine (OPV) may be contraindicated)

In addition, it should be noted that the Council of the Faculty of Homeopathy strongly supports the immunization programme.

19.3 Immunization in HIV-positive children

Current recommendations are that it is perfectly safe for HIV-infected children to receive:

- Measles, mumps, rubella (MMR)
- Oral polio (inactivated form may be given)
- Pertussis, diphtheria, tetanus, polio, typhoid, cholera, hepatitis B and Hib

They should not receive:

- BCG
- Yellow fever
- Oral typhoid

19.4 Additional information on vaccines

Vaccine	Type	Other specific contraindications*	Side-effects**	Comments
Diphtheria	Inactivated toxoid + adjuvant	As above	Swelling + redness common Malaise, fever, headache Severe anaphylaxis rare Neurological reactions very rare	
Tetanus	Inactivated toxoid + adjuvant NB *Bordetella pertussis* also acts as adjuvant	As above	Pain, redness, swelling common General reactions uncommon Malaise, myalgia, pyrexia Acute anaphylaxis and urticaria is common Peripheral neuropathy rare	
Pertussis	Killed *Bordetella pertussis* (as part of DTP) DTP containing acellular pertussis now available	As above + evolving neurological problem	Swelling and redness at injection site common Crying, fever with DTP or DT Persistent screaming and collapse now rare with current vaccines Convulsions and encephalopathy vv rare and link with vaccine itself contentious Much more common after disease than vaccination	
Polio	Live, attenuated OPV *or* Enhanced potency inactivated polio vaccine (eIPV)	As above + OPV Vomiting or diarrhoea Not at same time as oral typhoid vaccine Not for siblings and household contacts of immunosuppressed children Not within 3 weeks of immunoglobulin injection Contraindications Inactivated polio vaccine (IPV) Acute or febrile illness Extreme polymyxin B and neomycin sensitivity	Vaccine-associated polio in recipients of OPV and in contacts of recipients at rate of one of each per 2 million oral doses	Faecal excretion of vaccine virus lasts up to 6 weeks Contacts of recently immunized baby should be advised re need for strict personal hygiene, e.g. after nappy changes Babies on Special Care Baby Unit (SCBU) should be given IPV Recently immunized children may go swimming
Hib	Conjugate	As above	Local swelling and redness 10% — rate declines with subsequent doses	Disease incidence dramatically fallen since introduction in 1992
MMR	Live, attenuated	As above + allergy to neomycin or kanamycin	Malaise, fever, rash within 7–10 days, Parotid swelling 1% Febrile convulsion 1/1,000 Arthropathy/thrombocytopenia rare Theoretical risk of encephalitis but causal evidence lacking Encephalitis much more likely secondary to measles in unimmunized child All side-effects less common after 2nd dose	Medical Research Council and CSM concluded no link between MMR and autism or bowel disease. Separate vaccines may be harmful. Adverse publicity led to fall in uptake rates and consequent increased risk of measles outbreak

Vaccine	Type	Other specific contraindications*	Side-effects**	Comments
Men C	Conjugate (carrier proteins are diphtheria toxoid or tetanus toxoid derivatives	As above + hypersensitivity to vaccine components incl. diphtheria toxoid or tetanus toxoid	Swelling at injection site common particularly in older children Systemic symptoms incl. irritability and fever much more common in infants Headaches, dizziness	Protects against *N.meningitides* group C only If travelling abroad, should still receive meningococcal polysaccharide
BCG	Live, attenuated A and C vaccines	As above + positive sensitivity skin test to tuberculin protein Generalized septic skin conditions	Vertigo and dizziness occasional Immediate allergy/anaphylaxis rare Severe injection site problems usually due to poor injection technique Adenitis Lupoid-type local reaction (rare) Widespread dissemination of organism (v. rare)	If child has eczema give at eczema-free site Tuberculin skin test must be done 1st in all children over 3 months Reaction to tuberculin protein may be suppressed by: Infectious mononucleosis Other viral infection Live viral vaccines Hodgkin's Sarcoid Corticosteroids Immunosuppressant treatment or diseases

* Please refer to notes above for general contraindications to immunizations.

** All immunizations may be complicated by local or general side-effects as discussed above.

DTP, diphtheria + tetanus + pertussis; i.u., infectious unit; DT, diphtheria + tetanus; VV very, very; OPV, oral polio vaccine; Hib, *Haemophilus Influenzae* type b; MMR, measles, mumps, rubella; CSM, Committee on Safety of Medicines; Men C, meningitis C.

20. ADOPTION AND FOSTERING

20.1 Adoption

Adoption is about meeting the needs of a child and not prospective parents. When a child is adopted full parental rights are taken on by adopting parents and the child has all the rights of a natural child of those parents. Approximately 2,000 children per year are adopted in England, the majority of these being children over 4 years of age. Over half involve children being adopted by step-parents. Adoption of newborn babies is increasingly uncommon. Whilst infants and children from overseas are brought into the UK for adoption, it must be recognized that the legal complexities surrounding this area are immense.

In England and Wales social services and voluntary organizations act as adoption agencies. Prior to any child being adopted the following steps must occur:

- Freeing of child for adoption: baby/child's natural parents must give consent for adoption. Cannot be done until at least 6 weeks after birth for newborn infants. May not be required if parents deemed incapable of decision-making (e.g. severe mental illness).
- Meticulous assessment of prospective adoptive parents: carried out by social services. Very few absolute contraindications to adoption (certain criminal offences will exclude). Detailed medical history of prospective parents important to ensure they are physically able to look after child. Disabled adults are encouraged to adopt. Choice of family will ideally reflect birth heritage of child (i.e. ethnic origin).
- Application for adoption order: can be applied for as soon as the child starts living with prospective adoptive parents but it will not be heard for at least 3 months (for newborn infants the 3-month period begins at the age of 6 weeks).
- Adoption hearing: an Adoption Panel, including social workers and medical advisers consider both the needs of the child and prospective parents. May be contested. Decision on day as to whether Adoption Order to be granted.

Medical services are involved at two levels:

- In an advisory capacity to the adoption agency, e.g. scrutinizing reports, collecting further medical information if needed.
- Carrying out pre-adoption medicals — it is essential that prospective parents have all available information on, for example, health of both natural parents, pregnancy, delivery, neonatal problems, development, etc. so that they can make a fully informed decision about adopting the child. Any special needs of the child should be identified at such an examination and additional reports by psychiatrists/psychologists may be needed. Children with special needs usually thrive in secure family environments, but full medical information must be made available to prospective adopters.

There are no medical conditions in the child which absolutely contraindicate adoption.

20.2 Fostering

Foster care offers a child care in a family setting but does not provide legal permanency as parental rights remain with the natural parents, local authority or courts, depending on the legal circumstances. Different types of foster care include:

- Care of babies awaiting adoption
- Young children in whom return to parents is anticipated

For some children with strong natural family ties long-term fostering is appropriate.

Foster parents are selected by a foster panel and, as with adoption, their health and that of the children awaiting fostering is considered.

21. DISABILITY LIVING ALLOWANCE

Disability Living Allowance (DLA) is a tax-free, social security benefit for people with an illness or disability who need:

- Help with getting around
- Help with personal care
- Help with both of the above

Obviously all children need some help and supervision. Families can make a claim if the child needs more help and supervision than another child of the same age. The claim is not affected by the money the child or family already have. Children can only receive DLA for help getting around if they are 5 years old or over. The rate they get depends on the type of help or supervision they need. Children can only receive DLA for help with personal care if they are 3 months or over. The rate again depends on the amount of help and supervision the child needs.

Additional support funds

There are other sources of financial support, e.g. The Family Fund Trust, to help families with severely disabled children. The Family Fund Trust is funded by the national government and family's financial circumstances are taken into consideration when deciding whether to give support.

22. THE CHILDREN ACT 1989 AND HUMAN RIGHTS ACT 1998

22.1 Aims of the Children Act

This Act introduced extensive changes to legislation affecting the welfare of children. Its main aims included:

- Restructuring custody and access in divorce
- Moving towards a 'family court' handling all public and private proceedings about children
- Creating a single statutory code for the protection of children through the courts
- Promoting interagency co-operation in the prevention, detection and treatment of child abuse and neglect
- Making legal remedies more accessible whilst also encouraging negotiation, partnership and agreed solutions which avoid the need to resort to court

In all of the above, the Act stresses that the child's welfare is the paramount consideration. It provides a checklist of welfare parameters aiming to ensure that in planning for the child's protection and upbringing, full account is taken of his or her needs, wishes and characteristics.

Child protection issues contained in the Act

Social services have a duty to investigate if they have reasonable cause to suspect that a child has suffered, is suffering or is likely to suffer 'significant harm'. If investigation confirms the suspicion then the child may need to be accommodated by social services whilst matters are taken further. Parents of an accommodated child retain full parental responsibility, including the right to remove the child at any time. An emergency protection order may be available, enabling the child to be detained in hospital, if parents do not agree to voluntary admission.

Emergency Protection Order (EPO)

This replaced the 'Place of Safety Order' and may be needed if, for example, non-accidental injury is suspected. The order lasts a maximum of 8 days with a possibility of extension for a further 7. It may be granted by the court if one of the following is satisfied:

- There is reasonable cause to believe that the child is likely to suffer appreciable harm if not removed from their present accommodation
- Inquiries by local authority or an 'authorized person' are being frustrated by lack of access

In addition, a child likely to suffer significant harm may also be taken into **police protection** for 72 hours. This involves a decision internal to the police force, and in cases of extreme emergency is likely to be quicker than applying for an EPO.

A Care Order

This order confers parental responsibility on the social services (in addition to that of the parents) and usually involves removal from home, at least temporarily. It may be applied for in cases of non-accidental injury, where inquiries will take some time and where the child is not regarded as being 'safe' at home.

A Supervision Order

This gives social services the power and duty to visit the family and also to impose conditions, such as attendance at clinic, nursery, school or outpatient visits.

Both care and supervision orders may be taken out by a court if they are convinced that thresholds for appreciable harm to the child have been met. The court, however, is under duties to consider the full range of its power and not to make any order unless doing so would be better for the child than making no order. Whilst proceedings for either of these orders are pending, the court may make 8- and then 4-weekly cycles to allow time for the child's needs to be comprehensively assessed, and for parties to prepare their proposals for court.

Child Assessment Order (CAO)

This order may be used if there is a situation of persistent but non-urgent suspicion of risk. It is available if:

- Significant harm is suspected
- A necessary medical or other assessment would be unlikely or unsatisfactory without a court order

It therefore overrides the objections of a parent to whatever examination or assessment is needed to see whether the significant harm test is satisfied. In addition it may override the objection of a child who 'is of sufficient understanding to make an informed decision'. This order lasts up to 7 days.

Wardship

If insufficient powers are available via the Children Act then wardship via the High Court may be applied for. This gives the court virtually limitless powers and is used in exceptional circumstances, such as when a family objects to surgery or medical treatment because of religious reasons.

Despite all the above, the implementation of the Children Act has been associated with a significant reduction in the number of compulsory child protection interventions through the courts, in part due to greater social services' reliance on voluntary help and increased partnership with parents.

22.2 Human Rights Act 1998

This act requires that all UK law is interpreted in accordance with the European Convention of Human Rights so as to give effect to the requirements of the convention rights. The Act enables individuals to take action for breach of these rights which include:

- Article 2 — Right to Life
- Article 3 — Prohibition of torture
- Article 6 — Right to a fair trial
- Article 8 — Right to respect for private and family life

During child protection investigations there is potential conflict between the right of the child's family (Article 8) and the duties of the child protection team as they relate to Articles 2 and 3. Legal advice will need to be sought in situations of doubt.

23. CHILD ABUSE

Epidemiology

In Britain up to 100 children per year die as a result of non-accidental injuries. The incidence of non-accidental physical injury is around 1:2,000 children per year. In addition some reports suggest that by the age of 16 years up to 1:4 girls and 1:5 boys will have been sexually assaulted. Many victims, particularly those of sexual abuse do not come forward for many years. Sadly around 80% of these children are sexually abused by people they know.

Types of abuse

- **Physical injury** may be inflicted deliberately or by failure to provide a safe environment
- **Neglect,** e.g. inadequate provision of food
- **Emotional neglect**
- **Sexual abuse**
- **Potential abuse**, e.g. if another child previously harmed

Diagnosing child abuse

History

With any injury a careful history should be sought. The following should alert the clinician to the possibility of non-accidental injury:

- Discrepancy between history and injury seen
- Changing story with time or different people
- Delay in reporting
- Unusual reaction to injury
- Repeated injury
- History of non-accidental or suspicious injury in sibling
- Signs of neglect or failure to thrive

Social and family indicators of abuse

Factors commonly associated with child abuse include:

- Young, immature, lonely and isolated parents
- Poor interparental relationship
- Substance abuse in parent
- Parent who had rejection, deprivation or abuse in their childhood
- Parents with learning difficulties or difficult pregnancy
- Early illness in child
- Difficult behaviour in child

Examination

If non-accidental injury (NAI) without sexual abuse is suspected the child should be fully undressed and examined in a warm, secure environment by an appropriately experienced doctor. Careful charting of injuries is imperative.

Certain injuries are 'typical' in abuse:

- **Bruises** — Bruises are uncommon in children under 1 year, especially if not mobile; Bruises of different ages or finger-shaped bruises raise concerns, as do bruises on head, face and lumbar region (often finger marks), bruising around wrists and ankles (swinging), bruising inside and behind pinna (blow with hand), ring of bruises (bite mark)
- **Two black eyes**
- **Strap or lash marks**
- **Torn frenulum** — blow or force feeding
- **Perforated eardrum** — slap or blow to side of head
- **Small circular burns** — cigarette burn
- **Burns or scalds to both feet or buttocks**
- **Fractured ribs** — shaking
- **Epiphyses torn off** — swinging
- **Subdural haematoma** — shaking
- **Retinal haemorrhages** — shaking
- **Multiple injuries and injuries at different ages**

Potential pitfalls

Underdiagnosis much more common than overdiagnosis but beware of:

- Mongolian spots: most common in those of Asian origin; look like bruises, seen most commonly over buttocks
- Bleeding disorders: need FBC and clotting to exclude these if multiple bruises
- Underlying bony disorder: e.g. osteogenesis imperfecta or copper deficiency; if fractures present paediatric radiologist must be able to exclude former

Rough estimate of age of bruises

Accurate dating is not possible.

Age of bruise	Bruise appearance
<24 hours	Red or red/purple, swollen
1–2 days	Purple, swollen
3–5 days	Starting to yellow
5–7 days	Yellow, fading
>1 week	Yellow, brown, have faded

Healing of fractures

Fracture appearance	Average timing
Swelling of soft tissue resolves	2–10 days
Periosteal new bone	10+ days
Loss of fracture-line definition	14+ days
Soft callus	14+ days
Hard callus	21+ days
Remodelling	3+ months

It is not possible to date skull fractures

Management of suspected non-accidental injuries
- Put the interests of the child first
- Local protocols will be in place and should be adhered to
- If suspicion of NAI check local 'at risk' register
- History and examination should be done by senior, experienced paediatrician and well documented
- Additional information from school, GP, health visitor may be extremely helpful
- Skeletal survey and clotting may be needed
- Final diagnosis of NAI requires piecing together of information gleaned from many sources
- If NAI thought likely and child not ill enough to warrant hospital admission close liaison with social services/child protection team to discuss most appropriate place for child to be discharged to (see Child Protection issues in section 22.1 on Children Act)
- Social services will decide whether to call case conference (see below), at which whether to place child's name on 'at risk' register will be discussed

Case conference

This is a formal gathering of individuals with a legitimate interest in the child and family. It allows:

- Exchange of relevant information
- Decision as to whether abuse has taken place
- Decision on whether to place name on Child Protection Register
- Action plan for protecting child and helping family
- Identification of individuals to implement plan

Neglect

This may manifest as failure to thrive, failure of normal development or growth, or lack of normal emotional responses. Other causes need to be excluded, but typically the child progresses better in a hospital environment than at home.

Poisoning

Rare but consider if symptoms and signs difficult to explain. Blood and urine will need to be screened.

Munchausen's syndrome by proxy

In this condition a child receives medical attention for symptoms that have either been falsified or directly induced by their carer. Among the most common symptoms are bleeding, fever, vomiting, diarrhoea, seizures and apnoea. The doctor may be persuaded to order a range of increasingly complex investigations. Diagnosis is difficult and may involve in-patient observation. Once confirmed, social services and psychiatry services will need to be involved and a child protection conference convened.

Sexual abuse

Presentation
Sexual abuse presents in many ways:

- Allegations by child or adult (children rarely lie about this)
- Injuries to genitalia or anus (including bleeding or sexually transmitted disease (STD))
- Suspicious features including unexplained recurrent urinary tract infection (UTI), sexual explicitness in play, drawing, language or behaviour, sudden or unexplained changes in behaviour, e.g. sleep disturbance and loss of trust in individuals close to them, taking an overdose, running away from home.
- Psychosomatic indicators including recurrent headache, abdominal pain, enuresis, encopresis, eating disorders

Physical signs
The examination should take place in a quiet, child-centered room with appropriate facilities. Older children may prefer a doctor of the same gender. Consent is required prior to the examination and a forensic pack will be needed if the last assault was within 72 hours. The signs elicited must be taken in the context of the complete investigation. Careful documentation should be made in the form of sketches and sometimes photographs. As there is significant chance of coexisting physical abuse a full general examination should also be performed.

NB. It must be remembered that up to 50% of children subject to sexual abuse will have no abnormal physical signs.

The following should be looked for in girls:

- Reddening, bruising, lacerations and swelling of labia, perineum and vulva
- Presence of vaginal discharge (+comment on colour and amount). (NB on its own not strongly suggestive of sexual abuse)
- Hymenal opening — size (mm), margin, tears, scars (in prepubertal girl, hymenal opening >0.5 cm suspicious of sexual abuse, >1 cm even higher likelihood)
- Posterior fourchette — laceration/scars
- Vaginal examination ONLY in older girls if indicated

In boys, the following signs should be looked for:

- Penis — bruising, laceration, scars, burns
- Perineum — reddening, bruising
- Scrotum — bruising, reddening, burns

Anal examination
Examine young children on carer's knee and older children in left lateral position. Rectal examinations are rarely necessary and instead inspection should determine the presence or absence of acute signs such as:

- Swelling, reddening, bruising, haematoma, laceration or tears of anal margin
- Spasm, laxity and dilatation of anal sphincter
- Dilatation of perianal veins

Chronic signs should also be looked for including:

- Smooth thickened anal margin with shiny skin
- Chronic and acute fissures (single fissure unlikely to be significant)
- Spasm laxity and dilatation of anal sphincter
- Dilatation of perianal veins

In certain cases it may be appropriate to send swabs for:

- Gonorrhoea
- Trichomonas
- Chlamydia
- Herpes

And forensic samples to look for:

- Spermatozoa
- Semen
- Grouping of semen
- Saliva, etc.

Management of sexual abuse
The child must be believed and handled in a skilled and sensitive fashion. After completion of history and examination the points outlined in 'Management of NAI' should be followed.

Long-term legacy
The long-term problems associated with child sexual abuse include:

- Post-traumatic stress
- Suicidal behaviour
- Psychiatric illness
- Problems with relationships and sexual adjustment

24. SUDDEN INFANT DEATH SYNDROME (SIDS)

Definition

The definition of sudden infant death syndrome (SIDS) is 'the sudden death of an infant under one year of age which remains unexplained after the performance of a complete post-mortem examination and examination of the scene of death.'

Incidence
UK figures for 2000 — 0.4/1,000 live births

Many hypotheses have developed about the causes of SIDS. The search for an individual cause has shifted towards a more complex model. It seems likely that SIDS is due to an interaction of risk factors — developmental stage, congenital and acquired risks and a final triggering event.

Established risk factors for SIDS
- Age 4–16 weeks
- Prone sleeping position and side sleeping position*
- Overheating/overwrapping
- Soft sleeping surfaces
- Fever/minor infection
- Bed sharing with parents (contraindicated if parent has had alcohol)
- Maternal smoking (ante- and postnatal)**
- Low maternal age
- High birth order
- Low birth weight
- Preterm delivery ***
- Medical complications in the neonatal period
- Social deprivation
- Male sex
- Inborn errors of metabolism****

*The 'Back to Sleep' Campaign, whereby parents are educated re the protective effect of supine infant sleeping, is well documented to have led to a very significant drop in the incidence of SIDS in the UK over the last decade. Similar campaigns have also been successful in other countries such as New Zealand, Scandinavia and the USA.

**Smoking increases risk of SIDS by up to threefold. There is an increase in risk with increased likelihood of spontaneous apnoea and decreased ability to compensate after such an episode. Such effects are likely to be enhanced by intercurrent illness.

***Relative risk of SIDS with preterm delivery

Gestational age	Relative risk of SIDS
<28/40	3.6
28–31 weeks	4
32–33 weeks	2.4
34–36 weeks	1.7

Period for which ex preterm infants are at risk of SIDS is also longer than for term infants.

****Inborn errors of metabolism

Around 1% of cases of SIDS are likely to be due to the enzyme deficiency: medium-chain acyl Coenzyme A (CoA) dehydrogenase deficiency (MCAD). It is likely that other enzyme deficiencies contribute to SIDS in a subset of patients, especially those SIDS which occur at >6 months. Appropriate investigations should be initiated.

Other factors implicated in aetiology of SIDS

- *Helicobacter pylori* (leads to increase in ammonia production)
- Prolonged QT interval
- Small pineal gland with altered melatonin production
- Gastro-oesophageal reflux
- Paternal cannabis use

There is **no** hard evidence that antimony (a substance present in some cot mattresses) is implicated in SIDS. Similarly, whilst there used to be a seasonal variation in SIDS, this is now no longer observed.

Protective factors for SIDS
- Supine sleeping position
- Appropriate environmental temperature
- ? Pacifier use (may prevent baby sleeping deeply)

Practical guidance on management of sudden unexpected deaths in infancy
Each hospital should have its own protocol for dealing with SIDS, which should be adhered to. The following are, however, general guidelines:

- Contact consultant paediatrician immediately
- Ensure parents have a member of staff allocated to them and an appropriate room in which to wait
- Baby should be taken to appropriate area within A&E and **not** to the mortuary
- Initiate resuscitation unless it is evident baby has been dead for some time (e.g. rigor mortis or blood pooling)
- Parents should have option of being present during resuscitation with nurse supporting them throughout
- Take brief history of events preceding admission, including baby's past illnesses, recent health and any resuscitation already attempted; identify any predisposing factors for SIDS
- Consultant should decide, in consultation with parents, how long resuscitation should be continued for (it is usual to discontinue if there is no detectable cardiac output after 30 minutes)
- Once baby has been certified dead, consultant paediatrician should break news to parents, with support nurse present
- Explain to parents need to inform coroner and arrange post-mortem

Physical examination

Carry out by most senior paediatrician present as soon as resuscitation has been completed/abandoned. Need to record:

- Baby's general appearance, state of nutrition and cleanliness
- Weight, and position on centile chart
- Rectal temperature
- Marks from invasive or vigorous procedures such as venepuncture, cardiac massage
- Any other marks on skin
- Appearance of retinae
- Lesions inside mouth
- Any signs of injury to genitalia/anus

Further action within A&E

- Keep all clothing removed from baby in labelled specimen bags as it may assist the pathologist and may be needed for forensic examination
- Inform coroner's office and discuss collection of further lab specimens, take photographs and mementoes such as lock of hair or hand and footprints
- Arrange for skeletal survey
- Contact coroner and request them to instruct a specialist paediatric pathologist for the post-mortem
- Check Child Protection Register
- If any concerns re suspicious death contact police urgently

Taking of samples

In some centres all samples are taken at post-mortem, however in others some or all of the following should be taken within the A&E department:

- Blood for urea and electrolytes, FBC, blood culture, toxicology (clotted sample)
- Metabolic screen including amino and organic acids, oligosaccharides, blood spot on Guthrie card (for MCAD)
- Chromosomes (if dysmorphic)
- Nasopharyngeal aspirate, swabs (as appropriate) for bacteriology, Supra Pubic Aspirate (SPA) for urine microscopy, culture and sensitivity
- Consider skin and muscle biopsy

Support for family

- Ensure they have Foundation for Study of Infant Death leaflet and helpline number and Department of Health leaflet on post-mortem
- Offer to put in touch with local support organizations
- If mother was breast feeding discuss suppression of lactation
- If baby was a twin recommend admission/investigation of surviving twin
- Ensure family have telephone numbers of appropriate members of hospital team
- Offer to organize psychological support for older siblings
- Give details of counselling services
- Arrange transport home

Communication checklist
The following should be informed as soon as possible about baby's death.

- Coroner
- Coroner's officer
- Police
- Family doctor
- Health visitor
- Social worker
- Medical records
- Other paediatric colleagues previously involved in care

Follow-up arrangements
Ideally the paediatric consultant involved should organize to visit the family at home, as soon as is convenient for them. This allows more information on the family and baby to be obtained and also presents an opportunity for the parents to ask questions. Further follow-up visits should be organized, as necessary, and the post-mortem result should be discussed as soon as available.

25. ACCIDENT PREVENTION

Around 400 children per year die as a result of accidents in England and Wales and several thousand others suffer serious injuries. Consequently one of the Health of the Nation targets is to reduce deaths from such accidents by one-third by the year 2005.

Examples of how mortality and morbidity rates may be reduced include:

- Use of cycle helmets and car restraints (reduce severity of injury in road traffic accidents)
- Urban safety measures (e.g. crossing patrols, traffic redistribution schemes, improving safety on individual roads)
- Use of home safety devices (e.g. smoke detectors, stairgates, thermostat control of hot water)

Studies have established that educational programmes alone are not successful in preventing accidents and that to reduce accidents the educational material must be accompanied by:

- Targeting families most at risk of accidents
- Home visits
- Free distribution of devices such as smoke alarms

26. CHRONIC FATIGUE SYNDROME

This remains an ill-understood condition which may present to either paediatricians or psychiatrists. The cardinal symptoms are severe and disabling physical and mental fatigue lasting for more than 3 months. Symptoms are usually continuous, their effects on the individual manifest to a pathological degree and are rarely objectively confirmed. The diagnosis excludes known causes of chronic fatigue such as chronic illness and also excludes known psychological disease.

Aetiology

Whilst viruses such as Epstein–Barr and the enteroviruses are often implicated in the disease process, direct evidence of this is often hard to find. Case clustering does occur and whilst anecdotal cases have suggested immunization may be a trigger there is no direct evidence to support this theory. The aetiology is likely to be a combination of physical, psychological and behavioural factors. Often a trigger for the child's symptoms can be found.

Depression may be an associated feature, and the chronic course the disease takes makes psychological support and evaluation essential.

Initial assessment

All patients referred for consideration of the diagnosis require a full and thorough assessment with an appreciation of the reality of the child's symptoms and acknowledgement of their validity. A thorough history and examination should be taken, exploring precise symptomatology. Organic and psychological disease should be looked for. Of particular importance is determining the effect of the child's symptoms on their normal daily routine including activities at home and attendance at school.

Investigation

Organic disorders which should always be excluded include:

- Hypothyroidism
- Severe iron deficiency
- Recent Epstein–Barr virus (EBV) infection

Other investigations may be required if there are specific disease pointers.

Investigations should be done early on and, if possible, on one occasion only to prevent reliance on test results.

Management

Management is complex and requires the input of many professionals. It needs to be tailor-made for the individual child. Key points are:

- Facilitate the child and family to acknowledge the diagnosis, understand its implications and embark on a period of rehabilitation

- Assess current level of functioning by completing a daily programme to establish periods of eating, rest and activity
- Liaise closely with school/education authority
- Set goals:
  - Attendance at school is a key aim but gradual reintegration is usually required, with rest periods within school. Part days in school are preferable to exclusive home tuition.
  - Aim to increase activity levels by around 5% each week
- Encourage child to keep a diary
- Recognize early any predominant psychological symptoms including school phobia or depression and seek appropriate psychological or psychiatric help.

Pharmacological interventions such as corticosteroids and antidepressants (particularly SSRIs) have been used, but in a recent meta-analysis of treatments only physiotherapy (with a graded exercise programme) was shown to have a clearly beneficial effect. Cognitive techniques are used to assist patients to re-evaluate their understanding of the illness, combat depression and anxiety and look for underlying thoughts and assumptions that may contribute to disability.

Prognosis

The prognosis of chronic fatigue syndrome in children, in the absence of complications, is good. The onset of disease is more rapid and the response to therapy better than in adults, with a return to normal by 6–12 months after diagnosis in 80–90%.

Good prognostic factors in chronic fatigue syndrome

- Clearly defined trigger to illness
- Short duration of symptoms
- Supportive family with good interpersonal relationships
- Young age (adolescents overall do better than young or older adults)

27. FURTHER READING

Child and Adolescent Psychiatry — Modern Approaches, Rutter, Blackwell Science. 2002

Child Surveillance Handbook, Hall, D. Hill, P. Ellerman, D. Radcliffe Med. 1994

Immunisation against infant disease, HMSO 1996

www.sids.org.uk (Foundation of the Study of Infant Death).

Chapter 3

Clinical Pharmacology and Toxicology

Stephen R Tomlin and Michael Capra

CONTENTS

Clinical Pharmacology and Toxicology

1. PHARMACOKINETICS AND DYNAMICS

Pharmacokinetics is what the body does to a drug, pharmacodynamics is what the drug does to the body.

1.1   Absorption

- Liquid and intravenous forms of drugs (i.e. already in solution) are readily absorbed into the body's systemic circulation.
- Solid dosage forms (tablets and capsules) and suspensions must first be dissolved in the gastrointestinal tract (dissolution phase) before they can be absorbed, and thus absorption is slower.
- The term 'bioavailability' is applied to the rate and extent of drug absorption into the systemic circulation.

First-order kinetics

Oral absorption of drugs is often considered as demonstrating first-order kinetics. This is especially true with oral solutions. 'First-order kinetics' implies that the fractional rate of absorption is constant, thus absorption decreases the less there is left in the stomach. If a drug is absorbed at a constant rate independent of the amount left to absorb, then it is referred to as having 'zero-order kinetics'.

Ionization

Absorption of the majority of medicines is dependent on how ionized they are (their pK_a) and the acidity at the site of absorption. Drugs with acidic pK_as (for example: aspirin, phenoxymethylpenicillin (penicillin V)) will be mainly non-ionized in the acid stomach and thus readily absorbed. Phenobarbital being a weaker acid is better absorbed in the more alkaline intestine.

Neonates

Neonates (especially those who are premature) have reduced gastric acid secretion, therefore the extent of drug absorption is altered and less predictable.

At birth, drugs with an acidic pK_a will have decreased absorption. 24 hours after birth, acid is released into the stomach therefore increasing the absorption of acidic drugs. Normal adult gastric acid secretions are achieved by about 3 years of age.

Gastric motility is decreased during infancy, thus increasing the absorption of drugs that are absorbed in the stomach. However, drugs absorbed from the intestine will have a decreased or possibly delayed absorption.

Absorption and pK$_a$ of some drugs in adults and neonates

Drug	Neonatal oral absorption compared to adult	pK$_a$
Ampicillin	Increased	2.7
Penicillin	Increased	2.8
Phenytoin	Decreased	8.3
Paracetamol	Decreased	9.9
Diazepam	Same	3.7

1.2 Distribution

The concentration of a drug at various sites of action depends on the drug's characteristics and those of the tissue. Most drugs are water-soluble and will naturally go to organs such as the kidneys, liver, heart and gastrointestinal tract.

At birth, the total body water and extracellular fluid volume are much increased, and thus larger doses of water-soluble drugs are required on a mg/kg basis to achieve equivalent concentrations to those seen in older children and adults. This has to be balanced against the diminished hepatic and renal function when considering dosing.

	Pre-term	Full term	4–6 mths	1 y	>1 y	Adult
Extracellular fluid volume (%)	50	45	40	30	25	25
Total body water (%)	85	75	60	60	60	60
Fat content (%)	3	12	25	30	variable	18

Distribution is also affected by a decreased protein-binding capacity in newborns, and particularly in pre-term newborns, therefore leading to increased levels of the active free drug for highly protein-bound drugs.

- For example, phenytoin is highly protein-bound. But due to less protein binding in neonates (lower plasma protein levels and lower binding capacity) there is more free phenytoin than in older children and adults. Thus the therapeutic range for phenytoin in neonates is lower than in the rest of the general population as it is the free phenytoin that has the therapeutic action and can cause toxicity.
  - Therapeutic range for neonates = 6–15 mg/l
  - Therapeutic range for children and adults = 10–20 mg/l

The reduced protein binding is due to:

- low levels of plasma protein, particularly albumin
- qualitative differences in binding capacity
- competition with endogenous substances, particularly increased bilirubin after birth.

Volume of distribution

Distribution is measured by a theoretical volume in the body called the 'volume of distribution'. It is the volume that would be necessary to dilute the administered dose to obtain the actual plasma level within the body. The volume will be affected by the following characteristics (body size, body water composition, body fat composition, protein binding, haemodynamics and the drug characteristics). As a rule of thumb: drugs that are plasma protein-bound will mainly stay in the plasma and thus have a small volume of distribution; highly lipid-soluble drugs (especially in people with a high fat content) will have high volumes of distribution. Water-soluble drugs have increased volumes of distribution in neonates due to their increased total body water content.

The parameter can change significantly throughout childhood. Plasma albumin levels reach adult levels at approximately 1 year of age.

Blood–brain barrier

The blood–brain barrier in the newborn is functionally incomplete and hence there is an increased penetration of some drugs into the brain.

Transfer across the barrier is determined by:

- lipid solubility
- degree of ionization

Drugs that are predominantly unionized are more lipid-soluble and achieve higher concentrations in the cerebrospinal fluid (CSF). It is due to this increased uptake that neonates are generally more sensitive to the respiratory depressant effects of opiates than infants and older children.

Some drugs will displace bilirubin from albumin (for example: sulphonamides), so increasing the risk of kernicterus (encephalopathy due to increased bilirubin in the CNS – usually fatal) in at-risk neonates.

1.3 Half-life

Half-life is the time taken for the plasma concentration of a drug to decrease to half of its original value. Thus it follows that less drugs will be eliminated in each successive half-life.

- For example, theophylline:
  - if there is initially 250 mg in the body, after 1 half-life (4 h) 125 mg will remain; after 2 half-lives (8 h) there will be 62.5 mg left; and so on.

When a medicine is first given in a single dose, all the drug is at the absorption site and none is in the plasma. At this point, absorption is maximal and the rate of elimination is zero. As time goes on the rate of absorption decreases (first-order kinetics) and the rate of elimination increases. All the time that the absorption rate is higher than the elimination rate the plasma level will increase. When the two rates are equal, the concentration in the plasma will be at a maximum. After this point, the elimination rate will be higher and the levels will drop. A drug is said to be at 'steady state' after about 4–5 half-lives. So if multiple dosing is occurring the plasma levels at any particular point after a dose will always be the same.

1.4 Hepatic metabolism

Hepatic metabolism is generally slower at birth compared with adults. However, this increases rapidly during the first few weeks of life, so that in late infancy hepatic metabolism may be more effective than in adults.

The age at which the enzyme processes approach adult values varies with the drug and the metabolic pathway. For drugs such as diazepam, which are extensively metabolized by the liver, the decrease in half-life with age demonstrates this process.

	Pre-term babies	Full-term babies	Children
Diazepam half-life (h)	38–120	22–46	15–21

The hepatic metabolism process occurs either by sulphation, methylation, oxidation, hydroxylation or glucuronidation. Most hepatically metabolised drugs will undergo one or two of these processes.

Processes involving sulphation and methylation are not greatly impaired at birth, whereas those involving oxidation and glucuronidation are. It might be assumed that neonates would be at an increased risk of paracetamol toxicity; however, neonates use the sulphation pathway instead of glucuronidation and are able to deal with paracetamol as well (if not more efficiently) than adults.

Hydroxylation of drugs is deficient in newborns, particularly in pre-term babies, and this is the process that accounts for the huge variation in diazepam half-life as shown in the table above.

Grey-baby syndrome is a rare, but often fatal, toxic effect of chloramphenicol in neonates. It is due to the inability of the liver to glucuronidate the drug effectively in the first couple of weeks of life if correct doses are not given.

It is impossible to predict with any accuracy the possible toxic dose for a neonate and young infant even by applying all the above rules. For example, neonates unlike adults convert most theophylline to caffeine in the liver. Thus without dedicated studies we really are only guessing as to what toxic or non-toxic metabolites are being formed in this age group.

First-pass metabolism

Medication that is absorbed from the gastrointestinal tract goes straight to the liver before entering the systemic circulation. This is useful for some types of medication, which have to go to the liver to be activated (pro-drugs), e.g. enalapril. It is, however, limiting for medications that have to achieve good levels when given orally. Propranolol has a high first-pass metabolism, so quite large doses need to be given to achieve adequate systemic levels. Inhaled budesonide is often said to be relatively free of systemic side-effects because the steroid that is deposited in the throat and swallowed is almost entirely eliminated by first-pass metabolism.

1.5 Renal excretion

Drug excretion by the kidneys is mainly dependent on glomerular filtration and active renal tubule secretion. Pre-term infants have approximately 15% (or less) of the renal capacity of an adult, term babies have about 30% at birth, but this matures rapidly to about 50% of the adult capacity by the time they are 4–5–weeks-old. At 9–12 months of age, the infant renal capacity is equal to that of an adult.

1.6 Other clinical considerations

Many other factors influence drug handling and may alter an individual's response to a given dose.

Genetic considerations can lead to altered drug metabolism or altered responses, e.g.: glucose 6–phosphate dehydrogenase (G6PD) deficiency; succinylcholine sensitivity; acetylation status.

G6PD deficiency

This is a commonly inherited enzyme abnormality. It is an X-linked recessive disorder. Male homozygotes show significant drug-related haemolysis, but females only have minor symptoms. Anaemia is the most common presentation.

Main drugs to avoid:

- dapsone, nitrofurantoin, quinolones (ciprofloxacin, nalidixic acid, ofloxacin, norfloxacin), sulphonamides (co-trimoxazole), quinine, quinidine, chloroquine.

Succinylcholine sensitivity

Some people are extremely sensitive to the muscle relaxant succinylcholine. Serum pseudocholinesterase activity is reduced and the duration of action of the muscle relaxant (usually a few minutes) may be greatly increased, thus leading to apnoea (deaths have been reported). The incidence is about 1 in 2,500 of the population.

Acetylation status

Differences in the metabolism of isoniazid (INH) are seen in certain people and inherited as an autosomal recessive trait. People who are 'slow inactivators' have reduced activity of acetyltransferase, which is the hepatic enzyme responsible for the metabolism of INH and sulphadimidine (thus affects phenelzine and hydralazine metabolism). Toxic effects of such drugs may be seen in people who are 'slow acetylators'.

Slow acetylators are also predisposed to spontaneous and drug-induced systemic lupus erythematosus (SLE).

Examples of drugs that may induce SLE

Phenytoin	Isoniazid	Procainamide
Penicillin	Chlorpromazine	Tetracyclines
Hydralazine	Beta-blockers	Lithium
Sulphonamides	Clonidine	Methyldopa

Liver disease

Toxic substances normally cleared by the liver may accumulate in patients with liver impairment.

* Opioids and benzodiazepines may accumulate and cause central nervous system depression, thereby causing respiratory depression.
* Diuretics (loop and thiazide) may cause hypokalaemia.
* Rifampicin, which is excreted via the bile, will accumulate in patients with obstructive jaundice.
* Cirrhosis may cause hypoproteinaemia and thus reduce the number of binding sites for highly protein-bound drugs (e.g. phenytoin).
* Clotting factors are reduced in liver impairment, thus increasing the chances of bleeding in patients on warfarin.

Renal disease

* Nephrotoxic drugs will make any renal impairment worse by exacerbating the damage. Drugs that are renally excreted (most water-soluble drugs) will accumulate in renal impairment and the dosing intervals will need increasing to avoid toxicity.

Drugs that cause toxicity in severe renal impairment include:

* digoxin – cardiac arrhythmias, heart block
* penicillins/cephalosporins (high dose) – encephalopathy
* erythromycin – encephalopathy

Nephrotoxic drugs include:

* aminoglycosides (gentamicin, amikacin)
* amphotericin B
* non-steroidal anti-inflammatory drugs (e.g. diclofenac, indomethacin)

2. FORMULATION

Medicinal preparations often contain other ingredients (i.e. excipients) other than the medicine that is being prescribed. These adjuvants can have a pharmacological effect that needs to be taken into account when looking at medication consumption and assessing possible toxicity.

- Benzyl alcohol and methylparaben can displace bilirubin from albumin-binding sites, leading to exacerbation of jaundice. Benzyl alcohol may also cause a potentially fatal 'gasping syndrome'.
- Propylene glycol is a common solubilizing agent. In excess, it may cause severe toxicity including hyperosmolarity, lactic acidosis, dysrhythmias and hypotension.
- Polysorbate 20 and Polysorbate 80, which are used as emulsifying agents, have been associated with renal and hepatic dysfunction as well as hypotension (secondary to hypovolaemia), thrombocytopenia and metabolic acidosis.
- Lactose is a common additive, but rarely associated with severe toxicity. It may, however, be important if a child has lactose intolerance.
- Sugar and sorbitol are frequently added to liquid preparations for sweetness, which occasionally cause problems. Sugar can cause dental caries and sorbitol may cause diarrhoea.
- Alcohol is another common ingredient of many liquid pharmaceutical products and the quantity is often fairly significant. Products such as phenobarbital BP contains as much as 38% alcohol per 15 mg/5 ml. Equating this to a mg/kg quota, it wouldn't be that unusual to subject a neonate to the equivalent of an adult swallowing one or two glasses of wine.

3. PAEDIATRIC DOSING

Pharmacokinetic and pharmacodynamic data are seldom available for the paediatric population, this is because most medications are only licensed for adult use and have not undergone specific pre-marketing clinical studies in children. Data on therapeutic dosing for children are often anecdotal and based on case reports or very small population studies. New drugs are usually only studied in adult populations.

Part of the reasons for this are the stringent regulations put in place in 1962 following the thalidomide tragedy that had the effect of discouraging research. The legislation surrounding drugs' trials currently discourages trials in children, although in recent years there has been a call for more studies.

The surface area and the weight are the only common methods currently available to predict paediatric therapeutic doses from those used for adults.

Surface area

The surface area or percentage method for estimating doses is calculated as follows:

$$\frac{\text{Surface area of child (m}^2)}{1.76 \text{ m}^2} \times 100 = \text{per cent of adult dose;}$$

where: 1.76 m^2 is the average adult surface area.

Children are often said to tolerate or require larger doses of drugs than adults based on a weight basis, and the percentage method helps to explain this phenomenon. Body water (total and extracellular) is known to equate better with surface area than body weight. It thus seems appropriate to prescribe drugs by surface area if they are distributed through the extracellular fluid volume in particular.

Weight

$$\frac{\text{Adult dose (mg)}}{70 \text{ kg}} = \text{mg/kg dose;}$$

where: 70 kg is the average adult weight.

This method will give lower doses than the surface area method. It is far less accurate in clinical terms and is usually inappropriate for accurate therapeutic dosing. However, as it gives lower and thus safer estimates of what the toxic dose may be, it is a more practical and reasonably cautious method for extrapolating toxic doses.

Most paediatric doses given in textbooks are described in small age or weight groups on a mg/kg basis. However, these will often have been originally obtained from surface-area data and thus are larger than the adult dose divided by 70.

3.1 Clinical trials

Maximal tolerated dose

The term 'maximum tolerated dose' (MTD) is often used in clinical trials to help define the most appropriate therapeutic doses of a new drug. The MTD is the highest dose that is safe to administer to patients, and defines the upper limit of the usable dose range for efficacy studies.

Phase 1 trials and maximum tolerated dose
Dose-ranging schedules are applied to assess medication tolerance in Phase 1 trials, in which successive volunteers are exposed to increasing drug doses. In this way an indication of the maximum tolerated dose may be obtained. Clearly, it is important to determine whether the estimated therapeutic dose can be exceeded without mishap. If this dose is not determined, patients may be exposed to unsafe levels of medication or subtherapeutic doses of specific drugs. The upper end of the spectrum is characterized by the build-up of adverse

events that may outweigh the benefits to the patient. Towards this end of the spectrum we define the 'minimum intolerated dose' (MID) as the dose at which more than 50% of the patients in a study succumb to limiting adverse events or a medically unacceptable adverse event. The dose below this is defined as the MTD, and can be thought of as the maximum dose having an adverse-event profile in the population that is acceptable, based on indication-specific prospective criteria.

Although the MTD is a useful tool, for most drugs this value will only be available for adults. It will be necessary to extrapolate this dose for use in paediatrics.

4. PRESCRIBING OUTSIDE LICENCE

The unlicensed and off-label (licensed drugs being used outside their licence) use of medicines in children is widespread. It has been accepted by the Royal College of Paediatrics and Child Health (RCPCH) and the Neonatal and Paediatric Pharmacists Group (NPPG) that informed use of such medicines is necessary in paediatric practice when there is no suitable licensed alternative. Those who prescribe for a child should choose the medicine which offers the best prospect for that child, with due regard to cost. Legally, the prescriber is required to take full responsibility for such prescribing, which must be justifiable in accordance with a respectable, responsible body of professional opinion.

The choice of a medicine isn't therefore necessarily determined by its licence status, although it should take into account information made available as a consequence of licensing and contained in the Summary of Product Characteristics. This can be of only limited help when the medicine chosen is unlicensed or off-label, and the necessary information to support safe and effective prescribing must be sought elsewhere.

The national paediatric formulary 'Medicines for Children' written by the RCPCH and NPPG has been produced to meet the need for accessible sound information.

5. DRUG MONITORING

Most drugs have wide therapeutic windows and thus toxicity is unlikely at 'normal doses'. It is usually easy to see a medication effect, e.g. analgesics take away pain. There are, however, certain circumstances when it is important to measure drug levels to ensure that there are adequate levels for effect and/or that the levels are unlikely to cause toxicity.

A drug with a narrow therapeutic window has a narrow range between the drug concentration exhibiting maximum efficacy and minimum toxicity.

Medications that have narrow therapeutic windows are often monitored, as it is hard to predict that a dose for an individual patient will either be clinically effective or cause toxicity.

Common drugs for therapeutic drug monitoring

Phenytoin	Warfarin
Carbamazepine	Gentamicin
Phenobarbital	Vancomycin
Digoxin	Theophylline

Indications for monitoring:

- to confirm levels are not toxic and are at a level that is normally effective (usually checked once steady-state has been reached), e.g. gentamicin, vancomycin
- if toxicity is expected
- if external factors may have changed a level (change in renal/hepatic function, change in interacting concomitant medication)
- to check compliance

It is important to know that a drug is at a steady state when a level was measured and whether trough levels or peak levels are important.

6. INTERACTIONS

Many situations arise where interactions between different medications are important. Drugs may either inhibit or induce the liver enzyme systems, e.g.:

6.1 Drugs and the liver

Liver induction

- Will lead to treatment failure of:
  - warfarin, phenytoin, theophylline, oral contraceptive pill

- Caused by:
  - phenytoin, carbamazepine, barbiturates, rifampicin, chronic alcohol consumption, sulphonylureas

Liver inhibition

- Will lead to potentiation of:
  - warfarin, phenytoin, carbamazepine, theophylline, cyclosporin

- Caused by:
  - omeprazole, erythromycin, valproate, isoniazid, cimetidine, sulphonamides, acute alcohol consumption

Absorption interactions

Medication that changes the pH of the stomach or the motility of the stomach may vastly change the absorption of another medication (see Section 1.1).

Compatibility

When medications are administered, always be aware of their interactions before they enter the body. This is particularly important with parenteral medication. Many medications interact to produce non-effective products, toxic products or precipitates.

Examples of incompatible injections

- Amiodarone: precipitates in the presence of sodium ions
- Fat (in total parenteral nutrition): emulsifies when mixed with heparin
- Erythromycin: is unstable in acidic medium (glucose), so must be made up in sodium chloride
- Gentamicin: is partly inactivated by penicillin, so lines must be flushed between administrations

7. TOXICOLOGY

Each year 40,000 children attend A&E Departments with suspected poisonings. These poisoning incidents fall into three categories:

- Accidental – typically boys in the 1–4 years age group
- Intentional – usually teenage girls
- Deliberate – suspected if the signs cannot be explained in any other way

Principles of management include the following:

- Resuscitation if necessary
- Contact a national poisons unit for advice
- Induction of emesis (with ipecacuanha for example) is no longer indicated
- Consider limiting absorption of poison by:
    Activated charcoal – if ingestion is within 1 hour
    Gastric lavage – if a life threatening quantity of poison is ingested
- Acid, alkali or corrosive substances should be treated with caution – do not intervene with the above before seeking advice from the poisons unit.

7.1 Paracetamol

Levels of >250 mg/kg are likely to lead to severe liver damage.

Clinical features

- Nausea and vomiting are the only early symptoms although the majority of patients are asymptomatic
- Right subcostal pain may indicate hepatic necrosis

Management

- Activated charcoal if ingestion <4 hours
- Measure plasma paracetamol level at 4 hours or as soon as possible thereafter
- Acetylcysteine is possibly effective for up to 24 hours' post ingestion
- If patients are on enzyme-inducing drugs, treatment may need to be commenced at levels below the treatment line

7.2 Iron

Severity of poisoning is related to the amount of elemental iron ingested.

- 200 mg tablet of ferrous sulphate contains 65 mg elemental iron
- 300 mg tablet of ferrous gluconate contains 35 mg elemental iron

<20 mg/kg	toxicity unlikely
>20 mg/kg	toxicity may occur
>60 mg/kg	significant iron poisoning

Clinical features

1st stage
- Within a few hours
  - nausea and vomiting
  - abdominal pain
  - haematemesis

2nd stage
- 8 to 16 hours
  - apparent recovery

3rd stage
- 16 to 24 hours
  - hypoglycaemia
  - metabolic acidosis (due to lactic acid)

Late stage
- hepatic failure – 2 to 4 days

Management

- Initial treatment depends on the likelihood of toxicity >20mg/kg ingested?
- Plasma iron level
- Abdominal X-ray
  - No iron visible but > 20 mg/kg ingested
    - desferrioxamine orally
  - Iron in stomach: gastric lavage with desferrioxamine in the lavage fluid
  - Iron in intestine: desferrioxamine orally
    - picolax orally – bowel stimulant
- If >60 mg/kg ingested – administer parenteral desferrioxamine

7.3 Tricyclic antidepressants

Clinical features

- Depressed level of consciousness
- Respiratory depression
- Convulsion
- Arrhythmia
- Hypotension
- Anticholinergic effects: pupillary dilatation
  urinary retention
  dry mouth

Management

- Resuscitation
- Activated charcoal
- ECG monitoring
- Correct hypoxia and acidosis
- Treat secondary arrhythmias and convulsions

7.4 Aspirin overdose

Clinical features

In young children dehydration and tachypnoea. In older children and adults tachypnoea and vomiting with progressive lethargy. Tinnitus and deafness. Hypoglycaemia or hyperglycaemia can occur.

Three phases

Phase One

- May last up to 12 hours
- Salicylates directly stimulate the respiratory centre resulting in a respiratory alkalosis with a compensatory alkaline urine with bicarbonate sodium and potassium loss

Phase Two

- May begin straight away particularly in a young child and last 12–24 hours
- Hypokalaemia with as a consequence a paradoxical aciduria despite the alkalosis

Phase Three

- After 6–24 hours
- Dehydration, hypokalaemia and progressive lactic acidosis. The acidosis now predominating
- Can progress to pulmonary oedema with respiratory failure, disorientation and coma

Management

- Gastric lavage up to 4 hours. Activated charcoal for sustained release preparations. Level at 6 hours plotted on a normogram.
- Alkalisation of the urine to aid drug excretion, adequate fluids including bicarbonate sodium and potassium with close monitoring of acid base and electrolytes. Discuss with poisons centre.

7.5 Lead poisoning

Lead poisoning is uncommon but potentially very serious. It often results from pica (persistent eating of non-nutritive substances, e.g. soil) and is therefore more common in pre-school age children. Other causes include sucking/ingesting lead paint, lead pipes, discharge from lead batteries and substance abuse of leaded petrol.

Lead intoxication can be divided into acute and chronic effects, and results from its combination with and disruption of vital physiological enzymes.

Acute intoxication

- Reversible renal Fanconi-like syndrome

Chronic intoxication:

- Failure to thrive
- Abdominal upset: pain / anorexia / vomiting / constipation

- Lead encephalopathy: behavioural & cognitive disturbance drowsiness, seizures, neuropathies, coma
- Glomerulonehritis and renal failure
- Anaemia – microcytic / hypochromic, basophilic stippling of red cells

A co-existing iron deficiency is common which firstly further exacerbates the anaemia and secondly actually contributes to increased lead absorption. Basophilic stippling is due to inhibition of pyrimidine 5' nucleotidase and results in accumulation of denatured RNA.

Treatment involves

- Removing source
- Chelation: Mild-   Oral D-penicillamine
             Severe-   IV sodium calcium edetate (EDTA)
             Very severe- IM injections of dimercaprol to increase effect of EDTA.

Some US states implement universal screening for elevated lead levels in children.

Haematemesis occurs in iron poisoning; skin and hair changes are very common in arsenic intoxication.

7.6 Carbon monoxide

- Is a tasteless, odourless, colourless and non-irritant gas.
- Carbon monoxide binds to haemoglobin to form carboxyhaemoglobin which reduces the oxygen carrying capacity of the blood and shifts the oxygen dissociation curve to the left. The affinity of haemoglobin for carbon monoxide is 250 times greater than that for oxygen
- Endogenous production occurs and maintains a resting carboxyhaemoglobin level of 1-3%.
- Smoking increases carboxyhaemoglobin levels. Other sources of raised levels include car exhaust fumes, poorly maintained heating systems and smoke from fires.
- Clinical features of carbon monoxide poisoning occur as a result of tissue hypoxia. PaO2 is normal but the oxygen content of the blood reduced. Toxicity relates loosely to the maximum carboxyhaemoglobin concentration. Other factors including duration of exposure and age of the patient.

Maximum Carboxyhaemoglobin Concentration

10%	Not normally associated with symptoms
10–30%	Headache and dyspnoea,
60%	Coma, convulsions and death

Neuropsychiatric problems can occur with chronic exposure.

● Treatment of carbon monoxide is with 100% oxygen which will reduce the carboxyhaemoglobin concentration. Hyperbaric oxygen is said to reduce the carboxyhaemoglobin level quicker.

8. FURTHER READING

Applied Therapeutics: The Clinical Use of Drugs, sixth edition, Young, Y L and Koda Kimble, M A, Chapters 95 and 96. Lippincott Williams & Wilkins 2001.

Medicines for Children. Royal College of Child Health/Neonatal & Paediatric Pharmacists Group 1999.

Paediatric drug dosing, Maxwell, G W *Drugs* **37** 113–15, 1989.

Prescribing for infants and children. Rylance, G M, *British Medical Journal* **296**, 984–6 1988.

Principles of drug prescribing in infants and children: a practical guide, Watson, D, et al. *Drugs* **46**(2), 281–8 1993.

Chapter 4

Dermatology

Helen M Goodyear

CONTENTS

Dermatology

1. STRUCTURE AND FUNCTION OF THE SKIN

1.1 Structure of the skin

Epidermis

4 layers
- Stratum corneum — keratinization
- Stratum granulosum
- Stratum spinosum
- Stratum basale

Cells
- Keratinocytes (95%)
- Merkel cells
- Melanocytes
- Langerhans' cells

Marked regional variation in thickness of epidermis

Dermoepidermal junction
- A barrier and a filter

Dermis
- 15–20% of body weight
- Variable thickness — 5 mm back, 1 mm eyelids
- 2 protein fibres — collagen and elastin
- Supporting matrix/ground substance
  - proteoglycan (polysaccharide and protein)
- Rich blood supply

Cells
- Fibroblasts
- Mast cells
- Macrophages

Subcutaneous fat

Epidermal transit time: 52–75 days. Greatly decreased in hyperproliferative conditions, e.g. psoriasis
Palmoplantar skin: extra layer, stratum lucidum, present between stratum granulosum and stratum corneum
Two types of skin: glabrous skin on palms and soles and hair-bearing skin

1.2 Function of the skin

- **Barrier**: to the inward/outward passage of water and electrolytes
- **Mechanical**: depends on collagen and elastin fibres

- **Immunological**: cytokines, macrophages, lymphocytes and antigen presentation by Langerhans' cells
- **UV irradiation protection**: melanin is a barrier in the epidermis, protein barrier in the stratum corneum
- **Temperature regulation**: involves sweat glands and blood vessels in the dermis; heat loss by radiation, convection, conduction and evaporation
- **Sensory**: touch, pain, warmth, cold, itch
- **Respiration**: skin absorbs O_2 and excretes CO_2 accounting for 1–2% of respiration
- **Endocrine**: Vitamin D_3 synthesized in stratum spinosum and basale from previtamin D_3 due to UVB radiation

2. NEONATAL SKIN DISORDERS

2.1 Embryology

- **Nails**: forming from 8 to 9 weeks onwards
- **Hair**: synthesis from 17 to 19 weeks
- **Keratinization**: of epidermis from 22 to 24 weeks
- **Epidermis**: all layers present from 24 weeks
- **Preterm:** (24–34 weeks) have poor epidermal barrier with thin stratum corneum directly correlating to degree of prematurity; increased skin losses and absorption; within 2 weeks skin is the same as that of term infant
- **Dermis**: is less thick in neonate compared to adult; collagen fibre bundles smaller, elastin fibres immature, vascular and neural elements less well organized

2.2 Physiological lesions

- Cutis marmorata
- Physiological scaling
- Vernix caseosa
- Sebaceous gland hyperplasia
- Acrocyanosis (peripheral cyanosis)
- Harlequin colour change
- Sucking blisters
- Milia (large ones = pearls)
- Lanugo hairs in preterm baby

2.3 Differential diagnosis of vesiculopustular lesions

Transient rashes

- **Miliaria**: blockage of sweat ducts; vesicles (miliaria crystallina) or itchy red papules (miliaria rubra); first 2 weeks
- **Erythema toxicum neonatorum**: in first 48 hours; may recur beyond first month

- **Transient neonatal pustulosis melanosis**: superficial fragile pustules at birth, rupture easily leaving pigmented macule which lasts for up to 3 months
- **Infantile acropustulosis**: presents in first 3 months; recurrent crops of 1–4-mm vesicopustules usually on hands and feet; resolves by second to third year
- **Eosinophilic pustular folliculitis**: recurrent crops of papules on scalp, hands and feet; rare, usually males
- **Neonatal acne**: relatively common, resolves by 3 months

Infections and infestations — always take a swab to exclude *Staphylococcus aureus*/ Streptococcal infection and others in preterm infants or the immunocompromised. Scabies can occur in the first month of life.

Genetic and naevoid disorders

- **Epidermolysis bullosa**
- **Incontinentia pigmenti**: X-linked dominant, usually lethal in males; vesicular lesions in first 48 hours, verrucous lesions, streaky pigmentation and then atrophic pale lesions; associated with other abnormalities: **s**keletal, **e**ye, CNS and **d**entition (SEND)
- **Urticaria pigmentosa**: lesions in first year of life which urticate when rubbed; can present at birth; systemic involvement commoner if presents >5 years

2.4 Neonatal erythroderma

Causes of neonatal erythroderma

Skin disorders
- Seborrhoeic dermatitis
- Atopic eczema
- Psoriasis
- Ichthyosis
- Netherton's syndrome

Immunological disorders
- Omenn's syndrome
- Di George syndrome
- T-cell lymphoma
- Hypogammaglobulinaemia
- Graft vs. host disease

Metabolic/nutritional deficiencies
- Zinc deficiency
- Cystic fibrosis
- Protein malnutrition
- Multiple carboxylase deficiencies
- Amino acid disorders

2.5 Developmental abnormalities

- Amniotic bands
- Aplasia cutis congenita: isolated defect commonly on posterior scalp; associations include epidermolysis bullosa, limb defects, spinal dysraphism, trisomy 13, Goltz syndrome and Adams Oliver syndrome

2.6 Neonatal lupus erythematosus

Presents in first few weeks of life. Erythematous scaly rash, typically around the eyes. May be associated with congenital heart block.

3. BIRTHMARKS

3.1 Strawberry naevi (capillary haemangioma)

- Usually appear in first few weeks of life
- Commoner in preterm infants
- Precursor is an erythematous/telangiectatic patch +/– pale halo
- 3 phases: • proliferative (6–10 months)
             • stabilization
             • spontaneous resolution — pale centre initially
- Complications — ulceration, infection, bleeding, cardiac failure
- Treat if obstructs vital structures
- Often deep component: cavernous haemangioma

Multiple small diffuse haemangiomas in infants <3 months of age may be associated with visceral involvement, particularly liver; high mortality if untreated

Kasabach–Merritt syndrome: thrombocytopenia, rapidly enlarging haemangioma, micro-angiopathic haemolytic anaemia, localized consumption coagulopathy

3.2 Salmon patch (stork bite)

Nape of neck, upper eyelids, glabella; 10–20% in occipital region persist whilst others resolve spontaneously

3.3 Port wine stain (naevus flammeus)

- Present at birth
- Capillary malformation
- Associations • Sturge–Weber syndrome
               • Klippel–Trenaunay–Weber syndrome
- Persists throughout life
- Can treat with pulse dye laser

3.4 Sebaceous naevi

Present at birth; scalp/face; flat/slightly raised and hairless; can undergo neoplastic change after puberty

3.5 Melanocytic naevi

Present in 1–2% at birth. Congenital usually >5 mm, acquired <5 mm. Giant melanocytic naevi (bathing trunk naevi) have increased melanoma risk (4–14%). May be associated with neurocutaneous melanosis (EEG abnormalities, raised intracranial pressure (ICP) hydrocephalus and space-occupying lesion (SOL)).

4. DIFFERENTIAL DIAGNOSIS OF AN ITCHY, RED RASH

4.1 Atopic eczema

Affects 10–20% of children.

Multifactorial disease including

- Genetic factors: 70% of children have positive family history of atopy
- Immunological abnormalities: IgE dysregulation, skin immune abnormalities — altered cytokine secretion
- Altered pharmacological mechanisms

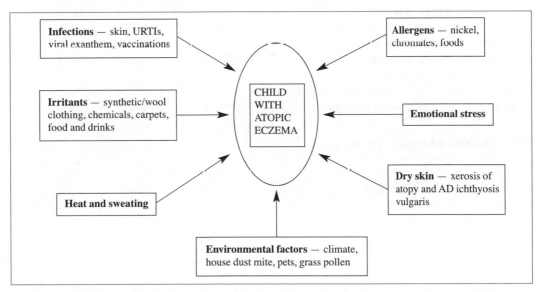

Exacerbating factors of atopic eczema (URTIs, upper respiratory tract infections; AD, autosomal dominant)

Features of atopic eczema

- **Age of onset**: usually in first 6 months, around 3 months most common
- **Site**: face/scalp initially, then flexures; extensor aspects may be involved
- **Erythematous macules/papules/plaques/oozing/crust formation**

143

Associated conditions

- Ichthyosis vulgaris
- Keratosis pilaris
- Food intolerance and allergy
- Pityriasis alba
- Juvenile plantar dermatosis
- Asthma
- Cataract

- **Tendency to secondary infection**: *Staphylococcus aureus*, Group A beta haemolytic Streptococcus, herpes simplex virus (HSV) (eczema herpeticum), warts, mollusca contagiosa
- **Skin colonization** with *S. aureus* in 90%
- **Lichenification**: chronic eczema
- **Resolves**: 50% by 6 years, 90% by 14 years

Differential diagnoses

- **Lichen simplex chronicus**: asymmetrical lesion, chronic rubbing and scratching
- **Infantile seborrhoeic dermatitis**: usually first 3 months, yellow greasy scales on scalp, forehead, napkin area and skin folds, lack of pruritus
- **Contact dermatitis**
- **Hyper IgE syndrome (Job's syndrome)**: IgE >2,000 IU/ml, recurrent cutaneous and sinopulmonary infections
- **Wiskott–Aldrich**: X-linked recessive, thrombocytopenia and recurrent pyogenic infections. Risk of malignancies, non-Hodgkin's lymphoma most common

Management of atopic eczema

General

- Avoid exacerbating factors
- Cut nails short, file edges
- Cotton clothes
- Non-biological washing powders (and avoid fabric softeners)

Topical treatments

- **Emollients** — bath oil once or twice daily, soap substitute, moisturizer qds (e.g. aqueous cream, emulsifying ointment). Any of the moisturizers can be used as soap substitutes. Use antiseptic bath oils, e.g. Dermol 600, Oilatum plus and emollients, e.g. Dermol 500 lotion if recurrent infection.
- **Steroid creams** — weakest strength possible applied twice daily to control the eczema. In general; 1% hydrocortisone if <2 years; moderate potency if needed, e.g. Eumovate, Betnovate 1 in 4 if >2 years. Never use potent, e.g. Betnovate, or very potent, e.g. Dermovate, in children except in specialized centres.

- **Bandages** — zinc impregnated, e.g. ichthopaste, worn with elasticated bandage such as Coban over the top. Change every 24–48 hours. Useful for chronic limb eczema.
- **Wet wraps** — Tubifast bandages of different sizes cut to make double body suit. Make first layer wet with either water or cream. Wear at night. Either emollients used under wraps, e.g. aqueous cream, or dilute steroid cream, e.g. Betnovate, 1 in 10 in aqueous cream.
- **Tacrolimus** (Protopic) 0.03% works on skin immune system, affecting cytokine release, new treatment for moderate or severe eczema. Use twice daily for 3 weeks then od.
- **Antihistamines** — use with caution in children <1 year.
- **Antibiotics** — consider a 10-day course if eczema flares up. Flucloxacillin +/– penicillin V or erythromycin. Beware of MRSA (methicillin-resistant *Staphylococcus aureus*) and resistance to erythromycin in some hospital-acquired *S. aureus*.
- **Aciclovir** — 1.5 g/m^2 per day intravenously for 5 days if eczema herpeticum. Oral aciclovir for HSV recurrences.
- **Diet** — avoid obvious trigger foods. Give 3-month trial of cows' milk protein-free diet if severe eczema <1 year. Involve Paediatric dietician.
- **Systemic therapy** — severe eczema unresponsive to above therapies. Use prednisolone, starting around 2 mg/kg to control eczema, then weaning down to lowest alternate day dose which controls eczema. Short course ciclosporin (up to 5 mg/kg per day) for 3–6 months also used, but monitoring renal and liver function carefully.
- **Alternative remedies** — many patients will use these, e.g. homeopathy, Chinese herbal medicine. Beware of potent steroid creams in Chinese herbal creams and monitor liver and renal function 3-monthly if taking herbs. Avoid in children <2 years.

4.2 Urticaria

Transient erythematous/oedematous itchy swellings of the dermis. Lasts few minutes to 24 hours. Clears leaving normal skin. 50% have angio-oedema (swelling of subcutaneous tissues). Histamine is the principal mediator released from mast cells.

Causes of urticaria

- **Infection**
  - Viral
  - Streptococcus
  - *Toxocara canis*

- **Food**
  - Cows' milk
  - Eggs
  - Nuts
  - Fish
  - Exotic fruits

- **Associated with systemic disease**

- **Drugs**
  - Penicillin/cephalosporins
  - Non-steroidal inflammatory drugs (NSAIDs)

- **Physical agents**
  - Cholinergic urticaria
  - Cold urticaria
  - Dermatographism

- **Idiopathic (50% cases)**

4.3 Infections and infestations

Scabies

Due to mite *Sarcoptes scabiei humanis.* The mite can survive for 24–36 hours off human host.

Variable intensely itchy skin eruption, about 1 month after infestation, is an immune response to the mite and includes:

- Burrows
- Excoriations
- Eczematization
- Papules
- Vesiculopustular lesions
- Bullae
- Secondary bacterial infection
- Nodules

Burrows common on palms, soles and sides of digits. Examine all family members if scabies is suspected. Treat all family at same time.

Management of scabies

- Use aqueous Malathion-based preparation, e.g. Derbac M (alcoholic-based preparation will sting)
- Treat all family members at the same time
- Two applications from the neck downwards at 24-hour intervals without washing. Get under nails and in skin creases. Reapply after hand washing. Caution if <1-year-old, applying for lesser time depending on age of child
- Apply to lesions on face if present (commoner if <1 year)
- Treat any secondary infection with systemic antibiotics
- Treat residual dry skin with emollients
- Wash all clothing, bedlinen and towels at the end of treatment

Viral infections

Tend to be maculopapular erythematous rashes which may be pruritic.

Tinea

Erythematous, circular scaly lesions with clearly defined margin. *Microsporum canis* fluoresces with UV light, *Trichophyton tonsurans* (of human origin, common in inner cities) does not. Take skin scrapings.

Impetigo

Superficially spreading skin infection characterized by yellowish-brown crust. May be bullous. Peaks in late summer and is commonest in children <5 years. Due to *Staphylococcus aureus* or Group A beta haemolytic Streptococcus. Treat with oral antibiotics.

Staphylococcal scalded skin syndrome

Due to exotoxin-producing Staphylococci. Localized infection becomes widespread after 24–48 hours. Characteristic signs are fever, skin tenderness, marked erythema, bullae and peeling of the skin. Treat with systemic antibiotics (flucloxacillin) and watch fluid balance.

Warts

Due to human papillomavirus (HPV). Commonest on hands and feet (plantar warts — verrucas) but occur at any site. Most resolve spontaneously but can last for several years.

Treat with salicylic acid–based wart paint, e.g. Salactol, applying each night and rubbing wart down with an emery board until wart is flat. May need to treat for 3 months or longer. Freezing with liquid nitrogen is effective but often requires multiple treatments at monthly intervals. Poorly tolerated in children <5 years.

Perianal warts

Usually innocently acquired but consider sexual abuse. Only treat if multiple and spreading. Use podophyllin 15%. May need surgery.

Mollusca contagiosa

'Water warts'. Due to poxvirus. Dome-shaped papules with an umbilicated centre. Spread by autoinoculation. Resolve spontaneously but can last for several years. Treatments tend to be associated with scarring.

NB. Both warts and mollusca contagiosa are commoner in children who are immunosuppressed and those with underlying skin disorders such as atopic eczema.

4.4 Psoriasis

- **Onset**: <2 years in 2% and at <10 years in 10% of cases
- **Increased epidermal turnover time**
- **Relapsing and remitting**: scaly rash, typically affects extensor surfaces and scalp (*Pityriasis amiantacea*)
- **Age of onset**: 5–9 years girls, 15–19 years boys
- **Genetic predisposition**: risk of psoriasis is 10% if first-degree relative affected, two psoriatic parents risk is 50%; 73% monozygotic and 20% dizygotic twins have concordant disease; HLA Cw6 (B13 and B17) linked to 9–15 times risk, HLA B27 associated with psoriatic arthropathy
- **Nail involvement**: pits, onycholysis, subungual hyperkeratosis; may precede onset of skin lesions
- **Arthropathy**: may be severe; higher incidence in patients with nail changes

Recognized types of psoriasis

- **Common plaque**: chronic psoriasis, psoriasis vulgaris
- **Guttate psoriasis**: (raindrop psoriasis) multiple small lesions on trunk

- **Flexural sites**: intertriginous areas
- **Erythrodermic psoriasis**
- **Pustular psoriasis**: acute generalized form or chronic localized to hands and feet

Provoking factors

- **Trauma** (Koebner phenomenon)
- **Infection**: streptococcal disease especially in throat in guttate psoriasis; may also play a role in chronic plaque psoriasis
- **Endocrine**: peaks at puberty (and menopause); gets worse in postpartum period
- **Sunlight**: usually beneficial but makes small number worse
- **Metabolic**: hypocalcaemia, dialysis
- **Drugs**: withdrawal of systemic steroids, beta blockers, antimalarials and lithium
- **Psychogenic factors**: stress
- **HIV**: psoriasis may appear for the first time or get dramatically worse

Differential diagnosis

- **Hyperkeratotic eczema**
- **Lichen planus**: flat-topped, purple polygonal papules with white reticulate surface (Wickham's striae); oral and nail changes may be present; rare in children; 90% resolve in 12 months
- **Pityriasis rosea**: larger herald patch, smaller lesions in Christmas tree distribution; clears in 6 weeks; linked to human herpes virus-7 (HHV 7)
- **Pityriasis lichenoides chronica**: excoriated papules on trunk and limbs in crops; lasts up to a few years

Management of psoriasis

- **Avoid triggering factors**
- **Treat Streptococcal infection**
- **Topical treatment**
  - Emollients
  - Tar-based bath emollients, e.g. Polytar
  - Tar and salicylic acid ointments
  - Vitamin D-derivative creams — calcipotriol (Dovonex) for mild to moderate psoriasis (up to 40% of skin area affected)
  - Mild-potency topical steroid creams with tar, e.g. Alphosyl HC for delicate areas, e.g. face, flexures, ears, genitals
  - Carefully supervised dithranol preparations, e.g. dithrocream
  - Topical retinoids used but unlicensed
- **Phototherapy** — UVB phototherapy if child old enough to comply. PUVA is contraindicated in young children.
- **Systemic therapy** — severe psoriasis, acute pustular psoriasis, e.g. methotrexate, ciclosporin, acitretin

5. BLISTERING DISORDERS

Causes of blistering disorders

- **Inherited**
  - Epidermolysis bullosa
  - Incontinentia pigmenti
  - Bullous ichthyosiform erythroderma

- **Drugs**
  - Fixed drug eruptions
  - Photosensitivity reaction
  - Sulphonamides
  - Barbiturates

- **Autoimmune**
  - Chronic bullous disease of childhood
  - Pemphigoid
  - Epidermolysis bullosa acquisita
  - Dermatitis herpetiformis
  - Pemphigus

- **Mechanobullous**
  - Trauma/friction
  - Burns
  - Insect bites/papular urticaria

- **Contact dermatitis**

- **Infection**
  - Bullous impetigo
  - Herpes simplex virus
  - Varicella/zoster
  - Hand, foot and mouth disease
  - Scabies

- **Neonatal disorders**
  - Infantile acropustulosis
  - Miliaria

- **Others**
  - Erythema multiforme
  - Stevens–Johnson syndrome
  - Henoch–Schönlein purpura
  - Porphyria
  - Toxic epidermal necrolysis
  - Hartnup's disease
  - Pachyonychia congenita

- **Dermatoses**
  - Eczema
  - Lichen planus

5.1 Epidermolysis bullosa (EB)

Heterogeneous condition. Need skin biopsy for definitive diagnosis. First trimester prenatal diagnosis is possible. Severe types at risk of nutritional deficiencies and anaemia.

There are three broad categories:

- **EB simplex:** mainly autosomal dominant (AD) — defect in basal layer of epidermis affecting keratins 5 and 14. Usually appears when child begins to crawl or walk, with blisters at friction sites, e.g. knees, hands and feet. Hair, teeth and nails not affected.
- **Junctional EB:** autosomal recessive (AR) — lethal and non-lethal variants. Mucous membranes can be severely affected and teeth are often abnormal. Laminin-5 defect. Raw denuded areas show little tendency to heal. Hoarseness due to laryngeal involvement.
- **Dystrophic EB:** AD and AR — subepidermal blister. Defect in collagen-VII production. Lesions heal with scarring. Hair and teeth are normal in dominant form, whilst involvement of mucous membranes, nails, hair and teeth may all be abnormal in recessive form. Web formation between digits leads to a useless fist. May develop squamous carcinoma.

5.2 Autoimmune blistering disorders

All rare. Listed in order of decreasing frequency.

Chronic bullous dermatosis of childhood
Usually >3 years, mean age 5 years. Tense blisters like a string of pearls usually on abdomen and buttocks. May present as genital blisters/erosions. 40% have mucous membrane involvement. Clears after 3 years. Linear basement membrane IgA.

Bullous pemphigoid
Can be <12 months. Palm and sole involvement common. 75% have mucous membrane changes. Lasts 2–4 years. Linear basement membrane IgG.

Dermatitis herpetiformis
Mean age 7 years. Affects buttocks, elbows, back of neck and scalp. Itchy. 15% resolve spontaneously. Skin changes can persist up to 18 months after gluten-free diet. IgA in papillary dermis.

Epidermolysis bullosa acquisita
Mechanobullous picture with blisters localized to areas of trauma. Remits in 2–4 years. Linear basement membrane IgG.

Pemphigus
Very rare. Flaccid blisters. Nikolsky's sign (a blister is induced by rubbing normal-appearing skin) positive. Mucous membrane involvement in vulgaris type, with stomatitis the presenting sign in 50% cases. Intercellular IgG.

6. ERYTHEMAS

6.1 Erythema multiforme

Acute self-limiting onset of symmetrical fixed red papules, some of which form target lesions. May blister. Can show Koebner phenomenon. May involve lips, buccal mucosa and tongue.

Causes of erythema multiforme

- **Infections**
  - Herpes simplex virus
  - Mycoplasma
  - Epstein-Barr virus
  - Chlamydiae
  - Orf
  - Deep fungal infections (histoplasmosis)

- **Underlying malignancy**

- **Drugs**
  - Sulphonamides
  - Penicillin

- **Collagen diseases**
  - Systemic lupus erythematosus (SLE)
  - Polyarteritis nodosa

Stevens–Johnson syndrome

Causes as for erythema multiforme.

- Severe erosions of at least two mucosal surfaces
- Prodromal respiratory illness
- Extensive necrosis of lips and mouth
- Purulent conjunctivitis
- Variable skin involvement — red macules, bullae, skin necrosis and denudation

6.2 Erythema nodosum

Nodular, erythematous eruption on extensor aspects of legs, less commonly on thighs and forearms. Regresses to bruises. Lasts 3–6 weeks.

Causes of erythema nodosum

- **Infections**
  - Streptococcus
  - Salmonella
  - Yersinia
  - Campylobacter
  - TB
  - Acnes
  - Chlamydia
  - Cat–scratch fever
  - Hepatitis B
  - Epstein–Barr virus
  - Mycoses

- **Gut disorders**
  - Ulcerative colitis
  - Crohn's disease

- **Malignancy**
  - Leukaemia
  - Lymphoma

- **Drugs**
  - Sulphonamides
  - Oral contraceptive pill

6.3 Erythema marginatum

Annular migratory erythema found in 10% of cases of rheumatic fever. Recurrent crops of lesions weekly. Active cardiac disease. Frequently precedes onset of migratory arthritis.

6.4 Erythema migrans

Lyme disease due to *Borrelia burgdorferi*. Red papule which develops with annular red ring around it.

7. PHOTOSENSITIVE DISORDERS

Causes of photosensitive disorders

- **Idiopathic**
  - Polymorphic light eruption
  - Actinic prurigo

- **Contact dermatitis** due to plants

- **SLE** — photosensitivity rash in 15–30%

- **Drugs**
  - Sulphonamides
  - Thiazides
  - Tetracycline

- **Genetic**

7.1 Genetic causes of photosensitivity

Phenylketonuria

AR. In addition to photosensitivity, skin changes include:

- Decreased pigmentation
- Eczema
- Fair hair
- Lightly pigmented eyes

Xeroderma pigmentosum

AR group of disorders due to DNA repair defect.

- Extreme photosensitivity
- Severe ophthalmological abnormalities
- Skin malignancies in childhood
- Neurological complications in 20%
- Freckling

Cockayne's syndrome

AD. Cells have increased sensitivity to UV light. Onset of symptoms is in the second year of life.

- Progressive neurological degeneration and growth failure
- Sensorineural hearing loss
- Skeletal abnormalities
- Dental caries
- Pigmentary retinopathy
- Cataracts

Trichothiodystrophy

AR. Hair has low sulphur content. Includes following defects 'PIBIDS':

- **P**hotosensitivity
- **I**chthyosis
- **B**rittle hair
- **I**ntellectual impairment
- **D**ecreased fertility
- **S**hort stature

Rothmund–Thomson syndrome

AR. Characterized by poikiloderma (atrophic pigmented telangiectasia) by end of first year.

- Sparse hair
- Skeletal dysplasia
- Short stature
- Cataract
- Hypogonadism
- Hypotrophic nails
- Increased risk of osteosarcoma and skin malignancy

Bloom's syndrome

AR.

- Growth retardation
- Immunodeficiency (IgA and IgM)
- Telangiectasia
- Pigmentary abnormalities
- Malignancies in third decade — leukaemia, lymphomas

Hartnup's disease

AR. Impaired amino acid transport in kidneys and small intestine. Most children asymptomatic.

- Photosensitivity with pellagra-like appearance is first sign
- Can form blisters

- Intermittent cerebellar ataxia
- Psychotic behaviour
- Mild mental retardation

Porphyrias

Group of diseases leading to accumulation of haem precursors. 5–aminolaevulinic acid (ALA) and porphobilinogen (PBG) have no cutaneous manifestations. Elevated porphyrins are associated with either acute photosensitivity or skin fragility with vesiculobullous and erosive lesions.

Erythropoietic protoporphyria (EPP)
Usually AD. Most common porphyria in children.

- Small pitted scars on nose and cheeks
- Burning/stinging sensation on exposed skin
- Photosensitivity less severe in adult life
- Gallstones in childhood
- Excess protoporphyrins in red cells and faeces (urine normal)

Congenital erythropoietic porphyria
AR. Presents at or shortly after birth. Acute episodes become less severe with time, leaving residual scarring, ulceration and marked deformity with sclerodactyly and loss of terminal phalanges.

- Severe photosensitivity
- Red staining of nappy
- Haemolytic anaemia
- Splenomegaly
- Hypertrichosis
- Teeth and bones may be red (fluoresce with UV light)

Porphyria cutanea tarda (PCT)
Familial or provoked by drugs, alcohol or infection.

- Skin fragility leading to vesicles/blisters and erosions
- Hypertrichosis
- Yellow/blue nails and onycholysis
- Systemic manifestations — anorexia, constipation, diarrhoea
- Urine dark brown

8. ICHTHYOSES

Disorders of keratinization, characterized by excessively dry and visibly scaly skin. Hereditary or associated with systemic disease.

8.1 Inherited ichthyoses

Ichthyosis vulgaris

AD. Variable range of expression; may affect in winter months only, affects 1:250. Fine, light scaling. Associated with keratosis pilaris and atopic eczema.

X-linked recessive ichthyosis (XRI, steroid sulphatase deficiency)

1:2,000 boys. Dark-brown scaling affecting limbs and trunk. Gene in Xp22.3 region.

- Cryptorchidism
- Corneal opacities
- Prolonged labour (placental sulphatase deficiency)

Lamellar ichthyoses

AD and AR. Large, dark, plate-like scales, reptilian appearance.

Bullous ichthyosiform erythroderma (BIE)

AD. Erythroderma and severe blistering at birth. Mutations in keratin 1 or 10.

Non-bullous ichthyosiform erythroderma

AR. Generalized fine scaling and erythroderma.

Associated congenital ichthyoses

Sjögren–Larsson syndrome
AR. Fatty alcohol oxidation defect in fibroblasts. Spastic di- or tetraplegia, mental retardation. Onset of neurological signs at 4–13 months of age.

Refsum's disease
AR. Phytanic acid oxylase defect.

- Retinitis pigmentosa
- Peripheral neuropathy
- Anosmia
- Sensory deafness
- Variable ichthyosis — ichthyosis vulgaris-type appearance

Associated steroid sulphatase deficiency
XRI can be associated with

- Kallmann's syndrome
- Pyloric stenosis
- Chondroplasia punctata
- Hypogonadism
- Mental retardation

Multiple sulphatase deficiency
AR. Lack of arylsulphatase A, B and steroid sulphatase.

- Neurodegenerative disease
- Coarse facies
- Hepatosplenomegaly
- Lumbar kyphosis

Trichothiodystrophy syndromes — Tay's syndrome and 'PIBIDS'
AR. Tay's do not have photosensitivity. Hair has decreased sulphur content.

Netherton's syndrome
AR.

- Neonatal erythroderma
- Ichthyosis linearis circumflexa
- Atopy
- Failure to thrive
- Recurrent infections
- Trichorrhosis invaginata — hair shaft abnormality

Happle's syndrome
XD (X-linked dominant). Conradi–Hunermann is AD and is now thought not to have cutaneous manifestations.

- Chondroplasia punctata
- Cicatricial alopecia
- Cataracts
- Short stature
- Follicular atrophoderma

KID syndrome
Mode of inheritance uncertain — ? AD or AR.

- **K**eratitis
- **I**chthyosis
- **D**eafness

Neutral-lipid storage disease (Chanarin–Dorfman syndrome)
AR. Fatty changes of the liver, variable neurological and ocular involvement. Multiple lipid vacuoles in monocytes and granulocytes.

CHILD syndrome
Congenital **h**emidysplasia, **i**chthyosiform erythroderma and **l**imb **d**efects.

8.2 Collodion baby

Yellow, shiny, tight film covering skin at birth. 10% have normal skin. Film shed at 1–4 weeks of life. Can persist for 3 months. Biopsy after day 14 is helpful.

Disorders presenting as collodion baby include:

- Gaucher's disease
- Lamellar ichthyosis
- Trichothiodystrophy
- Sjögren–Larsson syndrome
- Non-bullous ichthyosiform erythroderma
- Neutral-lipid storage disease
- Chondroplasia punctata
- Ichthyosis vulgaris
- Netherton's syndrome

Neonatal problems of collodion baby and harlequin ichthyosis (see below)

- Hypothermia
- Dehydration
- Hypernatraemia
- Cutaneous infection
- Poor sucking

May need up to 250 ml/kg per day fluids. Nurse in high-humidity incubator with up to 1-hourly application of white soft paraffin and liquid paraffin 50:50.

8.3 Harlequin ichthyosis

AR. Problems are the same as for collodion babies. Most of the survivors have non-bullous ichthyosiform erythroderma. Need continued high-intensity skin care and high-calorie feeds, otherwise fail to thrive. Use of retinoids (acitretin) is thought to account for increasing survival of these children.

Features of harlequin ichthyosis at birth

- Usually preterm
- Erythroderma
- Thick plate-like scales at birth — 'coat of armour'
- Deep red fissures
- Ectropion and eclabium (mouth pulled open with eversion of lips)
- Hands and feet have tightly bound digits. Tips may be necrotic.
- Nose and ears bound down
- Respiratory distress depending upon prematurity and the degree of restriction of chest movement

9. HAIR AND NAILS

9.1 Hair

The hair has cyclical periods of growth throughout life. The three phases are:

Anagen: growth phase
Catagen: intermediate phase
Telogen: resting usually 3 months before hair being shed

These phases occur randomly so that no one area is depleted of hair. Anagen lasts for variable lengths of time depending on site. Usually >3 years on the scalp.

Genetic causes of hair loss (diffuse)

- Ectodermal dysplasias — AD/AR. Group of disorders with two or more abnormalities including teeth, nails, sweat glands and other ectodermal structures
- Acrodermatitis enteropathica
- Netherton's syndrome
- Cockayne's syndrome
- Hair-shaft abnormalities — monilethrix, pili torti, Menkes' kinky hair syndrome (XR (X-linked recessive) — copper transport defect)
- Hartnup's disease
- Homocystinuria

Causes of non-scarring alopecia (hair loss)

- **Telogen effluvium**
- **Trichotillomania**
- **Trauma** from rubbing or traction from pony tails
- **Endocrine causes**: hypothyroidism, hypopituitarism
- **Drugs**: oral contraceptive pill
- **Loose anagen syndrome**: young girls; hair increases in density and thickness as child gets older.
- **Nutritional:** malnutrition, iron deficiency, zinc deficiency
- **Alopecia areata**
  - 2% prevalence. Usually >5 years.
  - Family history in 5–25%
  - Associated with autoimmune disorders (thyroiditis, vitiligo) and Down's syndrome
  - Scalp is normal in appearance; exclamation-mark hairs are characteristic
  - Outcome unpredictable; most children have small patchy hair loss and outlook is good; the more extensive the disease the worse the prognosis

Causes of scarring alopecia

- Aplasia cutis congenita
- SLE
- Fungal infection — tinea capitis, kerion
- Incontinenti pigmenti
- Pachyonychia congenita
- Epidermolysis bullosa
- Ichthyoses — CHILD syndrome, KID syndrome, syndromes with chondroplasia punctata

Causes of scalp scaling

- Seborrhoeic dermatitis
- Atopic eczema
- Fungal infection
- Psoriasis
- *Pityriasis amiantacea*
- Histiocytosis

Excessive hair growth
This is either androgen-independent 'hypertrichosis' or androgen-dependent 'hirsutism'.

Causes of hypertrichosis

- **Congenital**
  - Hypertrichosis lanuginosa
  - Cornelia de Lange syndrome
  - Rubenstein Taybi syndrome
  - Hurler's syndrome
  - Porphyria — EPP, PCT

- **Endocrine**
  - Hyper/hypothyroidism

- **Acrodynia** (mercury poisoning)

- **Focal lesions — Becker's naevus**

- **Drugs**
  - Ciclosporin
  - Minoxidil
  - Phenytoin
  - Diazoxide
  - Streptomycin
  - Acetazolamide

- **Head trauma**

- **Dermatomyositis**

Causes of hirsutism

- **Adrenal**
  - Congenital adrenal hyperplasia
  - Cushing's syndrome
  - Virilizing adrenal tumours

- **Turner's syndrome**

- **Ovarian**
  - Polycystic ovary syndrome
  - Ovarian tumours
  - Gonadal dysgenesis

9.2 Nails

Development begins at the 9th week of gestation and is complete after the 22nd week. Toenail development lags behind fingernails.

Nail changes — normal variants

Koilonychia: normal variant in early childhood due to thin nail-plate; commonly toenails; also associated with iron deficiency anaemia
Superficial longitudinal ridges: normal variant
Beau's lines: transverse depressions; can get at 1–2 months of age and with any severe illness which affects nail growth
Longitudinal pigmented bands: pigmented bands in dark-skinned children

Conditions affecting the nails

- **Acute paronychia**
- **Congenital malalignment of the big toe** (triangular shape to nail)
- **Atopic eczema**: pitting, Beau's lines, onycholysis
- **Parakeratosis pustulosa**: hyperkeratosis, onycholysis, pitting
- **Psoriasis:** nail pitting, onycholysis, salmon patches of nail-bed
- **Leuconychia:** liver disease, hypoalbuminaemia, hereditary and if punctate found following repetitive minor trauma
- **Twenty nail dystrophy**: many nails affected; spectrum of nail-plate surface abnormalities; may be associated with alopecia areata; regresses spontaneously
- **Lichen planus:** longitudinal ridging, pterygium
- **Nail–patella syndrome:** AD; nail hypoplasia, patella hypoplastic or absent, radial head abnormalities, iliac crest exostosis and nephropathy
- **Epidermolysis bullosa:** may be permanent nail loss
- **Pachyonychia congenita:** AD; severe nail-bed thickening due to hyperkeratosis; other features depend on type; include palmar plantar hyperkeratosis, cataracts, alopecia and bullae of palms and soles
- **Ectodermal dysplasias:** variable dystrophic nails depending on type
- **Alopecia areata:** nail pitting
- **Chronic mucocutaneous candidiasis:** nails are yellow–brown and are thickened; recurrence common due to underlying immune defects
- **Fungal infection**
- **Dystrophy:** CHILD syndrome, congenital erythropoietic porphyria
- **Hypothyroidism:** decreased nail growth, ridging and brittleness
- **Rothmund–Thomson:** hypotrophic nails
- **Pityriasis rubra pilaris:** half-and-half nail; thickened curved and terminal hyperaemia
- **Incontinentia pigmenti:** nail dystrophy in 40%

10. DISORDERS OF PIGMENTATION

Colour of the skin is due to melanin produced by melanocytes in the basal layer of the epidermis.

10.1 Causes of hypopigmentation

Causes of hypopigmentation

- **Nutritional deficiency**
  - Copper
  - Selenium
  - Kwashiorkor

- **Genetic**
  - Oculocutaneous albinism
  - Phenylketonuria
  - Homocystinuria
  - Apert's syndrome
  - Piebaldism
  - Waardenburg syndrome
  - Tuberous sclerosis
  - Menke's kinky hair syndrome
  - Epidermolysis bullosa (at sites of bullae)
  - Hypomelanosis of Ito (incontinentia pigmenti achromians of Ito)

- **Autoimmune**
  - Vitiligo

- **Infection**
  - Pityriasis versicolor
  - Vaccination sites

- **Trauma sites**

- **Post-inflammatory**
  - Eczema
  - Psoriasis

Chediak–Higashi syndrome

AR. Incomplete oculocutaneous albinism, photophobia and severe recurrent infections.

Vitiligo

Total loss of pigment. Often symmetrical. Spontaneous repigmentation uncommon. Associated with autoimmune disorders.

10.2 Causes of hyperpigmentation

Causes of hyperpigmentation

- **Genetic**
  - Incontinentia pigmenti
  - Goltz syndrome (focal dermal hyperplasia)
  - Peutz–Jeghers syndrome
  - Albright's syndrome
  - Xeroderma pigmentosum

- **Metabolic**
  - Liver disease
  - Haemochromatosis
  - Wilson's disease
  - Porphyria
  - CEP Congenital erythropoietic porphyria
  - Hepatic cutaneous porphyria

- **Infection**
  - Pityriasis versicolor

- **Drugs**
  - Minocycline
  - Tetracycline
  - AZT (Zidovudine)
  - Rifabutin
  - Clofazimine

- **Endocrine**
  - Addison's disease
  - Hyperthyroidism
  - Nelson's
  - Cushing's syndrome (ectopic ACTH production)

- **Nutritional**
  - Malabsorption
  - Pellagra (sun-exposed sites)
  - Kwashiorkor

- **Post-inflammatory**
  - Insect bites
  - Acne
  - Atopic eczema
  - Lichen simplex chronicus

Other pigmentary changes

Niemann–Pick type A

- Grey-brown/yellow–brown discoloration of sun-exposed areas

Metals

- Silver, bismuth and arsenic
- Slate-grey pigmentation

Mongolian blue spot

- Blue skin
- Typical site is lower back
- Common in Afro-Carribean and Asian babies
- Increased numbers of melanocytes deep in dermis
- Tends to disappear by 4 years of age

10.3 Disorders associated with multiple café-au-lait macules

- Neurofibromatosis type I (NFI)
- NFII (minority of patients)
- Piebaldism
- Ataxia telangectasia
- Multiple endocrine neoplasia
- Russell–Silver syndrome
- McCune–Albright syndrome
- Tuberous sclerosis
- Noonan's syndrome
- Bloom's syndrome
- Tay's syndrome

10.4 Skin changes associated with tuberous sclerosis

- Earliest changes are forehead plaques, Shagreen patch and hypomelanotic macules. Shagreen patch occurs typically in lumbar region but can be at top of leg.
- Facial angiofibromas (adenoma sebaceum): rare <2years. Present in 85% >5 years.
- Periungual fibromas: uncommon in first decade of life

11. MISCELLANEOUS DISORDERS

11.1 Granuloma annulare

Ring of firm skin-coloured papules. Usually asymptomatic. May follow non-specific trauma in 25%. 50% clear in 2 years. 40% have recurrent eruptions. Link to diabetes mellitus controversial. Always test urine for glucose.

11.2 Dermatitis artefacta

Self-inflicted lesions on sites readily accessible to patient's hands. Take a variety of forms including blisters.

11.3 Nappy rash

Irritant contact dermatitis

- Common
- Due to urine and faeces
- Interogenous areas characteristically spared
- May be infected with *Candida albicans* (satellite lesions and skinfold involvement)

Other causes

- Seborrhoeic dermatitis
- Atopic eczema
- Psoriasis
- Scabies
- Acrodermatitis enteropathica
- Langerhans' cell histiocytosis
- Kawasaki's disease
- Child abuse
- Blistering disorders

11.4 Acne

Affects face and upper trunk. Lesions include comedones, papules, pustules, nodules and cysts. Usually 10–16 years. May get neonatal acne and infantile acne. Investigate for underlying cause if acne appears for the first time between 1 and 7 years.

Treatment

- Topical — benzoyl peroxide 2.5% to 10%, topical retinoids, topical antibiotics
- Oral antibiotics — erythromycin, oxytetracycline (not if <12 years) taken bd
- Dianette (cyproterone acetate with ethinylestradiol) for females
- Isotretinoin (Roaccutane) vitamin A derivative for severe acne. Causes dry mucous membranes and may cause depression. Monitor lipids.

11.5 Spitz naevus

Pink/red, sometimes brown in colour. Benign lesion which can be difficult to distinguish from malignant melanoma. Excise if suspicious features, e.g. unusual pigmentation, rapid growth and size >1 cm.

11.6 Keloids

Hypertrophic scar extending beyond boundary of original wound. More common in pigmented skin. Intralesional injections of steroid (triamcinolone) may help. Tend to recur if surgically excised.

11.7 Acanthosis nigricans

Hyperpigmentation is the earliest feature ('dirty skin'), preferentially the flexures. May become hyperkeratotic and warty lesions elsewhere on the body. Occurs in families and is associated with obesity, syndromes of insulin resistance, hyperandrogenaemia and hypothyroidism.

12. FURTHER READING

Management of atopic eczema: McHenry PM, Williams HC, Bingham EA *BMJ* **310**:844, 1995.

Management of psoriasis in childhood: Burden AD. *Clin Exp Dermatol* **24**:341–5, 1999.

Pediatric Dermatology, Pediatric Clinics of North America. Volume 47(4), 2000.

Textbook of Pediatric Dermatology: Harper J, Oranje A, Prose N. Blackwell Scientific, 2000.

Chapter 5

Endocrinology

Heather Mitchell and Vasanta R Nanduri

CONTENTS

Endocrinology

1. HORMONE PHYSIOLOGY

1.1 Introduction

Hormones are chemical messengers produced by a variety of specialized secretory cells. Their effects may be:

- Via transport to a distant site of action (endocrine)
- A direct effect upon nearby cells (paracrine)

Plasma transport

- Most hormones are secreted into the systemic circulation, but those secreted from the hypothalamus are released into the pituitary portal system.
- Many hormones are bound to proteins when in the circulation. These binding proteins buffer against very rapid changes and act as a reservoir for the hormones — only free hormones can exert their biological action on tissues.

Examples of hormone-binding proteins

Hormone	Binding protein
Thyroxine	Thyroid-binding globulin
	Albumin
Testosterone/oestrogen	Sex hormone-binding globulin
Insulin-like growth factor-1	Insulin-like growth factor-binding proteins
Cortisol	Cortisol-binding protein

1.2 Hormone–receptor interactions

Types of hormone

There are three main types of hormones:

- Amine: catecholamines, serotonin (5–hydroxytryptamine, 5–HT)
- Steroid: cortisol, aldosterone, androgens, oestrogen, progesterone
- Peptide: growth hormone (GH), insulin, thyroxine

Amine and peptide hormones have short half-lives (minutes) and act on cell-surface receptors. Their secretion may be pulsatile and they often act via a second messenger (e.g. cyclic adenosine monophosphate (cAMP), calcium, etc.). Steroid hormones have longer half-lives (hours) and act on intracellular receptors. They act on DNA to alter gene transcription and protein synthesis. Thyroxine is the exception to this rule as it acts as a steroid hormone and binds to intracellular receptors.

Intracellular messengers

- Cyclic adenosine monophosphate (cAMP), e.g. glucagon, adrenocorticotrophic hormone (ACTH), luteinizing hormone (LH), follicle-stimulating hormone (FSH)
- Intracellular calcium, e.g. thyrotropin-releasing hormone (TRH), vasopressin, angiotensin II
- Tyrosine kinase, e.g. growth hormone (GH)

G-protein receptors

Hormone receptors linked to cAMP do not generate cAMP directly, but act via a G-protein receptor on the cell surface. The G-proteins may be inhibitory — G_i (e.g. somatostatin) or stimulatory — G_s (e.g. all other hormones) to the formation of adenylate cyclase. Hormones that use intracellular calcium as an internal messenger activate the cytoplasmic enzyme phospholipase C (PLC), which then releases inositol triphosphate from membrane phospholipids, which in turn releases calcium from stores in the endoplasmic reticulum.

Second messengers

Insulin-like growth factor-1 (IGF-1) and IGF-2 are GH-dependent peptide factors. They are believed to modulate many of the anabolic and mitogenic actions of GH. IGF-1 is important as a postnatal growth factor, whereas IGF-2 is thought to be essential for fetal growth.

Disorders of hormone–receptor interactions

- Syndromes of G-protein abnormalities:
  - McCune–Albright syndrome
  - pseudohypoparathyroidism

- Syndromes of receptor resistance:
  - Laron's syndrome
  - nephrogenic diabetes insipidus
  - androgen insensitivity syndrome
  - vitamin D-dependent rickets

1.3 Regulation

The effect and measured amount of a particular hormone in the circulation at any one time is the result of a complex series of interactions.

Control and feedback

Most hormones are controlled by some form of feedback. Insulin and glucose work on a feedback loop. Elevated glucose concentrations lead to insulin release, whereas insulin secretion is switched off when the glucose level decreases.

Receptor up- or down-regulation also occurs. Down-regulation leads to reduced sensitivity to a hormone and a reduced number of receptors after prolonged exposure to high hormone concentrations. A good example of this is the administration of intermittent gonadotropin-releasing hormone (GnRH), which induces priming and facilitates a large output of gonadotropins, while continuous GnRH leads to a downregulation of receptors and hence has a protective effect. However, this is not true of all pituitary hormones (e.g. ectopic ACTH secretion leads to receptor upregulation, which is the reverse process).

Patterns of secretion

- Continuous   e.g. thyroxine
- Intermittent:
    - pulsatile   e.g. FSH, LH, GH, prolactin
    - circadian   e.g. cortisol
    - stress-related e.g. ACTH
    - sleep-related   e.g. GH, prolactin

1.4 Investigation of hormonal problems

In view of the complexities of control on the concentration of a particular hormone and the various factors that influence its distribution and elimination, the use of a single random measurement of a hormone can be very difficult to interpret. The plasma levels vary throughout the day because of pulsatile secretion, environmental stress, or circadian rhythms. They are also influenced by the values of the substrates they control. It is therefore often hard to define a normal range and dynamic testing may be required.

- Blood hormone concentration measurements:
    - basal levels: those hormones in a steady state, e.g. thyroid function tests
    - timed levels: those hormones whose levels need to be interpreted with a normal range for the time of day, e.g. cortisol measured at 0000 h and 0800 h
    - stimulated: in suspected hormone deficiency, e.g. GH-stimulation tests
    - suppression: in conditions of hormone excess as hormone-producing tumours usually fail to show normal negative feedback, e.g. dexamethasone suppression test for suspected Cushing's disease
- Urine concentrations:
    - useful for identifying abnormalities in ratios of metabolites, e.g. diagnosis of the specific enzyme defect in congenital adrenal hyperplasia

2. HYPOTHALAMUS AND PITUITARY GLANDS

The hypothalamic–pituitary axis is of vital importance as it regulates many of the other endocrine glands in the body.

2.1 Anatomy

Hypothalamus

Extends from the preoptic area (anteriorly) to the mamillary bodies (posteriorly) and includes the 3rd ventricle. The hypothalamus has reciprocal connections with the frontal cortex and thalamus, and interacts with the limbic system and the brainstem nuclei involved in autonomic regulation where it differentiates into discrete nuclei. The axonal processes extend down into the median eminence where regulatory hormones are secreted into the portal circulation.

Pituitary gland

Situated inferior to the hypothalamus within the pituitary fossa, above the sphenoid sinus, medial to the cavernous sinuses which contain the internal carotid arteries and the IIIrd, IVth and VIth cranial nerves. It is the combined product of an outgrowth of ectoderm from the buccal mucosa and the downgrowth of neural tissue referred to as the 'infundibulum'. The anatomical relationships of the anterior and posterior pituitary glands are important as tumours may arise from and/or compress surrounding structures.

- Above: optic chiasm, pituitary stalk, hypothalamus
- Below: sphenoid sinus, nasopharynx
- Lateral: cavernous sinus, internal carotid arteries, III, IV, V, VI cranial nerves

- Anterior lobe: derived from an invagination of oral mucosa (Rathke pouch)
- Posterior lobe: derived from neuronal tissue and contains neurones from the hypothalamus

2.2 Hormone physiology of the anterior pituitary

Gonadotropins: (luteinizing hormone (LH)/and follicle-stimulating hormone (FSH))

Structure
LH and FSH are glycoproteins composed of an α- and a β-subunit. The α-subunits are identical to other glycoproteins within the same species, whereas the β-subunits confer specificity.

Function
In the male, Leydig cells respond to LH, which stimulates the first step in testosterone production. In the female, LH binds to ovarian cells and stimulates steroidogenesis.

FSH binds to Sertoli cells in the male and increases the mass of the seminiferous tubules and supports the development of sperm. In the female, FSH binds to the glomerulosa cells and stimulates the conversion of testosterone to oestrogen.

Regulation

Gonadotropin-releasing hormone (GnRH) is released in a pulsatile fashion, which stimulates the synthesis and secretion of LH and FSH. Expression and excretion of FSH are also inhibited by inhibin, a gonadal glycoprotein. This has no effect on LH. In the neonate there are high levels of gonadotropins and gonadal steroids. These decline progressively until a nocturnal increase occurs leading up to the onset of puberty (amplification of low-amplitude pulses).

Growth hormone (GH)

Structure

GH is a 191–amino acid peptide (22 kDa) secreted by somatotrophs. It circulates both in the unbound form and also bound to binding proteins, which are portions of the extracellular receptor domain.

Function

Growth hormone has direct effects on carbohydrate and lipid metabolism. The growth-promoting effects of GH are mediated by somatomedin C (otherwise known as IGF-1), which is produced in the liver cells following GH binding to cell-surface receptors and results in gene transcription. IGF-1 and IGF-2 are 70 amino acid peptides, structurally related to insulin. IGF-1 increases the synthesis of protein; RNA and DNA, increases the incorporation of protein into muscle and promotes lipogenesis. The IGFs are bound to a family of binding proteins (IGFBP-1 to -6) of which IGFBP-3 predominates. These binding proteins not only act as transporters for the IGFs, but also increase their half-life and modulate their actions on peripheral tissues.

Regulation

GH secretion is pulsatile, consisting of peaks and troughs. Nocturnal release occurs during non-dreaming or slow-wave sleep, shortly after the onset of deep sleep. There is a gradual increase in GH production during childhood, a further increase (with increased amplitude of peaks) during puberty secondary to the effect of sex steroid, followed by a post-pubertal fall. GH secretion is regulated by the hypothalamic peptides, growth hormone-releasing hormone (GHRH) and somatostatin, via the activation of G-protein receptors on the somatotrophs, increasing or reducing cAMP and intracellular Ca^{2+}. GHRH stimulates GH release, whereas somatostatin inhibits both GH synthesis and its release. GH and IGF-1 exert a tight feedback control on somatostatin, and probably also on GHRH.

Prolactin

Structure

Prolactin has a similar amino acid sequence to GH, and acts via the lactogenic receptor, which is from the same superfamily of transmembrane receptors as the GH receptor.

Function

Prolactin is responsible for the induction of lactation and cessation of menses during the puerperium. During the neonatal period, prolactin levels are high secondary to fetoplacental oestrogen. It then falls and remains consistent during childhood but there is a slight rise at puberty.

Regulation

Dopamine inhibition from the hypothalamus.

Thyroid-stimulating hormone (TSH)

Structure

TSH is a glycoprotein containing the same α-subunit as LH and FSH but a specific β-subunit.

Function

TSH is a trophic hormone and hence its removal reduces thyroid function to basal levels. It binds to surface receptors on the thyroid follicular cell and works via activation of adenylate cyclase to cause the production and release of thyroid hormone.

Regulation

TSH synthesis and release is modulated by thyrotropin-releasing hormone (TRH), which is produced in the hypothalamus and secreted into the hypophyseal portal veins, from where it is transported to the anterior pituitary gland. TRH secretion is influenced by environmental temperature, somatostatin and dopamine. Glucocorticoids inhibit TSH release at a hypothalamic level.

Adrenocorticotrophic hormone (ACTH)

Structure

ACTH is a 39–amino acid peptide cleaved from a large glycosylated precursor (pro-opiomelanocortin) which also gives rise to melanocyte-stimulating hormone (MSH) and β-endorphin.

Function

ACTH is responsible for stimulation of the adrenal cortex and in particular the production of cortisol. Hypothalamic control of its function is evident in the late-gestation fetus. ACTH plays a role in fetal adrenal growth.

Regulation

Corticotropin-releasing hormone (CRH) stimulates ACTH release via increasing cAMP levels. Arginine vasopressin (AVP) also stimulates ACTH release and potentiates the response to CRH.

2.3 The neurohypophysis and water regulation

The body maintains water balance by regulating fluid intake and output. There is a narrow range of normal serum osmolality between 280 and 295 mosmol/l.

Output

Controlled by:

- hypothalamic osmoreceptors and neighbouring neurones that secrete arginine vasopressin (AVP)
- concentrating effect of the kidney

Input

Controlled by:

- hypothalamic thirst centre

Arginine vasopressin (AVP)

Structure

Arginine vasopressin is a nonapeptide containing a hexapeptide ring. It is produced as a prohormone in the supraoptic and paraventricular nuclei. Action potentials from the hypothalamus cause its release from the posterior pituitary gland into the circulation.

Regulation

This is largely by the osmolality of extracellular fluid and haemodynamic factors. The release of AVP is modulated by stimulatory and inhibitory neural input. Noradrenaline (norepinephrine) inhibits AVP release and cholinergic neurones facilitate it.

Physiology

The normal mature kidney is able to produce urine in a concentration range of 60–1100 mosmol/kg. The ability to vary urine concentration depends on the spatial arrangements and permeability characteristics of the segments of the renal tubules.

AVP regulates the permeability of the luminal membrane of the collecting ducts. Low permeability in the presence of a low AVP concentration leads to dilute urine.

2.4 Pituitary disorders

Anterior pituitary

Congenital
- Agenesis of the corpus callosum
- Structural abnormalities:
  - septo-optic dysplasia
  - pituitary hypoplasia
- Idiopathic hormonal abnormalities:
  - isolated GH deficiency
  - idiopathic precocious puberty

Acquired

- Excess, e.g. intracranial tumours:
  - intracranial tumours
  - Cushing's disease — pituitary adenoma
- Deficiency, e.g. secondary to treatment with radiation or surgery:
  - pituitary damage
  - tumours
  - surgery
  - radiotherapy
  - trauma

Septo-optic dysplasia (De Morsier's syndrome)
A developmental anomaly of the midline structures of the brain. Classically characterized by:

- absence of septum pellucidum and/or corpus callosum
- optic nerve hypoplasia
- pituitary hypoplasia with variable pituitary hormone deficiencies (most commonly this is GH deficiency which may either be isolated or progress to an evolving endocrinopathy)

Treatment is by hormone replacement and management of visual difficulties.

Craniopharyngioma
This is one of the most common supratentorial tumours in children. It commonly presents with headaches and visual-field defects. On imaging, the tumour is frequently large and cystic. Treatment is by resection plus radiotherapy if initial resection is incomplete or recurrence occurs.

Post-operative hormonal deficiencies are common, involving both anterior and posterior pituitary hormones. Treatment is by hormonal supplementation. There is also the risk of hypothalamic damage. Remember: the hypothalamus is responsible for other effects that are not so easily treated by replacement therapy, e.g. temperature, appetite and thirst control. The obesity associated with hypothalamic damage (secondary to hyperphagia) is very difficult to manage and has a poor prognosis. The maintenance of fluid homeostasis in children with the combination of diabetes insipidus and adipsia (loss of thirst sensation) can be a challenge.

Acquired endocrine problems secondary to tumours and/or their treatment

- Short stature
- Pubertal delay or arrest
- Precocious puberty
- Thyroid tumours
- Infertility
- Hypopituitarism — isolated or multiple
- Gynaecomastia

Posterior pituitary

Diabetes insipidus

Defined as insufficient AVP causing a syndrome of polyuria and polydipsia. With an intact thirst mechanism copious water drinking maintains normal osmolalities. However, problems with the thirst mechanism or insufficient water intake lead to hypernatraemic dehydration.

It is important to remember that cortisol is required for water excretion. Therefore in children with both anterior and posterior pituitary dysfunction, there is a risk of dilutional hyponatraemia if they are cortisol-deficient and receiving DDAVP (1–deamino-8–D-arginine vasopressin) treatment. Hence the emergency management of the unwell child is to increase their hydrocortisone treatment and to stop their DDAVP.

Causes of diabetes insipidus

- Central: Craniopharyngioma
  Germinoma
  Langerhans cell histiocytosis (LCH)
  Idiopathic
  Trauma

- Nephrogenic: X-linked nephrogenic diabetes insipidus.
  Secondary to renal damage

Syndrome of inappropriate ADH (SIADH) secretion

Defined by the criteria of:

- water retention with hypo-osmolality
- normal or slightly raised blood volumes
- less than maximally dilute urine
- urinary sodium > sodium intake

Causes of SIADH

- CNS disorders: meningitis; abscess; trauma; hypoxic–ischaemic insult

- Respiratory tract disease: pneumonia; cavitation

- Reduced left atrial filling: drugs

- Malignancies: lymphoma; bronchogenic carcinoma; idiopathic

2.5 Investigation of hypothalamic and pituitary hormone disorders

Anterior pituitary stimulation tests

Many hormones (e.g. GH, LH and FSH) are secreted in a pulsatile fashion, and therefore a random measurement of the concentration of the circulating hormone is often inadequate for diagnosing a deficiency disorder.

Hormone measurement tests include:

- GH release/ACTH (via cortisol response):   Insulin tolerance test
- TSH/prolactin response: TRH test
- FSH/LH response: LHRH test

GH tests

Provocation tests of growth hormone are potentially hazardous. Insulin tolerance tests should only be performed in specialist centres because of the risk of severe hypoglycaemia. Other GH provocation tests include the use of glucagon, arginine and clonidine. Physiological tests of GH secretion include a 24–h GH profile and measurement of GH after exercise or during sleep.

Combined pituitary function test

The standard test involves the intravenous injection of either insulin or glucagon in combination with TRH and LHRH (in the pubertal child).

Blood samples are taken at 0 min (before stimulation), 20, 30, 60, 90 and 120 min.

Following insulin administration, a profound hypoglycaemia results in 20 min which needs to be corrected by the use of an oral glucose solution or the judicious use of i.v. 10% dextrose. (Remember: the rapid correction of hypoglycaemia with a hypertonic glucose solution can result in cerebral oedema.)

GH concentrations rise at 30 min following insulin, or 60–90 min following glucagon injection. A rise to over 20 mU/l rules out GH deficiency.

A normal TSH response to TRH is a rise at 20 min post-dose and then a fall by 60 min. A continued rise of TSH at 60 min implies hypothalamic damage. Secondary hypothyroidism is demonstrated by a low baseline TSH level, whereas primary hypothyroidism is associated with a raised TSH. A raised baseline prolactin level suggests a lack of hypothalamic inhibition of its release. Under normal circumstances following the administration of TRH, prolactin would be expected to rise at 20 min and then to be falling by 60 min.

In the absence of precocious puberty, the LHRH test will only demonstrate a rise in FSH and LH at 20 and 60 min during the first 6 months of life and in the peripubertal period. Raised baseline gonadotropin levels reflect gonadal failure.

Posterior pituitary function tests

- Paired urine and serum osmolalities
- Water deprivation test

The child is weighed in the morning and is then deprived of water for a maximum of 7 hours, during which time urine osmolality the child's weight, pulse rate and blood pressure are measured hourly. Plasma sodium levels and osmolality are measured every 2 hours.

The test is terminated if the patient's weight falls by 5% from the starting weight, serum osmolality rises (>295 mosmol/kg of water) in the face of an inappropriately dilute urine (<300 mosmol/kg) or if the patient becomes significantly clinically dehydrated/clinically unwell.

A diagnosis of diabetes insipidus (DI) may be made in the presence of a plasma osmolality >290 mosmol/kg of water with an inappropriately low urine osmolality.

The child is then given a dose of DDAVP and the urine and plasma osmolality are then measured. A rise in urine concentration confirms a diagnosis of central DI, whereas a child with nephrogenic DI will fail to concentrate urine after DDAVP.

2.6 Principles of management of hypothalamic–pituitary disorders

Treatment of anterior pituitary deficiencies

When specific hormones or their stimulating hormones are deficient then the actual hormone may be replaced, e.g.:

- Lack of GH response: replace with GH

However, if the deficient hormone is a trophic or regulatory hormone then it is the target hormone that is replaced, e.g.:

- Lack of TFT: replace with thyroxine
- Low gonadotropins: replace with testosterone in males, oestrogen in females
- ACTH: replace with hydrocortisone
- Vasopressin: replace with DDAVP

GH deficiency
The following are the licensed indications for treatment with GH. These recommendations have been endorsed by the National Institute for Clinical Excellence (NICE).

- Documented GH deficiency — congenital or acquired
- Turner's syndrome
- Chronic renal failure
- Prader–Willi syndrome

GH deficiency should be treated by a specialist who has experience of managing children with growth disorders. Most regimens involve daily injections with different doses of GH depending upon the indications. Close local/community liaison is required for this.

Panhypopituitarism
Replacement with GH, thyroxine, cortisol during childhood with induction and mainte-nance of puberty with the appropriate sex hormone (testosterone or estradiol). Parents of children who are cortisol- or ACTH-deficient should be given written instructions and training in the management of an acute illness and must have emergency supplies of i.m. hydrocortisone available at all times.

Treatment of posterior pituitary deficiencies

Central diabetes insipidus
Treatment with DDAVP (desmopressin) either as a nasal spray or tablets.

3. GROWTH

3.1 Physiology of normal growth

Prenatal

Factors influencing intrauterine growth

- Nutrition
- Genetic
- Maternal factors (smoking, blood pressure)
- Placental function
- Intrauterine infections
- Endocrine factors IGF-2

Postnatal growth

There are 3 principal phases of growth — infancy, childhood and puberty

Phases of postnatal growth	Factors
• Infancy	nutrition
• Childhood	GH (thyroxine)
• Puberty	sex hormones (GH)

Average growth during the pubertal phase is 30 cm (12 inches).

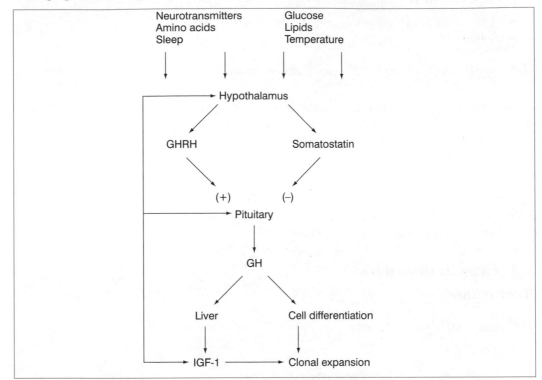

Growth axis

3.2 Assessment and investigation

The following parameters are important in the assessment of growth:

- Standing height
- Sitting height
- Head circumference
- Weight
- Skin-fold thicknesses
- Mid-arm circumference
- Pubertal status

Auxology

When measuring height, the optimal method is for the child to be measured by the same trained measurer, on the same equipment and at the same time of day on each occasion in order to minimize measurement error. A stadiometer should be used and supine height measured at <2 years of age and standing height at >2 years.

A child's height may be compared to the population using centile charts, and also considered in terms of his/her genetic potential by comparison with the mid-parental height.

Mid-parental height

- Add 12.6 cm to mother's height to plot on a boy's chart
- Subtract 12.6 cm if plotting a father's height on a girl's chart

- Mid-parental height is half-way between the plotted corrected parental heights

The measurement of skin-fold thicknesses (e.g. triceps, subscapular) gives important information about body fat distribution, which changes at different ages. For example, in puberty there is an increase in truncal fat but a reduction in limb fat. Mean arm circumference can be used to assess muscle bulk.

To estimate the rate at which a child is growing it is necessary to measure the height on two separate occasions (at least 4–6 months apart) and divide the change in height by the period of time elapsed. This is the height velocity and is expressed in cm/year. The height velocity can be plotted on standard reference charts.

3.3 Growth disorders

Short stature

Causes of short stature

- Familial

- Constitutional short stature, constitutional delay of growth and puberty

- Chronic illness:
  - congenital heart disease
  - respiratory disorders, e.g. cystic fibrosis
  - renal failure
  - malabsorption, e.g. coeliac disease, Crohn's disease
  - neurological, e.g. intracranial tumours

- Endocrine:
  - growth-hormone insufficiency
  - hypothyroidism
  - Cushing's syndrome

- Dysmorphic syndromes:
  - Turner's syndrome
  - Down's syndrome
  - low birth weight, e.g. Russell–Silver syndrome

- Skeletal dysplasia:
  - achondroplasia
  - hypochondroplasia
  - mucopolysaccharidoses
  - spondyloepiphyseal dysplasia

- Psychosocial/emotional deprivation

As a general rule, if a child has a normal growth rate then the cause of the short stature is in the past history, whereas a child with a low growth rate requires thought as to what current process(es) is causing the growth failure.

Familial short stature

This remains one of the commonest causes of short stature, whereby the child takes after the parents' heights and grows along a centile that is appropriate for their genetic potential.

Constitutional short stature

This is a condition commonly seen in teenage boys who have a combination of delay in growth and in puberty. There is often a history of a similar pattern of growth in male members of the family. Bone-age assessment (see below) is often the only investigation initially required and usually shows a delay. Children do reach their genetic potential, but later than their peers. Management consists primarily of reassurance and, in certain circumstances, the use of a short (<6 month) course of androgens to 'kick start' puberty.

NB: Constitutional delay of growth and puberty should not be diagnosed in girls without thorough investigation.

Common syndromes associated with short stature

Achondroplasia

- Inheritance:
  - autosomal dominant (but 50% new mutations)
- Clinical features:
  - megalocephaly
  - short limbs
  - prominent forehead
  - thoracolumbar kyphosis
  - midfacial hypoplasia
  - short stature
- Radiology:
  - diminishing interpeduncular distances between L1 and L5
- Complications:
  - short stature
  - dental malocclusion
  - hydrocephalus
  - repeated otitis media

Hypochondroplasia

- Definition:
  - rhizomelic short stature distinct from achondroplasia
- Inheritance:
  - probable allelic autosomal dominant disorder

- Clinical features:
  - affected persons appear stocky or muscular
  - usually recognized from 2 to 3 years of age
  - wide variability in severity
- Radiology:
  - no change in interpeduncular distances between L1 and L5
- Complications:
  - short stature

Mucopolysaccharidoses (MPS)

- Inheritance:
  - autosomal recessive, X-linked recessive
- Clinical features — depend on type of MPS:
  - short spine and limbs
  - coarse facial features
  - reduced intelligence and abnormal behaviour in some forms
  - Hurler's syndrome — shortened lifespan
  - marked skeletal abnormalities and severe short stature in Morquio's syndrome

Russell–Silver syndrome

- Inheritance:
  - sporadic
- Definition:
  - syndrome of short stature of prenatal onset
  - occurrence is sporadic and aetiology is unknown
- Clinical features:
  - short stature of prenatal onset
  - limb asymmetry
  - short incurved 5th finger
  - small triangular face
  - café-au-lait spots
  - normal intelligence
  - bluish sclerae in early infancy

Turner's syndrome

- Definition:
  - a syndrome with a 45XO (or XO/XX or rarely XO/XY) karyotype associated with short stature, ovarian dysgenesis and dysmorphic features
- Inheritance:
  - sporadic
- Clinical features:
  - neonatal:
    - lymphoedema of hands and feet

- facial/skeletal:
  - short stature (mean adult height is 142 cm); widely spaced nipples, shield-shaped chest; prominent, backward-rotated ears; squint, ptosis; high arched palate; low posterior hairline, webbed neck; wide carrying angle; short 4th metacarpal; hyperconvex nails
- neurological: specific space–form perception defect
- endocrine: autoimmune diseases (hypothyroidism); type 2 diabetes; infertility and pubertal failure
- associations: horse-shoe kidneys; coarctation of the aorta; excessive pigmented naevi

Turner's syndrome needs to be excluded in all girls whose height is below that expected for the mid-parental centile as not all girls with Turner's syndrome show the classical phenotype.

Assessment of a child with short stature
Measure and plot the child's and parents' height and see if child is growing along predicted centile for genetic potential. Assess pubertal status according to Tanner stages (see below, section 4.2). In teenage boys who are not yet in puberty, a constitutional delay is the most likely.

History and clinical examination should identify an obvious chronic illness, which should then be specifically investigated. Features of recognized dysmorphic syndromes should be looked for. A child who is disproportionate should undergo skeletal survey to rule out a skeletal dysplasia.

Investigation of short stature
If above ruled out, need:

- Full blood count
- Urea and electrolytes, CRP
- Coeliac antibodies screen
- Thyroid function tests
- Karyotyping
- IGF-1 levels
- Bone age
- GH provocation tests

Bone age
This is a measure of the maturation of the epiphyseal ossification centres in the skeleton. Bone age proceeds in an orderly fashion and therefore defines how much growth has taken place and the amount of growth left. A delayed bone age may be caused by constitutional delay of growth and puberty, GH deficiency or hypothyroidism. An advanced bone age is caused by precocious puberty, androgen excess (e.g. congenital adrenal hypoplasia, CAH) and GH excess.

Tall stature

Causes of tall stature in childhood

- Familial tall stature
- Constitutional obesity
- Precocious puberty
- Androgen excess:
  - Congenital adrenal hyperplasia
- GH excess
- Thyrotoxicosis
- Syndromes:
  - Cerebral gigantism
  - Marfan's syndrome
  - Klinefelter's syndrome

Familial tall stature

This is a child of tall parents whose height is following a centile line above, yet parallel, to the 97th centile, which is appropriate for the predicted mid-parental centile.

Constitutional obesity

Remember: if a child is tall and fat it is most probably due to constitutional obesity. These children often have a slightly advanced bone age and go into puberty relatively early (not precocious) and thus end up appropriate (or slightly tall) for parents' heights.

Syndromes of tall stature

Marfan's syndrome

- Inheritance:
  - autosomal dominant
- Clinical features:
  - skeletal:
    - arachnodactyly
    - tall stature
    - scoliosis
    - high arched palate
    - pectus excavatum/carinatum
    - joint hypermobility
  - CNS:
    - learning disabilities
  - ocular:
    - lens dislocation
  - cardiovascular system:
    - aortic dissection
    - mitral valve prolapse

- respiratory:
  - pneumothorax

Klinefelter's syndrome

- Definition:
  - karyotype 47XXY
- Inheritance:
  - sporadic
- Clinical features:
  - tall and slim
  - cryptorchidism
  - gynaecomastia
  - mental retardation
  - azoospermia and infertility
  - immature behaviour

Sotos syndrome (cerebral gigantism)

- Inheritance:
  - sporadic
- Clinical features:
  - birth weight and length >90th centile
  - excessive linear growth during the first few years (which characteristically falls back)
  - head circumference is proportional to length
  - large hands and feet
  - large ears and nose
  - intellectual retardation
  - clumsiness

Assessment of a child with tall stature

Measure child and parents' heights and compare with weight. Assess pubertal status. History and clinical examination should identify an obvious cause or syndrome that can then be investigated.

Investigation of tall stature

- Thyroid function
- Bone age
- Skeletal survey
- Karyotype

4. PUBERTY AND INTERSEX DISORDERS

4.1 Physiology of normal puberty

The clinical manifestations of normal pubertal development occur secondary to sequential changes in endocrine activity.

Hormonal control of puberty

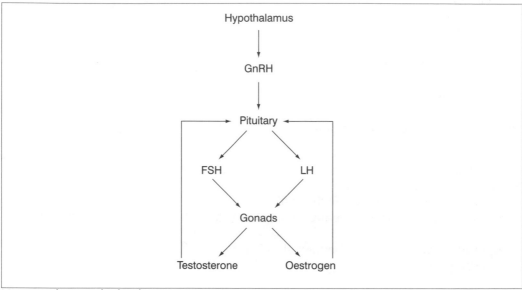

Hormonal control of puberty

The pulsatile release of GnRH from the hypothalamus leads to the secretion of LH and FSH from the gonadotropin cells of the pituitary gland.

In the male, Leydig cells respond to LH, which stimulates the first step in testosterone production. In the female, LH binds to ovarian cells and stimulates steroidogenesis. FSH binds to Sertoli cells in the male where it increases the mass of the seminiferous tubules and supports the development of sperm. In the female, FSH binds to the glomerulosa cells and stimulates the conversion of testosterone to oestrogen.

Sex steroids
Testosterone is produced by the Leydig cells of the testes. It is present in the circulation bound to sex-hormone binding globulin (SHBG). Free testosterone is the active moiety at target cells. Testosterone is then either converted to dihydrotestosterone (DHT) by 5α-reductase or to oestrogen by aromatase. Both DHT and testosterone attach to nuclear receptors, which then bind to steroid-responsive regions of genomic DNA to influence transcription and translation.

Oestrogen is produced by the follicle cells of the ovary. The main active form of oestrogen is oestradiol. This circulates bound to SHBG and causes growth of the breasts and uterus, the female distribution of adipose tissue and it also increases bone mineralization.

Inhibin
Inhibin is a glycoprotein produced by Sertoli cells in males and granulosa cells in females.

SHBG
Androgens reduce SHBG formation, and oestrogens stimulate its formation. Therefore increased free testosterone levels magnify androgen effects.

Hormonal regulation

In the presence of GnRH the gonadotropins are controlled by the sex steroids and inhibin. LH and FSH levels are under the influence of negative feedback mechanisms in both the hypothalamus and pituitary. Inhibin inhibits FSH only and acts at the level of the pituitary.

Positive feedback also occurs during mid-puberty in females. Increased oestrogen primes gonadotropins to produce LH until, at a critical stage at the middle of the menstrual cycle, a large surge is released causing ovulation.

4.2 Clinical features of normal puberty

The physical changes of pubertal development may be described by an objective method derived by Tanner:

Male genitalia development
Stage 1   Pre-adolescent
Stage 2   Enlargement of scrotum and testes and changes in scrotal skin
Stage 3   Further growth of testes and scrotum; enlargement of penis
Stage 4   Increase in breadth of penis and development of glans; further growth of scrotum and testes
Stage 5   Adult genitalia in shape and size

Female breast development
Stage 1   Pre-adolescent
Stage 2   Breast-bud formation
Stage 3   Further enlargement and elevation of breast and papilla with no separation of their contours
Stage 4   Projection of areola and papilla to form a secondary mound above the level of the breast
Stage 5   Mature stage with projection of papilla only

Pubic hair
Stage 1   Pre-adolescent
Stage 2   Sparse growth of long, slightly pigmented, downy hair
Stage 3   Hair spread over junction of the pubes, darker and coarser

Stage 4   Adult-type hair, but area covered is smaller
Stage 5   Adult in quantity and type

Axillary hair
Stage 1   No axillary hair
Stage 2   Scanty growth
Stage 3   Adult in quantity and type

Puberty starts on average at age 12 years in boys and 10 years in girls. As nutrition and health improve, the age of onset of puberty is becoming earlier with each generation.

In the male, acceleration in growth of the testes (from a prepubertal 2 ml volume) and scrotum are the first sign of puberty. This is followed by reddening and rugosity of scrotal skin, later by development of pubic hair, penile growth and axillary hair growth.

A 4 ml testicular volume signifies the start of pubertal change. Peak height velocity occurs with testicular volumes of 10–12 ml.

In the female, the appearance of the breast bud and breast development is the first sign of puberty. It is due to production of oestrogen from the ovaries. This is followed by the development of pubic and axillary hair, which is controlled by the adrenal gland. Peak height velocity coincides with breast stage 2–3. Menarche occurs late at breast stage 4, by which stage growth is slowing down. Most girls have attained menarche by age 13 years.

Body composition

Prepubertal boys and girls have equal lean body mass, skeletal mass and body fat. The earliest change in puberty is an increase in lean body mass.

Growth spurt

The pubertal growth spurt is the most rapid phase of growth after the neonatal period. This is an early event in girls and occurs approximately 2 years earlier than in boys, i.e. at a mean age of 12 years. The mean height difference between males and females of 12.5 cm is due to the taller male stature at the time of pubertal growth spurt and increased height gained during the pubertal growth spurt.

Adrenarche

Adrenal androgens, dehydroepiandrosterone sulphate (DHEAS) and androstenedione rise approximately 2 years before gonadotropins and sex steroids rise. Adrenarche begins at 6–8 years of age and continues until late puberty. Control of this is unknown. Adrenarche does not influence onset of puberty.

Gynaecomastia

Gynaecomastia is physiological and occurs in 75% of boys to some degree (usually during the first stages of puberty), but most regress within 2 years. Management is by reassurance, support and weight loss if obesity is a factor.

Causes of gynaecomastia

- Normal puberty (common)
- Obesity (common)
- Klinefelter's syndrome
- Partial androgen insensitivity

4.3 Abnormal puberty

- Early (precocious):
  - <9 years in boys
  - <8 years in girls
- Discordant (abnormal pattern)
- Delayed:
  - >14 years in boys
  - >13 years in girls

Precocious puberty

Definition
Central precocious puberty is consonant with puberty (i.e. occurs in the usual physiological pattern of development but at an earlier age). It is due to premature activation of the GnRH pulse generator. In girls, often no underlying cause is found; however, this is almost always pathological in males.

Causes of true precocious puberty (gonadotropin-dependent)

- Idiopathic
- CNS tumour
- Neurofibromatosis
- Septo-optic dysplasia — in this rare condition precocious puberty may occur in the presence of deficiencies of other pituitary hormones (see section 2.4).

Causes of gonadotropin-independent precocious puberty

- McCune–Albright syndrome (usually due to ovarian hypersecretion)
- Testicular/ovarian tumours
- Liver or adrenal tumours — may cause virilization

Useful tests for the investigation of precocious puberty

- Oestradiol
- Androgens, including 17–hydroxyprogesterone
- Luteinizing hormone-releasing hormone (LHRH) stimulation test
- Bone age
- Pelvic ultrasound scan
- Brain magnetic resonance imaging (MRI)
- Abdominal computed tomography (CT) if adrenal/liver tumour suspected

Management of precocious puberty

Gonadotropin-releasing hormone analogues (GnRHa) may be used to halt the progression of puberty. Children who enter puberty early are tall initially, but end up as short adults due to premature closure of epiphyses. Although GH has been used in addition to GnRHa, there is no clear evidence that final height is improved.

Discordant puberty (abnormal pattern)

- Breast development only — gonadotropin-independent precocious puberty, e.g. McCune–Albright syndrome
- Inadequate breast development, e.g. gonadal dysgenesis, Poland anomaly
- Androgen excess — pubic hair, acne, clitoral enlargement, e.g. congenital adrenal hyperplasia (CAH), Cushing's disease, polycystic ovarian syndrome (PCO), adrenal neoplasm
- Inadequate pubic hair, e.g. androgen insensitivity, adrenal failure
- No menarche, e.g. polycystic ovaries/absent ovaries or uterus
- No growth spurt, e.g. hypothalamic–pituitary disorders, skeletal dysplasias

Premature thelarche

- Usually in girls aged between 1 and 3 years
- Isolated breast development (never more than stage 3)
- No other signs of puberty
- Normal growth velocity for age
- Normal bone age
- Prepubertal gonadotropin levels
- Progress to puberty at normal age

Delayed puberty

Definition

No signs of puberty at an age when pubertal change would have been expected.

Causes of delayed puberty

- Constitutional delay of growth and puberty
- Hypothalamic or pituitary disorders:
  - hypogonadotrophic hypogonadism
  - idiopathic
  - pituitary tumours
  - post-central irradiation
  - post-intracranial surgery
  - post-chemotherapy
- Anorexia nervosa
- Systemic disease
- Kallman's syndrome — hypogonadotrophic hypogonadism with anosmia
- Gonadal dysgenesis:
  - Turner's syndrome
- Hypothyroidism

Investigation of delayed puberty in boys

In otherwise well boys with short stature and delayed puberty the most likely cause is constitutional delay. Initially this requires no investigations apart from that of bone age. If after a trial of treatment there is no progression of puberty, further investigations may be needed including:

In boys:

- LH, FSH, testosterone
- LHRH test
- karyotyping

In girls:

- karyotyping
- LH, FSH, oestrogen
- LHRH test
- pelvic ultrasound

Treatment

Constitutional delay:

- reassurance
- androgens: oxandrolone orally daily or depot testosterone injection monthly
- reassess at 4–6 months

Other causes of delayed puberty:

- treat underlying cause
- induce and maintain puberty with testosterone in boys, ethinylestradiol in girls

4.4 Intersex disorders

Classification

- Virilized female
- Inadequately virilized male
- True hermaphrodite

Causes of a virilized female

- Androgens of fetal origin
- Congenital adrenal hyperplasia (CAH)
- Androgens of maternal origin
- Drugs/maternal CAH
- Tumours of ovary or adrenal gland
- Idiopathic

Causes of an inadequately virilized male

- XY gonadal dysgenesis
- LH deficiency
- Leydig cell hypoplasia
- Inborn errors of testosterone synthesis
- 5α-reductase deficiency
- Androgen insensitivity

Useful investigations

- Karyotyping
- 24–h urine steroid profile
- Pelvic ultrasound
- 17–OH progesterone (day 3)
- LH/FSH testosterone/dihydrotestosterone
- Human chorionic gonadotropin (HCG) test

Management of a child with an intersex disorder

Requires multidisciplinary assessment and management involving endocrinology, paediatric urology, gynaecology and psychology input.

5. THE ADRENAL GLAND

5.1 Anatomy

The adrenals are triangular in shape and located at the superior pole of the kidneys. Each adrenal gland comprises a cortex, arising from mesoderm at the cranial end of the mesonephros, and a medulla, which arises from neural crest cells.

The cortex consists of 3 zones:

- zona glomerulosa   produces aldosterone
- zona fasciculata   produces cortisol/androstenedione
- zona reticularis   produces DHEAS

5.2 Physiology

Cortex

The adrenal cortex has three principal functions:

- Glucocorticoid production (cortisol)
- Mineralocorticoid production (aldosterone)
- Androgen production (testosterone, androstenedione)

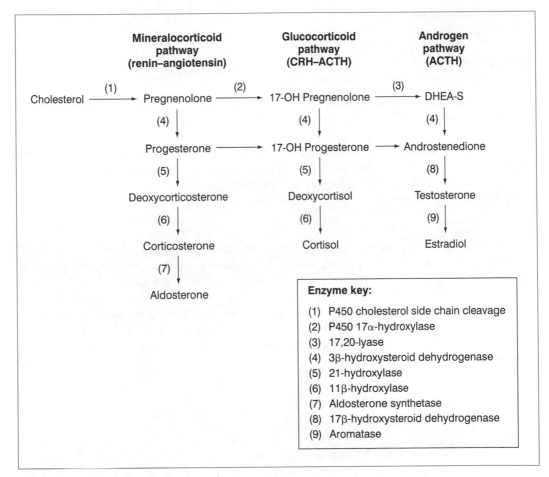

Pathways of adrenal hormone synthesis

Glucocorticoids

Cortisol is the principal glucocorticoid. It:

- plays a vital role in the body's stress response
- is an insulin counter-regulatory hormone increasing gluconeogenesis, hepatic glycogenolysis, ketogenesis
- is necessary for the action of other hormones, e.g. noradrenaline (norepinephrine), adrenaline (epinephrine), glucagon
- influences other organ physiology:
  - normal blood vessel function
  - cardiac and skeletal muscle
  - nervous system
  - inhibition of the inflammatory response of tissues to injury
  - secretion of a water load

Cortisol secretion is under pituitary control from ACTH. ACTH has a circadian rhythm, being at its lowest at midnight and rising in the early morning. There is also a negative feedback loop from cortisol. ACTH acts via cAMP and causes a flux of cholesterol through the steroidogenic pathway.

Mineralocorticoids

Aldosterone has the main mineralocorticoid action:

- It increases sodium reabsorption from urine, sweat, saliva and gastric juices in exchange for potassium and hydrogen.

The secretion of aldosterone is primarily regulated by the renin–angiotensin system, which is responsive to electrolyte balance and plasma volumes. Hyponatraemia and hyperkalaemia can also have a direct aldosterone stimulatory effect. ACTH can produce a temporary rise in aldosterone but this is not sustained.

Renin

Renin is a glycoprotein synthesized in the juxtaglomerular apparatus, and stored as an inactive proenzyme in cells of the macula densa of the distal convoluted tubule. Its release is stimulated by reduced renal perfusion, hyperkalaemia and hyponatraemia.

Renin hydrolyses angiotensin to form angiotensin I (an α_2-globulin synthesized in the liver). This is converted to angiotensin II by angiotensin-converting enzyme (ACE). ACE is present in high concentrations in the lung, but is also widely distributed in the vasculature for local angiotensin II release.

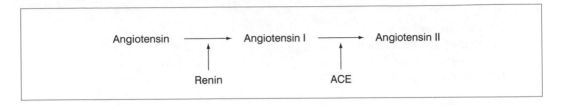

Adrenal androgens

These include testosterone, androstenedione and DHEAS. Secretion varies with age and, although responsive to ACTH, do not always parallel the cortisol response.

5.3 Disorders of the adrenal gland

Medulla

Phaeochromocytoma

Catecholamine-secreting tumours. Malignancy is uncommon, but 10% are bilateral. Catecholamine excess leads to sustained hypertension. Phaeochromocytomas are associated with von Recklinghausen's disease, von Hippel–Landau disease and syndromes of multiple endocrine neoplasia (MEN).

Investigation

- MIBG (metaiodobenzylguanidine) isotope scans
- Plasma and urine catecholamine measurement

Management

The management of phaeochromocytoma is by surgical excision. Pre-operative management requires both α- and β-adrenoceptors blockade in order to prevent an acute hypertensive crisis or cardiac dysrhythmias.

Cortex

Adrenal insufficiency

Causes

- Primary:
  - idiopathic
  - congenital adrenal hyperplasia
  - adrenal haemorrhage
  - Addison's disease:
    - TB
    - autoimmune disease
  - iatrogenic

- Secondary:
  - pituitary hypoplasia
  - isolated ACTH deficiency
  - panhypopituitarism
  - tumour, e.g. craniopharyngioma

Addison's disease

- Definition:
  - adrenal hypofunction
- Aetiology:
  - autoimmune
  - secondary to TB
  - associated with adrenal leucodystrophy
- Presentation:
  - often with non-specific symptoms of tiredness and abdominal pain
  - may present with collapse related to a salt-losing crisis

Investigation of adrenal cortical insufficiency

- Synacthen test, which assesses the ability of the stimulated adrenal glands to mount a hormone response. A dose of synthetic ACTH is given and the cortisol level measured after 30 and 60 min. A normal adrenal response would be a cortisol level >450–550 nmol/l at 30 min.
- A 24–h blood cortisol profile assesses the natural secretion from the adrenal gland. This would be expected to show the normal diurnal rhythm of cortisol secretion, with an increase in the morning and a nadir at midnight.

Treatment
Glucocorticoid and mineralocorticoid replacement using hydrocortisone and fludrocortisone, respectively

Adrenal steroid excess (Cushing's syndrome)

Causes

- Primary: adrenal tumour
- Secondary: pituitary ACTH-secreting tumour; ectopic ACTH production
- Iatrogenic: exogenous administration of steroids

- Definition:
  - a syndrome of cortisol excess. Cushing's disease is the term used when this is secondary to a pituitary ACTH-producing tumour (adenoma).
- Clinical features:
  - obesity — central distribution of fat — buffalo hump
  - purple striae
  - hypertension
  - osteoporosis
  - hypogonadism
  - growth failure

- Investigations:
  - 24–h urine cortisol
  - 24–h profile (loss of circadian rhythm, no suppression of midnight cortisol level)
  - dexamethasone suppression test
  - MRI brain/CT adrenals
- Treatment:
  - treat underlying cause

Congenital adrenal hyperplasia

- Aetiology:
  - deficiency of one of the enzymes in biosynthetic pathway of the adrenal cortex. The classical type is deficiency of the enzyme 21–hydroxylase.
- Pathophysiology:
  - in classical CAH, there is a block in the production of cortisol and aldosterone with a build up of the 17–hydroxyprogesterone, the enzyme's precursor. The continuing ACTH drive leads to the precursors being directed along the androgen biosynthetic pathway causing virilization.
- Presentation:
  - ambiguous genitalia (in girls with 21–hydroxylase deficiency, and occasionally in boys with 3β-hydroxysteroid dehydrogenase deficiency)
  - salt-losing crisis and hypotension
  - hypertension may occur in 11β hydroxylase deficiency
  - precocious puberty (in boys)
  - virilization
- Investigation:
  - karyotyping
  - 17–OH progesterone (17–OHP)
  - urine steroid profile (metabolite pattern will help in diagnosing specific enzyme block)
  - adrenal androgen levels
  - bone age in older children

Treatment

- Hydrocortisone and fludrocortisone to replace the deficient steroids but also to suppress the ACTH drive to the adrenal androgens. Growth is a good method of monitoring replacement therapy. Children who grow excessively fast with increased height velocity are either getting inadequate doses or may be non-compliant. 17–OHP levels are also useful for monitoring treatment.
- It is important to teach parents to recognize signs of illness and to be able to administer emergency hydrocortisone.
- Additional sodium chloride replacement is also required during the first year of life and electrolytes may need to be monitored over this period.
- Surgery may be required in females with virilization.

6. THE THYROID GLAND

6.1 Anatomy

The thyroid gland is formed from a midline outpouching of ectoderm of the primitive buccal cavity which then migrates caudally. It consists of follicles made of colloid surrounded by follicular cells and basement membrane. Thyroid hormone is synthesized at a cellular level and stored in thyroglobulin, a glycoprotein that is the main constituent of the colloid. Between the follicular cells are the parafollicular cells (C cells) which are of neurogenic origin and secrete calcitonin.

6.2 Physiology

The function of the thyroid gland is to concentrate iodine from the blood and return it to peripheral tissues in the form of thyroid hormones (thyroxine; tetra-iodothyronine, (T4) and tri-iodothyronine (T3)). In blood, the hormones are linked with carrier proteins, e.g. thyroxine-binding globulin and prealbumin. T4 is metabolized in the periphery into T3 (more potent) and reverse T3 (less potent).

Hormonogenesis

1. Iodide trapping by the thyroid gland
2. Synthesis of thyroglobulin
3. Organification of trapped iodine as iodotyrosines (mono-iodotyrosine (MIT) and di-iodotyrosine (DIT)).
4. Coupling of iodotyrosines to form iodothyronines and storage in the follicular colloid
5. Endocytosis of colloid droplets and hydrolysis of thyroglobulin to release T3, T4 and mono- and di-iodothyronine.
6. Deiodination of MIT and DIT with intrathyroid recycling of the iodine

Thyroid hormone acts by penetrating the cell membrane and then binding to a specific nuclear receptor. It modulates gene transcription and mRNA synthesis. This leads to increased mitochondrial activity.

Functions of thyroid hormone

Thyroid hormone has multiple physiological actions. It is required for somatic and neuronal growth. Other actions include thermogenesis, stimulation of water and ion transport, acceleration of substrate turnover, amino acid and lipid metabolism. It also potentiates the actions of catecholamines.

Regulation

Thyroid hormone release is regulated by thyroid-stimulating hormone (TSH) and iodine levels. TSH has both immediate and delayed actions on thyroid hormone secretion.

- Immediate actions:
  - stimulates binding of iodide to protein
  - stimulates thyroid hormone release
  - stimulates pathways of intermediate metabolism
- Delayed action (several hours):
  - stimulates trapping of iodide
  - stimulates synthesis of thyroglobulin

Physiological variations in iodide modulate trapping by the thyroid membrane.

Iodide inhibits the stimulation of cAMP by TSH and pharmacological doses block organification.

6.3 Disorders of thyroid function

Hypothyroidism

Causes of hypothyroidism

- Primary:
  - congenital:
  - thyroid dysgenesis
  - agenesis
  - hypoplasia
  - ectopic gland
  - biosynthetic defects

  - acquired:
    - autoimmune
    - post-surgery
    - post-cervical irradiation
    - systemic disorders
    - iodine deficiency
    - iodine overload

- Secondary:
  - congenital:
    - congenital pituitary abnormalities
    - receptor resistance
  - acquired:
    - post-cranial irradiation
    - post-tumour
    - post-surgery

Screening for congenital hypothyroidism

TSH is measured as part of the newborn screening programme performed between the 5th and 7th day of life. A blood spot from a heel prick is put on to a filter paper. Concentrations of TSH of over 10 mU/l are picked up by this test and abnormal results are immediately notified by the test centre to the relevant local hospital/specialist unit or the GP.

This screening programme detects >90% of cases of congenital hypothyroidism. Those due to secondary (pituitary causes) can not be picked up as TSH levels are low.

Hyperthyroidism

Causes of hyperthyroidism

- Autoimmune thyroiditis, e.g. Graves' disease
- Diffuse toxic goitre
- Nodular toxic goitre
- TSH-induced
- Factitious

Graves' disease

This is a multisystem, autoimmune disorder involving the eyes, hyperthyroidism and a dermopathy. There is an increased incidence in adolescence and is 6–8 times more common in girls than in boys. Thyroid-stimulating immunoglobulin may be demonstrated.

Thyroid neoplasia

This usually presents as solitary nodules, of which 50% are benign adenomas or cystic lesions. The prevalence of malignancy in childhood is 30–40% and the risk increases following radiation to the neck during infancy or early childhood. Hyperfunctioning adenomas are rare and most (90%) are well-differentiated follicular carcinomas.

Medullary carcinoma may occur as part of the MEN II (hyperparathyroidism and phaeochromocytoma) syndrome.

6.4 Investigation and management of thyroid disorders

Investigation

- Baseline blood tests:
  - free T4/T3/TSH measurements
- Stimulation tests:
  - TRH test
- Thyroid ultrasound scan
- Radionuclide scans

In primary hypothyroidism, T4 will be low and associated with a raised TSH. In hyperthyroidism, T4 will be raised and TSH suppressed.

In secondary hypothyroidism, T4 will be low in association with a low TSH. Further investigation is with a TRH test. This involves the injection of TRH followed by measurement of TSH at 30 and 60 minutes post-dose. In an individual with normal thyroid function, TSH would rise at 30 min but fall by 60 min. However, in patients with hypothalamic dysfunction, TSH would have continued to rise at 60 min post-injection.

'Sick thyroid syndrome' refers the scenario of a variety of abnormalities on thyroid function testing in an unwell patient but which spontaneously resolve as the illness improves. Usually this is a normal free T4 level with raised TSH.

Management of thyroid disorders

Hypothyroidism

- Replacement of thyroid hormone deficiency is with once-daily oral thyroxine tablets.
- Babies with congenital hypothyroidism should be started on thyroxine replacement as early as possible to limit damage to the developing brain. Outcome is usually good. However, intrauterine damage can not be completely corrected for and detailed psychometric testing may detect specific deficits.
- Initial doses start at 25 mcg per day with a gradual increase over the years.
- The dose may be monitored by assessing the free T4 and TSH levels at regular intervals.

Hyperthyroidism

- Initial medical treatment:
  - suppression of thyroid hormone secretion using specific antithyroid treatments, e.g. carbimazole, propylthiouracil
  - blunting the peripheral effects of the thyroid hormones using α-blockade, e.g. propranolol
- Definitive treatment:
  - this is contemplated if there has been no remission in symptoms on medical treatment, and may involve subtotal thyroidectomy and radioactive iodine

Radioactive iodine is becoming an increasingly popular choice for teenagers.

7. GLUCOSE HOMEOSTASIS

7.1 Physiology

The concentration of glucose in the blood is maintained by a balance between food intake or glucose mobilization from the liver and glucose utilization. Homeostatic mechanisms keep this within a narrow range.

In the fed state, insulin release is stimulated by a raised glucose and amino acid concentration. It is also stimulated by gut hormone release. In the fasting state, blood glucose concentrations fall and insulin production is turned off under the influence of somatostatin. A low glucose concentration is sensed by the hypothalamus, which regulates pancreatic secretion and stimulates the release of the counter-regulatory hormones glucagon, ACTH, GH, prolactin and catecholamines.

Actions of insulin

- Liver:
  - conversion of glucose to glycogen
  - inhibits gluconeogenesis
  - inhibits glycogenolysis
- Peripheral:
  - stimulates glucose and amino acid uptake by muscle
  - stimulates glucose uptake by fat cells to form triglycerides

Actions of the counter-regulatory hormones

- Inhibition of glucose uptake
- Stimulation of amino acid release by muscle
- Stimulation of lipolysis to release free fatty acids which can be oxidized to form ketones
- Stimulation of gluconeogenesis and glycogenolysis

7.2 Diabetes mellitus

Causes

Causes of diabetes mellitus

- Progressive loss of islet-cell function
- Insulin resistance
- Iatrogenic, e.g. post-pancreatic surgery

The most common cause of diabetes in childhood is type 1 autoimmune diabetes, although type 2 diabetes is increasingly being reported in association with obesity in teenagers. Type 2 diabetes is a combination of α-cell failure and insulin resistance.

Epidemiology

- UK — annual incidence is 20 per 100,000 children
- In many countries the incidence is rising, in some the incidence in children <5 years of age is increasing.
- Diabetes under 1 year of age is extremely rare. Incidence increases with age. Minor peak at age 4–6 years, major peak at 10–14 years
- No clear pattern of inheritance
- Increased risk if 1 family member is affected

Physiology of diabetes in β-cell failure

Low insulin level ultimately leads to ketoacidosis through the following mechanisms:
- liver glycogen mobilization to form glucose
- muscle protein breakdown to form free amino acids
- adipose tissue breakdown of triglycerides to form free fatty acids which are α-oxidized to form ketone bodies

Clinical effects

As the blood glucose level increases, the glucose in the glomerular filtrate exceeds the ability of the proximal tubules to reabsorb it. This leads to glycosuria. Polyuria then occurs, since the loop of Henle is unable to concentrate the urine because the renal tubules are insufficiently hyperosmolar. Extracellular volume depletion leads to thirst and polydipsia.

Diagnosis

- Glycosuria — >55 mmol/l
- Hyperglycaemia — random glucose >11.1 mmol/l, fasting glucose >7.6 mmol/l
- Ketonuria — >4 mmol/l

Glucose tolerance test not routinely necessary for diagnosis.

Diabetic ketoacidosis (DKA)
Most common presenting feature of diabetes. Commonest cause of diabetes-related deaths in children.

Definition

- Glycosuria, ketonuria, hyperglycaemia
- pH <7.3, bicarbonate <15 mmol/l
- 5% or more dehydrated, vomiting, drowsiness

Principles of management of DKA

- Rehydration (slowly over 48 h) to prevent large fluid shifts and the risk of cerebral oedema. An initial fluid bolus can be used to resuscitate the child. Normal fluid requirements are calculated as maintenance + 10% deficit given evenly over 48 h.
  - **Rule of thumb**:
    - 6 ml/kg per h for children weighing 3–9 kg
    - 5 ml/kg per h for children weighing 10–19 kg
    - 4 ml/kg per h for children weighing >20 kg
  - This usually covers ongoing losses, but if excessive they need replacement.
  - Initial fluid is 0.9% saline.
  - When blood glucose down to 12–15 mmol/l change to fluid containing glucose, e.g. 4% glucose + 0.45% saline.
- Intravenous insulin 0.05–0.1 IU/kg per h with the rate of infusion adjusted according to the blood glucose concentration
- Monitoring of glucose
- Replacement of potassium and monitoring of electrolytes

Long-term management of diabetes

- Subcutaneous insulin — with a combination of short/rapid-acting insulins and a long-acting insulin. The insulin may be delivered via a b.d. or q.d.s. regimen or continuously via an insulin pump. The usual requirement is insulin 1 IU/kg/day.
- Diet containing adequate protein, small amounts of fat and complex carbohydrate with regular food intake.

The aims of management are to normalize blood glucose concentrations to prevent acute hypoglycaemia and to reduce the risk of long-term complications developing. Monitoring is by capillary glucose measurements, glycated haemoglobin (Hb A1C) and screening for complications. Evidence shows that the more intensive treatment and monitoring regimens lead to a reduced risk of complications. These children are best managed by a multidisciplinary team including a paediatrician, dietician, diabetic nurse and ideally a psychologist.

Long-term complications increase with time (>10 years from onset of diabetes). They include nephropathy, retinopathy and neuropathy. All children with diabetes should have an annual review which include 24h urine collection for microalbuminuria and ophthalmology assessment.

7.3 Hypoglycaemia

Causes of hypoglycaemia

- Inadequate glucose production:
  - counter-regulatory hormone deficiencies
  - glycogen storage disease
  - enzyme deficiency, e.g. galactosaemia

- Excessive glucose consumption; i.e. hyperinsulinism:
  - transient
  - infant of a diabetic mother
  - Beckwith–Wiedemann syndrome

- Persistent:
  - persistent hyperinsulinaemic hypoglycaemia of infancy
  - insulinoma
  - exogenous insulin

Investigation of hypoglycaemia

Blood taken for a diagnostic screen is only useful if taken when the patient is hypoglycaemic (glucose <2.6 mmol/l) and should include the following:

- Blood:
  - glucose
  - insulin (C peptide)
  - cortisol
  - GH
  - lactate
  - free fatty acids
  - amino acids
  - ketone bodies (β-hydroxybutyrate and acetoacetate)
- Urine:
  - organic acids

In hypoglycaemic states in the absence of ketones it is important to look at the free fatty acids (FFA). Normal FFA suggests hyperinsulinism and raised FFA suggests a fatty-acid oxidation defect. Hypoglycaemia in the presence of urinary ketones suggests either a counter-regulatory hormone deficiency or an enzyme defect in the glycogenolysis or gluconeogenesis pathways.

(For further information please refer to Chapter 12, *Metabolic Medicine*)

8. BONE METABOLISM

8.1 Physiology of calcium and phosphate homeostasis

- Principal regulators of calcium concentrations:
  - vitamin D (and its active metabolites)
  - parathyroid hormone (PTH)
  - calcitonin
- Regulators of phosphate concentrations:
  - main regulator is vitamin D
  - less strictly controlled than calcium

Vitamin D

Vitamin D_3 (cholecalciferol) is produced in the skin from a provitamin as a result of exposure to ultraviolet light. Excess sunlight converts provitamin D to an inactive compound thus preventing vitamin D intoxication. Vitamin D is also ingested and is a fat-soluble vitamin. Vitamin D is converted to its active form by 1,25–hydroxylation.

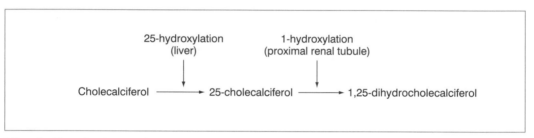

Vitamin D activation pathway

Vitamin D:
- Increases intestinal absorption of calcium
- Increases osteoclastic bone resorption
- Inhibits PTH secretion and hence increases 1α-hydroxylation

Parathyroid hormone

The PTH gene is located on chromosome 11. Active PTH is cleaved from a prohormone and then secreted by the parathyroid glands. Low calcium, cortisol, prolactin, phosphate and vitamin D all affect PTH secretion, but maximal PTH secretion occurs at a calcium concentration of <2 mmol/l.

Immediate effects of PTH

- Reduction in renal calcium excretion. It promotes calcium reabsorption in the distal tubule by stimulating the 1α-hydroxylation of vitamin D

- Promotion of phosphaturia by inhibiting phosphate and bicarbonate reabsorption in the proximal tubule
- Mobilization of calcium from bone — together with vitamin A, the osteoblasts are stimulated to produce a factor that activates osteoclasts to mobilize calcium

Delayed effects of PTH

- Promotion of calcium and phosphate absorption from gut

Calcitonin

Produced by the C cells of the thyroid gland and synthesized as a large precursor molecule. Its primary functions are:

- inhibition of bone resorption
- thought to interact with gastrointestinal hormones to prevent post-prandial hypercalcaemia

8.2 Disorders of calcium and phosphate metabolism

Hypocalcaemia

Causes of hypocalcaemia

- Transient neonatal hypocalcaemia
- Dietary
- Malabsorption
- Vitamin D deficiency
- Hypoparathyroidism
- Pseudohypoparathyroidism

Causes of hypoparathyroidism

- Parathyroid absence or aplasia
- Di George syndrome (thymic abnormalities/cardiac defects/facial appearances)
- Autoimmune
- Associated with multiple endocrinopathy
- Iatrogenic — post-thyroid surgery

Pseudohypoparathyroidism

- Clinical features:
  - mental retardation
  - short stature
  - characteristic facies
  - shortening of 4th and 5th metacarpal and metatarsal
  - ectopic calcification

- Aetiology:
  - due to end-organ resistance
- Associations:
  - TSH resistance and raised TSH levels

Pseudopseudohypoparathyroidism
Phenotypic features of pseudohypoparathyroidism are present but are not associated with the biochemical abnormalities.

Hypercalcaemia

Clinical features are non-specific, often with anorexia, constipation, polyuria, nausea and vomiting in a child with failure to thrive.

Causes of hypercalcaemia

- Low PTH:
  - vitamin D intoxication
  - infantile hypercalcaemia
  - transient
  - William's syndrome
  - associated with tumours
- High PTH:
  - primary hyperparathyroidism
  - familial hypocalciuric hypercalcaemia

Rickets

Causes of rickets

- Hypocalcaemic:
  - calcium deficiency:
    - dietary
    - malabsorption
  - vitamin D deficiency:
    - dietary
    - malabsorption
    - lack of sunlight
    - liver disease
    - anticonvulsants
    - biosynthetic defect of vitamin D
    - 1α-hydroxylase deficiency
    - liver disease
    - renal disease
  - defective vitamin D action

- Phosphopenic:
  - renal tubular loss
    - isolated, e.g. X-linked hyphosphataemia
    - mixed tubular, e.g. Fanconi's syndrome
- Abnormal bones
- Renal osteodystrophy

8.3 Investigations of bone abnormalities

- Calcium, phosphate, alkaline phosphatase
- Creatinine
- 1,25–vitamin D, 25–vitamin D, vitamin D concentrations
- PTH
- Urinary calcium, phosphate, creatinine and cAMP
- X-rays
- Technetium bone scan/bone mineral density

9. MISCELLANEOUS ENDOCRINE DISORDERS

9.1 Obesity

Obesity is the excessive accumulation of fat. This may be due to an increase in size or in the number of adipocytes. There is no threshold value at which fatness becomes pathological.

Causes of obesity

- Nutritional:
  - simple obesity/constitutional obesity
- Syndromes:
  - Down's
  - Laurence–Moon–Biedl
  - Prader–Willi
- Endocrine:
  - hypothalamic damage
  - hypopituitarism, GH deficiency
  - hypogonadism
  - hypothyroidism
  - Cushing's syndrome
  - pseudohypoparathyroidism
  - hyperinsulinism
  - iatrogenic
    - glucocorticoids
    - oestrogens

- Inactivity
- Psychological disturbances

In general, simple constitutional obesity is associated with tall stature in childhood, whereas endocrine causes of obesity tend to be associated with short stature or a reduction in height velocity.

Consequences of obesity

- Childhood:
  - insulin resistance and abnormal glucose tolerance
  - pickwickian syndrome
  - orthopaedic problems
  - obstructive sleep apnoea
  - increased cardiac diameter
- Adulthood — above +:
  - hyperlipidaemia
  - hypertension
  - diabetes
  - increased risk of death from cardiovascular disease

Syndromes associated with obesity

Prader–Willi

- Genetics:
  - deletion from paternally derived long arm of chromosome 15q
- Clinical features:
  - neonatal hypotonia
  - feeding difficulties in the newborn period
  - obesity (food-seeking behaviour)
  - hypogonadism
  - tendency to diabetes mellitus
  - strabismus
  - facial features:
    - narrow forehead
    - olive-shaped eyes
    - antimongoloid slant
    - carp mouth
    - abnormal ear lobes
  - orthopaedic:
    - small, tapering fingers
    - congenital dislocation of the hips
    - retarded bone age

- IQ:
  - reduced, usually 40–70
- behavioural difficulties:
  - food-seeking
- endocrine:
  - insulin resistance

Laurence–Moon–Biedl

- Clinical features:
  - mental retardation
  - obesity — marked by 4 years of age
  - retinitis pigmentosa/strabismus
  - polydactyly/clinodactyly
  - moderate short stature
  - hypogonadism
- Associations:
  - renal abnormalities
  - diabetes insipidus

Beckwith–Wiedemann

- Clinical features:
  - large birth weight
  - transient hyperinsulinism
  - macrosomia
  - linear fissures on ear lobes
  - umbilical hernia/exomphalos
  - hemihypertrophy
- Associations:
  - Wilms' tumour

Assessment of the obese child

- Height, weight and pubertal assessment
- Body mass index (BMI): BMI = wt (kg)/ht $(m)^2$; in children, the BMI should be compared to BMI centile charts as a person's BMI varies during different phases of childhood. For adults the following ranges are used:
  - 20–25   healthy
  - 25–30   overweight
  - 30–40   clinically obese
  - >40   morbidly obese
- Identification of an underlying cause:
  - thyroid function tests
  - cortisol measurements at midnight and 0800 h

- Evidence of complications:
  - respiratory function
  - orthopaedic problems
  - blood pressure
  - fasting lipids
  - oral glucose tolerance test

Management of obesity

- Identification and treatment of underlying cause
- Dietary measures
- Increased exercise
- Psychological support

9.2 Multiple endocrine neoplasia syndromes

Autosomal dominant syndromes: genetic counselling is available for families

- Type I (Wermer's syndrome): pancreatic (gastrinoma, insulinoma)/pituitary/parathyroid
- Type II (Sipple's syndrome): medullary thyroid cancer/parathyroid/ phaeochromocytoma

Patients with MEN IIb have additional phenotypic features — marfanoid habitus, skeletal abnormalities, abnormal dental enamel, multiple mucosal neuromas

9.3 Autoimmune polyglandular syndromes

- Type 1   Addison's disease, chronic mucocutaneous candidiasis, hypoparathyroidism
- Type 2   Primary hypothyroidism, primary hypogonadism, type I diabetes, pernicious anaemia, Addison's disease, vitiligo

10. FURTHER READING

Clinical Paediatric Endocrinology, Brook, Charles GD (ed.); PC, Hindmarsh (ed), 4th edition, Blackwell Science, 2001.

Effect of intensive diabetes treatment on the development and progression of long-term complications in adolescents with insulin-dependent diabetes mellitus: Diabetes Control and Complications Trial. *Journal of Pediatrics* **125**, 177–88.

Growth reference charts for use in the United Kingdom. Wright, CM, Booth, IW, Buckler, JMH, *et al.* (2002). *Archives of Disease in Childhood* **86**, 11–14.

Handbook of Endocrine Investigations in Children, Hughes IA; Wright 1989.

Managing intersex. Creighton, S and Minto, C (2001). *British Medical Journal* **323**, 1264–6.

Optimization of thyroxine dose in congenital hypothyroidism. Hindmarsh, PC (2002). *Archives of Disease in Childhood* **86**, 73–5.

Chapter 6

Evidence-based Medicine, Clinical Governance and Consent

Robert A Wheeler

CONTENTS

Evidence-based Medicine, Clinical Governance and Consent

1. BACKGROUND

Until the early 1980s, the quality of care in NHS hospitals was the responsibility of the Health Authorities. By the late 1970s, clinical audit was recognized as a means of measuring quality and had become quickly absorbed into the training requirements of doctors. With the advent of the hospital Trusts, politicians took renewed interest in quality issues. The Conservative administration had already coined the phrase 'Clinical Governance' by 1996; the advent of the New Labour government in 1997 confirmed Clinical Governance (CG) as the byword for quality assurance and enforcement.

A White Paper followed[1], translating the concept into several national developments, with a mission to set or enforce standards. These included the National Institute for Clinical Excellence (NICE), the Commission for Health Improvement (CHI) and National Service frameworks, the latter to 'drive up' the quality of services for specific groups of patients (e.g. cardiac, cancer) by setting national standards and describing service modules. Several other apparently disparate concepts were drawn into this initiative: Appraisal/assessment of doctors; Integrated Care or Managed Pathways; Evidence-based Practice.

By late 1998, when interested parties had recovered from the onslaught of novel watchdogs, words and concepts, a steady stream of contradictory literature had begun to flow at national and local level, all trying to make sense of what 'Clinical Governance' actually meant.

The Government's slickest definition appeared in the White Paper[2]:

> 'The means by which organizations are accountable for continuously improving the quality of their services and safeguarding high standards of care by creating an environment in which excellence in clinical care will flourish.'

The Scottish Office[3] was even more illuminating:

> 'Corporate accountability for clinical performance.'

Trusts, Royal Colleges and clinicians were being pressed to incorporate CG into their business plans as a matter of real political urgency, with not the least idea of what to do next. There was also considerable open dissent. Some pundits dismissed the initiative as

219

political expediency, all re-packaging and spin, whilst their colleagues were genuinely offended at what they saw as a slur on their previous lifelong commitment to maintain quality care.

However, from the confusion appeared some recurring themes, elements of CG that were manageable and possibly interrelated.

Glossy flow diagrams from the Defence Societies began to appear, linking elements such as Audit, Evidence and Risk, although the RCPCH as late as autumn 1999 could only define its 'Blueprint for Clinical Governance' as 'Accountability for clinical performance.'

The Government, perhaps reacting to the confusion established a Clinical Governance Support Team, together with a help-line, in November 1999.

Generally, pundits began to tease out simple and workable plans for implementation, e.g. four pillars: Clinical effectiveness, Professional development, Quality improvement and Risk management[4]. Trusts took rather a wider view, incorporating the patient's experience, research and information technology into the CG package.

But how to translate it all into real life?

2. IMPLEMENTATION

What follows is a recipe for establishing Clinical Governance.

It is immediately evident that not all the pillars of CG can be addressed at once. It is prudent to establish a list of the most important elements, then to prioritize. Risk management, Education/appraisal, Clinical performance and Evidence base forms a realistic starting point.

2.1 Risk management

A risk describes anything which may put the patient, clinician or parent in harm's way. This may be as specific as the risk of injecting the wrong chemotherapy into the spine, or as banal as ensuring that the doors to the outpatient's department do not trap children's fingers. Risks can thus come from the spectrum of practice, and the principle of management is to identify them before they cause damage.

A formal 'Risk assessment exercise' can be run throughout the unit, effectively taking a clip-board through the entire department, noting all possible potential problems. Since this is even more tedious than it sounds, Risk 'tools' have been developed; series of minutiae-type questions designed to discover any potential hazards, whether emanating from clinical practice or health and safety issues.

This is actually more exciting than it sounds. If, by use of the risk assessment it is possible to demonstrate that one's colleagues are overworked and overtired, then this is undoubtedly a significant risk: a Clinical Governance issue. Bearing in mind that the Chief Executive bears ultimate responsibility for CG matters; your use of the risk tool has promptly and legitimately transferred the burden of an 'hours' issue to the management.

A 'risk assessment' performed carefully, accurately and on a yearly basis gives a good foundation of predicting (prospectively) the risks a unit faces. Equally, immediate retrospective data is acquired by Critical incident reporting. In this way, any mishap, which a member of staff subjectively considers a risk, can be reported promptly. Examples of critical incidents include: a staff nurse feeling the ward is unsafe; prescribing errors by undertrained or overtired doctors; or medical equipment malfunction.

Such reports are collated and reviewed on a monthly basis by senior medical, nursing and administrative staff. Some reports are dismissed as frankly trivial; for others a simple 'local' solution is obvious, whilst more fundamental flaws in the system may require such fundamental change as to merit consideration by the Trust Board.

The attraction of such reporting is that it encourages staff to be freely critical, which tends to expose weaknesses in practice, which would otherwise go unrecognized.

There are other sources of these risk data. Complaints from distressed or injured patients, whether relating to domestic or clinical issues, serve to highlight hazards. Nationally recognized risks can also be contemplated: Do you have safeguards against imperfect consent for research procedures? Are your neonatal central venous catheter tips in a safe site?

Risk management thus means identifying risks prospectively or retrospectively, then finding a solution for them. If the solution is not immediately available to the clinician, then the risk (and the liability) is passed to the management.

2.2 Education/appraisal

Having indicated that only one topic can realistically be addressed at a time, this section of CG can be run in parallel with other activities. Continuing education for doctors is now mandatory, and in the future is likely to be reflected in demands for dedicated fixed consultant education sessions. Colleges have already recognized that education comes in various forms; formal teaching, courses, private reading, preparing lectures and research, amongst others.

Assessment and Appraisal are prominent on the political agenda, hence the anxiety of the General Medical Council to produce a workable formula. It is clear that assessment (which is a mere observation; a measuring of attendance, workload, waiting times, educational target fulfilment) is a great deal easier to perform than appraisal (a process of valuation, estimating the worth and quality of clinical activity).

This is because the individual can perform assessment themselves; it may involve tedious and time-consuming data collection and form filling, but it is an objective exercise. Appraisal, however, can only be performed by an outsider, who shares enough of the appraisee's training to allow pertinent questions to be asked, and relevant feedback to be given.

Appraisal is equally time consuming, but potentially threatening and more subjective than assessment.

As the GMC found out in 1999/2000, there is substantial resistance to these processes within the profession, partly on grounds of principle, partly because of practicality of process, time and cost. Nevertheless, local units are increasingly attempting to put assessment and appraisal in place; many already have systems operating, although they will recognize the need for modification as experience of these processes accrues.

2.3 Clinical performance

The much-publicized medical errors of recent years, together with a logarithmic rise in medical negligence litigation has led to calls for measurement of clinical performance. At its most simplistic, it has afforded the Government an opportunity to publish 'league tables' for Trusts in areas such as cardiac mortality. Whilst recognized as grotesque oversimplifications, this has led to the call for individual practitioners to publish their 'results'.

The response has been to answer this call with audit; i.e. establishing a 'gold standard', measuring whether the local unit is at variance with the standard, modifying practice to improve results and then re-measuring (re-audit) to ensure that the modification has achieved the desired result.

Any conceivable clinical intervention has potential for audit and it has been a highly satisfactory tool as a measure of clinical performance, provided it is used appropriately and correctly.

Audit programmes can be integrated with other aspects of CG. If a clinical intervention is identified as a risk either by Risk assessment, by Critical incident reporting or as the result of a cluster of similar complaints, then this gives an ideal opportunity for audit. At present, audit remains the single most effective method of performance measurement. Isolated specialties such as cardiac surgery have developed national databases of results, allowing unit comparison, but this obviously demands close integration and co-operation within a professional specialty. The advantage of audit is that it can be performed equally well in isolation, as long as a 'gold standard' for comparison can be identified.

To maintain enthusiasm for audit within a department is quite a different matter, partly because some doctors see this as a merely self-fulfilling process. A pragmatic approach is a rolling audit, where a topic is chosen which continually poses a clinical challenge; the adherence to the unit protocol for the management of bronchiolitis would be a recurring theme.

An audit can be set up along the usual lines, but then the re-audit phases, together with retrospective comparisons and prospective protocol adjustment, can be undertaken by successive generations of junior staff. In this way, audit becomes an integrated part of the working routine, not dependent on additional enthusiasm or drive by the medical team. Ideally, a combination of rolling 'routine' audit, with additional audits reacting to risks should run simultaneously.

2.4 Evidence base

Medicine is currently largely practised by consensus, with some reference to preceding experience. Consensus implies a broad agreement between practitioners, but the details of their treatment plans may vary markedly, based on their training and experience.

An example can be drawn from the management of vesicoureteric reflux (VUR); in 2001, a substantial number of surgeons were advocating surgical intervention for grade 2/3 VUR, whilst equally vociferous nephrologists insisted on antibiotic treatment alone. The consensus between these two recognizable specialist groups only existed on the basis of an agreement to disagree.

However, this exposes doctors to the charge that practices are inconsistent, varying between individuals in one centre, or between centres across the nation. Inconsistency generates uncertainty, leading to claims that some patients are suffering because of an inferior treatment, or that opportunities are being lost when relatively rare conditions are treated so differently that no conclusions can be drawn as to which treatment may be more appropriate. It is easy to sympathize with these arguments, from a patient's point of view. Surely there must be a best way to treat a disease, so why doesn't every hospital do it like that?

The simple answer to consistency is the use of guidelines and protocols. Once agreed, these at least ensure local certainty that a specific diagnosis is treated similarly by all practitioners, accepting the need for flexibility to deal with anomalous circumstances. National protocols are obviously more difficult to agree, as they represent loss of local sovereignty, which doctors are traditionally loathe to accept. In fields where treatment regimens are necessarily complex, such as paediatric oncology, the need for nationally agreed protocols is obvious; the UKCCSG (United Kingdom Children's Cancer Study Group) is a good example of how this can be made to work. Taking this one step further, UKCCSG has an increasingly close liaison with the equivalent European SIOP (Société International Oncologie Pediatrique), making international protocols a reality. Thus consistency of treatment across national boundaries is achievable, but still unusual. However, despite consistency, has the agreed protocol any evidential basis?

Current protocols are still largely based on precedent. There has been substantial work to provide evidence for the therapies we employ, notably the Cochrane Library. However, there is a great temptation to equate evidence with published work, and these are quite clearly not the same thing. If the demand for evidence-based medicine is rigorous, it follows that every aspect of every intervention is founded on a prospective randomized controlled trial of adequate size and power to achieve statistical significance.

A review of the Cochrane data, and the Clinical Evidence compendium[5] updated every 6 months shows how few therapies are based on 'proof'. Furthermore, in the present climate where ethical considerations make it increasingly difficult to perform clinical trials, it seems most unlikely that we will ever replace precedent with evidence.

An interesting associated issue is the Integrated Care Pathway (ICP). This describes a protocol or guideline which is created in a modular form, which details the treatment of a specified diagnosis from the first point of medical contact to discharge from medical care. This means that the whole process is dissected into the constituent actions, the available evidence for that action ascertained and verified, then all the parts are reconstituted into the ICP. If this sounds like a huge undertaking, you are still underestimating the effort involved.

Take an admission for observation in a child with a head injury.

- Seen by a paramedic...
- ABC sequence plus collar...evidence for benefit?
- A&E admission, Skull X-ray...evidence for benefit?
- Admission for neurological observation...evidence for benefit?
- Detained in hospital for 12 hours...evidence for benefit?

And so it goes on. You may consider this a banal example; but if one considers the modular dissection of an admission with urinary tract infection, it is not hard to see why 2 years is a reasonable estimate for the time it takes to write the relevant ICP.

This has led to many CG groups effectively despairing of producing ICPs within the foreseeable future. If pressed by the Trust management, the solution would be to purchase an appropriate 'off the shelf' ICP and customize it for local use. It can also be seen, with the paucity of 'gold standard' research with which to support the individual modules, how difficult it may be to write such a document; there will still need to be a firm reliance on consensus medicine.

2.5 Interaction

However, it can also be seen how these various elements of Clinical Governance interact, giving endless opportunities for flow diagrams and presentations.

If you start with risk, many topics will be generated that will merit further study, many by audit...a measure of the unit's performance. The audit will demand a 'gold standard' for comparison, which can (possibly) be supplied from the available evidence base. Obtaining this evidence or the consensus view may well be the appropriate use of a consultant's private study time, i.e. Continued medical education.

Once the 'gold standard' has been determined, it can be incorporated as a module within the appropriate Integrated Care Pathway. This may then be subject to rolling audit, etc.

The other three elements of CG will need to be addressed in the fullness of time.

Research governance has grown to the status of a chapter in itself; patient satisfaction and the governance aspects of IT have yet to evolve to a stage where they can be understood.

In summary, many see the advent of Clinical Governance as a statement of the blindingly obvious. However, with the political climate changing away from favouring doctors, the above model does allow CG to be implemented in a useable form, which is recognizable as a coherent plan by any agency choosing to scrutinize the working practices of a unit. It will allow the risks that we all face to be recognized, corrected and learned from as an automatic function, which may yet confer benefit on both doctors and their patients. Although resources will be required to deliver the CG agenda, no new money has been identified to fund it. However, future health planning may well be based upon information derived from the CG process.

3. CONSENT

Consent is required before any intervention, because society opposes the uninvited touch. At its simplest, the outstretched hand, preliminary to a handshake, by implication invites touching. However, the patient who consults their doctor does not assume that their very presence in the consulting room gives the doctor licence to touch them. The uninvited touch is, historically, an act of common assault. However, it is not the avoidance of this rather dramatic accusation that drives most contemporary doctors to obtain consent, although very occasionally the charge is still made.

What is far more relevant is the concept of negligence, where the doctor fails to deliver a reasonable standard of care to the patient, to whom there is undoubtedly a duty to provide such care. Obtaining consent implies that the doctor has provided all necessary information for the patient to make an informed decision. Often, the only record of this provision is the signed consent form. This document thus acts as a shield against a claim of assault, and objective evidence that some formal provision of information has occurred.

There are two excellent documents concerning consent[6,7] which provide comprehensive guidelines to issues surrounding consent.

The main questions to be considered when obtaining informed consent may be summarized:

When is consent required?

Consent is required for any intervention.

Who should obtain consent?

The senior clinician treating the patient.

In what form should consent be taken?

There is no legal requirement for written consent, which can equally be verbal or by acqui-escence provided the patient is correctly informed. However, a written document, which is signed by the patient, forms a piece of objective evidence that consent has been taken. Furthermore, if the document also records the details of the information given, it increases the certainty that relevant issues have been discussed. If the consent is verbal, it would be prudent to record the circumstances, witness topics discussed and outcome in the clinical notes.

From whom should consent be obtained?

To consent to treatment, an individual must have the capacity (i.e. intelligence and under-standing) fully to understand what treatment is being proposed.

It is assumed that a person of 16 years has such capacity, but in the period between 16 and 18 years, if the person is incapacitated, their parents may consent on their behalf.

A child of less than 16 years may give consent if capacity can be established, but the test is relatively rigorous. The child would need to understand the purpose and nature of the pro-posed treatment, to understand the risks, benefits and alternatives, and to understand the consequences of not undergoing the treatment. Furthermore, the child must be able to remember the information for long enough to make a considered decision. These criteria were established during The 'Gillick' case and form the basis of 'Gillick competence'.

Whilst it is accepted that a child with capacity can agree to a treatment, refusal of therapy, particularly if for life-threatening disease, clearly gives more difficulty, and advice should be sought from social services and the hospital legal department (e.g. a child with anorexia nervosa refusing tube feeds).

Either of the married parents may give consent on behalf of their child, but only the mother can normally consent if they are not married. It is irrelevant when the parents married, as long as the marriage occurred before the consent is given.

Legal guardians or the court may also consent on the behalf of children in some circumstances.

What if parents refuse consent?

The child is the patient, not the parents. If a parent refuses to give permission for a treatment which is neither life saving nor preventing deterioration, the treatment must be postponed. It will then be necessary to re-evaluate whether the benefit of the treatment outweighs the disadvantage of alienating the parents. If the treatment is still deemed necessary, legal advice should be obtained, which may lead to an approach to the court for directions.

If the proposed treatment is to save life or prevent deterioration of health, the doctor's obli-gation, on the basis of the child's best interests, is to deliver the treatment. Provided this treatment would be viewed as appropriate and the standard of care satisfactory, a subsequent court action would be very likely to support the doctor who overrides the parents' wishes in these circumstances. However, except in the most extreme circumstances, a second or senior opinion should always be sought and the hospital's legal services alerted.

In both the elective and emergency situation, referral to the hospital's Clinical Ethics Committee may help clarify the issues and provide support for doctors in this very difficult and unusual situation. Such a referral will probably come to be seen as a mandatory step by the courts within the next few years.

In the absence of a parent, when a child is unable to consent because of illness or lack of capacity, can the doctor treat in the emergency situation?

If emergency treatment is necessary, the doctor may treat on the basis of the child's best interests, which include the necessity to save life and avoid a significant deterioration in health. However, the views of the parents and the child (if known), the likelihood of improvement with treatment and the necessity to avoid restricting future treatment options where possible must all be considered in this situation.

What information should be provided to obtain informed consent?

The amount of information clearly depends upon the circumstances, and a balance between denying the patient relevant information and causing undue alarm must be found. Topics to be considered would include the certainties of diagnosis; the options for treatment (including non-treatment); a balanced opinion of the likely outcome of these options; and the purpose, risks, benefits and side-effects of the intervention. The General Medical Council (GMC) would also recommend ensuring that the name of the senior clinician is reiterated, together with a reminder that withdrawal from the treatment continues to be an option.

4. References

1. *The New NHS–Modern, Dependable.* SS DoHealth. London, The Stationery Office 1997.
2. *A First Class Service.* SS DoHealth. London, The Stationery Office 1998.
3. *Guidance on Clinical Governance* Scottish Office DoHealth. 1998.
4. *A Strategic Approach to Implementing Clinical Governance* Dale RF, Croft AM ARCSE 1999 81 248–250.
5. Clinical Evidence Barton S. Ed. *BMJ* Issue 4 2000.
6. *Reference guide to consent for examination or treatment,* DoHealth 2001 www.doh.gov.uk/consent
7. *Report of the consent working party March 2001,* Medical Ethics Dept, BMA London.

Chapter 7

Gastroenterology and Nutrition

Mark Beattie

229

Gastroenterology and Nutrition

1. BASIC ANATOMY AND PHYSIOLOGY

1.1 Anatomy

Oesophagus

Outer longitudinal and inner circular muscle layers with myenteric plexus in-between. Mucosa is lined by stratified squamous epithelium. Adult length 25 cm.

Stomach

Lined by columnar epithelium. Chief cells produce pepsin. Parietal cells produce gastric acid and intrinsic factor. 3 litres a day of secretions in adults. Gastric acid secretion is stimulated by vagal stimulation, gastrin and histamine via H_2 receptors on parietal cells. Secretion is inhibited by sympathetic stimulation, nausea, gastric acidity and small intestinal peptides. Blood supply from coeliac axis.

Small intestine

Main function is absorption, mostly in the duodenum and jejunum apart from bile salts and vitamin B_{12} which are absorbed in the terminal ileum. Blood supply from mid-duodenum onwards is the superior mesenteric artery. Adult length 2–3 metres.

Colon

Functions primarily for salt and water reabsorption. Blood supply from superior mesenteric artery until the distal transverse colon and then the inferior mesenteric artery after that. Approximately 1 m long in adults.

Pancreas

Retroperitoneal. Endocrine (2% of tissue mass) and exocrine function (98%). Blood supply from coeliac axis.

1.2 Digestion

Carbohydrate digestion

- Carbohydrates are consumed as monosaccharides (glucose, fructose, galactose), disaccharides (lactose, sucrose, maltose, isomaltose) and the polysaccharides (starch, dextrins, glycogen).

- Salivary and pancreatic amylase break down starch into oligosaccharides and disaccharides. Pancreatic amylase aids carbohydrate digestion but carbohydrate digestion is not dependent upon it.
- Disaccharidases (maltase, sucrase, lactase) in the microvilli hydrolyse oligo- and disaccharides into monosaccharides:
  - Maltose into glucose
  - Isomaltose into glucose
  - Sucrose into glucose and fructose
  - Lactose into glucose and galactose
- Monosaccharides are then absorbed, glucose and galactose by an active transport mechanism and fructose by facilitated diffusion.

Protein digestion

- In the stomach, gastric acid denatures protein and facilitates the conversion of pepsinogen into pepsin.
- Trypsin, chymotrypsin and elastase, secreted as the inactive precursors, are produced by the exocrine pancreas. Enterokinase (secreted in the proximal duodenum) activates trypsin and trypsin further activates trypsin, chymotrypsin and elastase.
- These proteases convert proteins into oligopeptides and amino acids in the duodenum.
- The small intestine absorbs free amino acids and peptides by active transport which then enter the portal vein and are carried to the liver.

Fat digestion

- Entry of fats into the duodenum causes release of pancreozymin–cholecystokinin which stimulates the gallbladder to contract.
- Hydrolysis of triglycerides by pancreatic lipase takes place.
- Free fatty acids, glycerol and monoglycerides are emulsified by bile salts to form micelles which are then absorbed along the brush border of mucosal cells.
- Short-chain fatty acids enter the portal circulation bound to albumin. Long-chain fats are re-esterified within the mucosal cells into triglycerides which combine with lesser amounts of protein, phospholipid and cholesterol to create chylomicrons.
- Chylomicrons enter the lymphatic system and are transported via the thoracic duct into the bloodstream

Pancreatic function

The pancreas secretes more than a litre of pancreatic juice per day, which is bicarbonate-rich and contains enzymes for the absorption of carbohydrate, fat and protein. Faecal elastase is a commonly used screen for pancreatic function.

Gut hormones

The main gut hormones are:

Gastrin — stimulated by vagal stimulation, distension of the stomach. Stimulates gastric acid, pepsin and intrinsic factor. Stimulates gastric emptying and pancreatic secretion.
Secretin — stimulated by intraluminal acid. Stimulates pancreatic bicarbonate secretion,

inhibits gastric acid and pepsin secretion and delays gastric emptying.

Cholecystokinin–pancreozymin — stimulated by intraluminal food. Stimulates pancreatic bicarbonate and enzyme secretion. Stimulates gallbladder contraction, inhibits gastric emptying and gut motility.

Other gut hormones include:

Gastric inhibitory peptide	Stimulated by glucose, fats and amino acids; inhibits gastric acid secretion, stimulates insulin secretion and reduces motility
Motilin	Stimulated by acid in the small bowel; increases motility
Pancreatic polypeptide	Stimulated by a protein-rich meal; inhibits gastric and pancreatic secretion
Vasoactive intestinal peptide (VIP)	Neural stimulation; inhibits gastric acid and pepsin secretion; stimulates insulin secretion; reduces motility

Enterohepatic circulation

Bile is produced by the liver and stored in the gallbladder. It is secreted into the duodenum following gallbladder contraction (stimulated by cholecystokinin–pancreozymin release). Bile acids aid fat digestion. They are formed from cholesterol. Primary bile acids are produced in the liver. Secondary bile acids are formed from primary bile acids through conjugation with amino acids by the action of intestinal bacteria. Primary and secondary bile acids are deconjugated in the intestine, reabsorbed in the terminal ileum and transported back to the liver bound to albumin for recirculation.

2. NUTRITION

2.1 Breast feeding

Breast feeding and infection

10% of the protein in mature breast milk is secretory IgA. Lymphocytes, macrophages, proteins with non-specific antibacterial activity and complement are also present. There have been many studies in the Third World to show that infants fed formula milk have a higher mortality and morbidity particularly from gastrointestinal infection. In the UK, studies have been done which show:

- Breast feeding for more than 13 weeks reduces the incidence of gastrointestinal and respiratory infections
- The response to immunization with the Hib vaccine is higher in breast-fed than formula-fed infants
- The risk of necrotizing enterocolitis in low birth-weight babies is lower in those who are breast fed

Breast feeding and allergy

The incidence of atopic eczema in infants born to atopic mothers is reduced by breast feeding. Overall, however, there is no definitive proven reduction in atopy apart from this specific circumstance.

Breast feeding and neurological development

Although there are confounding variables which make study of this subject difficult, there is work that suggests that neurological development is enhanced in breast-fed infants.

Breast feeding and diabetes

Infants who are breast fed have a reduced risk of developing diabetes.

Breast feeding and infantile colic

There is no good evidence to show that breast feeding reduces the incidence of infantile colic.

Contraindications to breast feeding

Maternal drugs and breast feeding are discussed elsewhere (see Chapter 13, Section 5.3).

- With regard to TB; infants can be immunized at birth with isoniazid-resistant BCG and treated with a course of isoniazid.
- With regard to HIV; the virus has been cultured from breast milk and is transmitted in it. In the Western world this makes breast feeding contraindicated, as it will increase the perinatal transmission rate. The problem is not so straightforward in the developing world where the risks of bottle feeding are high due to contaminated water supplies.

Term and preterm formula

The principal differences are that preterm formula contains more electrolytes, calories and minerals. All of the following are higher in preterm than term formula; energy, protein, carbohydrate, fat, osmolality, sodium, potassium, calcium, magnesium, phosphate and iron.

Human (breast) milk and cows' milk

The energy content is the same. Human milk contains less protein than cows' milk — the cows' milk having much higher casein content. The fat, although different qualitatively, is the same in amount. Human milk contains more carbohydrate. Cows' milk contains more of all the minerals except iron and copper.

2.2 Iron

- Dietary sources include cereals, red meat (particularly liver) fresh fruit, green vegetables.

- Absorbed from the proximal small bowel. Vitamin C, gastric acid and protein improve absorption. 5–10% of dietary iron is absorbed.
- Deficiency causes hypochromic microcytic anaemia. Associated with poor appetite and reduced intellectual function.
- Common causes include poor diet — particularly prolonged or excess milk feeding, chronic blood loss, malabsorption.
- Low serum iron, high transferrin suggests deficiency. Low iron, low transferrin suggests chronic disease. Ferritin is an indicator of total body stores but is also an acute-phase reactant.
- Treatment is directed against the underlying cause. Dietary advice and iron supplements, of which numerous commercial preparations are available, are indicated in most patients. Side-effects of iron supplements include abdominal discomfort and constipation. They can be fatal in overdose.

2.3 Folate

- Dietary sources include liver, green vegetables, cereals, orange, milk, yeast and mushrooms. Excessive cooking destroys folate.
- Absorbed from the proximal small bowel
- Deficiency causes megaloblastic anaemia, irritability, poor weight gain and chronic diarrhoea. Thrombocytopenia can occur.
- The serum folate reflects recent changes in folate status and the red cell folate is an indicator of the total body stores
- Treatment of deficiency is with oral folic acid
- Folate levels are not affected by the acute-phase response.

Causes of folate deficiency

- Reduced intake
- Coeliac disease
- Tropical sprue
- Blind-loop syndrome
- Congenital folate malabsorption (autosomal recessive)
- Increased requirements (infancy, pregnancy, exfoliative skin disease)
- Increased loss (haemodialysis)
- Methotrexate
- Trimethoprim
- Anti convulsants
- Oral contraceptive pill

2.4 Vitamin B$_{12}$

- Dietary sources include foods of animal origin, particularly meat
- Absorbed from the terminal ileum facilitated by gastric intrinsic factor.
- Deficiency causes megaloblastic anaemia, low vitamin B$_{12}$, increased methyl-malonic acid in the urine.

- Clinical features include anaemia, glossitis, peripheral neuropathy, subacute combined degeneration of the cord, optic atrophy.
- Causes include pernicious anaemia (rare in childhood), gastric- and parietal-cell antibodies are usually positive.
- Other causes of vitamin B_{12} deficiency include poor intake (vegan diet) and malabsorption, e.g. blind-loop, post-resection.
- Treatment is with vitamin B_{12} usually given im initially 1–2 times a week then 3-monthly. Folic acid is also needed.

2.5 Zinc

- Dietary sources include beef, liver, eggs and nuts
- Deficiency occurs secondary to poor absorption rather than poor intake
- Clinical features include anaemia, growth retardation, periorofacial dermatitis, immune deficiency, diarrhoea
- Responds well to oral zinc

Acrodermatitis enteropathica

- Autosomal recessive inheritance.
- Basic defect is impaired absorption of zinc in the gut.
- Presents with skin rash around the mouth and peri-anal area, chronic diarrhoea at the time of weaning and recurrent infections. The hair has a reddish tint, alopecia is characteristic. Superinfection with Candida is common as are paronychia, dystrophic nails, poor wound healing and ocular changes (photophobia, blepharitis, corneal dystrophy).
- Diagnosis is by serum zinc levels and the constellation of clinical signs. This is difficult as the serum zinc is low as part of the acute-phase response. Measurement of white cell zinc levels is more accurate. The plasma metallothionein level can also be measured. Metallothionein is a zinc-binding protein that is decreased in zinc deficiency but not in the acute-phase response.
- Zinc deficiency in the newborn can produce a similar clinical picture.
- The condition responds very well to treatment with oral zinc.

2.6 Fat-soluble vitamins

Vitamin A

- Deficiency causes night blindness, poor growth, xerophthalmia, follicular hyperplasia and impaired resistance to infection
- Excess causes carotenaemia, hyperostosis with bone pain, hepatomegaly, alopecia and desquamation of the palms. Acute intoxication causes raised intracranial pressure.
- Dietary sources are milk, fat, fruit and vegetables, egg and liver.
- Vitamin A has an important role in the resistance to infection particularly at mucosal surfaces. In the Third World where vitamin A deficiency is endemic, vitamin A reduces the morbidity and mortality associated with severe measles.

Vitamin E

- Is an antioxidant
- Found in green vegetables and vegetable oils
- Deficiency causes ataxia, peripheral neuropathy and retinitis pigmentosa

Abetalipoproteinaemia

- Autosomal recessive inheritance.
- Pathogenesis is failure of chylomicron formation with impaired absorption of long-chain fats with fat retention in the enterocyte.
- Malabsorption occurs from birth.
- Presents in early infancy with failure to thrive, abdominal distension and foul smelling, bulky stools.
- Symptoms of vitamin E deficiency (ataxia, peripheral neuropathy and retinitis pigmentosa) develop later.
- Diagnosis is by low serum cholesterol, very low plasma triglyceride level, acanthocytes on examination of the peripheral blood film, absence of betalipoprotein in the plasma.
- Treatment is by substituting medium-chain triglycerides for long-chain triglycerides in the diet. Medium-chain triglycerides (MCT) are absorbed via the portal vein rather than the thoracic duct. In addition, high doses of the fat-soluble vitamins (A, D, E and K) are required. Most of the neurological abnormalities are reversible if high doses of vitamin E are given early.

Vitamin K

- Is contained in cows' milk, green leafy vegetables and pork. There is very little in breast milk.
- Deficiency in the newborn period presents as haemorrhagic disease of the newborn. This usually presents on day 2 or 3 with bleeding from the umbilical stump, haematemesis and malaena, epistaxis or excessive bleeding from puncture sites. Intracranial bleeding can occur. Diagnosis is by prolongation of the prothrombin and partial thromboplastin times with the thrombin time and fibrinogen levels being normal. Treatment is with fresh-frozen plasma and vitamin K.
- There is no proven association between intramuscular vitamin K and childhood cancer

2.7 Malnutrition

It is essential to think about the pathogenesis of malnutrition when assessing nutrition and looking at nutritional supplementation. Malnutrition can only result from:

- Inadequate intake or excessive losses
- Increased metabolic demand without increased intake
- Malabsorption

One or all of these may contribute to malnutrition in an individual.

A good example is cystic fibrosis

1. Pancreatic malabsorption causing increased losses

2. Increased energy needs
    Chronic cough
    Dyspnoea   } causing increased needs
    Recurrent infection
    Inflammation

3. Reduced intake
    Anorexia
    Vomiting   } resulting in reduced intake
    Psychological problems

All these together result in an energy deficit. All of these factors need to be considered when nutritional supplementation is considered.

2.8 Protein-energy malnutrition

Marasmus and kwashiorkor

Marasmus is characterized by muscle wasting and depletion of the body fat stores. Kwashiorkor is characterized by generalized oedema with flaky or peeling skin and skin rashes. Most children with malnutrition — rare in the Western world, exhibit a combination of the two. Micronutrient deficiencies are common in these children.

3. FAILURE TO THRIVE

Failure to thrive refers to the failure to gain weight at an adequate rate. It is common in infancy. It occurs because of one or a combination of the following:

- Failure of carer to offer adequate calories
- Failure of the child to take sufficient calories
- Failure of the child to retain adequate calories

Clearly this can be organic or non-organic. Insufficient calories may be offered as a consequence of parental neglect or because of a failure of the carer to appreciate the calorie requirements of the child. Insufficient calories may be taken as a consequence of feeding difficulties (for example, cerebral palsy) or increased needs (for example, cystic fibrosis) and calories may not be retained because of absorptive defects or loss because of vomiting or diarrhoea.

The investigation of failure to thrive is generally only fruitful when specific pointers to organic problems are elucidated in the history or on physical examination.

The management of non-organic failure to thrive requires health-visitor input and often dietary assessment. In difficult cases hospital admission is indicated for evaluation and to ensure an adequate weight gain can be obtained if sufficient calories are given.

3.1 Organic causes of failure to thrive

This list provides examples only and is by no means exhaustive.

Organic causes of failure to thrive

Gastrointestinal	Coeliac disease, cows' milk, protein intolerance, gastro-oesophageal reflux
Renal	Urinary tract infection, renal tubular acidosis
Cardiopulmonary	Cardiac disease, cystic fibrosis, bronchopulmonary dysplasia
Endocrine	Hypothyroidism
Neurological	Cerebral palsy
Infection/immunodeficiency	HIV, malignancy
Metabolic	Inborn errors of metabolism
Congenital	Chromosomal abnormalities
ENT	Adenotonsillar hypertrophy

3.2 Nutritional supplementation

Nutritional supplementation should be with the help of a dietician. It is essential, however, to have some background information and to:

- Treat underlying pathology which may be a factor
- Assess the child's requirements
- Give additional calories either by increasing the calorie density of feed or giving feed by a different route, e.g. nasogastric tube, gastrostomy tube or parenterally

Enteral nutrition refers to that given either directly (by mouth) or indirectly (via nasogastric tube or gastrostomy) into the gastrointestinal tract. Parenteral nutrition is given either into the peripheral or central veins, usually the latter.

It may be helpful to consider specific scenarios:
A 6-month-old infant has congenital heart disease and is failing to thrive — comment on his nutritional status. What nutritional supplementation would you recommend?

In this infant the poor nutritional state will be as a consequence of increased metabolic demands and poor intake secondary to breathlessness. Supplementation would be by increasing the calorie density of feeds and consideration of other methods of administration such as via a nasogastric tube. It is obviously also of importance to maximize medical therapy of the heart disease.

This 6-month-old infant has bronchopulmonary dysplasia and severe failure to thrive. Comment on possible causes.

In this infant the above applies. In addition, other factors may be relevant such as chronic respiratory symptoms, gastro-oesophageal reflux and neurodevelopmental issues. Supplementation would be by increasing calorie density and considering using a nasogastric tube or gastrostomy to give feed. In addition, investigation for problems like gastro-oesophageal reflux may be considered.

This 13-year-old boy has cerebral palsy. Comment on his nutritional status. What strategies could be used to improve his nutrition? Why do you think his nutritional status is so poor?

This child's principal problem is likely to be with intake, either because of reflux or secondary to bulbar problems or both. In addition to nutritional supplements, this child may benefit from help with feeding practices including the involvement of a dietician, speech and language therapist, occupational therapist and neurodevelopmental paediatrician. Other medical problems may be relevant such as recurrent chest infections secondary to aspiration, intractable fits. Consideration needs to be given to nasogastric tube or gastrostomy tube feeding if appropriate. In some instances a fundoplication will also be required.

This boy has cystic fibrosis. Comment on his nutritional status. What can be done to help?

The additional factor in this child is malabsorption for which pancreatic supplementation is required. Children with cystic fibrosis often dislike food and need either a nasogastric tube or gastrostomy to help with administration. The energy requirements are high and calorie supplementation with energy-dense supplements is required.

3.3 Diseases for which enteral nutrition may be indicated

- **Gastrointestinal**
  - Short-bowel syndrome
  - Inflammatory bowel disease
  - Pseudo-obstruction
  - Chronic liver disease
  - Gastro-oesophageal reflux
  - Glycogen storage disease types I and III
  - Fatty-acid oxidation defects

- **Neuromuscular disease**
  - Coma and severe facial and head injury
  - Severe mental retardation and cerebral palsy
  - Dysphagia secondary to cranial nerve dysfunction, muscular dystrophy or myasthenia gravis

- **Malignant disease**
  - Obstructing disease
  - Head and neck
  - Oesophagus
  - Stomach
  - Abnormality of deglutition following surgical intervention
  - Gastrointestinal side-effects from chemotherapy and/or radiotherapy
  - Terminal supportive care

- **Pulmonary disease**
  - Bronchopulmonary dysplasia
  - Cystic fibrosis
  - Chronic lung disease

- **Congenital abnormalities**
  - Tracheo-oesophageal fistula
  - Oesophageal atresia
  - Cleft palate
  - Pierre Robin syndrome

- **Other**
  - Anorexia nervosa
  - Cardiac cachexia
  - Chronic renal disease
  - Severe burns
  - Severe sepsis
  - Severe trauma

3.4 Gastrostomy tube feeding

Gastrostomy tubes are generally inserted endoscopically (percutaneous endoscopic gastrostomy) and the complications are few.

Indications

- In chronic disease with nutritional impairment, e.g. cystic fibrosis, bronchopulmonary dysplasia
- For nutritional therapy, e.g. Crohn's disease
- Difficulties with feeding, e.g. cerebral palsy, particularly with an associated bulbar palsy
- In severe gastro-oesophageal reflux with a fundoplication
- Children dependent upon nasogastric feeding for any other reason

3.5 Total parenteral nutrition (TPN)

It is important to use the gut, and in infants and children where supplementary feeding is required the gut should be used where possible. Complete exclusion of luminal nutrients is associated with atrophic changes in the gut, reduced pancreatic function, biliary stasis and bacterial overgrowth. It is not usually necessary to use for less than 5 days except in the extreme preterm. There is no indication to start TPN as an emergency, although the addition of even small amounts of nitrogen as amino acids can reverse catabolism of muscle mass.

Indications

Neonates

Absolute indications:
- Intestinal failure (short gut, functional immaturity, pseudo-obstruction)
- Necrotizing enterocolitis

Relative indications:
- Hyaline membrane disease
- Promotion of growth in preterm infants
- Possible prevention of necrotizing enterocolitis

Older infants and children

Intestinal failure:
- Short gut
- Protracted diarrhoea
- Chronic intestinal pseudo-obstruction
- Post-operative abdominal or cardiothoracic surgery
- Radiation/cytotoxic therapy

Exclusion of luminal nutrients:
- Crohn's disease

Organ failure:
- Acute renal failure or acute liver failure

Hypercatabolism:
- Extensive burns
- Severe trauma

Complications of central venous catheter insertion

Sepsis
Air embolism
Arterial puncture
Arrhythmias
Chylothorax
Haemothorax
Pneumothorax
Haemo/hydropericardium
Malposition of catheter
Nerve injury
Central venous thrombosis
Thromboembolism
Extravasation from fractured catheter
Tricuspid valve damage
Catheter tethering

Complications of TPN

Phlebitis
Infection
Hypo- and hyperglycaemia
Electrolyte disturbance
Fluid overload
Hypophosphataemia
Anaemia
Thrombocyte and neutrophil dysfunction
Trace-element deficiencies
Trace-element excess
Vitamin deficiencies
Hyperammonaemia
Essential fatty-acid deficiency
Cholestasis and hepatic dysfunction
Metabolic acidosis
Hypercholesterolaemia
Hypertriglyceridaemia
Granulomatous pulmonary arteritis

Some of the consequences of trace-element abnormalities described during parenteral nutrition

Trace element	Deficiency	Excess
Zinc	Periorofacial dermatitis Immune deficiency Diarrhoea Growth failure	
Copper	Refractory hypochromic anaemia Neutropenia Osteoporosis Subperiosteal haematoma Soft tissue calcification	
Selenium	Cardiomyopathy Skeletal myopathy, pain and tenderness Pseudoalbinism	
Chromium	Glucose intolerance Peripheral neuropathy Weight loss	Renal and hepatic impairment
Manganese	Lipid abnormalities Anaemia	Liver toxicity Damage to basal ganglia
Molybdenum	Tachycardia Central scotomata Irritability Coma	
Aluminium		Anaemia Osteodystrophy Encephalopathy

3.6 Short-bowel syndrome

- Intestinal failure secondary to massive resection

Management

- Maintain normal growth and development
- Promote intestinal adaptation
- Prevent complications

- Establish enteral nutrition
- Total parenteral nutrition

Factors that influence outcome

- Ileum adapts better than jejunum
- Better prognosis if ileocaecal valve present
- Better outcome if colon present
- Coexistent disease, e.g. enteropathy
- Presence of liver disease is an adverse risk factor

Outcome

- <30 cm of small bowel is usually associated with the need for long-term nutritional support
- Bowel lengthening procedure or small-bowel transplantation are options

3.7 Nutritional supplements

This needs to be done in conjunction with a trained paediatric dietician. It is useful to be aware of some of the products available.

General principles

- Normal infant feeds or milk contain 0.7 kCal/ml (2.92J/ml)
- Feeds can be concentrated, e.g. 15% feeds, 4 scoops in 100 ml (normal 1 scoop in 30 ml)
- Carbohydrate supplements can be used — usually as glucose polymer, e.g. Maxijul, Polycal
- Carbohydrate and fat supplements can be used, e.g. Duocal
- Feeds with a higher calorie density can be used, e.g. Infatrini (under age 1) 1 kCal/ml (4.18J/ml), Nutrini (over age 1) 1 kCal/ml (4.18J/ml), Nutrini extra 1.5 kCal/ml (6.28J/ml)
- Special feeds can be used, e.g. hydrolysed-protein formula feeds, soya-based feeds, lactose-free feeds, MCT-based feeds
- Supplements can be given, e.g. Fortisip (1.5 kCal/ml) (6.28J/ml), Fortijuice (1.5 kCal/ml) (6.28J/ml), Fortipuds — there are many commercially available products

4. FOOD INTOLERANCE

It is important to distinguish allergy and intolerance. An allergy implies an immune-mediated reaction to food antigen (protein). Classically this is by IgE-mediated, type I hypersensitivity. The signs of this include anaphylaxis, urticaria and atopic dermatitis. Intolerance implies a reaction to food taken either in small quantity or in excess. It is a non-specific term. Examples range from symptoms due to a non-IgE-mediated immune reaction to food, such as coeliac disease, through to symptoms induced by simple overindulgence. An intolerance doesn't necessarily need to be to a protein and includes, for example, lactose intolerance.

4.1 Cows' milk protein intolerance

There is a wide spectrum of clinical features induced by cows' milk protein and the condition is not always well defined, leading to concerns about under- and over-diagnosis.

Clinical spectrum of cows' milk protein intolerance

- Acute type 1-mediated hypersensitivity
- Delayed-onset hypersensitivity
- Cows' milk sensitive enteropathy
- Cows' milk allergic colitis
- Non-specific symptoms ?attributable to cows' milk

It is the latter group that presents the most difficulty and includes a wide variety of symptoms including colic, generalized irritability, chestiness, recurrent upper respiratory tract symptoms and constipation. Diagnosis is dependent on the clinical manifestations. A good history and, if possible, dietetic assessment is essential. To strictly diagnose allergy the Goldmann criteria should be met, which are that the attributable symptoms disappear on removal of the offending antigen and recur when it is reintroduced. Skin-prick testing and IgE radioallergosorbent testing (RAST) is sometimes useful. They test type I-mediated hypersensitivity. A negative result does not exclude allergy and a positive result can be seen in children who tolerate cows' milk protein without a problem. If either an enteropathy or colitis is suspected then it is useful to get histological confirmation.

Management

- Milk exclusion with a milk substitute. Soya preparations are commonly used and are palatable. There is, however, a cross-reactivity between cows' milk and soya protein of up to a third and so hydrolysed protein formula feeds are preferred.
- A hydrolysed protein is one which is broken down into oligopeptides and peptides. A hydrolysed protein milk formula is therefore one which does not contain whole protein. An elemental formula is a hydrolysed protein formula in which the protein is broken down into amino acids. Examples of hydrolysed protein formulae include Pregestimil, Nutramigen, Prejomin, Pepti-junior. Neocate and elemental EO28 are elemental formulas.
- Other conditions in which hydrolysed protein formula feeds are used include enteropathies, e.g. post-gastroenteritis, post-necrotizing enterocolitis, short-gut syndrome, severe eczema, Crohn's disease.
- The natural history of cows' milk intolerance is resolution with 80–90% back on a normal diet by the third birthday. It is sensible to challenge regularly. This will depend on the child's presentation. It is usual to organize challenges in hospital, particularly if the initial reaction was severe, because of the risk of anaphylaxis.
- Children with a past history of anaphylaxis or severe respiratory symptoms following allergen ingestion require an adrenaline pen for use either in the home or school setting in the event of accidental exposure to the offending food antigen.

It is common in children with milk allergy to see reactions to other foods, the most common of which are soya, egg, wheat and peanut.

Skin-prick testing and IgE RAST are most useful in children with peanut, nut and egg allergy.

4.2 Peanut allergy

Peanut and nut allergies are seen with increasing frequency. It is important to remember that peanuts are a vegetable rather than a true nut. 60–80% of children with peanut allergy are also allergic to other nuts. Reactions vary from mild urticaria to life-threatening anaphylaxis. Skin-prick testing is useful with a high sensitivity and specificity. It is important to get the diagnosis right, lots of children have non-specific reactions during childhood and are labelled 'peanut-allergic'. Peanut avoidance is difficult and dietetic support is essential. Food contamination in food production, i.e. nuts not in ingredients, but may have traces because of cross-contamination from other food production lines, is common. There is some controversy about whether all nuts should be avoided in peanut-allergic patients and about whether peanut oils should be given. The natural history suggests children with early-onset allergy may grow out of it, although older children with symptomatic reactions are more likely to persist. Active management involves challenging peanut skin-prick-negative children. This is clearly not without risk and needs to be done in an inpatient setting with facilities for resuscitation.

Common other nuts that cause allergic reactions include brazil nut, cashew nut, hazelnut, walnut, almond and pistachio nut.

4.3 Food-induced anaphylaxis

Children who have had an anaphylactic reaction are at increased risk of a second reaction after second exposure, for which there is a significant mortality. These children benefit from an adrenaline pen. It is important that such children and their families are taught properly about the indications for use of the pen and subsequent action that should be taken. The school and all the main carers need to be involved. A medic-alert bracelet is useful. Children should also keep antihistamines in the house. These are appropriate for minor reactions and some units advocate their use prior to potential accidental exposure.

It is essential to be aware of the guidelines for the management of an anaphylactic reaction and the reader is referred to the most recent Paediatric Advanced Life Support/Advanced Paediatric Life Support (PALS/APLS) guidelines for this.

4.4 Carbohydrate intolerance

Disorders of disaccharide absorption

Primary
Congenital alactasia
Congenital lactose intolerance
Sucrose–isomaltase deficiency

Secondary (acquired)
Post-enteritis (rotavirus), neonatal surgery, malnutrition
Late-onset lactose intolerance

Disorders of monosaccharide absorption

Primary
Glucose–galactose malabsorption

Secondary (acquired)
Post-enteritis, neonatal surgery, malnutrition

Lactose intolerance

Carbohydrate intolerance is usually lactose intolerance and usually acquired. The deficient enzyme is the brush-border enzyme lactase which hydrolyses lactose into glucose and galactose. The intolerance will present with characteristic loose explosive stools. The diagnosis is made by looking for reducing substance in the stool following carbohydrate ingestion. The test used is the Clinitest tablets (which detect reducing substance in the stool), the detection of more than 0.5% is significant. Formal confirmation of which is the offending carbohydrate is through stool chromatography. Treatment is with a lactose-free formula in infancy and a reduced lactose intake in later childhood.

Following gastroenteritis, carbohydrate intolerance can be either to disaccharides or monosaccharides. It is usually in children who have been infected with rotavirus. Both types of intolerance are usually transient and both respond to removal of the offending carbohydrate. Both mono- and disaccharide intolerance will result in the reducing substances in the stool being positive.

Glucose–galactose malabsorption

This is a rare autosomal recessively inherited condition, characterized by rapid-onset watery diarrhoea from birth. This responds to withholding glucose (stopping feeds) and relapses on reintroduction. The diagnosis is essentially a clinical one. Reducing substances in the stool will be positive and small-bowel biopsy and disaccharide estimation normal. Treatment is by using fructose as the main carbohydrate source. Fructose is absorbed by a different mechanism to glucose and galactose.

Sucrase–isomaltase deficiency

This is a defect in carbohydrate digestion, with the enzyme required for hydrolysis of sucrose and alpha-limit dextrins not present in the small intestine. Symptoms of watery diarrhoea and/or failure to thrive develop after the introduction of sucrose or complex carbohydrate into the diet.

- Symptoms can be very mild
- Reducing substances in the stool negative (non-reducing sugar)

Diagnosis is by stool chromatography. Management is by removal of sucrose and complex carbohydrate from the diet.

Hydrogen breath testing

The hydrogen breath test looks for carbohydrate malabsorption. The principle is that mal-absorbed carbohydrate will pass to the colon where it is metabolized by bacteria and hydrogen gas released. The gas is then absorbed and released in the breath. If there is a peak it suggests carbohydrate malabsorption. An early peak raises the possibility of bacterial overgrowth. Lactulose, which is a non-absorbable carbohydrate, can be given to ensure the colonic flora can metabolize carbohydrate and to assess transit time.

Other tests of gastrointestinal function

Xylose tolerance test

- Indirect method used to assess small-bowel absorption
- Xylose is a carbohydrate; a load (15 mg/m^2, max 25 g) is ingested and a blood level taken at 1 hour, a level of less than 25 mg/dl is suggestive of carbohydrate malabsorption
- The test is neither sensitive nor specific
- False-positive results are obtained in pernicious anaemia and when there is gut oedema

Faecal alpha-1 antitrypsin

- Serum protein, not present in the diet
- Same molecular weight as albumin
- Faecal levels reflect enteric protein loss (e.g. protein-losing enteropathy)

Faecal calprotectin

- Neutrophil protein
- Stable in faeces
- Found in both adults and children to be a simple and non-invasive measure of bowel inflammation

Faecal elastase

- Pancreas specific enzyme which is stable during intestinal transport
- Stable in faeces
- Reliable indirect marker of pancreatic function
- False-positives in short gut and bacterial overgrowth

5. GASTRO-OESOPHAGEAL REFLUX

Gastro-oesophageal reflux is common and implies passage of gastric contents into the lower oesophagus. It is a normal physiological phenomenon. It is common in infancy and also seen in older children and adults particularly after meals. It is secondary to transient relaxation of the lower oesophageal sphincter not associated with swallowing.

Differential diagnosis of gastro-oesophageal reflux

- Infection, e.g. urinary tract infection, gastroenteritis
- Intestinal obstruction, e.g. pyloric stenosis, intestinal atresia, malrotation
- Food allergy and intolerance, e.g. cows' milk allergy, soy allergy, coeliac disease
- Metabolic disorders, e.g. diabetes, inborn errors of metabolism
- Psychological problems, e.g. anxiety
- Drug-induced vomiting, e.g. cytotoxic agents
- Primary respiratory disease, e.g. asthma, cystic fibrosis

Symptoms and signs of gastro-oesophageal reflux disease

- **Typical**
  - Excessive regurgitation/vomiting
  - Nausea
  - Weight loss/failure to thrive
  - Irritability with feeds, arching, colic/food refusal
  - Dysphagia
  - Chest/epigastric discomfort
  - Excessive hiccups
  - Haematemesis/anaemia — iron-deficient
  - Aspiration pneumonia
  - Oesophageal obstruction due to stricture

- **Atypical**
  - Wheeze/intractable asthma
  - Cough/stridor
  - Apnoea/apparent life-threatening events/sudden infant death syndrome (SIDS)
  - Cyanotic episodes
  - Generalized irritability
  - Sleep disturbance
  - Neurobehavioural symptoms — breath holding, Sandifer syndrome, seizure-like events
  - Worsening of pre-existing respiratory disease
  - Secondary, e.g. post-surgery

Investigation of gastro-oesophageal reflux

The natural history of mild gastro-oesophageal reflux is resolution and many patients can be managed symptomatically with antacids and thickeners. More significant cases need further investigation particularly if there are symptoms or signs of oesophagitis. There are various investigations available which need to be considered in conjunction with the clinical picture:

- Barium radiology — not particularly sensitive or specific but will pick up anatomical problems such as malrotation or stricture

- pH study — 'gold standard' for acid reflux, but unless dual pH recording is performed (i.e. simultaneous oesophageal and gastric pH monitoring) will miss alkaline reflux
- Nuclear medicine 'milk' scan which will assess acid or alkali reflux following a physiological meal, assess gastric emptying and it is possible to do a 24-hour film to look for evidence of aspiration (technetium-99m radioscintigraphy)
- Upper GI endoscopy with biopsy

Scoring system for pH monitoring

- % of time pH <4 (reflux index)
- Number of episodes >5 minutes
- Duration of the longest episode
- Total number of reflux episodes

% of time pH <4

- Mild reflux 5–10
- Moderate reflux 10–20
- Severe 20–30

Management of gastro-oesophageal reflux

General measures
Functional reflux does not require specific treatment

Simple measures

- Explanation and reassurance
- Review of feeding, posture
- Review of feeding practice, e.g. too frequent feeds, large volume feeds
- Use of feed thickeners or an anti-reflux milk

Older children

- Lifestyle and diet
- Avoid excess fat, chocolate, tea, coffee, gaseous drinks
- Avoid tight-fitting clothes

Specific treatment

Antacids
Acid suppression
- H_2 blockers, e.g. ranitidine
- Proton-pump inhibitors, e.g. omeprazole, lansoprazole

Prokinetic drugs
- Metoclopramide
- Domperidone
- Erythromycin
- Cisapride

251

Cisapride is no longer licensed for use in children because of anxieties about potential cardiotoxicity. It can still be used on a named patient basis, although seldom is.

Step-up approach to the treatment of gastro-oesophageal reflux

Step 1 Lifestyle changes
Step 2 Antacids /thickeners/H$_2$ blockers/?prokinetics
Step 3 Proton-pump inhibitors
Step 4 Add prokinetics if not already tried/consider change in diet
Step 5 Surgery

Surgery is required for reflux resistant to medical treatment. High-risk groups include those with neurodisability or intractable respiratory symptoms exacerbated by reflux.

5.1 Differential diagnosis of reflux oesophagitis

- Cows' milk allergic oesophagitis
- Candidal oesophagitis
- Chemical oesophagitis from caustic ingestion
- Crohn's disease

5.2 Feeding problems in cerebral palsy

- Feeding difficulties may be secondary to bulbar weakness with oesophageal incoordination, primary or secondary aspiration or reflux oesophagitis.
- Additional factors such as mobility of the patient, degree of spasticity, nutritional state and the presence of other conditions such as constipation are also relevant.
- Children require careful multidisciplinary assessment by a feeding team including dietetics, speech and language therapy, occupational therapy and the neurodevelopmental paediatrician. A video barium assessment of the swallow is often indicated.
- Gastro-oesophageal reflux disease is common and should be treated aggressively.
- Attention to nutrition is of key importance and many children benefit from a feeding gastrostomy with or without an anti-reflux procedure.

5.3 Barrett's oesophagus

- Presence of metaplastic columnar epithelium in the lower oesophagus
- Thought to be a consequence of long-standing gastro-oesophageal reflux
- Increase in the risk of adenocarcinoma of the oesophagus
- Rare in childhood
- Requires aggressive medical treatment, regular endoscopic assessment and because the risk of malignancy is felt to relate to the extent of persistent exposure of the distal oesophagus to acid, surgery is often considered

Notes

- Barium swallow assesses the oesophagus
- Barium meal assesses the stomach and proximal duodenum
- Barium meal and follow-through assess the stomach and small bowel to the terminal ileum
- Small-bowel meal (administered via an nasojejunal tube assesses the small bowel only)
- Barium enema assesses the colon
- A video barium can be used to assess the swallow and check for primary aspiration

6. PEPTIC ULCER DISEASE

6.1 *Helicobacter pylori* infection

Helicobacter pylori is a Gram-negative organism. Infection is usually acquired in childhood. Prevalence rates, however, are very variable. Persistent infection causes a chronic gastritis which may be asymptomatic. There is a strong relationship between Helicobacter infection and peptic ulceration in adults. *H. pylori* is also a carcinogen. There is no proven association between Helicobacter infection and recurrent abdominal pain. Transmission is faeco-oral and familial clustering is common.

Diagnosis is by the following:

- Serology — usually reverts to negative within 6–12 months of treatment
- Rapid urease tests — C-13 breath test, CLO test
- Histology
- Culture (difficult)

Treatment is indicated for gastritis or peptic ulceration. There are various regimes. The most common used in children is omeprazole, amoxicillin and metronidazole for 2 weeks. Outcome following treatment is variable.

6.2 Other causes of antral gastritis and peptic ulceration

- Anti-inflammatory drugs
- Crohn's disease
- Zollinger–Ellison syndrome
- Autoimmune gastritis (adults)

6.3 Zollinger–Ellison syndrome

Gastrin-producing tumour of the endocrine pancreas, presenting with gastric acid hyper-secretion resulting in fulminant and intractable peptic ulcer disease.

7. CHRONIC DIARRHOEA

Chronic diarrhoea refers to diarrhoea that has persisted for more than 2–3 weeks. Children with chronic diarrhoea and failure to thrive need further assessment, as the underlying cause may be a malabsorption.

Common causes include:
* Coeliac disease
* Food intolerance
* Cystic fibrosis
* Infections/immunodeficiency
* Inflammatory bowel disease

In children with chronic diarrhoea who are thriving, alternative diagnosis such as constipation, carbohydrate intolerance and toddler's diarrhoea should be considered. Chronic constipation is a common cause presenting as apparent diarrhoea which is in fact overflow soiling.

Protracted diarrhoea/intractable diarrhoea of infancy

Refers to persistent diarrhoea starting in infancy and is less common.

Examples include:

Congenital microvillous atrophy

* Intractable diarrhoea which is present from birth
* Pathology is ultrastructural abnormality at the microvillous surface
* Long-term nutritional support with total parenteral nutrition is required

Glucose–galactose malabsorption

* See Section 4.4

Congenital chloride diarrhoea

* Autosomal recessive
* Severe watery diarrhoea starting at birth — often past history of polyhydramnios
* Serum sodium and chloride are low with a high stool pH and stool chloride
* Treatment is with sodium and potassium chloride supplements
* Prognosis is good if diagnosis is made early

Autoimmune enteropathy

- Protracted diarrhoea presenting in infancy associated with the presence of circulating autoantibodies against intestinal epithelial cells
- Severe villous atrophy with an inflammatory infiltrate
- Associated with other autoimmune conditions
- Treatment is with immunosuppression

Small-bowel biopsy

- Usually performed through a gastroscope — previously via a Crosby capsule
- Coeliac disease results in total villous atrophy with characteristic features (see later); partial villous atrophy, which is less commonly seen has a wide differential diagnosis

Differential diagnosis of partial villous atrophy

- Coeliac disease
- Transient gluten intolerance
- Cows' milk sensitive enteropathy
- Soy protein sensitive enteropathy
- Gastroenteritis and post-gastroenteritis syndromes
- Giardiasis
- Autoimmune enteropathy
- Acquired hypogammaglobulinaemia
- Tropical sprue
- Protein energy malnutrition
- Severe combined immunodeficiency (SCID)
- Antineoplastic therapy

7.1 Coeliac disease

The prevalence is between 1:1000 and 1:2000 in the UK, higher in Northern Europe. There are associations with HLA B8, DR7, DR3 and DQw2. There is an increased incidence in first-degree relatives (approximately 1:10). Intolerance is to gliadin in gluten which is present in wheat, rye, barley and oats.

Coeliac disease presents after 6 months of age (i.e. after gluten has been introduced into the diet). Chronic diarrhoea and poor weight gain (short stature in older children) generally occur. Other features include anorexia, lethargy, generalized irritability, abdominal distension and pallor. Atypical presentations with less-specific symptoms including recurrent abdominal pain are increasingly common and picked up early with the advent of antibody screening. With family screening, silent (i.e. disease in the absence of overt symptoms) coeliac disease is increasingly recognized.

Diagnosis is by small-bowel biopsy (endoscopic duodenal or jejunal). The characteristic features on biopsy are of subtotal villous atrophy, crypt hypertrophy, intraepithelial lymphocytosis and a lamina propria plasma-cell infiltrate. It is of crucial importance that the child's gluten intake is adequate at the time of the biopsy otherwise a false-negative result may be obtained.

Treatment is with a gluten-free diet for life. There is a long-term risk of small-bowel lymphoma and other gastrointestinal malignancies if the diet is not adhered to. The gluten-free diet itself has no long-term complications, although in the young child its use should be supervised by a paediatric trained dietician.

The standards for the diagnosis of coeliac disease are set out by the European Society of Paediatric Gastroenterology. Diagnosis is confirmed by characteristic histology and a clinical remission on a gluten-free diet. There are indications for a subsequent gluten challenge and these include initial diagnostic uncertainty and when the diagnosis is made under the age of 2 years. The latter being because at that age there are other causes of a flat jejunal biopsy (see above). A gluten challenge involves an initial control biopsy on a gluten-free diet followed by a period on gluten with a repeat biopsy after 3–6 months and then again after 2 years, sooner if symptoms develop. The response to a challenge can be monitored by antibody screening. There are reports of late relapse following gluten challenge.

Antibody testing in the screening of children with failure to thrive or other gastrointestinal symptoms in whom coeliac disease is a possibility and in the ongoing management of children with coeliac disease is helpful. The biopsy, however, does at the moment remain the 'gold standard' for diagnosis.

Antibody tests available:

- IgG anti-gliadin
- IgA anti-gliadin
- IgA anti-reticulin
- IgA anti-endomysial

The IgA anti-endomysial antibody is the most sensitive and specific and is currently the 'gold standard'. However false-negatives occur in children who are IgA-deficient. This means IgA levels should be done routinely alongside the endomysial antibody test.

The IgA anti-endomysial antibody will turn negative in a child with coeliac disease on a gluten-free diet. This can be used as a marker of compliance.

The most recent test that has become available is the IgA antibody to tissue transglutaminase.

Associations of coeliac disease

- Increased incidence of small-bowel malignancy, especially lymphoma
- Increased incidence of IgA deficiency
- Increased incidence of autoimmune thyroid disease, pernicious anaemia and diabetes mellitus (HLA B8 associations)
- Dermatitis herpetiformis

7.2 Cows' milk protein sensitive enteropathy

Implies enteropathy secondary to cows' milk protein and improves following withdrawal of cows' milk protein with a longer term history of resolution in most cases (see earlier).

7.3 Giardiasis

- Is a protozoal parasite which is infective in the cyst form. Also exists in the trophozoite form. Found in contaminated food and water.
- Clinical manifestations vary; can be asymptomatic, acute diarrhoeal disease, chronic diarrhoea. Partial villous atrophy is occasionally seen.
- Diagnosis is by stool examination for cysts or examination of the duodenal aspirate at small-bowel biopsy
- Treatment is with metronidazole and is often given blind in suspicious cases.

7.4 Cystic fibrosis

This subject is well covered in Chapter 17, *Respiratory*. It is important to remember the GI manifestations.

Gastrointestinal manifestations of cystic fibrosis

- **Pancreatic**
  - Insufficiency occurs in up to 90%
  - Pancreatitis
  - Abnormal glucose tolerance in up to 10% by the second decade
  - Diabetes mellitus

- **Intestinal**
  - Meconium ileus
  - Atresias
  - Rectal prolapse
  - Distal obstruction syndrome
  - Strictures ?secondary to high-dose pancreatic supplementation

- **Hepatobiliary**
  - Cholestasis in infancy
  - Fatty liver
  - Focal biliary fibrosis
  - Multilobular cirrhosis

- **Abnormalities of the gallbladder**
  - Cholelithiasis
  - Obstruction of the common bile duct

7.5 Schwachman–Diamond syndrome

- Autosomal recessive
- Incidence 1:20–200,000
- Main features — pancreatic insufficiency, neutropenia and short stature
- Other features include metaphyseal dysostosis, mild hepatic dysfunction, increased frequency of infections, further haematological abnormalities (including thrombocytopenia, increased risk of malignancy)

7.6 Bacterial overgrowth (small bowel)

- Repeated courses of antibiotics are a risk factor.
- Stasis causes bacterial proliferation with the emergence of resistant strains.
- Malabsorption results with steatorrhoea and fat-soluble vitamin malabsorption
- Diagnosis is by a high index of suspicion — particularly in patients with risk factors, e.g. previous GI surgery, short-bowel syndrome. Hydrogen breath testing may be useful. Radioisotope-labelled breath testing may also have a role. Barium radiology if obstruction is suspected. Culture of the duodenal juice.
- Treatment involves appropriate management of the underlying cause. Metronidazole, which is effective orally and intravenously, is the antibiotic of first choice. Probiotics have been used.

7.7 Intestinal lymphangiectasia

- Functional obstruction of flow of lymph through the thoracic duct and into the inferior vena cava
- Leads to fat malabsorption and a protein-losing enteropathy
- Treatment is with medium-chain triglycerides — absorbed directly into the portal vein
- Can be primary or secondary to other causes of lymphatic obstruction

8. RECURRENT ABDOMINAL PAIN

Recurrent abdominal pain is very common in childhood, affecting up to 10% of the school-age population. In the majority of cases the aetiology is non-organic. The condition is more common in girls than boys and a family history is common. The pain is usually periumbilical and rarely associated with other gastrointestinal symptoms such as diarrhoea, blood per rectum or weight loss.

Abdominal pain accompanied by other symptoms is suggestive of organic pathology. Night pain is suggestive of oesophagitis or peptic ulceration. Diarrhoea with blood per rectum suggests a colitis and diarrhoea associated with weight loss a malabsorption syndrome.

Children with chronic abdominal pain lasting for longer than 3 months should have a basic blood screen, including inflammatory markers and coeliac disease serology.

There are three syndromes:

- Isolated paroxysmal abdominal pain
- Abdominal pain associated with symptoms of dyspepsia
- Abdominal pain associated with altered bowel habit

Factors that suggest an organic cause:

- Age <5 years
- Constitutional symptoms — fever, weight loss, poor growth, joint symptoms, skin rashes
- Vomiting — particularly if bile stained
- Pain that awakens the child from sleep
- Pain away from the umbilicus +/– referred to back/shoulders
- Urinary symptoms
- Family history of inflammatory bowel disease, peptic ulcer disease
- Perianal disease
- Occult or gross blood in the stool
- Abnormal screening blood tests

8.1 Functional abdominal pain

This implies non-organic pain. It is more common in girls than boys. Children are usually older than 5 years. Peak age 8–9 years. Pain is usually gradual onset, variable severity with symptom-free periods, periumbilical, lasts 1–3 hours, type of pain (e.g. burning, stabbing) unclear, rarely causes a child to wake from sleep, not usually related to meals, activity or bowel movement. Loose diagnostic criteria is three or more episodes in 3 months. Pain interferes with normal activity, e.g. results in time off school. Extraintestinal symptoms common (e.g. headache). Family history common. Child often offered positive reinforcement for symptoms.

Normal examination. Normal investigations.

Associations

- Timid, nervous anxious characters
- Perfectionists — over-achievers
- Increased number of stresses and more likely to internalize problems than other children, but no increase in the risk of depression or other psychiatric problems when compared with children with organic pain
- School absence common — may be a degree of school refusal — may be issues at school

Remember children with organic pathology can suffer from non-organic pain and children with non-organic pain can also have organic pathology.

Management of functional abdominal pain

1. Positive diagnosis
2. Education
3. Realistic expectation of treatment

- Pain is real not psychogenic or imaginary
- Goal of management cannot be total freedom from pain
- Support the child
- Avoid environmental reinforcement
- Review associated symptoms (e.g. headache)
- Dietary triggers (fibre, lactose, chocolate)
- Lifestyle issues, e.g. exercise, school attendance
- Diary of symptoms occasionally useful in severe cases

A number of children in this group benefit from the diagnostic label 'irritable bowel syndrome'. A number of children with recurrent abdominal pain in childhood go on either to develop migraine or recurrent tension headache as adults.

9. INFLAMMATORY BOWEL DISEASE

The recent British Paediatric Surveillance Unit survey suggests the incidence of inflammatory bowel disease in children under 16 is 5:100,000, with Crohn's disease being twice as common as ulcerative colitis.

9.1 Crohn's disease

Crohn's disease is a chronic inflammatory disorder of bowel involving any region from mouth to anus. The inflammation is transmural with skip lesions. There has been an increase in incidence over the past 10 years. 10–15% of cases present in childhood, usually in the second decade. The commonest presenting symptoms are abdominal pain, diarrhoea and weight loss. Growth failure with delayed bone maturation and delayed sexual development is common. The diagnosis is made on the basis of clinical symptoms, raised inflammatory indices and diagnostic tests including barium radiology, gastroscopy and colonoscopy with biopsy. White cell scanning is not useful as a diagnostic test as it is not sufficiently sensitive, particularly in small-bowel disease. Treatment is difficult as the disease often runs a chronic relapsing course. The aim of management is to induce a disease remission and facilitate normal growth and development.

The most widely used treatment in children is enteral nutrition, used as an exclusion diet for up to 8 weeks followed by a period of controlled food reintroduction. The type of enteral nutrition used varies and can be either elemental (protein broken down into peptide chains or amino acids) or polymeric (whole protein). This induces remission in up to 90% of patients. Maintenance is with 5 ASA derivatives and continued nutritional support. Unfortunately disease relapse is common and either repeated courses of enteral nutrition or corticosteroids are usually required. Corticosteroid dependence or resistance can occur and additional immunosuppression or surgery is indicated. The most commonly used additional immunosuppressive agent is azathioprine which will reduce steroid requirements in 60–80%, and in many of those patients induce a long-term remission. Important toxicity includes the risk of myelosuppression and so regular blood counts are required. Other medications tried include thalidomide, methotrexate and monoclonal antibodies to tumour necrosis factor-alpha. Surgical resection is indicated for disease resistant to medical therapy particularly if there is growth failure, although there is a high risk of recurrence following surgery.

Extraintestinal manifestations of Crohn's disease

- Joint disease in 10% — ankylosing spondylitis rarely
- Skin rashes — erythema nodosum, erythema multiforme, pyoderma gangrenosum
- Liver disease (rare in childhood) — sclerosing cholangitis, chronic active hepatitis, cirrhosis
- Uveitis
- Osteoporosis

9.2 Ulcerative colitis

- Ulcerative colitis is an inflammatory disease limited to the colonic and rectal mucosa. It is the more distal bowel that is the most involved. Inflammation is neither pan-enteric or transmural as is seen in Crohn's disease. A backwash ileitis into the terminal ileum is often seen. The characteristic histology in the colon is of mucosal and submucosal inflammation with goblet-cell depletion, cryptitis and crypt abscesses but no granulomas. The inflammatory change is usually diffuse rather than patchy.
- Aetiology is unknown. Disease is more common in females than males.
- The gut disease can be mild, moderate or severe. The symptoms of colitis are diarrhoea, blood per rectum and abdominal pain. Systemic disturbance can accompany more severe disease; tachycardia, fever, weight loss, anaemia, hypoalbuminaemia and leucocytosis.
- Although unusual, the disease can present with predominantly extraintestinal manifestations including growth failure, arthropathy, erythema nodosum.
- The presentation can be more indolent with occult blood loss, non-specific abdominal pain, cholangitis and raised inflammatory indices.
- Complications of ulcerative colitis include toxic megacolon, growth failure, cholangitis, carcinoma, non-malignant stricture. The cancer risk reflects the disease severity and duration of disease. Regular screening is carried out in adult life.
- Diagnosis is by endoscopy and biopsy with the classical histological features being shown. A small number of children have an indeterminate or unclassified colitis. The differential diagnosis of colitis is wide and a list of the causes of a non-infective and an infective colitis are listed overleaf. It is, for example, crucial to exclude infection in a child presenting with acute colitis which, particularly if the disease is of short duration, is more likely.

Management is with 5 ASA derivatives, local or systemic steroids, azathioprine to reduce steroid toxicity in steroid-dependent patients. Surgical resection is indicated in resistant cases. Surgery is a colectomy with ileostomy. Reversal is possible in early adult life by ileoanal anastomosis and pouch formation.

Management of toxic colitis involves intravenous fluids, antibiotics and corticosteroids.

Differences between Crohn's disease and ulcerative colitis

Crohn's	Ulcerative colitis
Panenteric	Colon only
Skip lesions	Diffuse
Transmural	Mucosal
Granulomas	Crypt abscesses
Perianal disease	

Colitis can be indeterminate, i.e. the histological features are consistent with inflammatory bowel disease but not diagnostic of either Crohn's disease or ulcerative colitis.

9.3 Differential diagnosis of colitis

Causes of infective colitis

Salmonella spp.
Shigella spp.
Campylobacter pylori
Escherichia coli 0157 (and other *E. coli*)
Clostridium difficile (pseudomembranous colitis)
Yersinia spp.
Tuberculosis
Cytomegalovirus
Entamoeba histolytica

Causes of a non-infective colitis

Ulcerative colitis
Crohn's disease
Necrotizing enterocolitis
Microscopic colitis
Behçet's disease
Food allergic colitis
Enterobius vermicularis

9.4 Pseudomembranous colitis

- Occurs secondary to *Clostridium difficile* — Gram-positive anaerobe
- Risk factor is disruption of the normal intestinal flora by antibiotics

- Clinical features vary from asymptomatic carriage to life-threatening pseudomembranous colitis
- Pathogenesis is through toxin production
- Treatment is with vancomycin (oral) or metronidazole (i.v. or oral); probiotics may have a role
- Relapse rate is 15–20%

9.5 Behçet's syndrome

- Orogenital ulceration with/without non-erosive arthritis, thrombophlebitis, vascular thromboses or CNS abnormalities including meningoencephalitis
- Treatment of orogenital ulceration is often unsatisfactory, however local and/or systemic steroids may be used acutely
- Other drugs that have been used in prophylaxis include azathioprine and thalidomide

10. GASTROINTESTINAL BLEEDING

Can present as haematemesis (usually upper GI source), malaena (partially digested blood) or frank blood per rectum.

10.1 Causes of gastrointestinal bleeding

- Anal fissure
- Volvulus
- Intussusception
- Peptic ulcer
- Polyp
- Meckel's diverticulum
- Inflammatory bowel disease
- Haemolytic–uraemic syndrome
- Infective colitis
- Henoch–Schönlein purpura
- Vascular malformation
- Oesophagitis/varices
- Epistaxis/swallowed blood — including swallowed maternal bood in the neonatal period
- Necrotizing enterocolitis
- Haemorrhagic disease of the newborn
- Trauma/sexual abuse

10.2 Intussusception

- Peak incidence aged 6–9 months. Male to female ratio 4:1.

- Usually presents with spasmodic pain, pallor and irritability. Vomiting is an early feature and rapidly progresses to being bile stained. Passage of blood-stained stools often occurs and a mass is frequently palpable. The presentation, however, is often atypical.
- The intussusception is usually ileocaecal, the origin being either the ileocaecal valve or the terminal ileum.
- An identifiable cause is commoner in those who present later — Meckel's, polyp, reduplication, lymphosarcoma and Henoch–Schönlein purpura being examples.
- Diagnosis is usually on clinical grounds. Confirmation is by plain abdominal X-ray, ultrasound or air-enema examination.
- Treatment is either with air-enema reduction if the history is short or surgically at laparotomy. Resuscitation with saline is often required. Contraindications to air enema include peritonitis and signs of perforation.

10.3 Meckel's diverticulum

- Remnant of the vitellointestinal duct
- Present in 2% of individuals
- 50% contain ectopic gastric, pancreatic or colonic tissue
- Distal ileum on the anti-mesenteric border within 100 cm of the ileocaecal valve and is around 5–6 cm long
- Presents with intermittent, painless blood per rectum; bleeding can be quite severe and may require a blood transfusion; other presentations include intussusception (commoner in older males), perforation and peritonitis
- The technetium scan is used to look for ectopic gastric mucosa

10.4 Polyposis

Juvenile polyps

85% of polyps seen in childhood. Present at age 2–6 years with painless blood per rectum. Most polyps are solitary and located within 30 cm of the anus. Not premalignant.

Peutz–Jeghers syndrome

Autosomal dominant inheritance. Diffuse gastrointestinal hamartomatous polyps associated with hyperpigmentation of the buccal mucosa and lips. Premalignant.

Gardener's syndrome and familial adenomatous polyposis coli

Best considered together. Both conditions are inherited as an autosomal dominant. Gardener's syndrome is familial adenomatous polyposis plus bony lesions, subcutaneous tumours and cysts. Both conditions carry a very high risk of colonic carcinoma and prophylactic colectomy at the end of the second decade is advised.

11. GASTROENTERITIS

Gastroenteritis remains a common problem. The majority of cases can be managed at home. Oral rehydration therapy is the mainstay of treatment, with rapid rehydration over 4–6 hours with reassessment and the early reintroduction of normal feeds after that. Breast feeding should not be stopped. Antimicrobials are only of use in very specific circumstances. Antidiarrhoeal agents are of no use. Complications such as carbohydrate intolerance and chronic diarrhoea and failure to thrive are relatively rare.

Composition of oral rehydration solution (ORS)

Oral rehydration therapy (ORT), which has probably saved more children's lives world-wide than any other medical intervention, remains the mainstay of treatment. WHO-ORS contains 90 mmol/l of sodium and is specifically designed for cholera treatment. European ORS contain between 35 and 60 mmol/l sodium with varying concentrations of glucose and potassium. There remains controversy over the best combination but it would appear that all of the available formulations are effective and safe. Home-made solutions, usually with an excess of salt, put children at risk of hypernatraemic dehydration.

Causes of gastroenteritis

- **Unknown**: In both the developed and undeveloped world, no pathogens are identified in up to 50% of cases, even when the condition is fully investigated
- **Viral**: Rotaviruses (commonest), adenovirus, small-round viruses, and astroviruses
- **Bacterial**: Campylobacter (commonest), *Shigella* spp., *Salmonella* spp., enteropathogenic *E.coli*, enterotoxigenic *E.coli* 0157:H7 (rare but associated with haemolytic–uraemic syndrome), *Vibrio cholerae*, *Yersinia enterocolitica*
- **Protozoa**: Cryptosporidium (particularly in the immunocompromised host), Giardia which has a varied presentation from the asymptomatic carrier state to chronic diarrhoea with growth failure, *Entamoeba histolytica* (amoebic dysentery)

Differential diagnosis

This is potentially wide and includes many other potential conditions including:

- Other infections, e.g. otitis media, tonsillitis, pneumonia, septicaemia, urinary tract infection, meningitis
- Gastro-oesophageal reflux
- Food intolerance
- Haemolytic–uraemic syndrome
- Intussusception
- Pyloric stenosis
- Acute appendicitis
- Drugs, e.g. laxatives, antibiotics

Assessment of dehydration

% Dehydration	Severity	Clinical features
3		Undetectable
3–5	Mild	Slightly dry mucous membranes
5	Moderate	Decreased skin turgor, slightly sunken eyes, depressed fontanelle, circulation preserved
10	Severe	All above more marked, drowsiness, rapid weak pulse, cool extremities, capillary refill time greater than 2s
12–14	Moribund	

Children with 10% dehydration usually require intravenous fluid resuscitation

Remember:

- <3% dehydration is clinically not apparent
- A normal capillary refill time (<2 seconds) makes severe dehydration very unlikely (measured by pressing the skin and measuring the time taken for the skin to re-perfuse)
- Useful signs include reduced skin turgor, dry oral mucosa, sunken eyes and altered conscious level

Hospital admission should be considered when:

- Diagnosis is unclear/complications have arisen, e.g. carbohydrate intolerance (see earlier)
- Home management fails/unable to tolerate fluids/persistent vomiting
- Severe dehydration
- Significant other medical condition, e.g. diabetes, immunocompromised
- Poor social circumstances
- Hydration difficult to assess, e.g. obesity
- Inability to reassess

11.1 Post-gastroenteritis syndromes

Acute gastroenteritis usually resolves in 7–10 days. Chronic diarrhoea is defined as diarrhoea lasting >3 weeks, particularly if associated with poor weight gain/weight loss (should be referred for investigation). The continuing diarrhoea may be secondary to a second infection or reflect the 'unmasking' of another pathology, for example coeliac disease, cows' milk protein intolerance or cystic fibrosis.

12. CONSTIPATION

Childhood constipation is common. Most children do not have an underlying cause and their constipation is functional.

Many factors can trigger constipation including:

- Intercurrent illness with poor fluid and food intake
- Perianal pathology such as anal fissure or streptococcal infection resulting in stool withholding
- Difficult early toilet training resulting in stool withholding

If associated with a mega rectum then soiling is common. A plain abdominal X-ray may be helpful in the assessment of such patients with the potential to assess severity and extent. This can be helpful particularly in the obese patient when clinical assessment is often difficult. The soiling occurs because the normal sensory process of stool being in the rectum, resulting in distension and the urge to defecate, is lost when the rectum is permanently distended. This should be distinguished from encopresis in which stool is passed in to the pants at inappropriate times and in inappropriate places with no underlying constipation — the latter being a primarily psychological problem.

Underlying physical causes need to be considered for the purpose of the exam, including Hirschsprung's disease, endocrine causes such as thyroid disease and meconium ileus equivalent or distal intestinal obstruction syndrome seen in children with cystic fibrosis.

Hirschsprung's disease is very rare in children who have at some stage of their life had a normal bowel habit and usually presents in the neonatal period.

Most constipation is short term and is readily treated with bulk and/or stimulant laxatives.

The management of chronic functional constipation is more difficult and often requires a multidisciplinary approach. Many factors are often involved in perpetuation of the problem including local pathology such as anal fissure, lower abdominal pain, poor diet, poor fluid intake, lack of exercise, previous difficult toileting experiences, and psychosocial problems. High doses of stimulant and bulk laxatives are required, usually for a prolonged period. Enema therapy, which can reinforce difficult toileting experiences, should be reserved for the more difficult cases. An essential part of management is explanation and reassurance and practical advice and support in the institution of a toileting regimen. Children need to sit on the toilet regularly, this is best 15–30 minutes after meals.

Commonly used laxatives include lactulose, sodium docussate, Senokot, sodium picosulphate.

Constipation is common in children with nocturnal and diurnal enuresis and treatment of the constipation frequently results in a significant improvement in the wetting.

12.1 Perianal streptococcal infection

- Common cause of perianal redness
- Can present as constipation or perianal pain
- Secondary to group A Streptococcus
- Treatment is with penicillin, there may be a need for continuing laxatives

Other causes of perianal soreness

- Poor perineal hygiene
- Soiling/encopresis
- Threadworm infestation
- Lactose intolerance (acidic stool)
- Anal fissure
- Sexual abuse (rare)

12.2 Hirschsprung's disease

- Absence of ganglion cells in the myenteric plexus of the most distal bowel
- Males > females. 1 in 5,000. Gene on chromosome 10
- Long-segment Hirschsprung's disease is familial with equal sex incidence
- Associated with Down's syndrome; high frequency of other congenital abnormalities
- Usually presents in infancy, failure to pass meconium with presentation in the older child being rare — the diagnosis in this group usually being chronic functional constipation; most children with Hirschsprung's will have never had a normal bowel habit
- Enterocolitis commonly can occur before or after surgery
- Definitive test = rectal biopsy to confirm the absence of ganglion cells in the sub mucosal plexus; histochemistry will demonstrate excessive acetylcholinesterase activity and the absence of ganglion cells
- Surgery is excision, usually with temporary colostomy followed by pull-through at a later stage
- Ultrashort-segment Hirschsprung's disease is very rare and can present significant diagnostic difficulty

13. MISCELLANEOUS

13.1 Pyloric stenosis

Projectile non-bilious vomiting, onset between 3 weeks and 5 months of age.

- Infant presents hungry and with weight loss
- First-born males more commonly affected
- Palpable pyloric tumour and visible gastric peristalsis present
- Mild unconjugated hyperbilirubinaemia and hypochloraemic, hypokalaemic metabolic alkalosis occurs

- Ultrasound confirms the diagnosis
- Treatment is by pyloromyotomy (Ramstedt's procedure) after correction of the electrolyte and acid–base disturbance

13.2 Appendicitis

- Most common surgical emergency in childhood
- Rare under age 1 year
- Peaks in adolescence
- Many normal appendices are removed
- 30% diagnosed after perforation
- Pain, vomiting and fever; raised white cell count is common
- Right iliac fossa pain with rebound tenderness (McBurney's point) is the classical presentation but atypical presentations are common; pelvic appendicitis is commonly diagnosed late
- Differential diagnosis includes urinary tract infection, mesenteric adenitis (common), constipation, Henoch–Schönlein purpura, Meckel's diverticulum
- Ultrasound can be useful but is not sensitive or specific
- Management is appendicectomy

13.3 Pancreatitis

Acute pancreatitis

Common causes in childhood include:

- Infections, e.g. mumps, coxsackieviruses, EBV, hepatitis A, HIV
- Biliary tract disease, e.g. choledochal cyst, choledocholithiasis
- Trauma
- Multisystem disease, e.g. SLE, Kawasaki's disease, haemolytic–uraemic syndrome, inflammatory bowel disease
- Drugs, e.g. azathioprine, 5 ASA derivatives
- Metabolic and systemic diseases, e.g. cystic fibrosis, metabolic disease, malnutrition and refeeding, diabetes mellitus, hyperlipidaemia

Symptoms can be non-specific with abdominal pain, tenderness, nausea, vomiting, low-grade fever and reduced bowel sounds with distension. Acute haemorrhagic pancreatitis (rare) can be fulminant at presentation and has a high mortality. Serum amylase is typically elevated 4–5 times above normal. Serum lipase can be measured. CRP is useful prognostically and to monitor progress. Ultrasound +/– CT/MRI can be helpful. Management is generally supportive with adequate fluids and analgesia. An underlying cause should be sought. Pancreatic pseudocyst is a rare complication and surgical drainage may be necessary.

NB. A raised amylase does not necessarily signify pancreatitis. It can occur with salivary gland pathology, other intra-abdominal pathology including biliary tract disease, peptic ulceration, peritonitis, intestinal obstruction and appendicitis, and in more systemic disease such as acidosis, renal insufficiency and drug ingestion.

Chronic pancreatitis

This is usually hereditary (autosomal dominant, positive family history) or due to congenital abnormalities of the pancreatic or biliary duct system. Other causes include hyperlipidaemia and cystic fibrosis.

13.4 Ascites

Not obvious clinically in up to 50%. Clinical features include abdominal distension with bulging of the flanks, protrusion of the umbilicus, scrotal swelling, fluid thrill, shifting dullness. Differential diagnosis is wide and includes cirrhosis, congestive cardiac failure, nephrotic syndrome, protein-losing enteropathy.

14. LIVER DISEASE

14.1 Physiology of bilirubin metabolism

Red blood cells are phagocytosed by the reticuloendothelial system. Bilirubin is formed from the catabolism of haem. Transported to liver bound to albumin. Bilirubin is then conjugated with glucuronic acid by glucuronyl transferase in the liver and excreted in the bile. Bacterial metabolism of bilirubin in the bowel leads to formation of urobilinogen, some of which enters the enterohepatic circulation and is excreted in the bile.

Biliary obstruction leads to conjugated hyperbilirubinaemia which is excreted in the urine rather than stool and leads to pale stools and dark urine.

14.2 Neonatal jaundice

Causes of unconjugated hyperbilirubinaemia in the neonatal period

Physiological
Breast milk
Sepsis
Haemolysis   Rhesus incompatibility
                      ABO incompatibility
                      Hereditary spherocytosis
                      Glucose 6-phosphate dehydrogenase deficiency
                      Pyruvate kinase deficiency
Polycythaemia/bruising
Hypothyroidism
Galactosaemia
Cystic fibrosis including meconium ileus
Crigler–Najjar syndrome
Gilbert's syndrome

Crigler–Najjar syndrome

- Type I (autosomal recessive) is due to complete absence of uridine diphosphate (UDP) glucuronyl transferase in the liver. Jaundice presents soon after birth and rapidly progresses to toxic levels (kernicterus). Untreated, death usually occurs by the end of the first year. Diagnosis is by estimation of hepatic UDP glucuronyl transferase activity in a specimen obtained by needle liver biopsy. Repeated exchange transfusions and phototherapy aid short-term survival. The only long-term therapeutic option is liver transplantation.
- Type II (autosomal dominant) is less severe and responds to treatment with phenobarbital. Kernicterus is unusual.

Gilbert's syndrome

- Gilbert's syndrome is defined as unconjugated hyperbilirubinaemia with no evidence of haemolysis and normal liver function tests. If done the liver biopsy is normal.
- The prevalence is 6%. The condition is more common in males than females. Inheritance is autosomal dominant with incomplete expression.
- The pathogenesis is unclear but probably represents a mild functional deficiency of the enzyme UDP glucuronyl transferase.
- The clinical picture is of mild fluctuating jaundice (serum bilirubin 30–50 μmol/l) aggravated by infection, exertion and fasting. Of some diagnostic use, the condition improves with phenobarbital and worsens with nicotinic acid.

Conjugated hyperbilirubinaemia in the neonatal period

Infectious — hepatitis A, B, C, cytomegalovirus (CMV), rubella, herpes simplex
Metabolic — cystic fibrosis, tyrosinaemia, galactosaemia, fructosaemia
Intrahepatic — Alagille's syndrome, congenital hepatic fibrosis
Extrahepatic — biliary atresia, choledochal cyst, inspissated bile syndrome
Toxic — TPN-related, sepsis, urinary tract infection, drugs
Endocrine — hypopituitarism, hypothyroidism
Miscellaneous — intestinal obstruction

Dubin–Johnson and rotor syndromes

Dubin–Johnson syndrome
Autosomal recessive. Presents with conjugated hyperbilirubinaemia and bilirubinuria. It is due to a reduced ability to transport organic anions such as bilirubin glucuronide into the biliary tree. Black pigmentation of the liver on biopsy. Life expectancy is normal. Jaundice is exacerbated by alcohol, infection and pregnancy.

Rotor syndrome
Autosomal recessive. Presents with conjugated hyperbilirubinaemia. It is due to a deficiency in organic anion uptake as well as excretion. No black pigment in the liver. Normal life expectancy. Jaundice exacerbated by alcohol, infection and pregnancy. Sulphabromopthalein excretion test is abnormal.

14.3 Extra-hepatic biliary atresia

Currently, biliary atresia is the commonest indication for liver transplantation in childhood. Most of this is extrahepatic biliary atresia. The incidence 1 in 8,000 to 20,000 live births. The disorder is thought to be acquired. Presents as neonatal cholestasis. Investigation is complex and any infant with prolonged jaundice which is predominantly conjugated needs to be referred to a liver centre for further assessment. Treatment is with a portoenterostomy (Kasai procedure). The outcome is much better if surgery is carried out before 3 months of age. Post-operatively there is a high risk of cholecystitis and children need intravenous antibiotic therapy if unwell. A proportion go on to get chronic liver disease and a number require transplantation.

Intrahepatic biliary atresia

This is less common and can be either syndromic or non-syndromic. Alagille's syndrome is an example worth remembering.

Alagille's syndrome

- Paucity of intrahepatic bile ducts
- Characteristic facies — prominent forehead, wide-apart deep-set eyes, small pointed chin
- Vertebral arch defects/hemivertebrae butterfly vertebra
- Renal tract anomalies
- Embryotoxon (slit lamp for cornea)
- Growth retardation
- Mental retardation
- Hypoglycaemia
- Heart disease — usually peripheral pulmonary stenosis

Alpha-1 antitrypsin deficiency
Autosomal recessive phenotype determined by Pi (protease inhibitor) typing. The condition presents with cholestasis in infancy, cirrhosis in childhood and chronic obstructive pulmonary disease in early adult life.

15. ACUTE HEPATITIS

15.1 Hepatitis A

- RNA virus. Diagnosis is by detection of the hepatitis A virus IgM. Transmission is faeco-oral. There is no carrier state and fulminant hepatic failure is very rare (<0.1%). The liver function however may be abnormal for up to 1 year.
- Prevention is by either passive or active immunization. Passive immunization is with immunoglobulin which lasts for 3–6 months. Active immunization is with a live attenuated virus. Booster immunization being required after 12–18 months.
- Clinical symptoms are initially non-specific and include anorexia, nausea, fatigue and fever associated with epigastric pain and tender hepatomegaly. The icteric phase then

develops with jaundice, pale stools and dark urine. Sometimes there is pruritus, depression and persistent jaundice with raised transaminases for a prolonged period. The prothrombin time should be monitored. A raised prothrombin time raises the possibility of severe hepatic necrosis or decompensation of underlying liver disease.

15.2 Hepatitis B

- Is a DNA virus. Diagnosis is by detection of the hepatitis B surface antigen (HBsAg). HBeAg-positive patients carry a larger virus load and are more infectious. Acute and ongoing chronic infection is associated with anti-HBcIgM (where c = core). Anti-Hbe and Anti-HBs antibodies appear as an effective immune response develops. All HBsAg-positive subjects are infective.
- Transmission is parenteral, percutaneous in blood or contaminated fluid.
- The perinatal transmission rate is dependent upon the maternal serology. If mother is HBsAg +ve and HBeAg –ve the risk is 12–25%. If mother is HBsAg +ve and HBeAg +ve the risk is 90%.
- The younger the age at infection the less the likelihood of symptomatic liver disease but the greater the risk of prolonged viral carriage. 90% of infants infected in the first year of life become chronic carriers.
- Clinically the disease is often asymptomatic but an acute hepatitic picture can develop with acute liver failure in <1%. The risk of fulminant hepatitis is increased by co-infection with hepatitis D. In those with a typical hepatitic picture the chronic carrier rate is low.
- Chronicity results in an increased risk of cirrhosis and hepatocellular carcinoma. Males are more likely to become chronic carriers than females. Chronically infected children have a 25% lifetime risk of cirrhosis or hepatocellular carcinoma.
- Prevention is by both active and passive immunization
- Interferon-alpha is a recognized treatment of chronic infection

Vertical transmission of hepatitis B

- Vertical transmission is thought to account for 40% of hepatitis B world-wide.
- The hallmark of ongoing infection is the presence of HBsAg. The presence of antibody to HBsAg alone suggests successful immunization; its presence along with anti-HBcAg suggests resolved infection.
- Mainly thought to occur around the time of birth.
- Risk of transmission is increased to a rate of > 90% if the mother is HBeAg-positive.
- Hepatitis B immunoglobulin given at birth alone reduces the risk of vertical transmission.
- The effect of giving active immunization (hepatitis B vaccine at birth, 1 and 6 months) and passive immunization with hepatitis B immunoglobulin is additive.
- Protection is achieved in 93% of neonates.
- Active immunization does not seem to be affected by transmitted maternal IgG.

15.3 Hepatitis C

- RNA virus. Transmission is either perinatal or parenteral. The vertical transmission rate is 9%, higher in HIV-positive mothers. Diagnosis is usually by serology with the detection of the anti-HCV antibody. Blood and blood products for transfusion have been screened since 1990.
- Infection is usually asymptomatic or an acute hepatitis can occur. Fulminant hepatitis is uncommon but can occur. HCV RNA detection establishes the presence of viraemia confirming infection and infectivity. Persistence of HCV RNA indicates continuing infection.
- Chronic infection is common (prevalence 0.2–0.7% in Northern Europe, 1–2% in Southern Europe and Japan) with the development of cirrhosis and hepatocellular carcinoma in a number of cases, after an interval of 10–15 years.
- Treatment with interferon-alpha has been given. No vaccine is available.

15.4 Hepatitis D

- RNA virus. Parenteral transmission.
- Can only replicate in the presence of hepatitis B virus, and so can only occur in hepatitis B carriers.
- Diagnosis is by detection of antihepatitis D antibodies and HbsAg in the serum.
- Presentation can be asymptomatic, with acute hepatitis or fulminant hepatic failure.
- Successful eradication requires high-dose interferon.

15.5 Hepatitis E

- RNA virus. Epidemics occur in developing countries. UK infection is usually in travellers from endemic areas. Transmission is faeco-oral.
- The clinical course of hepatitis E infection is similar to hepatitis A. Complete recovery from acute infection occurs. Chronic infection has not been described, although acute fulminant hepatic failure can occur and is more common during pregnancy.
- Diagnosis is by serology. No vaccine treatment or prophylaxis is available.

16. CHRONIC LIVER DISEASE

16.1 Portal hypertension

The cardinal feature of portal hypertension is splenomegaly. Portal hypertension does not necessarily imply liver disease. If there are no clinical or biochemical features of liver disease and the liver is not enlarged, portal vein obstruction is the most likely cause.

Clinical features of portal hypertension

- Splenomegaly
- Cutaneous portosystemic shunts (caput medusae — flow from the umbilicus, venous hum above the umbilicus, haemorrhoids)
- Ascites, hypoalbuminaemia, increased incidence of infections
- Liver small or hepatomegaly
- Failure to thrive, reduced muscle bulk

As a consequence of the portosystemic shunts:
- Gastrointestinal haemorrhage (oesophageal varices, internal haemorrhoids)
- Encephalopathy

As a consequence of the large spleen (hypersplenism):
- Thrombocytopenia
- Anaemia
- Leucopenia

The commonest causes of portal hypertension are:
- Cirrhosis
- Portal vein obstruction
- Congenital hepatic fibrosis
- Hepatic vein outflow obstruction

Causes of portal hypertension

Pre-hepatic

Portal vein thrombosis

Intrahepatic

Pre-sinusoidal	Neoplasia	
	Schistosomiasis	
	Hepatic cyst	
Sinusoidal	Cirrhosis	Biliary atresia
		Neonatal hepatitis
		Alpha 1 antitrypsin deficiency
Post-sinusoidal	Veno-occlusive disease	

Post-hepatic

Budd–Chiari syndrome
Right ventricular failure
Constrictive pericarditis

Portal vein obstruction

50% no obvious aetiology, probably a developmental defect. Other causes include congenital abnormalities of the portal vein, intra-abdominal sepsis and umbilical catheterization in the neonatal period. Presentation is usually either with asymptomatic splenomegaly or life-threatening bleeding. Occasionally the presentation can be with failure to thrive.

Congenital hepatic fibrosis

Autosomal recessive. Child looks well. Large hard liver with well-preserved liver function. Large spleen secondary to portal hypertension. Large polycystic kidneys (75%).

16.2 Chronic hepatitis

Chronic hepatitis implies continuing inflammation, necrosis and fibrosis that can lead to cirrhosis. The commonest causes are hepatitis B and C, autoimmune liver disease and chronic drug induced hepatitis.

Presentation can be minor, insidious, acute or fulminant.

Autoimmune liver disease

- This encompasses disorders of the liver associated with circulating autoantibodies in which the inflammatory response targets either the parenchyma (autoimmune hepatitis) or the biliary tree (sclerosing cholangitis)
- Variable in presentation
- Usually responsive to anti-inflammatory and immunosuppressive therapy

16.3 Drug-induced liver disease

Includes direct hepatotoxicity (e.g. paracetamol) and adverse drug reactions.

- NSAIDs
- Antimicrobials including antituberculous drugs
- Anticonvulsants
- Anticancer drugs
- Immunosuppressive drugs

16.4 Cirrhosis

- Biliary tract disorders
  - Biliary atresia
  - Choledochal cyst
  - Congenital hepatic fibrosis
  - Cystic fibrosis
  - Sclerosing cholangitis

- Genetic and metabolic causes
  - Alpha-1 antitrypsin deficiency
  - Wilson's disease
  - Glycogen storage disease

- Infection
  - Hepatitis B and C
  - CMV

- Autoimmune disease

- Drugs and toxins — alcohol

- Nutrition
  - TPN

Clinical features of cirrhosis

- Failure to thrive
- Clubbing
- Anaemia
- Jaundice (variable)
- Palmar erythema
- Xanthelasma
- Spider naevi
- Large hard or small impalpable liver
- Encephalopathy

Complications of cirrhosis

- Portal hypertension
- Bleeding diatheses
- Increased susceptibility to infections
- Hyperdynamic circulation
- Ascites
- Spontaneous bacterial peritonitis
- Pulmonary hypertension
- Hepatoma
- Malnutrition
- Gallstone formation
- Renal failure
- Hepatic encephalopathy
- Endocrine changes
- Impaired hepatic metabolism of drugs and hormones

Management of cirrhosis

- If possible determine the cause and treat the underlying condition.
- Minimize further liver damage.
- Diet containing adequate protein and essential fatty acids, trace elements and vitamins for growth and normal activities; plus adequate calorie intake. Monitor prothrombin time and fat-soluble vitamin status.
- Ascites best dealt with by restricting salt intake and/or diuretics.
- Children with alimentary bleeding should be admitted, even if small for assessment as they may have a slow initial bleed followed by a massive bleed. Should have an i.v. line, cross-match and think of the cause.
- Bacterial peritonitis should be sought early and managed aggressively with appropriate antibiotics.
- Hepatic encephalopathy; prevent the accumulation of ammonia, remove/correct identifiable precipitating factors, improve liver function by reducing protein intake, antibiotics — neomycin and lactulose
- Hepatorenal failure is usually a terminal event requiring liver transplantation.

16.5 Wilson's disease (hepatolenticular degeneration)

- Incidence 1:500,000. Autosomal recessive inheritance. Gene known and is on chromosome 13.
- The pathology is as a consequence of decreased biliary excretion of copper and impaired caeruloplasmin production. Caeruloplasmin is the plasma protein which transports copper.

Effects

Liver	Chronic active hepatitis, portal hypertension and fulminant hepatic failure
Brain	Progressive lenticular degeneration due to copper deposition; Psychiatric disorders
Cornea	Kayser–Fleischer rings
Lens	Sunflower cataract
Kidney	Renal tubular disorders
Blood	Haemolysis

- The hepatic presentation can be as asymptomatic hepatomegaly, acute hepatitis, chronic active hepatitis, portal hypertension (ascites, oedema, variceal haemorrhage) or fulminant hepatic failure. The lenticular degeneration usually presents with tremor.
- Diagnosis is by a low plasma caeruloplasmin level and high urinary copper excretion. The latter can occur in other forms of hepatitis and a liver biopsy is often required. In equivocal cases the increased copper excretion after chelation with D-penicillamine is of diagnostic importance.
- Untreated, the condition is fatal. Treated, the prognosis is good. Treatment is with oral penicillamine as a copper-binding agent in conjunction with a low copper diet. Patients on penicillamine require vitamin B_6 supplements as it is an antimetabolite. Other drugs include triethylene tetramine hydrochloride and zinc.
- The condition does not present under the age of 5 years.

16.6 Liver transplantation

- Indications
  1. Endstage chronic disease — likelihood of death within 12 months or evidence of deterioration which will worsen the prognosis for liver transplantation
  2. Unacceptable quality of life
  3. Fulminant or subacute liver failure — age <2 years or INR >4
  4. Metabolic disorders, e.g. Wilson's, alpha-1 antitrypsin, galactosaemia
  5. Liver tumours

- 90% 2-year survival; 64–75% 5-year survival
- Lifelong immunosuppression
- Supply of suitable donors major limiting factor
- Can split organ between recipients or use one part of liver from a related donor
- Complications
  - Major surgery
  - Long-term antirejection drugs
  - Rejection — worse in first month but may occur any time

16.7 Causes of hepatomegaly

Differential diagnosis of hepatomegaly

Infection
Hepatitis A
Hepatitis B
EBV infection

Storage disorders

Fat
Cystic fibrosis
Obesity
Malnutrition
TPN

Lipid
Gaucher's disease

Glycogen
Glycogen storage disease

Infiltration
Primary liver tumours
Secondary tumour, e.g. lymphoma, leukaemia, neuroblastoma

Obstructive
Hepatic vein thrombosis
Congestive cardiac failure

Miscellaneous
Wilson's disease
Alpha-1 antitrypsin deficiency
Congenital hepatic fibrosis

Idiopathic
Very large liver
Storage disorder
Reticuloendothelial disease, e.g. leukaemia
Gross fatty change
Malignancy
Congestive cardiac failure

Differential diagnosis of splenomegaly

Infection
Bacterial, viral or protozoal
Septicaemia
Infectious mononucleosis
Malaria

Autoimmune disease
Juvenile chronic arthritis
SLE

Haemolytic disorders
Hereditary spherocytosis
Sickle-cell anaemia (early)

Neoplastic
Acute leukaemia
Hodgkin's disease

Disordered splenic flow
Portal hypertension
Cirrhosis
Cardiac failure

Infiltration
Gaucher's disease

Extramedullary haemopoiesis
Thalassaemia

17. FURTHER READING

Diseases of the Liver and Biliary System in Childhood: Kelly DA. 1st edition. Blackwell Science 1999.

Diseases of the Small Intestine in Childhood: Walker-Smith JA, Murch SH. 4th edition. Isis Medical Media 1999.

Forfar and Arneil's Textbook of Paediatrics: Campbell AGM, Macintosh N (eds), 5th edition, Chapter 11. Churchill Livingstone 1998.

Paediatric Gastrointestinal Disease: Wyllie R, Hyams JS (eds). 2nd edition. WB Saunders 1999.

Chapter 8

Genetics

Louise C Wilson

CONTENTS

Genetics

1. CHROMOSOMES

Within the nucleus of somatic cells there are 22 pairs of autosomes and one pair of sex chromosomes. Normal male and female karyotypes are 46,XY and 46,XX, respectively. The normal chromosome complement of 46 chromosomes is known as **diploid**. Genomes with a single copy of each chromosome or three copies of each are known, respectively, as **haploid** and **triploid**. A karyotype with too many or too few chromosomes, where the total is not a multiple of 23, is called **aneuploid**.

Chromosomes are divided by the centromere into a short '**p**' arm ('**petit**') and long '**q**' arm. **Acrocentric** chromosomes (13, 14, 15, 21, 22) have the centromere at one end.

Lyonization is the process whereby in a cell containing more than one X chromosome, only one is active. Selection of the active X is usually random and each inactivated X chromosome can be seen as a Barr body on microscopy.

Mitosis occurs in somatic cells and results in two **diploid** daughter cells with nuclear chromosomes which are genetically identical both to each other and the original parent cell.

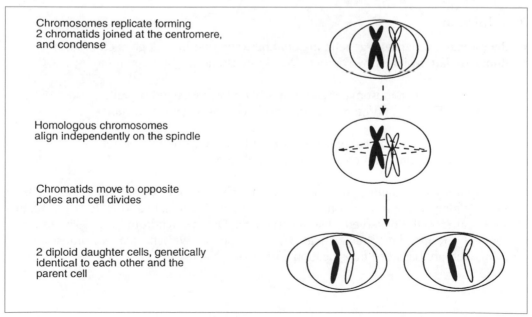

Chromosomes replicate forming 2 chromatids joined at the centromere, and condense

Homologous chromosomes align independently on the spindle

Chromatids move to opposite poles and cell divides

2 diploid daughter cells, genetically identical to each other and the parent cell

Mitosis

Meiosis occurs in the germ cells of the gonads and is also known as **'reduction division'** because it results in four **haploid** daughter cells, each containing just one member (homologue) of each chromosome pair and all genetically different. Meiosis involves two divisions (**meiosis I and II**). The reduction in chromosome number occurs during meiosis I and is preceded by exchange of chromosome segments between homologous chromosomes called **crossing over**. In males the onset of meiosis and spermatogenesis is at puberty. In females, replication of the chromosomes and crossing over begins in fetal life, but the oocytes remain suspended prior to the first cell division until just before ovulation.

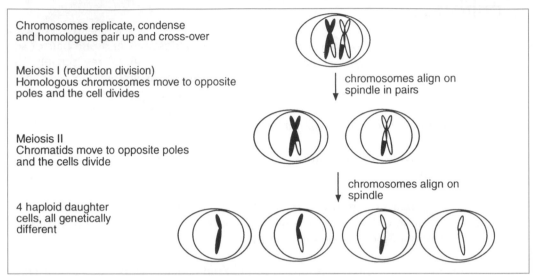

Meiosis

Translocations

- **Reciprocal**: exchange of genetic material between non-homologous chromosomes
- **Robertsonian**: fusion of two acrocentric chromosomes at their centromeres, e.g. (14;21)
- **Unbalanced:** if chromosomal material has been lost or gained overall
- **Balanced:** if no chromosomal material has been lost or gained overall

Carriers of balanced translocations are usually phenotypically normal but are at increased risk for having offspring with chromosomal imbalance.

Carriers of a Robertsonian translocation involving chromosome 21 are at increased risk of having offspring with translocation Down's syndrome. For female and male (14;21) translocation carriers, the observed offspring risks for Down's syndrome are 15% and 5%, respectively. Remember, they can also have offspring with normal chromosomes or offspring who are balanced translocation carriers like themselves.

1.1 Common sex chromosome aneuploidies

Turner's syndrome (karyotype 45,X)

This affects 1:2,500 liveborn females, but it is a frequent finding amongst early miscarriages. Patients are usually of normal intelligence. They have streak ovaries which result in failure of menstruation, low oestrogen with high gonadotrophins, and infertility. Normal secondary sexual characteristics may develop spontaneously or be induced with oestrogens. Short stature throughout childhood with failure of the pubertal growth spurt is typical. Final height can be increased by early treatment with growth hormone.

Features of Turner's syndrome

- Webbed or short neck
- Low hairline
- Shield chest with widely spaced nipples
- Cubitus valgus (wide carrying angle)
- Cardiovascular abnormalities particularly aortic coarctation in 10–15%
- Renal anomalies (e.g. horseshoe kidney, duplicated ureters, renal aplasia) in approximately 1/3
- Non-pitting lymphoedema in approximately 1/3

Triple X syndrome (karyotype 47,XXX)

This affects 1:1,000 newborn females. These patients show little phenotypic abnormality but tend to be of tall stature. Whilst intelligence is typically reduced compared to siblings, it usually falls within normal or low-normal limits, however mild developmental and behavioural difficulties are more common. Fertility is normal but the incidence of early menopause is increased.

Klinefelter's syndrome (karyotype 47,XXY)

This affects 1:600 newborn males. Phenotypic abnormalities are rare pre-pubertally, other than a tendency to tall stature. At puberty, spontaneous expression of secondary sexual characteristics is variable but poor growth of facial and body hair is common. The testes are small in association with azoospermia, testosterone production around 50% of normal and raised gonadotrophins. Gynaecomastia occurs in 30% and there is an increased risk of male breast cancer. Female distribution of fat and hair and a high-pitched voice may occur but are not typical. Intelligence is generally reduced compared to siblings but usually falls within normal or low-normal limits. Mild developmental and behavioural problems are more common.

47,XYY males

This affects 1:1,000 newborn males. These males are phenotypically normal but tend to be tall. Intelligence is usually within normal limits but there is an increased incidence of behavioural abnormalities.

1.2 Common autosomal chromosome aneuploidies

Down's syndrome (trisomy 21)

Down's syndrome affects 1:700 live births overall and is usually secondary to meiotic non-disjunction (failure of the chromosomes to segregate correctly in meiosis) during oogenesis, which is commoner with increasing maternal age. Around 5% of patients have an underlying Robertsonian translocation, most commonly between chromosomes 14 and 21. Around 3% have detectable **mosaicism** (a mixture of trisomy 21 and karyotypically normal cells) usually resulting in a milder phenotype.

Phenotypic features of Down's syndrome

- Brachycephaly
- Upslanting palpebral fissures, epicanthic folds, Brushfield spots on the iris
- Protruding tongue
- Single palmar crease, 5th finger clinodactyly, wide sandal gaps between 1st and 2nd toes
- Hypotonia and moderate mental retardation

Common features of Down's syndrome

- Cardiovascular malformations in 40%, particularly atrioventricular septal defects (AVSD)
- Gastrointestinal abnormalities in 6%, particularly duodenal atresia and Hirschprung's disease
- Haematological abnormalities, particularly acute lymphoblastic leukaemia (ALL), acute myeloblastic leukaemia (AML) and transient leukaemias
- Hypothyroidism
- Cataracts in 3%
- Alzheimer's disease in the majority by 40 years of age

Edward's syndrome (trisomy 18)

This affects 1:6,000 newborns. This typically causes intrauterine growth retardation, a characteristic facies, prominent occiput, overlapping fingers (2nd and 5th overlap 3rd and 4th), rockerbottom feet (vertical talus) and short dorsiflexed great toes. Malformations, particularly congenital heart disease, diaphragmatic hernias, renal abnormalities and dislocated hips, are more common. Survival beyond early infancy is rare but associated with profound mental handicap.

Patau syndrome (trisomy 13)

This affects 1:5,000 newborns (will be lower with antenatal screening). Affected infants usually have multiple malformations including holoprosencephaly and other CNS abnormalities, scalp defects, microphthalmia, cleft lip and palate, post-axial polydactyly, rocker-bottom feet, renal abnormalities and congenital heart disease. Survival beyond early infancy is rare and associated with profound mental handicap.

1.3 Microdeletion syndromes

The term 'microdeletion' refers to a chromosome deletion which is too small to see on standard karyotyping. Microdeletions usually involve two or more adjacent (contiguous) genes. They can be detected using specific fluorescent probes (**f**luorescent *in situ* **h**ybridization, **FISH**).

Examples of microdeletion syndromes:

- **Di George syndrome** (parathyroid gland hypoplasia with hypocalcaemia, thymus hypoplasia with T-lymphocyte deficiency, congenital cardiac malformations particularly interrupted aortic arch and truncus arteriosus, cleft palate, learning disability) due to microdeletions at 22q11. There appears to be an increased incidence of psychiatric disorders, particularly within the schizophrenic spectrum. The condition is also known as velocardiofacial syndrome, Shprintzen syndrome and by the acronym CATCH 22 (an unpopular name which is falling into disuse).
- **William's syndrome** (supravalvular aortic stenosis, hypercalcaemia, stellate irides, mental retardation) due to microdeletions involving the elastin gene on chromosome 7
- **WAGR syndrome** (association of **W**ilms tumour, **a**niridia, **g**enitourinary abnormalities and mental **r**etardation) due to deletions of chromosome 11p13
- **Smith–Magenis syndrome** (association of mental retardation, self-injurious behaviours and marked sleep disturbance) due to a microdeletion on chromosome 17

Microdeletions can involve any part of any chromosome and collectively are likely to underlie a significant proportion of undiagnosed mental handicap and/or malformation syndromes. Screening for microdeletions at the tips (telomeres) of the chromosomes is available in specialized centres.

2. MENDELIAN INHERITANCE

2.1 Autosomal dominant (AD) conditions

These result from mutation of one copy of a gene carried on an autosome. All offspring of an affected person have a 50% chance of inheriting the mutation. Within a family the severity may vary (**variable expression**) and known mutation carriers may appear clinically normal (**reduced penetrance**). Some conditions, such as achondroplasia and NF1, frequently begin *de novo* through new mutations arising in the egg or (more commonly) sperm.

Examples of autosomal dominant (AD) conditions

Achondroplasia
Ehlers–Danlos syndrome (most)
Facioscapulohumeral dystrophy
Familial adenomatous polyposis coli
Familial hypercholesterolaemia
Tuberous sclerosis
Gilbert's syndrome

Huntington's chorea
Marfan's syndrome
Neurofibromatosis types 1 and 2 (NF1–2)
Noonan's syndrome
Porphyrias (except congenital erythropoietic which is AR)
von Willebrand's disease

*Conditions pre-fixed 'hereditary' or 'familial' are usually autosomal dominant

2.2 Autosomal recessive (AR) conditions

These result from mutations in both copies of an autosomal gene. Where both parents are carriers each of their offspring has a 1 in 4 (25%) risk of being affected, and a 50% chance of being a carrier.

Examples of autosomal recessive (AR) conditions

Alkaptonuria
Ataxia telangiectasia
β-thalassaemia
Congenital adrenal hyperplasias
Crigler–Najjar (severe form)
Cystic fibrosis
Dubin–Johnson
Fanconi anaemia
Galactosaemia
Glucose 6-phosphatase deficiency
   (von Gierkes)**

Glycogen storage diseases
Homocystinuria
Haemochromatosis
Mucopolysaccharidoses (all except Hunter's syndrome)
Oculocutaneous albinism
Phenylketonuria
Rotor (usually)
Sickle-cell anaemia
Spinal muscular atrophies
Wilson's disease
Xeroderma pigmentosa

**Do not confuse with glucose 6-phosphate dehydrogenase deficiency (favism) which is XLR
Most metabolic disorders are autosomal recessive — remember the exceptions

2.3 X-linked recessive (XLR) conditions

These result from a mutation in a gene carried on the X chromosome and affect males because they have just one gene copy. Females are usually unaffected but may have mild manifestations as a result of unfavourable lyonization. This form of inheritance is characterized by the following:

- NO MALE-TO-MALE TRANSMISSION (an affected father passes his Y chromosome to all his sons)
- All daughters of an affected male are carriers (an affected father passes his X chromosome to all his daughters)

- Sons of a female carrier have a 50% chance of being affected and daughters have a 50% chance of being carriers

Examples of X-linked recessive (XLR) conditions

Alport's syndrome (usually XLR; some AR forms)
Becker muscular dystrophy
Duchenne muscular dystrophy
Fabry's disease
Fragile X syndrome
Glucose 6-phosphate dehydrogenase deficiency (favism)

Haemophilias A and B (Christmas disease)
Hunter's syndrome (MPS II)
Lesch–Nyhan disease
Ocular albinism
Red–green colour blindness
Testicular feminization syndrome
Wiskott–Aldrich syndrome

2.4 X-linked dominant (XLD) conditions

These are caused by a mutation in one copy of a gene on the X chromosome but both male and female mutation carriers are affected. Because of lyonization, females are usually more mildly affected and these disorders are frequently lethal in males. For the reasons outlined above:

- There is no male-to-male transmission
- All daughters of an affected male would be affected
- All offspring of an affected female have a 50% chance of being affected

Examples of X-linked dominant (XLD) conditions

Goltz syndrome
Incontinentia pigmenti

Rett syndrome
Vitamin D-resistant rickets

3. MOLECULAR GENETICS

3.1 DNA (deoxyribonucleic acid)

DNA is a **double-stranded** molecule composed of purine (adenine + guanine) and pyrimidine (cytosine and thymine) bases linked by a backbone of covalently bonded **deoxyribose sugar** phosphate residues. The two antiparallel strands are held together by hydrogen bonds which can be disrupted by heating and re-form on cooling:

- **Adenine (A) pairs with thymine (T)** by 2 hydrogen bonds
- **Guanine (G) pairs with cytosine (C)** by 3 hydrogen bonds

3.2 RNA (Ribonucleic acid)

DNA is **transcribed** in the nucleus into messenger RNA (mRNA) which is **translated** by ribosomes in the cytoplasm into a polypeptide chain. RNA differs from DNA in that it is:

- **Single stranded**
- Thymine is replaced by **uracil**
- The sugar backbone is **ribose**

3.3 Polymerase chain reaction (PCR)

This is a widely used method for generating large amounts of the DNA of interest from very small samples. PCR can be adapted for use with RNA providing the RNA is first converted to DNA.

PCR is a method by which a small amount of target DNA (the template) is selectively amplified to produce enough to perform an analysis. This might be the detection of a particular DNA sequence such as that belonging to a pathogenic micro-organism or an oncogene, or the detection of differences in genes such as mutations causing inherited disease. Therefore the template DNA might consist of total human genomic DNA derived from peripheral blood lymphocytes or it might consist of a tumour biopsy or a biological fluid from a patient with an infection.

In order to perform PCR, the sequence flanking the target DNA must usually be known so that specific complementary oligonucleotide sequences, known as primers, can be designed. The two unique primers are then mixed together with the DNA template, deoxyribonucleotides (dATP, dCTP, dGTP, dTTP) and a thermostable DNA polymerase (Taq polymerase, derived from an organism which inhabits thermal springs).

- In the initial stage of the reaction the DNA template is heated (typically for about 30 seconds) to make it single stranded. As the reaction cools the primers will anneal to the template if the appropriate sequence is present.
- The reaction is then heated to 72°C (for about a minute) during which time the Taq DNA polymerase synthesises new DNA between the two primer sequences, doubling the copy number of the target sequence.
- The reaction is heated again and the cycle is repeated. After 30 or so cycles (each typically lasting a few minutes) the target sequence will have been amplified exponentially.

The crucial feature of PCR is that to detect a given sequence of DNA it only needs to be present in one copy (ie. one molecule of DNA): this makes it extremely powerful.

Clinical Applications of PCR

- Mutation detection
- Single cell PCR of in vitro fertilised embryo to diagnose genetic disease before implantation

- Detection of viral and bacterial sequences in tissue (Herpes Simplex Virus in CSF, Hepatitis C, HIV in peripheral blood, meningococcal strains).

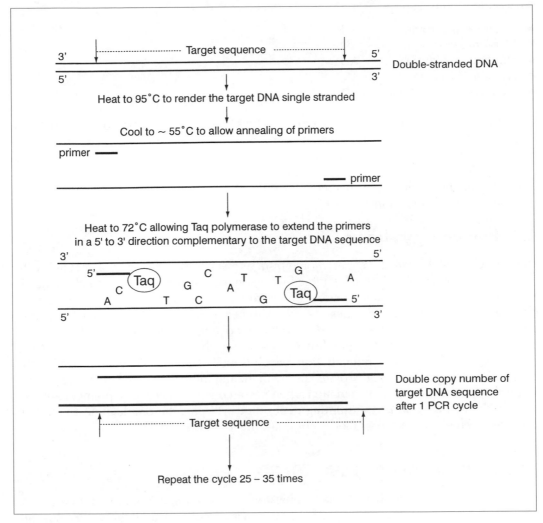

Polymerase chain reaction

3.4 Reverse Transcription PCT (rt PCR)

This is a modification of conventional PCR used to amplify messenger RNA (mRNA) sequence in order to look at the expression of particular genes within a tissue. mRNA is single-stranded, unstable, and is not a substrate for Taq DNA polymerase. For that reason it must be converted to complementary DNA (cDNA) using reverse transcriptase, a retroviral enzyme, which results in a double stranded DNA copy of the original RNA sequence. PCR can then be performed in the normal way.

4. TRINUCLEOTIDE REPEAT DISORDERS

These conditions are associated with genes containing stretches of repeating units of three nucleotides and include:

- Fragile X syndrome   XLR
- Myotonic dystrophy   AD
- Huntington's chorea   AD
- Freidreich's ataxia   AR
- Spinocerebellar ataxias   AD

In normal individuals the number of repeats varies slightly but remains below a defined threshold. Affected patients have an increased number of repeats, called an **expansion**, above the disease-causing threshold. The expansions may be unstable and enlarge further in successive generations causing increased disease severity (**'anticipation'**) and earlier onset, **e.g. myotonic dystrophy**, particularly congenital myotonic dystrophy following transmission by an affected mother.

4.1 Fragile X syndrome

This causes mental retardation, macro-orchidism and seizures and is often associated with a cytogenetically visible constriction ('fragile site') on the X chromosome. The inheritance is X-linked but complex. Among controls there are between 6 and 55 stably inherited trinucleotide repeats in the *FMR1* gene. People with between 55 and 230 repeats are said to be premutation carriers but are unaffected. During oogenesis in female premutation carriers, the triplet repeat is unstable and may expand into the disease-causing range (230 to >1,000 repeats) known as a '**full mutation**' which is methylated, effectively inactivating the gene. All males and around 50% of females with the full mutation are affected. The premutation does not expand to a full mutation when passed on by a male. Male premutation carriers are known as '**normal transmitting males**' and will pass the premutation to all their daughters (remember they pass their Y chromosome to all their sons).

5. MITOCHONDRIAL DISORDERS

Mitochondria are **exclusively maternally inherited**, deriving from those present in the cytoplasm of the ovum. They contain copies of their own **circular 16.5-kilobase chromosome** carrying genes for several respiratory-chain enzyme subunits and transfer RNAs (tRNAs). Mitochondrial genes differ from nuclear genes in having no introns and using some different aminoacid codons. Within a tissue, or even a cell, there may be a mixed population of normal and abnormal mitochondria known as **heteroplasmy**. Different proportions of abnormal mitochondria may be required to cause disease in different tissues, known as a **threshold effect**. Disorders caused by mitochondrial gene mutations include:

- **MELAS** (**m**itochondrial **e**ncephalopathy, **l**actic **a**cidosis, **s**troke-like episodes)
- **MERRF** (**m**yoclonic **e**pilepsy, **r**agged **r**ed **f**ibres)
- Mitochondrially inherited diabetes mellitus and deafness
- Leber's hereditary optic neuropathy (NB. Other factors also contribute)

6. GENOMIC IMPRINTING

For most genes both copies are expressed, but for some genes either the maternally or paternally derived copy is preferentially used, a phenomenon known as **genomic imprinting**. The best examples are the Prader–Willi and Angelman syndromes, both caused by either cytogenetic deletions of the same region of chromosome 15q or by **uniparental disomy** of chromosome 15 (where both copies of chromosome 15 are derived from one parent with no copy of chromosome 15 from the other parent).

Prader–Willi	**Angelman**
Clinical Neonatal hypotonia and poor feeding Moderate mental handicap Hyperphagia + obesity in later childhood Small genitalia	'Happy puppet', unprovoked laughter/ clapping Microcephaly, severe mental handicap Ataxia, broad-based gait Seizures, characteristic EEG
Genetics 70% deletion on paternal chromosome 15 25–28% maternal uniparental disomy 15 (i.e. no paternal contribution) 2–5% imprinting centre defect	80% deletion on maternal chromosome 15 2–3% paternal uniparental disomy 15 (i.e. no maternal contribution) 2–5% imprinting centre defect 10–15% mutations in the *UBE3A* gene remainder unknown

Other imprinting disorders

Russell–Silver syndrome
Prenatal onset growth retardation, relative macrocephaly, triangular facies, asymmetry, 5th finger clinodactyly and normal IQ associated with maternal uniparental disomy for chromosome 7 in a proportion. The cause in the remainder is not yet known.

Beckwith–Wiedemann syndrome
Prenatal-onset macrosomia, facial naevus flammeus, macroglossia, ear lobe creases, pits on the ear helix, hemihypertrophy, nephromegaly, exomphalos (omphalocele) and neonatal hypoglycaemia. There is an increased risk of Wilms', adrenocortical and hepatic tumours in childhood. The condition appears to result from abnormalities of chromosome 11p15 which contains several imprinted genes including the *IGF-2* (insulin-like growth factor 2) gene.

7. IMPORTANT GENETIC TOPICS

This section includes short notes on conditions that form popular exam topics.

7.1 Ambiguous genitalia (see also Chapter 5 *Endocrinology*)

Normal development of the reproductive tract and external genitalia

A simplified outline is shown below.

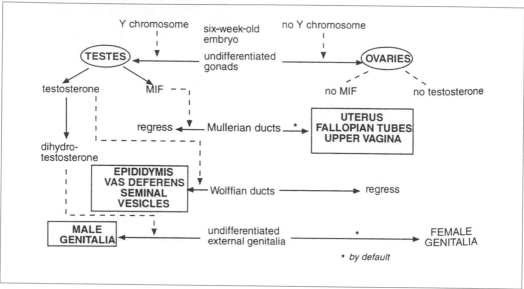

Outline of the normal development of the reproductive tract and external genitalia

The 6-week embryo has undifferentiated gonads, Mullerian ducts (capable of developing into the uterus, Fallopian tubes and upper vagina), Wolffian ducts (capable of forming the epididymis, vas deferens and seminal vesicles) and undifferentiated external genitalia.

In the presence of a Y chromosome the gonads become testes which produce testosterone and Mullerian inhibiting factor (MIF). Testosterone causes the Wolffian ducts to persist and differentiate and, after conversion to dihydrotestosterone (by 5α-reductase), masculinization of the external genitalia. MIF causes the Mullerian ducts to regress.

In the absence of a Y chromosome the gonads become ovaries which secrete neither testosterone nor MIF. In the absence of testosterone the Wolffian ducts regress and the external genitalia feminize. In the absence of MIF, the Mullerian ducts persist and differentiate.
The causes of **ambiguous genitalia** divide broadly into those resulting in undermasculinization of a male fetus, those causing masculinization of a female fetus, and those resulting from mosaicism for a cell line containing a Y chromosome and another which doesn't. They are summarized in the diagram on page 295.

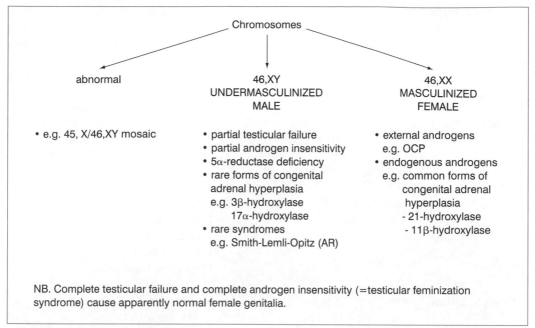

Ambiguous genitalia — outline of causes

7.2 Cystic fibrosis (CF)

This results from mutations in the *CFTR* (cystic fibrosis transmembrane regulator) gene. Around 85–90% of CF mutations in North European Caucasians are detectable on current mutation screening, but detection rates in other populations are lower. The *ΔF508* mutation (deletion of three nucleotides coding for a phenylalanine residue) alone accounts for 75% of mutations in Caucasians. Because a proportion of mutations is not currently detectable, negative molecular testing cannot exclude a diagnosis of cystic fibrosis. See also *Respiratory* Chapter 17.

7.3 Duchenne and Becker muscular dystrophy (See also Chapter 15, *Neurology*.)

These result from different mutations within the dystrophin gene on chromosome Xp21.

Important distinguishing features of Duchenne and Becker muscular dystrophy		
	Duchenne	**Becker**
Immunofluorescent dystrophin on muscle biopsy	Undetectable	Reduced/abnormal
Wheelchair dependence	95% at <12 years	5% at <12years
Mental handicap	20%	rare

7.4 Neurofibromatosis (NF)

There are two forms of NF which are clinically and genetically distinct:

	NF1	NF2
Major features	≥6 café-au-lait patches (CALs) Axillary/inguinal freckling Lisch nodules on the iris Peripheral neurofibromas	Bilateral acoustic neuromas (vestibular schwannomas) Other cranial and spinal tumours
Minor features	Macrocephaly Short stature	CALs (usually <6) Peripheral schwannomas Peripheral neurofibromas Deafness/tinnitus/vertigo Lens opacities/cataracts

Complications	Plexiform neuromas
	Optic glioma (2%)
	Other cranial and spinal
	  tumours
	Pseudarthrosis
	  (especially tibial)
	Renal artery stenosis
	Phaeochromocytoma
	Learning difficulties
	Scoliosis
	Spinal cord and nerve compressions
	Malignant change/sarcomas
		Spinal cord and nerve
		  compressions
		Malignant change/sarcomas

Gene	Chromosome 17	Chromosome 22

7.5 Tuberous sclerosis (TS)

There are at least two separate genes which cause TS, on chromosomes 9 and 16.

Clinical features of tuberous sclerosis

- **Skin/nails**
  - Ash-leaf macules
  - Shagreen patches (especially over the lumbosacral area)
  - Adenoma sebaceum (facial area)
  - Subungual/periungual fibromas

- **Eyes**
  - Retinal hamartomas

- **Heart**
  - Cardiac rhabdomyomas, detectable antenatally, usually regressing during childhood

- **Kidneys**
  - Renal cysts

- **Neurological**
  - Seizures
  - Mental handicap

- **Neuroimaging**
  - Intracranial calcification (periventricular)
  - Subependymal nodules
  - Neuronal migration defects

7.6 Marfan's syndrome

This results from mutations in the fibrillin gene on chromosome 15. Intelligence is usually normal. Mutation screening for Marfan's syndrome is not available outside a research setting (due to the size of the gene and the family-specific nature of the mutations) and the diagnosis remains a clinical one.

Clinical features of Marfan's syndrome

- **Musculoskeletal**
  - Tall stature with disproportionately long limbs (dolichostenomelia)
  - Arachnodactyly
  - Pectus carinatum or excavatum
  - Scoliosis
  - High, narrow arched palate
  - Joint laxity
  - Pes planus

- **Heart**
  - Aortic root dilatation and dissection
  - Mitral valve prolapse

- **Eyes**
  - Lens dislocation (typically up)
  - Myopia

- **Skin**
  - Striae

Homocystinuria (See Chapter 12 *Metabolic Medicine.*)
This is most commonly due to cystathione-β-synthase deficiency and causes a Marfan-like body habitus, lens dislocation (usually down), mental handicap, thrombotic tendency and osteoporosis. Treatment includes a low methionine diet +/– pyridoxine.

7.7 Noonan's syndrome

This is an autosomal dominant condition. Around 50% have mutations of the PTPN11 (protein tyrosine phosphatase SHP-2) gene on chromosome 12. The karyotype is usually normal.

Clinical features of Noonan's syndrome

- **Cardiac**
  - Pulmonary valve stenosis
  - Hypertrophic cardiomyopathy
  - Septal defects (ASD, VSD)
  - Branch pulmonary artery stenosis

- **Musculoskeletal**
  - Webbed or short neck
  - Pectus excavatum or carinatum
  - Widely spaced nipples
  - Wide carrying angle (cubitus valgus)
  - Short stature in 80%

- **Other features**
  - Ptosis
  - Low-set and/or posteriorly rotated ears
  - Small genitalia and undescended testes in boys
  - Coagulation defects in 30% (partial factor XI:C, XIIC, and VIIIC deficiencies, von Willebrand's, thrombocytopenia)
  - Mild mental retardation in 30%

7.8 Achondroplasia

A short-limb skeletal dysplasia resulting from autosomal dominant mutations in the *FGFR3* (fibroblast growth factor receptor 3) gene on chromosome 4. There is a high new mutation rate. Important complications are hydrocephalus, brainstem or cervical cord compression resulting from a small foramen magnum, spinal canal stenosis, kyphosis and sleep apnoea.

7.9 CHARGE association

A sporadic malformation syndrome including:

Colobomas
Heart malformations
Atresia of the choanae
Retardation of growth and development (mental handicap)
Genital hypoplasia (in males)
Ear abnormalities (abnormalities of the ear pinna, deafness)

Cleft lip/palate and renal abnormalities are also common.

7.10 VATER (VACTERL) association

A sporadic malformation syndrome including:

Vertebral abnormalities
Anal atresia +/– fistula
Cardiac malformations
Tracheo oesophageal fistula
Renal anomalies, **r**adial ray defects
Limb anomalies, especially radial ray defects

7.11 Pierre Robin sequence

This is the association of micrognathia and cleft palate. In some definitions glossoptosis is included to form a triad. It may occur in isolation or be part of an underlying syndrome, most commonly Stickler syndrome (in around a third), but also including velocardiofacial (deletion 22q11) and Treacher–Collins syndromes.

7.12 Potter sequence

Oligohydramnios as a result of renal abnormalities, urinary tract obstruction or amniotic fluid leakage may lead to secondary fetal compression with joint contractures (arthrogryposis), pulmonary hypoplasia and squashed facies known as the Potter sequence.

8. GENETIC TESTING

Genetic tests are broadly divided into cytogenetic tests (karyotyping and FISH tests) and molecular genetic tests which involve analysing DNA for sequence changes (mutations). Most DNA tests use the polymerase chain reaction (PCR) as a preliminary step to enrich the sample for the specific DNA sequence to be analysed. As a general rule, tests for single gene (Mendelian) disorders will be DNA-based. There is a huge list of conditions for which molecular genetic testing is available in specialized laboratories.

Commoner conditions for which molecular genetic (DNA) testing is available:

- Angelman syndrome
- Charcot–Marie–Tooth (HMSN1)
- Cystic fibrosis
- Duchenne/Becker muscular dystrophy
- Fragile X syndrome
- Friedreich's ataxia
- Huntington's chorea
- Myotonic dystrophy
- Prader–Willi syndrome
- Spinal muscular atrophy
- Spinocerebellar ataxias

8.1 Prenatal testing

- **CVS or CVB** (chorionic villus sampling or biopsy): a small piece of placenta is taken either transabdominally or transvaginally. CVS testing can be safely performed from 10 to 11 weeks' gestation.
- **Amniocentesis**: amniotic fluid is taken, containing cells derived from the surfaces of the fetus and amniotic membranes. Amniocentesis is usually performed from 15 to 16 weeks' gestation.
- **Cordocentesis**: A method of obtaining fetal blood which can be performed from 18 weeks' gestation.

Each procedure carries a small risk of miscarriage. Chromosome and DNA testing can be performed on any of the above types of sample.

In general, where the chromosomal abnormality or specific DNA mutation in a family is known, it is possible to offer a prenatal test for it. For families with a genetic disorder for which the gene is known (e.g. Duchenne muscular dystrophy) but where their family-specific mutation is not known, antenatal genetic testing may still be possible using genetic linkage (gene tracking). Testing for many metabolic disorders is still based on enzyme or biochemical analysis performed on CVS or amniocentesis samples.

8.2 Family screening for genetic disorders

Whenever an individual is diagnosed with a genetic disorder, thought should be given to the risks that other family members may have inherited the condition or have an increased risk of affected offspring. This is particularly important for chromosome translocations and X-linked disorders. It is also important for autosomal recessive disorders where consanguineous unions are likely, or where the carrier frequency is high in members of the same ethnic group.

8.3 Dysmorphic syndromes

These are recognizable patterns, usually involving mental handicap and/or malformations. There may be a characteristic-associated facial appearance. It is worth knowing some dysmorphic terminology to describe a child if you are asked to — e.g. brachycephaly (flattening of the back of the skull), 5th finger clinodactyly (incurved little fingers), micrognathia (small mandible), synophrys (eyebrows meeting in the mid-line), posteriorly rotated ears, upslanting palpebral fissures. However, you should remember that individual dysmorphic features are common in the general population (e.g. single palmar creases) and usually only become significant when they are numerous and associated with physical disability or mental handicap. Don't rush into guessing a diagnosis. It is more important that you make an accurate assessment than name the specific syndrome.

Dysmorphic syndromes that you may be asked about include:

- Down's syndrome
- Turner's syndrome
- CHARGE association
- VATER association
- Beckwith–Wiedemann syndrome
- NF1
- Tuberous sclerosis
- Marfan's syndrome
- Achondroplasia
- Russell–Silver syndrome
- Angelman syndrome
- Prader–Willi

Other conditions not outlined previously include:

- **Goldenhar syndrome**
  Facial asymmetry, malformed ear(s) and deafness, pre-auricular tags, epibulbar dermoid cysts, cervical vertebral abnormalities, congenital cardiac defects, structural renal malformations, occasional radial or intracranial abnormalities, IQ usually normal.
- **Treacher–Collins syndrome**
  Micrognathia, hypoplastic zygomatic arches, malformed ears and deafness, lower eye-lid colobomas, cleft palate, face usually symmetrically affected, IQ usually normal.
- **Cornelia de Lange**
  (A much overdiagnosed syndrome!) — growth retardation, microcephaly, synophrys, generalized hirsutism, limb defects ranging from proximally placed thumbs to ectrodactyly (lobster-claw deformity), severe developmental delay.
- **Crouzon syndrome**
  A variable autosomal dominant craniosynostosis syndrome characterized by premature closure of the coronal sutures, mid-facial hypoplasia, proptosis secondary to shallow orbits and a beak-shaped nose. Intelligence is usually normal and there is no syndactyly. It results from mutations in the *FGFR2* (fibroblast growth-factor receptor 2) gene.
- **Apert syndrome**
  A severe craniosynostosis syndrome with mid-facial hypoplasia, prominent eyes, a beak-shaped nose, a high, narrow and sometimes cleft palate, and syndactyly of digits 2–5 (sometimes including the thumb) to give characteristic 'mitten' hands and feet. Around 50% have some degree of mental handicap. It is autosomal dominant resulting from specific mutations in the *FGFR2* gene, although most are new (*de novo*) mutations.
- **Rubinstein–Taybi syndrome**
  A mental retardation syndrome associated with microcephaly, down-slanting palpebral fissures, hypertelorism, mild ptosis, a characteristic nose with protruding columella and broad medially deviated thumbs and halluces. The condition usually results from *de novo* autosomal dominant deletions or mutations involving the *CBP* (CREB transcription-factor binding protein) gene on chromosome 16p13.

- **Cockayne syndrome**
  A progressive neurological disorder characterized by failure to thrive, deep-set eyes, cataracts, retinopathy, sensorineural deafness, central and peripheral demyelination with loss of skills, and cutaneous sun sensitivity. Cockayne syndrome is autosomal recessive and diagnosed by demonstrating abnormal DNA repair and recovery of RNA synthesis in fibroblasts after UV irradiation.

- **Poland syndrome**
  A sporadic malformation characterized by syndactyly and shortening of the fingers of one hand together with ipsilateral absence of part of pectoralis major (usually the sternal head). Ipsilateral rib defects and absence of the nipple or breast may also occur.

- **Fetal alcohol syndrome**
  Most affected infants are of low birth weight with hypotonia and jitteriness in the neonatal period. Associated features include failure to thrive, developmental delay, mild–moderate microcephaly, short palpebral fissures, a smooth philtrum, thin upper lip and small dysplastic 5th finger nails. Around a third have cardiac abnormalities, most commonly VSD.

- **Klippel–Feil syndrome**
  This describes the sporadic association of a short neck and low posterior hairline with fusions of the cervical vertebrae. Neck webbing, torticollis, high (Sprengel) shoulder, deafness (conductive or sensorineural), VSD, cleft palate and renal anomalies may also occur.

- **Aicardi syndrome**
  This is an X-linked dominant condition which is presumed embryonic lethal in males. In females it is characterized by infantile spasms often with asynchronous burst-suppression on EEG, chorioretinopathy, agenesis of the corpus callosum and other abnormalities including microphthalmia and vertebral anomalies. The gene involved is not yet known.

9. FURTHER READING

ABC of Clinical Genetics: Kingston H M, 3rd edition. BMJ Publishing 2002.

Practical Genetic Counselling: Harper PS, 5th edition. Butterworth Heinemann 1998.

Smith's Recognizable Patterns of Human Malformation: Jones K L, 5th edition. WB Saunders 1997.

Chapter 9

Haematology and Oncology

Michael L Capra

CONTENTS

Haematology and Oncology

1. HAEMOGLOBIN (Hb)

1.1 Haemoglobin synthesis

Erythropoietic activity is regulated by erythropoietin, a hormone secreted by the peritubular complex of the kidney (90%), the liver and elsewhere (10%). Stimulus to erythropoietin production is the oxygen tension within the kidney. Mitochondria of the developing erythroblast are the main sites for the synthesis of haem.

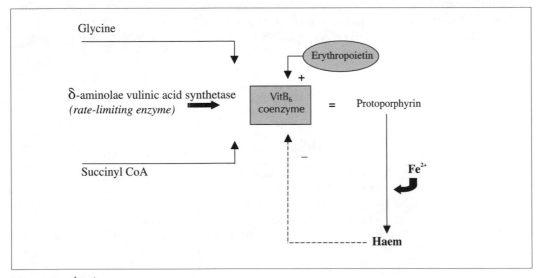

Haem synthesis

- The cofactor vitamin B_6 is stimulated by erythropoietin and inhibited by haem
- The Fe^{2+} is supplied by circulating transferrin
- Globin chains, comprising a sequence of polypeptides, are synthesized on ribosomes
- A tetramer of four globin chains, each with its own haem group attached, is formed to make a molecule of haemoglobin

1.2 Red cell physiology

The 8-μm diameter red cell has three challenges, to:

- pass through the microcirculation of capillaries (diameters of 3.5 μm)
- maintain Hb in the reduced state
- maintain an osmotic equilibrium despite a high concentration of protein (5x that of plasma)

It achieves this by:

- the protein, spectrin, which enables it to have a flexible biconcave-disc shape;
- generating reducing power in the form of nicotinamide adenine dinucleotide (NADH) from the Embden–Meyerhof pathway and NADPH (reduced NADP) from the hexose monophosphate shunt; this reducing power is vital in preventing oxidation injury to the red cell and for reducing functionally dead methaemoglobin (oxidized haemoglobin) to functionally active, reduced haemoglobin (see figure below);
- generating energy in the form of ATP from the Embden–Meyerhof pathway; this energy is utilized to drive the cell membrane Na^+/K^+ pump to exchange 3 ions of intracellular Na^+ for 2 ions of K^+ thus maintaining an osmotic equilibrium;
- generating 2,3-diphosphoglycerate (2,3-DPG) to reversibly bind with haemoglobin to maintain the appropriate affinity for oxygen.

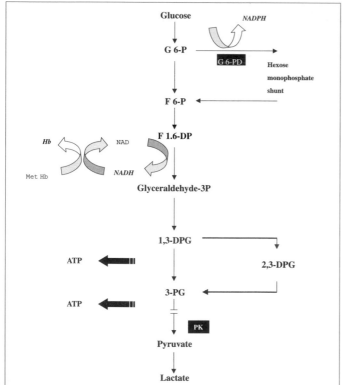

The Embden–Meyerhof and associated pathways

F 6-P, fructose 6-phosphate;
F 1,6-DP, fructose 1,6-diphosphate;
Met Hb, methaemoglobin;
PK, protein kinase.

1.3 Oxygen-dissociation curve

When oxygen is unloaded from a molecule of oxygenated haemoglobin, the β chains open up allowing 2,3-DPG to enter. This results in the deoxygenated haemoglobin having a low affinity for oxygen, preventing haemoglobin from stealing the oxygen back from the tissues. This 2,3-DPG-related affinity for oxygen gives the oxygen-dissociation curve its nearly sinusoidal appearance rather than that of a straight line.

Factors that cause this dissociation curve to shift are summarized in the figure below.

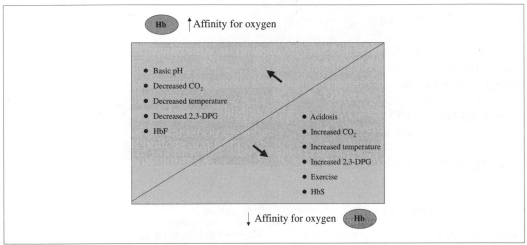

Factors shifting the oxygen-dissociation curve HbF, fetal haemoglobin; HbS, sickle-cell haemoglobin.

Shift of the curve by changes in the blood CO_2 is important to enhance oxygenation of the blood in the lungs and also to enhance release of oxygen from the blood to the tissues. This is the *Bohr effect.*

As CO_2 diffuses from the capillaries into the alveoli within the lungs, PCO_2 is reduced and the pH increases. Both of these effects cause the curve to shift left and upwards. Therefore the quantity of oxygen that binds with the haemoglobin becomes considerably increased, thus allowing greater oxygen transport to the tissues. When the blood reaches the capillaries the exact opposite occurs. The CO_2 from the tissues diffuses into the blood, decreasing the pH and causing the curve to shift to the right and downwards; that is the curve shifts to the right in the tissues and to the left in the lungs.

2. HAEMOGLOBIN ABNORMALITIES

These result from the synthesis of an abnormal haemoglobin (haemoglobinopathy) or a decreased rate of synthesis of normal α- or β-globin chains (thalassaemia). The chain structure is determined from a pair of autosomal genes. The genes for β-, σ- and γ-chains are carried on chromosome 11, while chromosome 16 carries the α-chain. Haemoglobinopathy and thalassaemia genes are allelomorphic (different genes can occupy the same locus on a chromosome) — the reason why mixed haemoglobinopathies can occur in one patient. For example, HbS and thalassaemia may occur in one patient.

2.1 Thalassaemia

Thalassaemia results from a genetically determined imbalanced production of one of the globin chains. α-, β-, σ- and γ-globin chains make up normal fetal and adult Hb in the following combinations:

- Fetal Hb: HbF $\alpha_2 + \gamma_2$

  Hb Barts γ_4

- Adult Hb: HbA $\alpha_2 + \beta_2$ (97%)

  HbA$_2$ $\alpha_2 + \sigma_2$ (2.5%)

Haemoglobin types in the different haemoglobinopathies

Disease	Genes	Haemoglobin type present
Sickle-cell disease	*S/S*	S + F
Sickle-cell trait	*S/A*	S + A
Hb C disease	*C/C*	C
Hb C trait	*C/A*	C + A
Hb D disease	*D/A*	D
Hb E disease	*E/A*	E + F
Sickle-cell — Hb C disease	*S/C*	S + C + F
Sickle-cell — thalassaemia	*S/β⁺*	S + F (also A if *β⁺*, if *β⁰* then no A)
Hb C — thalassaemia	*C/β⁺*	C + F (also A if *β⁺*, if *β⁰* then no A)
Hb E — thalassaemia	*E/β⁺*	E + F (also A if *β⁺*, if *β⁰* then no A)

Clinical management of thalassaemia

Safe blood transfusion programmes with effective iron-chelation therapy have transformed the outlook for children with thalassaemia.

Red cell transfusions

The aim here is to eliminate the complications of anaemia and ineffective erythropoiesis, which will allow the child to grow and develop normally. The decision to commence on a transfusion programme can be difficult, but generally the recommendation is to start when the haemoglobin concentration is ≤6.0 g/dl over 3 consecutive months. The desired maintenance Hb level is around 9.5 g/dl, with care being taken not to increase the iron burden too much.

Chelation treatment

The challenge here is to balance the complications of iron overload with the complications of the desferrioxamine — the chelating agent of choice. When to initiate chelation therapy remains unclear, but it is recommended to perform a liver biopsy after 1 year of a transfusion programme to establish the iron burden. Serum ferritin, although helpful, is not entirely accurate especially at the high levels seen in such patients.

Bone marrow transplantation

Remains an option in severe β-thalassemia, but this treatment option must be carefully balanced against the morbidity (and significant mortality) associated with allogeneic transplantation.

2.2 Sickle-cell disease

- Primarily affects people of African, Afro-Caribbean, Middle Eastern, Indian and Mediterranean descent
- In parts of Africa, 30% of the population have sickle-cell trait
- Is caused by a single-base mutation of adenine to thiamine, resulting in a substitution of valine for glutamic acid (at the 6th codon) on the β-globin chain
- HbS is insoluble and forms crystals when exposed to low oxygenation tension
- The symptoms of anaemia are mild relative to the severity of the anaemia, as HbS shifts the oxygen-haemoglobin curve to the right (see figure on p. 309)
- Presents after the age of 6 months — the time at which the production of haemoglobin should have switched from fetal to adult Hb
- The clinical picture is variable, although usually it is one of a chronic severe haemolytic anaemia punctuated by crises
- Crises may be visceral, aplastic, haemolytic and painful (see below) and are precipitated by infection, acidosis, dehydration and deoxygenation from whatever cause
- Patients are susceptible to infections with *Pneumococcus*, *Haemophilus* and *Salmonella* spp.

Sickle-cell disease (SCD) — clinical entities and appropriate management

Acute painful episodes (vaso-occlusive crises)

- Most frequent complication of SCD
- Common sites include bone and abdomen
- Pathophysiology: ischaemic tissue injury from the obstruction of blood flow by sickled erythrocytes
- Precipitating factors: infection, fever, acidosis, hypoxia, dehydration, sleep apnoea and exposure to extremes of heat and cold
- Diagnosis is based strictly on the history and clinical findings only

Treatment includes the following:

- Pain relief
- Antibiotic treatment if fever present and blood culture

- Ensure patient is adequately hydrated-intravenous fluid is recommended
- Check haematological parameters and crossmatch blood

Acute chest syndrome

Is responsible for up to 25% of all deaths in children with SCD. Aetiology is variable and may include both infectious and non-infectious causes (pulmonary infarction, hypoventilation secondary to rib/sternal infarction, fat embolism, pulmonary oedema secondary to fluid overload).

Treatment includes:

- Pain relief
- Oxygen
- Hydration

Intravenous antibiotic (3rd generation cephalosporin initially, add erythromycin for the child ≥5 years as *Mycoplasma* spp. may be present). Consider blood transfusion if the Hb level is ≥1.5 g/dl less than baseline. If severe and condition deteriorating, an exchange transfusion is indicated.

Aplastic crisis

Occurs when red cell production is temporarily reduced while the ongoing haemolytic process continues — resulting in severe anaemia. Parvovirus is usually the aetiological agent. The haemoglobin can fall to 3 g/dl and is the cause of presentation — malaise, lethargy, syncope and congestive heart failure. Urgent transfusion is necessary, but must be performed slowly as the patient may develop cardiac failure acutely.

Acute splenic sequestration crisis

Is characterized by pooling of large quantities of red blood cells in the spleen with sudden enlargement of the spleen and a precipitous decline in haemoglobin. Occurs most commonly in infants and young children between 6 months and 5 years. Treatment will be in the form of a blood transfusion and of any underlying causes.

Stroke

Stroke occurs in 5–10% of people with SCD, with the highest risk being between the ages of 1 and 9 years. Treatment should follow the general principles for sickle-cell disease — infection, oxygen, hydration and blood parameters. In addition, an exchange transfusion is indicated as soon as possible.

2.3 Other haemoglobinopathies

Sickle-cell trait

Individuals are usually asymptomatic as long as they are maintained with good oxygenation — an important point during anaesthesia.

Hb C disease

- Due to a substitution of lysine for glutamic acid in the β-globin chain at the same point as the substitution in Hb S
- Milder clinical course than Hb S
- Prevalent in West Africa

Hb D and Hb E disease

- Hb D is prevalent on the North-West coast of India, while Hb E is in South-East Asia — and both demonstrate mild anaemia only

Sickle-cell — Hb C disease

- Typically has a similar clinical picture to that of Hb S, although less infection and less crises are described
- Associated with avascular necrosis of the femoral head and vascular retinal changes

3. BLOOD GROUP ANTIBODIES

Approximately 400 red blood cell group antigens have been described, of which the ABO and rhesus (Rh) groups are of major clinical significance. Kell, Duffy, Kidd and Lutheran groups occasionally cause reactions, while the remaining groups rarely do.

3.1 ABO system

This consists of three allelic genes — *A, B* and *O*. Each gene codes for a specific enzyme that will result in the production of a carbohydrate residue. This residue will attach itself onto one of the three respective lipid and sugar chains — H-antigen, A-antigen and B-antigen chains on the red cell membrane. The *O* gene is an amorph and therefore does not transform the H antigen.

The *A* gene encodes for a carbohydrate residue that will attach itself to the end of the A-antigen chain, thereby blocking the distal glycoprotein antigenic portion. Similarly, the *B* gene encodes for a carbohydrate residue that will block the antigenic portion of the chain (see figure overleaf).

ABO blood groups

Group	O	A	B	AB
Genotype	*OO*	*AA* or *AO*	*BB* or *BO*	*AB*
Antigens	O	A	B	AB
Naturally occurring antibodies	anti A anti B	anti B	anti A	none
Frequency in the UK	46%	42%	9%	3%

A, B, AB and O blood groups

Group O

Group A

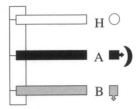

O antigen present but both A and B have no carbohydrate to cover the immunogenic distal portions of their chains. Anti-A and anti-B will therefore be produced.

A carbohydrate called A antigen has been produced to sit on the distal portion of A. B remains exposed therefore immunogenic — anti-B will be produced.

Group B

Group AB

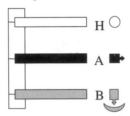

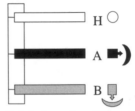

A carbohydrate called B antigen has been produced to sit on the distal portion of B. A remains exposed therefore immunogenic — anti-A will be produced.

Carbohydrates A and B have been produced to sit on the distal portions of A and B. No immunogenic distal portions are exposed therefore no antibodies will be produced.

A, B, AB and O blood groups

4. ANAEMIA

Anaemia can be classified by decreased substrate, abnormal production and destruction of red cells, as below.

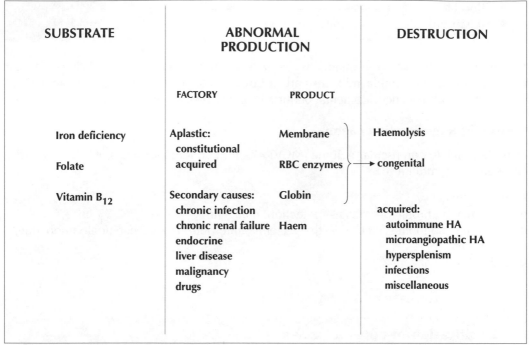

Working classification of anaemia

4.1 Iron deficiency anaemia

The major part of body iron is in the form of haem — essential for the delivery of oxygen to the tissues. Iron can exist in both the reduced (electron gain) or oxidized (electron loss) state, the vital property for electron-transfer reactions. A useful mnemonic is *LEO = loss of an electron is oxidation*. As iron is a major constituent of many important respiratory chain enzymes it is therefore directly involved in the production of cellular energy in the form of ATP. Deficiency of iron results in widespread non-haematological effects: for example, reduced CNS higher functions, diminished T-cell function and cell-mediated immunity as well as diminished muscle performance.

● Iron deficiency anaemia (Hb <11 g/dl) occurs in 10 to 30% of preschool children living in inner cities in the UK

Causes of iron deficiency

- Dietary insufficiency, e.g. unfortified milk
- Increased physiological requirement — infancy/adolescence
- Blood loss — gastrointestinal
- Malabsorption — coeliac disease

The most common reason in infancy is the early weaning to cows' milk. Giving an infant iron-supplemented formula milk instead of cows' milk not only prevents anaemia but reduces the decline in developmental performance observed in those given only cows' milk.

Causes of a microcytic anaemia

Definition: mean corpuscular volume (MCV) <72 fl in children <2 years or <78 fl in older children (fl = femtolitres).

- Iron deficiency
- Anaemia of chronic disorders — infection, malignancy
- Disorders of globin synthesis — thalassaemia trait, homozygous haemoglobinopathies
- Lead poisoning
- Sideroblastic anaemia

4.2 Aplastic anaemia

Classification of aplastic anaemia

- Constitutional (30%)
  - Fanconi's anaemia
  - Familial marrow aplasia in association with hand anomalies, deafness, ataxia, immune deficiencies
  - Dyskeratosis congenita
    - ectodermal dysplasia, X-linked
  - Shwachman–Diamond syndrome
    - pancreatic insufficiency
  - Amegakaryocytic thrombocytopenia
  - Reticular dysgenesis
- Acquired
  - Idiopathic — majority of cases
  - Drugs, e.g. acetazolamide, chloramphenicol
  - Infections, e.g. Epstein–Barr virus (EBV), viral hepatitis, parvovirus
  - Toxins, e.g. glues, dichlorodiphenyltrichloroethane (DDT)
  - Paroxysmal nocturnal haemoglobinuria

Steroids and/or anti-thymocyte globulin (ATG) have some beneficial effects in a few cases. The prognosis is invariably poor in severe cases, with bone marrow transplantation the only viable treatment option available.

4.3 Hereditary haemolytic anaemias (HHA)

For an understanding of HHA, one has to consider the membrane, red cell enzyme and haemoglobin defects involved.

Membrane defects

Hereditary spherocytosis

- Commonest hereditary HA in north Europeans
- Autosomal dominant
- Complex defect, but involves the spectrin structural protein
- Diagnosis made on appearances of blood film — the presence of spherocytes by demonstrating that the cells are osmotically active by using the osmotic fragility test
- The serum bilirubin and lactate dehydrogenase (LDH) may be elevated
- Treatment, by splenectomy, is reserved for severe cases

Hereditary elliptocytosis

- Usually autosomal dominant
- Most cases are asymptomatic

Red cell enzyme defects

Although a deficiency of any enzyme involved in the Embden–Meyerhof pathway may cause haemolysis, the two most commonly occurring deficiencies are:

Glucose 6-phosphate dehydrogenase (G6PD) deficiency

- G6PD helps to maintain glutathione in a reduced state, thus protecting the red cell from oxidative injury
- X-linked
- Different mutations of the gene are all found in different racial groups — Black Africans: 10% incidence, Mediterranean races: up to 35%
- Neonatal jaundice may be first sign
- Precipitating causes include infections, acidosis, favism, drugs
- Diagnose by assaying G6PD enzyme

Drugs to avoid in G6PD deficiency

- Analgesics/antipyretics: aspirin, probenecid
- Antimalarials: chloroquine
- Sulfonamides: dapsone
- Antibiotics: co-trimoxazole, nitrofurantoin, nalidixic acid, chloramphenicol
- Cardiovascular drugs: procainamide
- Miscellaneous: ascorbic acid, methyldopa, urate oxidase

Pyruvate kinase (PK) deficiency

- Deficiency of PK blocks the Embden–Meyerhof pathway — see figure on p. 308
- PK deficiency causes a rise in 2,3-DPG, thus a shift to the right on the oxygen-dissociation curve and consequent improvement in oxygen availability (figure on p. 309). Patients can therefore tolerate very low Hb levels.
- Autosomal recessive
- Infections, especially parvovirus, can produce dramatic haemolysis
- Splenectomy may be beneficial

4.4 Haemoglobin defects

See also Section 2, *Haemoglobin abnormalities*

Autoimmune haemolytic anaemia (AIHA)

- Coombs test (antihuman globulin) positive (see page 319)
- Uncommon in childhood, but if present is usually due to an intercurrent infection — predominantly viral but occasionally mycoplasma in origin
- In the older child, AIHA may be a manifestation of a multisystem disease, e.g. systemic lupus erythematusus (SLE)
- Causes include drugs (high-dose penicillin), infections (non-specific viral, measles, varicella, EBV), multisystem disease (SLE, rheumatoid arthritis) and lymphoproliferative disease (Hodgkin's lymphoma)
- Can be divided into warm and cold types depending on the temperature at which the causative cell-bound antibody is best detected
      Warm (usually IgG) — multisystem disease
      Cold (usually IgM) — infective causes

Microangiopathic haemolytic anaemia

- A rapidly developing haemolytic anaemia with fragmented red cells and thrombocytopenia
- Occurs in haemolytic–uraemic syndrome (HUS) and thrombotic thrombocytopenic purpura (TTP)

Hypersplenism

- The red cell lifespan is decreased by sequestration in an enlarged spleen for whatever cause

Infections

- Malaria
- Septicaemia

Miscellaneous

- Burns
- Poisoning
- Hyperphosphataemia
- A-betalipoproteinaemia

The Coombs (anti-globulin) test

Anti-human globulin (AHG) is produced in many animal species following the injection of human globulin. When AHG is added to human red cells that have been coated (sensitized) by immunoglobulin or complement components, agglutination of the red cells will occur, indicating a positive test.

There are two antiglobulin tests:

Direct antiglobulin test

This is used to detect antibody or complement on the red cell surface where sensitization has occurred *in vivo*.

A positive test occurs in:

- Haemolytic disease of the newborn
- Autoimmune haemolytic anaemia
- Drug-induced immune haemolytic anaemia
- Haemolytic transfusion reactions

Indirect antiglobulin test

This is used to detect antibodies that have coated the red cells *in vitro*. It is a two-staged procedure. The first stage involves incubation of test red cells with serum. The second stage involves washing these red cells with saline to remove free globulins. AHG is then added to the washed red cells. Agglutination implies that the original serum contained antibody, which has coated the red cells *in vitro*.

This indirect antiglobulin test is used in the following circumstances:

- Routine cross-matching procedures — to detect antibodies in the patient's serum that will be directed towards the donor red cells
- Detecting atypical blood group antibodies in serum during screening procedures
- Detecting blood group antibodies in a pregnant woman
- Detecting antibodies in serum in autoimmune haemolytic anaemia

5. THE WHITE CELLS: PHAGOCYTIC CELLS

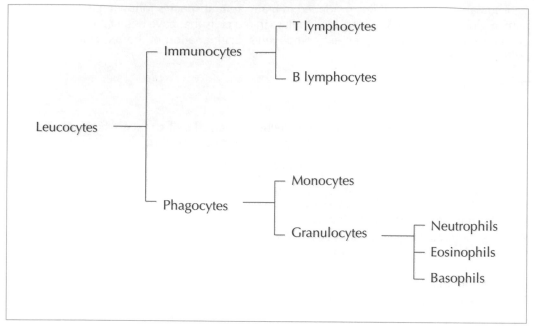

White cells or leucocytes can broadly be classified into groups.

The primary function of the white cells, in conjunction with immunoglobulins and complement, is to protect the body against infection.

Granulocytes and monocyte cells comprise the phagocytic (myeloid) group of white cells. They originate from a common precursor cell. It takes between 6 and 10 days for the precursor cell to undergo mitosis and maturation within the bone marrow. The immature neutrophil remains in the bone marrow as a reserve pool until required in peripheral blood. Bone marrow normally contains more myeloid than erythroid precursors — in a ratio of up to 12:1 and between 10 and 15 times more the number of granulocytes than in peripheral blood. Granulocytes spend only a matter of hours within the bloodstream before going into tissues. There are two pools of cells within the bloodstream — the circulating pool (what is included in the blood count) and the marginating pool (not included in the blood count as these cells adhere to the endothelium).

Formation, proliferation, differentiation and function

Growth factors are produced in stromal cells (endothelial cells, fibroblasts and macrophages) and from T lymphocytes. Under the influence of specific growth factors — stem-cell factor, IL (interleukin) -1, IL-3 and IL-6, a haematopoietic stem cell is produced. Granulocyte–monocyte colony-stimulating factor (GM-CSF) increases the commitment of this stem cell to differentiate into a phagocyte. Further differentiating and proliferating stimulus from G-CSF is required for neutrophil, from IL-5 for eosinophil and from M-CSF for monocyte production.

In addition, growth factors affect the function of the mature myeloid cells:

- Optimizing phagocytosis, superoxide generation and cytotoxicity in the neutrophil
- Optimizing phagocytosis, cytotoxicity and production of other cytokines in the monocyte
- Increasing membrane integrity and surface-adhesion properties of target cells
- GM-CSF can immobilize phagocytes at local sites of inflammation thereby causing accumulation at these sites

5.1 Neutrophils

Neutropenia

Neutropenia is defined as a reduction of the absolute neutrophil count below the normal for age.

The normal range of neutrophils for children at different ages

Age	Total WBC × 10^9/l		Neutrophils × 10^9/l		%
	Mean	Range	Mean	Range	
Birth	18	9.0 – 30	11	6.0 – 26	61
1 week	12	5.0 – 21	5.5	1.5 – 10	45
1 month	10.8	5.0 – 19.5	3.8	1.0 – 9	35
6 months	11.9	6.0 – 17.5	3.8	1.0 – 8.5	32
1 year	11.4	6.0 – 17.5	3.5	1.5 – 8.5	31
6 years	8.5	5.0 – 14	4.3	1.5 – 8	51
16 years	7.8	4.5 – 13	4.4	1.8 – 8	57

Neutropenia can be divided according to the severity, indicating the likely clinical consequences:

- Mild   1.0 – 1.5 (10^9/l)   Usually no problem
- Moderate   0.5 – 1.0 (10^9/l)   Clinical problems more common
- Severe   <0.5   (10^9/l)   Potentially severe and life-threatening, especially if prolonged beyond a few days

Bacterial infections such as cellulitis, superficial and deep abscess formation, pneumonia, septicaemia are the commonest problems associated with isolated neutropenia, while fungal, viral and parasitic infections are relatively uncommon.

The typical inflammatory response may be greatly modified with poor localization of infection, resulting in a greater tendency for infection to disseminate.

Although challenging in some cases, it is important to identify the cause of the neutropaenia (see overleaf) especially for the two following reasons:

- The clinical significance of the neutropenia will depend upon whether or not there is underlying marrow reserve
- Identifying the cause can help in predicting the duration of the neutropenia and therefore subsequent management

Marrow suppression (decreased production) will usually cause a severe neutropenia. The majority of children treated with chemotherapy will be in this group. Increased consumption or sequestration will cause mild to moderate neutropenia.

Causes of neutropenia

Decreased marrow production

Congenital
Kostmann's syndrome
Reticular dysgenesis

Acquired
Aplastic anaemia
Fanconi's anaemia
Drug suppression
Cyclical neutropenia
Vitamin B_{12}, folate, copper deficiency
Chronic benign neutropenia
Myelofibrosis
Osteopetrosis

Export
Metabolic conditions:
    Propionic, isovaleric and
    methylmalonic acidaemia
    Hyperglycinaemia

Consumption
Autoimmune antibodies
Neonatal isoimmune haemolytic disease
Infection/endotoxaemia

Sequestration
Immune complexes
Viral
SLE
Felty's syndrome
Sjögren's syndrome
Hypersplenism

Associated with immune deficiency
X-linked hypogammaglobulinaemia
Selective immunoglobulin deficiency states

Associated with phenotypical abnormal syndromes
Shwachman's syndrome
Chediak–Higashi syndrome
Cartilage hair hypoplasia
Dyskeratosis congenita

The risk of infection is directly proportional to the duration of neutropenia. If the duration of neutropenia is predicted to be prolonged, preventive measures against possible future infective episodes may be considered, for example:

- Good mouth care and dental hygiene
- Prophylaxis against *Pneumocystis* spp. (co-trimoxazole)
- Prophylaxis against fungal infections (fluconazole)
- Prophylaxis against recurrent herpes simplex infection (aciclovir)
- Regular throat and rectal swabs looking for Gram-negative colonization
- Dietary avoidance of unpasteurized milk and salads
- Avoidance of inhaling building/construction dust because of the risk of acquiring Aspergillus infection

Neutrophilia

The neutrophil count can be increased in one of the following three ways:

- Increased production of neutrophils as a result of increased progenitor cell proliferation or an increased frequency of cell division of committed neutrophil precursors
- Prolonged neutrophil survival within the plasma due to impaired transit into tissues
- Increased mobilization of neutrophils from the marginating pools or bone marrow

Acute neutrophilia

Neutrophils can be mobilized very quickly, within 20 minutes after they have been triggered, from the marginating pool. A stress response (acute bacterial infection, stress, exercise, seizures and some toxic agents) releases adrenaline (epinephrine) from endothelial cells which decreases neutrophil adhesion. This results in the neutrophils adhering to the endothelial lining of the vasculature (the marginating pool) being dragged into the circulation.

The bone marrow storage pool responds somewhat slower (a few hours) in delivering neutrophils in response to endotoxins, released from micro-organisms, or complement.

Corticosteroids may inhibit the passage of neutrophils into tissues, thereby increasing the circulating number.

Chronic neutrophilia

The mechanism in chronic neutrophilia is usually an increased marrow myeloid progenitor-cell proliferation. The majority of reactions last a few days or weeks. Infections and the chronic inflammatory conditions (e.g. juvenile chronic arthritis, Kawasaki's disease) are the predominant stimulators of this reaction. Less common causes include, for example, malignancy, haemolysis or chronic blood loss, burns, uraemia and post-operative states.

Splenectomy or hyposplenism may result in a reduced removal of increased neutrophils from the circulation.

5.2 Eosinophils

Eosinophils enter inflammatory exudates and have a special role in allergic responses, in defence against parasites and in removal of fibrin formed during inflammation. Eosinophils are proportionately reduced in number during the neonatal period. The causes of eosinophilia are extensive but some of the major causes are:

- Allergic diseases, e.g. asthma, hay fever, urticaria
- Parasitic diseases, e.g. worm infestation
- Recovery from infection
- Certain skin diseases, e.g. psoriasis, dermatitis herpetiformis
- Pulmonary eosinophilia
- Drug sensitivity
- Polyarteritis nodosa
- Hodgkin's disease

5.3 Basophils

Basophils, the least common of the granulocytes, are seldom seen in normal peripheral blood. In tissues they become mast cells. They have attachment sites on their cell membrane for IgE — which, when attaching, will cause degranulation to occur resulting in the release of histamine.

5.4 Monocytes

Monocytes, the largest of the leucocytes, spend a short time in the bone marrow and an even shorter time in the circulation (20–40 hours) before entering tissues where the final maturation to a phagocyte takes place. A mature phagocyte has a lifespan of months to years.

6. THE WHITE CELLS: LYMPHOCYTES

Lymphocytes, divided into T and B lymphocytes, are the immunologically active cells which aid the phagocytes to defend the body from an infective or other foreign invasion by aiding specificity.

Formation

The bone marrow and thymus are the two primary sites in which lymphocytes are produced, not by specific antigens but by non-specific cytokines. Thereafter they undergo specific transformation in secondary or reactive lymphoid tissue — the lymph nodes, spleen, the circulating lymphocytes and the specialized lymphoid tissue found in the respiratory and gastrointestinal tracts.

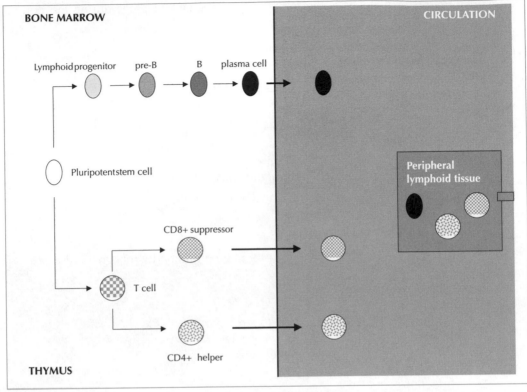

Diagrammatic illustration of immunocyte production

T cells are produced in the bone marrow and undergo transformation in the thymus, whereas the exact location in which the B lymphocytes are transformed remains unknown.

In peripheral blood 80% of the lymphocytes are T cells, while only 20% are B. T cells are responsible for cell-mediated immunity (vs. intracellular organisms and transplanted organs). B cells and plasma cells (differentiated B cells) are responsible for humoral immunity by producing immunoglobulins.

7. PLATELETS

Megakaryocytes, produced in the bone marrow, develop into platelets by a unique process of cytoplasm shedding. As the megakaryocyte matures the cytoplasm becomes more granular, these granules develop into platelets and are released into the circulation as the cytoplasm is shed.

Platelet production is under the control of growth factors, particularly thrombopoeitin and IL-6, while GM-CSF and IL-3 have megakarocyte colony-stimulating factor (MG-CSF) properties.

325

The main function of platelets is the formation of mechanical plugs during the normal haemostatic response to vascular injury.

7.1 Thrombocytopenia

A useful classification of thrombocytopenia is tabled below.

Thrombocytopenia — causes

- **Impaired production**
  - Congenital
  - TAR (thrombocytopenia and absent radius) syndrome
  - Fanconi's anaemia
  - Wiskott–Aldrich syndrome
  - Acquired
    - Aplastic anaemia
    - Bone marrow replacement, for example infiltration by malignant disease

- **Decreased platelet survival**
  - Immune-mediated
    - Immune (idiopathic) thrombocytopenic purpura (ITP)
    - Neonatal isoimmune thrombocytopenia
    - Alloimmune neonatal thrombocytopenia
    - Neonatal ITP
    - Infections
    - Drug-induced
    - Autoimmune disorders (e.g. SLE)
    - Malignancy

  - Non-immune-mediated
    - Disseminated intravascular coagulation (DIC)
    - Haemolytic–uraemic syndrome (HUS)
    - Thrombotic thrombocytopenia purpura (TTP)
    - Kasabach–Merritt syndrome
    - Cyanotic congenital heart disease
    - Liver disease
    - Drug-induced
    - Miscellaneous

7.2 Immune thrombocytopenic purpura (ITP)

Immune thrombocytopenic purpura (ITP) is a generic term used to describe an immune-mediated thrombocytopenia that is not associated with drugs or other evidence of disease. It is not a specific condition in that the cause and pathology are poorly understood. It may follow a viral infection or immunization and is caused by an inappropriate response of the immune system.

ITP does not have a predictable course, although it usually follows a benign self-limiting course. Approximately 20% of cases, in older girls predominantly, fail to remit over 6 months (chronic ITP).

Investigations

- A bone marrow biopsy is not indicated in a typical case, but when the diagnosis is uncertain it is a necessity
- Autoantibodies against platelet surface glycoprotein can be commonly detected, although they are neither a useful diagnostic test nor a useful prognostic indicator

Management

- No clear benefit of inpatient management.
- Written information about ITP, sensible advice (avoidance of contact sports, what to do in the event of an accident, etc.) and a contact person to call are usually sufficient.
- Treatment to raise the platelet count is not always required as the few remaining platelets, even if profoundly low in number ($<10 \times 10^9/l$), function more efficiently. The risk of serious bleeding from ITP as compared to the thrombocytopenia related with marrow failure syndromes, is low.
- Less than 1% of cases suffer an intracranial haemorrhage. In a recent national audit in the UK (performed over a 14-month period in 1995) no intracranial bleeds were reported in 427 patients.

Treatment includes the following modalities:

Intravenous immunoglobulin (IVIG)

The treatment of choice in severe haemorrhage as it raises the platelet count the fastest — usually within 48 hours. The most practical and effective administration of IVIG is a single dose of 0.8 gs/kg, although side-effects are common at this dose. Traditionally, 0.4g/kg/day has been given over 5 days.

Side-effects with IVIG are common and, as IVIG is a pooled blood product, a risk of viral transmission does exist.

Steroids

Given at a dose of 1–2 mg/kg daily for up to 2 weeks. Evidence has been shown that a higher dose of 4 mg/kg for 4 days may raise the platelet count as quickly as IVIG.

Anti-D

This has shown to be effective in children who are Rh-positive. It is a rapid single injection, although it may cause significant haemolysis.

Splenectomy

Rarely required and is only indicated in a patient with chronic ITP who has significant bleeding unresponsive to medical treatment. The failure rate after splenectomy is at least 25%.

Platelet transfusions are generally not indicated in ITP as it is a consumptive disorder.

Other agents

Vincristine, cyclophosphamide and cyclosporin have all been used with varying degrees of success. The combination of cyclophosphamide and rituximab (an anti-CD2O antibody) is currently demonstrating promising results.

Neonatal isoimmune thrombocytopenia

Babies may be born thrombocytopenic as a result of the transplacental passage of maternal antiplatelet antibodies. This can occur in two ways.

Alloimmune neonatal thrombocytopenia (ANT)

- Maternal antibodies are produced as a result of direct sensitization to fetal platelets (analogous to haemolytic disease of the newborn).
- Nineteen human platelet alloantigen (HPA) systems have been documented, the most important one (resulting in 85% of ANT cases) is HPA-1a. Only 3% of the population does not express HPA-1a, therefore if a mother does not express HPA-1a the chances of her partner expressing HPA-1a is high — resulting in an HPA-1a positive fetus. Only 6% of such mothers will become sensitized, and then not all sensitized mothers will produce a thrombocytopenic baby.
- Antibodies against HPA-1a are IgG and therefore can cross the placenta, bind to fetal platelets and decrease their survival time.
- Not only is it possible but it is common that ANT occurs in the first born.
- The diagnosis of ANT is suspected when a low platelet count is demonstrated in an otherwise healthy term neonate with a normal clotting screen.
- Treatment is in the form of an urgent platelet transfusion if severe (platelet count <20 x 10^9/l) as the risk of an intracerebral bleed is high in the first few days of life.
- Treatment of the fetus with periumbilical transfusions of immunologically compatible platelets (maternal platelets can be used) or maternal infusions of IgG and/or corticosteroids are possible — but not without significant risks.
- Genetic counselling, identification of the paternal genotype (heterozygous for HPA-1 results in a 50% chance of a positive genotype fetus) and close liaison between the haematologist, obstetrician and neonatologist is essential.

7.3 Neonatal isoimmune thrombocytopenia

- Occurs in babies born to mothers with active or previous ITP
- Clinically identical presentation to ANT but treatment is different, in that maternal platelets cannot be used as they will be consumed
- Maternal steroid therapy prior to delivery may improve the fetal platelet count

Drug-induced thrombocytopenia

An immune thrombocytopenia may occur with the following commonly prescribed drugs:

- Sodium valproate
- Phenytoin
- Carbamazepine

- Co-trimoxazole
- Rifampicin
- Heparin (non-immune mechanisms also possible)

7.4 Functional abnormalities of platelets

Before classifying these abnormalities it is important to understand the normal function of platelets. In order to achieve haemostasis, platelets undergo the following reactions of adhesion, secretion or release reaction, aggregation and procoagulation.

Adhesion

Adhesion of platelets to subendothelial lining requires interactions between platelet membrane glycoproteins, elements of vessel wall (e.g. collagen) and adhesive proteins such as von Willebrand factor (vWF) and fibronectin.

Release reaction

Collagen exposure results in the release or secretion of the contents of platelet granules: fibrinogen, serotonin, ADP, lysosomal enzymes, heparin-neutralizing factor. The cell membrane releases an arachidonate derivative which transforms into thromboxane A_2 — a stimulus for aggregation as well as being a powerful vasoconstrictor.

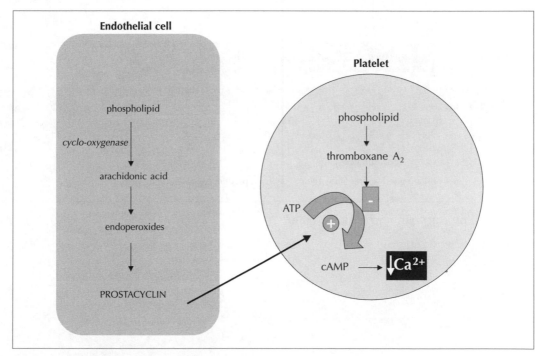

Production of prostacyclin and thromboxane

Aggregation

The contents of the platelet granules, specifically ADP and thromboxane A_2, cause additional platelets to aggregate at the site of injury.

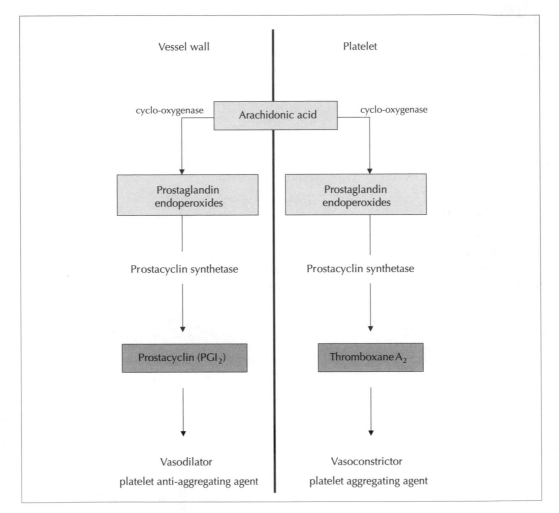

Function of prostacyclin and thromboxane

Platelet procoagulation activity

After secretion and aggregation have taken place a phospholipid (platelet factor 3) becomes exposed on the platelet membrane, thereby making itself available for its surface to be used as a template for two important coagulation protein reactions — the conversion of factor X to X_a and prothrombin to thrombin. These reactions are Ca^{2+}-dependent.

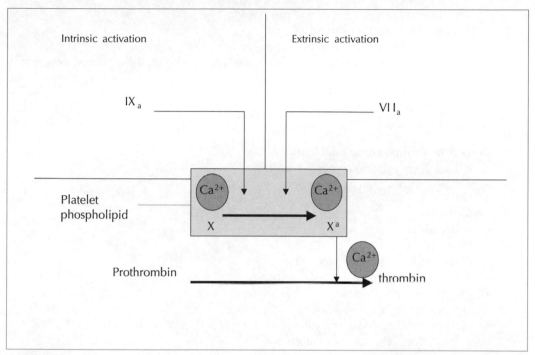

Procoagulant activity

Functional platelet abnormalities — classification

- **Congenital**
  Defects of platelet membrane
    - e.g. Glanzmann's thrombasthenia
      - *rare, autosomal recessive, failure to aggregate*
      - *normal platelet count and morphology*
      - Bernard–Soulier syndrome
      - *rare, autosomal recessive, failure of adhesion*
      - *no receptor to bind to vWF. Giant platelets, moderate platelet count reduction*

  Deficiency of storage granules
    - e.g. Wiskott–Aldrich syndrome
      - Chediak–Higashi syndrome

  Defects of thromboxane deficiency
    - e.g. thromboxane synthetase deficiency
      - cyclo-oxygenase deficiency

- **Acquired**
  - Renal failure
  - Liver failure
  - Myeloproliferative disorders
  - Acute leukaemia, especially myeloid
  - Chronic hypoglycaemia
  - Drugs
  - Aspirin, non-steroidal anti-inflammatory drugs (NSAIDs), penicillin, cephalosporin, sodium valproate

Investigations

- A prolonged bleeding time and normal or moderately reduced platelet count are the characteristic hallmarks of a congenital/hereditary platelet disorder (or von Willebrand's disease)
- Platelet size followed by tests of aggregation and secretion in response to ADP, collagen, arachidonate and ristocetin will be necessary

8. BLOOD FILM

8.1 Approach to a blood film at MRCPCH level

Is the pathology in the red or white blood cell?

This is the first and vital question you need to ask yourself when presented with a blood film to interpret. Apart from the accompanying history being important in helping you to answer this question, the other clue will be the number of white cells seen. If there is an abundance of white cells the likelihood that the pathology will be in the white cells is very high, and I will go as far as to say that acute lymphoblastic leukaemia will be top of your differential diagnosis. If only an occasional white cell is seen then red cell pathology is likely. Platelet pathology will be unlikely at MRCPCH level — the only real possibility is one of giant platelets (same size as a red cell, or bigger) in the Bernard–Soulier syndrome.

Red cell pathology?

Once you have decided on red cell pathology then look at the following parameters:

Shape

- Sickle-shaped cells as in sickle-cell disease
- Fragments of red cells (e.g. Helmet cells, etc.) indicative of microangiopathic haemolysis such as in the haemolytic–uraemic syndrome.
- All different shapes, i.e. poikilocytosis as in thalassaemia, sickle-cell, iron deficiency anaemia.

Size

- Small cells or microcytosis in iron deficiency anaemia
- Large cells or macrocytosis in vitamin B_{12} and/or folate-deficient anaemia
- Different sizes: anisocytosis (haemoglobinopathies, anaemias)

Amount of central pallor in red cell

- No central pallor: spherocytosis (hereditary spherocytosis, haemolytic conditions, burns for example)
- Large central pallor: hypochromic anaemia
- 'Halo' central pallor: target cells (haemoglobinopathies, hyposplenism)

Red cell inclusions

- Malaria: most commonly *Plasmodium falciparum*, seen as a 'signet-ring' inclusion
- Howell-Jolly bodies: remnants of nuclear fragments, seen in hyposplenism
- Heinz bodies: denatured haemoglobin, resulting from oxidant stress (e.g. G6PD) or haemolysis; can only be seen with special stain, so if normal stain then it is most likely a Howell–Jolly body
- Basophilic stippling: multiple small inclusions in a red cell — e.g. lead poisoning

White cell pathology?

The abundance of white cells is most likely to be leukaemia at the MRCPCH level. A lymphoblast cell is recognized by its size (large), with a large nucleus taking up nearly the entire cells with only a rim of cytoplasm remaining (in contrast, a mature neutrophil has a multilobed small nucleus). The morphological differentiation between acute lymphoblastic leukaemia (ALL) and acute myeloid leukaemia (AML) is not realistic at this level, but remember the relative incidence of each, 4:1, respectively.

9. COAGULATION

A representation of the coagulation cascades is shown below. It consists of an extrinsic pathway (tissue thromboplastin is the initiator) and the intrinsic pathway (what happens in the blood when it clots away from the body). These two pathways share a common final pathway resulting in the production of a fibrin clot.

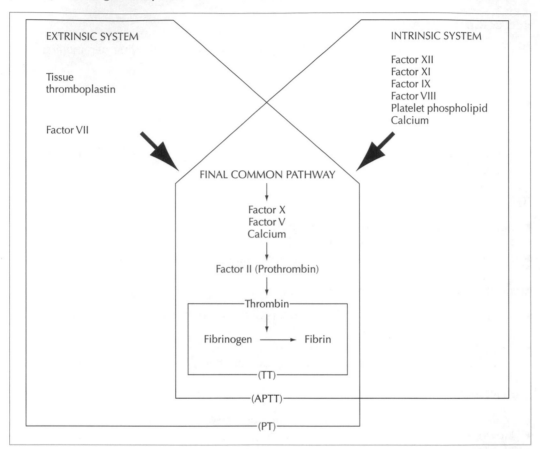

Representation of the coagulation cascades

The system can be divided into boxes, each box representing one of the following three basic screening tests of coagulation:

- **Prothrombin time** (PT) measures the extrinsic system and common pathway
- **Activated partial thromboplastin time** (APTT) measures the intrinsic system and common pathway
- **Thrombin time** (TT) measures the final part of the common pathway, it is prolonged by the lack of fibrinogen and by inhibitors of this conversion, e.g. heparin and fibrin degradation products.

9.1 Natural anticoagulants

It is important that thrombin is limited to the site of injury. This is achieved by circulating inhibitors of coagulation:

- Antithrombin III — the most potent inhibitor, heparin potentiates its effect markedly
- Protein C inhibits factors Va and VIIIa and promotes fibrinolysis
- The action of protein C is enhanced by protein S

9.2 Coagulation disorders

Haemophilia A (factor VIII deficiency or absence)

- Levels of factor VIII in carriers are variable due to random inactivation of the X chromosome (lyonization). As a result, DNA probes are now recommended to detect carrier status.
- Prolonged APTT and factor VIII clotting assay reduced.
- Bleeding time and prothrombin times are normal.
- Vasopressin (DDAVP) may be useful in releasing endogenous factor VIII from its stores in mild haemophilia. Tranexamic acid, by inhibiting fibrinolysis, may be useful.

Haemophilia B (factor IX deficiency or absence), Christmas disease

- Exactly the same as above, except factor IX is involved rather than factor VIII
- Incidence is one-fifth that of haemophilia A

von Willebrand's disease

von Willebrand's disease (vWD) is a more complicated entity compared to haemophilia A or B and is generally poorly described — hence often overlooked in clinical practice. It therefore deserves an in-depth explanation.

von Willebrand factor (vWF), is an adhesive glycoprotein encoded by a gene on chromosome 12. It is produced by endothelial cells and by platelets. vWF has two main functions, to:

- stabilize and protect circulating factor VIII from proteolytic enzymes
- mediate platelet adhesion

vWD will therefore result when the synthesis of vWF is reduced or when abnormal vWF is produced.

The clinical presentation of vWD will include the following:

- Mucous membrane bleeding
- Excess bleeding following surgical/dental procedures
- Easy bruising

Three types (at least) have been described:

- **Type 1**
  - Most common, accounts for at least 70% of vWD
  - Due to a partial deficiency of vWF
  - Autosomal dominant

- **Type 2**
  - Due to abnormal function of vWF

- **Type 3**
  - Due to the complete absence of vWF

Often, can be mistaken for haemophilia A, as factor VIII levels will be low as there is no vWF to protect factor VIII from proteolysis. Laboratory results are important in distinguishing the types of vWD and the differentiation from haemophilia. In vWD type 1 the following results will be expected:

Platelet count	N
Bleeding time	N / ↑
Factor VIII	↓
vWF	↓
Ristocetin cofactor activity	↓

Ristocetin, an antibiotic, is now confined to laboratory-only use after it was documented to cause significant thrombocytopenia. Ristocetin, when added to a patient's plasma, will bind vWF and platelets together causing platelet aggregation (hence, the clinical thrombo-cytopenia). In the absence of vWF, no platelet aggregation will be seen (vWF type 3). In the presence of decreased vWF, diminished aggregation will ensue (vWD type 1). Hence, when faced with the clinical picture of haemophilia A (bruising, normal platelet count, slightly increased bleeding time and a decreased factor VIII), the ristocetin cofactor test will be able to differentiate between vWD (decreased) and haemophilia A (normal).

Haemorrhagic disease of the newborn

- Vitamin K-dependent factors are low at birth and fall further in breast fed infants in the first few days of life
- Other factors associated with this deficiency include:
  - Liver-cell immaturity
  - Lack of gut bacterial synthesis of the vitamin K
  - Low quantities in breast milk
- Haemorrhage is usually between day 2 and day 4 of life
- PT and APTT are both abnormal, while the platelet count and fibrinogen levels are normal. Fibrin degradation products (FDP's) will not be detected.
- Treatment is with vitamin K, either administered intramuscularly at birth or orally on day 1, followed by interval dosing thereafter
- Prophylactic vitamin K remains controversial — see further reading

10. MALIGNANT PATHOLOGY

- There are 1,200 new cases of malignancy diagnosed each year in the UK in children under 15 years of age (an incidence of 1 in 600 children <15 years)
- The relative incidence rates for the different tumour types is illustrated below
- Leukaemia, together with lymphoma, account for nearly 50% of all cases
- Brain and spinal cord tumours are the most commonly occurring solid tumours
- Overall, childhood cancer is about one-third more common in boys than girls

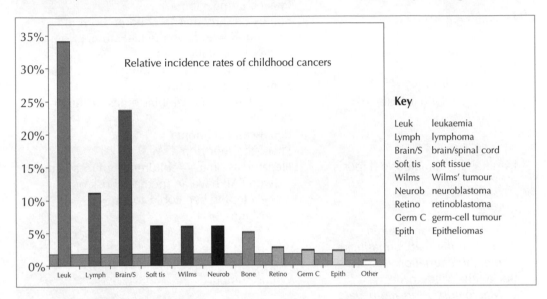

Relative incidence rates of childhood cancers

Key

Leuk	leukaemia
Lymph	lymphoma
Brain/S	brain/spinal cord
Soft tis	soft tissue
Wilms	Wilms' tumour
Neurob	neuroblastoma
Retino	retinoblastoma
Germ C	germ-cell tumour
Epith	Epitheliomas

Environmental factors predisposing to cancer

- Ultraviolet radiation — skin cancer, particularly malignant melanoma
- Ionizing radiation
    - Preconceptual paternal exposure — remains controversial
    - *In-utero* exposure — increased incidence of leukaemia
    - Postnatal exposure — leukaemia
- Electromagnetic fields — remains controversial

Syndromes/conditions predisposing to cancer

Syndrome	Cancer
Down	Acute leukaemia
	20 times more susceptible than population
Neurofibromatosis type 1	Brain tumours, including optic glioma
	Juvenile myelomonocytic leukaemia
	Phaeochromocytoma
Li–Fraumeni	Soft tissue sarcomas in children born to families who have the Li–Fraumeni syndrome (mutation of p53)
Klinefelter	Germ-cell tumours, including dysgerminoma
Tuberous sclerosis	Benign tumours in organs
von Hippel–Lindau disease	Cerebellar haemangioblastomas — multiple
	Retinal angiomas
	Renal-cell carcinoma
	Phaeochromocytoma
Familial adenomatous polyposis (FAP)	Hepatoblastoma — children born to a parent with FAP have an increased risk of developing hepatoblastoma
WAGR *Wilms' tumour, aniridia genitourinary abnormalities, mental retardation*	Wilms' tumour
Beckwith–Weidemann *Macroglossia, organomegaly Omphalos, hemihypertrophy*	Wilms' tumour
Denys–Drash *Pseudohermaphroditism Wilms' tumour, nephrotic syndrome*	Wilms' tumour
Perlman *Phenotypically similar to Beckwith–Weidemann*	Wilms' tumour
Xeroderma pigmentosum	Basal- and squamous-cell skin carcinoma
Ataxia telangiectasia	Leukaemia and B-cell lymphoma

10.1 Leukaemia

The leukaemias can be divided into acute and chronic leukaemia. Chronic leukaemia accounts for less than 5% of all leukaemias in childhood — all of these cases would be chronic myeloid leukaemia (CML) as CLL does not exist in childhood.

- In acute leukaemia, a differentiating white cell undergoes a structural and/or numerical change in its genetic make-up, causing a failure of further differentiation and dysregulated proliferation and clonal expansion

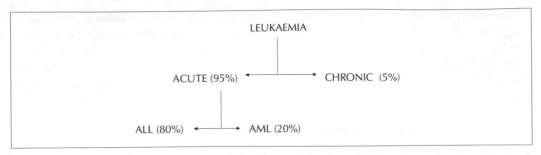

- Aetiology remains unknown, although associations or risk factors have been identified;
  - Chromosomal breakage or defective DNA repair mechanisms (e.g. Fanconi's anaemia, ataxia telangiectasia)
  - Chemotherapy — second tumour effect
  - Immunodeficiency syndrome, for example Wiskott–Aldrich
  - Trisomy 21
  - Identical twin, especially if twin contracted leukaemia in infancy
  - Ionizing radiation
- Clinical presentation is related to bone marrow failure and possibly to extramedullary involvement

Acute lymphoblastic leukaemia (ALL)

Acute lymphoblastic leukaemia (ALL) is divided into B-cell or T-cell ALL depending on what cell line (determined by immunophenotyping) the clone lies. The figure above illustrates this clearly. The majority of cases (>80%) originate from the B-cell line with common ALL (cALL), arising from the lymphoid progenitor cell, being the commonest. About 15% are T-cell ALL with 2% demonstrating mixed lineage. cALL has the most favourable prognosis out of all the immunophenotypes.

Poor prognostic signs in ALL include:

- Presenting white cell count (WCC) greater than $50 \times 10^9/l$
- Outside the age range 2–9 years
- Males do less well than females
- Some chromosomal translocations, including the presence of the Philadelphia chromosome
- Normal diploid number of chromosomes in blast cell (hyperdiploidy carries a more favourable prognosis).
- Afro-Caribbean ethnicity
- CNS disease

The poor risk or prognostic factors above are now used to tailor treatment, i.e. a child with a high WCC will get more intensive treatment than if the WCC had been normal. Treatment is in the form of intensification blocks with ongoing maintenance therapy in between. Central nervous system-directed treatment is a vital component of treatment, as lymphoblasts can be protected from standard chemotherapy by being on the 'other-side' of the blood–brain barrier. In standard risk this will comprise intrathecal chemotherapy at regular intervals; but for higher risk children, high-dose intravenous methotrexate (at sufficient dose to cross the blood–brain barrier) or cranio–spinal radiotherapy may be required. The latter is the most effective in sterilizing the CNS of lymphoblasts, but it has a high price to pay in that the neurocognitive side-effects can be profound. Treatment overall is over a 2-year period, although currently there is evidence to suggest that a 3-year regimen produces superior results. The 5-year survival rate for standard-risk ALL is now approximately 80%.

Acute myeloid leukaemia (AML)

- Is divided into seven subtypes depending on morphology (FAB — French, American, British classification) and immunophenotyping characteristics — M1 to M7
- Chromosomal abnormalities occur in at least 80% of cases, with translocations the most common
- Treatment is with a more intensive, but shorter chemotherapy regimen than that used for ALL.
- Bone marrow transplantation remains controversial, as the reduced remission rates with this modality need to be weighed up together with the increased mortality of the transplantation procedure
- 5-year survival figures are now in excess of 50%

10.2 Lymphoma

Two types of lymphoma are recognized: non-Hodgkin's lymphoma (NHL) and Hodgkin's disease (HD). In NHL the originating cell is either a B or T lymphocyte or an immature form thereof, while in HD the originating cell is not clear. It is thought, but not proven, that the Hodgkin's cell or its derivative, the Reed–Sternberg cell, derives from lymphoid tissue.

Non-Hodgkin's lymphoma (NHL)

- NHL is the term adopted to describe a heterogeneous group of malignant proliferations of lymphoid tissue
- Burkitt's lymphoma is derived from a mature B cell
- NHL is derived from the same T- and B-lineage lymphoid cells as ALL, but an important difference exists between these two entities

In ALL, 80% of cases are pre-B cell-derived; while 20% in T cell-derived. In NHL this is reversed, with pre-B cell-derived tumours being very rare.

The following sites are commonly affected, in descending order of frequency:

- Abdomen — usually with B-cell disease
- Mediastinum — typically T cell in origin
- Head and neck — no specific cell

Classification of NHL remains challenging and controversial. Chemotherapy is the mainstay of treatment as NHL is a systemic disease, despite the apparent local sites of disease.

Hodgkin's disease (HD)

- The EBV-related causal hypothesis remains unproven
- Painless cervical lymphadenopathy is the most frequent presenting symptom
- An open surgical nodal biopsy is necessary to examine lymph node architecture and stromal cellular elements
- Chemotherapy and/or radiotherapy remain the treatment modalities of choice and the focus of current trials; similar results are produced from each modality, but chemotherapy can decrease fertility and radiotherapy can cause significant neck and chest muscle atrophy

10.3 Tumour-lysis syndrome

- High-count ALL (especially T cell) and B-NHL have the potential of bulky disease — a high cell mass, which will undergo lysis with treatment, resulting in the intracellular contents of potassium, phosphate and nuclear debris being released into the circulation
- Blast cells have four times the amount of phosphate of normal white cells
- Uric acid crytals and phosphate (precipitating out with calcium) crystals may cause acute renal failure and the following:
  - Fluid overload ↑
  - Phosphate ↑
  - Potassium ↑
  - Urea and creatinine ↑
  - Calcium ↓

Treatment involves:

- Hyperhydration
- Uric acid-lowering agents — allopurinol or uricozyme
- Treatment of hyperkalaemia
- Consideration of fluid filtration or dialysis

10.4 Tumours of the CNS

- The anatomical grouping together of brain tumours masks their diverse biological differences
- Brain tumours in children tend to be located in the posterior fossa, in the midline, have greater differentiation and slightly better survival figures than their counterparts in adults
- Brain tumours as a general rule do not metastasize out of the CNS
- They are notorious to diagnose because of their varied and often non-specific presentations. The mean time from onset of symptoms to diagnose is 5-months.

Presenting symptoms of brain tumours

Presenting symptoms	% of children
Vomiting	65
Headache	64
Changes in personality and mood	47
Squint	24
Out-of-character behaviour	22
Deterioration of school performance	21
Growth failure	20
Weight loss	16
Seizures	16
Developmental delay	16
Disturbance of speech	11

Astrocytoma

- Most commonly occurring brain tumour
- Range from low-grade (benign) tumours, usually in the cerebellum, to high-grade (malignant) tumours, usually supratentorial and brainstem
- The glioblastoma multiforme tumour has a near-fatal prognosis

Medulloblastoma (primitive neuroectodermal tumour (PNET) occurring in the cerebellum)

- 20% of brain tumours
- The most commonly occurring high-grade tumour
- Commonly metastasizes within the CNS, and it is the one tumour that can metastasize out of the CNS
- Prognosis is in the region of a 50% 5-year survival

Brainstem glioma

- 20% of brain tumours
- Can either be diffuse (e.g. diffuse pontine glioma) or local
- Less than 10% survival

Craniopharyngioma

- 8% of all brain tumours
- Situated in the suprasellar region predominantly
- Presenting features may be in the form of raised intracranial pressure, visual disturbances, pituitary dysfunction and psychological abnormalities
- Treatment remains controversial but usually involves surgery and/or radiotherapy

10.5 Retinoblastoma

Retinoblastoma may be:

Hereditary

- 40%
- Deletion of a tumour-suppressor gene at chromosome 13q14

- Behaves in an autosomal dominant fashion (with a high degree of penetrance) but requires inactivation of remaining allele at the cellular level
- Usually multifocal disease
- Early onset (mean — 10 months)
- Increased risk of developing a second primary tumour

or Sporadic

- 60%
- Unifocal
- Late onset (mean 18 months)

10.6 Neuroblastoma

- An aggressive tumour of the sympathetic chain (neural crest origin)
- Presenting symptoms often non-specific and can mimic commonly occurring conditions; symptoms are due to the numerous possible tumour sites, metastases and the associated metabolic disturbances (due to catecholamine secretion: sweating, pallor, diarrhoea, hypertension)
- Urinary and plasma catecholamine metabolites (vanillyl mandelic acid (VMA) and homovanillic acid (HVA) may be raised

Prognostic factors are:

- Tumour stage
- Age (inversely proportional)
- Histopathology
- Molecular biology: presence of the following confers increased risk:
  - N-*myc* amplification
  - 1p deletion
  - serum ferritin ↑
  - LDH ↑
- Stage 4S — local primary tumour with dissemination to liver, skin or bone marrow occurring in infancy; 85% will regress

10.7 Wilms' tumour (nephroblastoma)

- Presents in a well child with a painless (or minimal discomfort) abdominal mass, haematuria and hypertension (independently or collectively)
- Intensity of treatment is relative to the staging and the histology of the tumour
- Very good overall prognosis — in excess of 90% 5-year survival

10.8 Bone tumours

Osteosarcoma

- Twice as common as Ewing's sarcoma
- Predominantly in the metaphyses of long bones, 50% occurring in the femur

- Presentation peaks in teenage years, suggesting a relationship between rapid bone growth and tumour formation
- 80% of all patients develop lung metastases

Ewing's sarcoma

- Occurs more commonly in flat bones (e.g. pelvis, ribs, vertebra) than osteosarcoma, although long bones can be affected
- Can be extraosseous in rare cases

10.9 Soft tissue sarcomas

These are a group of tumours derived from contractile, connective, adipose and vascular tissue. Rhabdomyosarcoma (RMS) is the most common of these, arising from cells destined to be striated muscle cells. RMS can occur anywhere in the body, with the common sites being genitourinary, parameningeal and orbit.

10.10 Malignant germ-cell tumours

Tumours derived from germ cells (cells giving rise to gonadal tissue) can be gonadal (30%) or extragonadal cells (70%).

- Extragonadal sites are the sacrococcygeal region, retroperitoneum, mediastinum, neck and the pineal area of the brain.
- As gonadal tissue can give rise to any cell type, tumours derived from such cells may express any cell line in any stage of differentiation. This gives rise to range of tumours, from an undifferentiated embryonal carcinoma to a benign and fully differentiated mature teratoma.
- Serum markers α-fetoprotein and β-HCG are useful in diagnosing and monitoring disease state.

10.11 Hepatoblastoma

- Hepatoblastoma, an embryonal tumour of the liver, occurs in an otherwise normal liver (compared to hepatocellular carcinoma) and presents in children under the age of 2 years generally
- An association between familial adenomatous polyposis and hepatoblastoma exists

10.12 Langerhans-cell histiocytosis

- Langerhans cells are bone marrow-derived cells of the macrophage/monocyte series which migrate to the epidermis. Here they function as potent antigen-presenting cells.
- What causes Langerhans cells to be pathological remains unknown. Is it a reactive disease with a chronic relapsing course, or is it due to uncontrolled proliferation (clonal entity)?

- The excess Langerhans cells deposit in the skin and other organs where they cause inflammatory tissue damage as a result of the release of cytokines and prostaglandins.
- Without a known pathogenesis, treatment is challenging. Chemotherapy has been used, to some effect, in controlling disease.

10.13 Role of bone marrow transplantation

The three broad areas in which bone marrow transplantation is a possibility, are to:

- replace a missing enzyme, e.g. mucopolysaccharidosis, adrenoleucodystrophy
- restore bone marrow function following high-dose or bone marrow ablative chemotherapy, e.g. chemotherapy for neuroblastoma
- treat and/or immunomodulate a disease process, e.g. acute myeloid leukaemia, juvenile chronic myeloid leukaemia — CML (now myelomonocytic — JMML), high-risk ALL (e.g. Philadelphia chromosome +ve)

Bone marrow transplant can be:

- Autologous – patient receives his/her own bone marrow
- Allogeneic – patient receives donated marrow from either a sibling (matched related donor) or an unrelated donor (matched unrelated donor — MUD)

The technique of harvesting peripheral-blood stem cells from a patient prior to ablative chemotherapy, and returned post-chemotherapy, now provides an alternative to bone marrow harvesting. Currently, the use of cord-blood stem cells is becoming an option for bone marrow transplant.

10.14 Late effects of cancer treatment

Chemotherapy

Second malignancies
Leukaemia and lymphoma are the two most likely secondary malignancies to occur — particularly AML with topoisomerase II inhibitors (e.g. etoposide) while alkylators (e.g. nitrogen mustard, cyclophosphamide) may cause either.

Cardiac
Cardiomyopathy is the most likely complication particularly with anthracycline-containing chemotherapy, which is commonly used in treating solid tumours and, to a lesser extent, leukaemia. This toxicity is exacerbated by thoracic radiotherapy.

Reduced fertility or infertility
Diminished fertility potential with increasing cumulative doses of alkylating chemotherapy (particularly with procarbazine, which at high doses will render all males infertile), for example in Hodgkin's disease.

Pulmonary

Pulmonary fibrosis may result from bleomycin chemotherapy used, for example, in Hodgkin's disease and germ-cell tumours.

Neurocognitive

There is insufficient data at present to claim a definite association between chemotherapy and neurocognitive difficulties, although this may very well exist. Methotrexate is the one exception where an association has been made.

Auditory

Otoxicity may result from platinum-containing agents, for example, cisplatinum and carbo-platinum, used commonly in the treatment of CNS and other solid tumours.

Renal

Decreased renal function as measured by the glomerular filtration rate (GFR) may be caused by the same platinum-containing agents as above. In addition, a Fanconi's syndrome with electrolyte abnormalities may result from numerous chemotherapeutic agents.

Radiotherapy

The developing child is extremely susceptible to the damaging effects of radiotherapy, particularly in the following areas:

- Neurocognitive — especially in the younger child
- Endocrine abnormalities — particularly growth and hypothyroidism
- Second malignancies — particularly sarcomas and lymphoma
- Musculoskeletal atrophy
- Organ damage — for example, cardiac, lung, gastrointestinal

11. FURTHER READING

Idiopathic thrombocytopenic purpura: Bolton-Maggs PHB. *Arch Dis Child* **83**(220-222), 2000.

Iron supplemented formula milk related to reduction in psychomotor decline in infants from inner city areas: Williams J, Wolff A, Daly A, MacDonald A, Aukett A, Booth I. Randomised study *BMJ* **318**(693-698), 1999.

Paediatric Haematology: Lilleyman J, Hann I, Blanchette V (editors). Churchill Livingstone 2000.

Paediatric Oncology: Pinkerton CR, Plowman PN (editors). Chapman and Hall Medical 1997.

Management of severe alloimmune thrombocytopenia in the newborn: Ouwehand WH, Smith G, Ranasinghe E. *Arch Dis Child* Fetal Edition **82**(F173-75), 2000.

Patterns of care and survival for children with acute lymphoblastic leukaemia diagnosed between 1980 and 1994: Stiller CA, Eatock EM. *Arch Dis Child* **81**(202-208), 1999.

The vitamin K debacle – cut the Gordian knot but first do no harm (Annotations): Tripp JH, McNinch AW. *Arch Dis Child* **79**(295-297), 1998.

Chapter 10

Immunology

Bobby Gaspar and Waseem Qasim

CONTENTS

Immunology

1. INTRODUCTION

Immunity against specific infectious agents is brought about by a complicated set of inter-actions between host and pathogen which, under normal circumstances, maintains an ade-quate balance between the two. From early in life humans come into contact with a wide variety of infectious agents including bacteria, fungi and viruses. Some of these become commensals, some cause troublesome infections in the neonatal period, some are pathogenic throughout childhood, whilst others remain significant pathogens throughout life. Increased susceptibility to infectious diseases occurs in individuals with a wide variety of abnormalities including anatomical, metabolic, haematological, oncological and immunological abnormalities.

The immune system can be divided into specific and non-specific components. Non-specific immunity refers to the first-line of defence against pathogens which, if breached, leads to the specific or adaptive immune response being activated. This first-line of defence consists of a variety of components including mechanical barriers (e.g. skin), secretions (e.g. tears), mucus in the respiratory tract and gut, bile and enzymes in the gastrointestinal tract, acidity of urine and gastric acid fluid and the normal commensals of the skin and gut which prevent colonization with pathogenic organisms. Second-line, non-specific mechanisms include complement components which bind to phagocytic receptors found on cells, and particularly neutrophils and macrophages, which may interact with antigens in a non-specific way.

Specific immunity is divided into humoral and cellular responses. Humoral immunity refers to the production of antibody specific for an invading pathogen or antigen, while cellular immunity is mediated via cells of the immune system. Lymphocytes are central to both arms of the specific immune system. B lymphocytes produce antibodies and present antigens to T lymphocytes. T lymphocytes themselves may act as cytotoxic cells killing virally infected cells, or as helper cells providing help or suppression to other cells involved or recruited into the specific immune response.

The crucial difference between the specific and non-specific arms of the immune system is the ability of the specific arm to develop memory. This immunological memory allows the rapid mobilization of specific immune mechanisms on the second and subsequent chal-lenges with a particular antigen such as a virus. This response may be mediated via the humoral (antibody) or cellular (T cell) system. Either way, the consequence of memory is the protection from recurrent infection with the same antigen. Memory is learnt during the development of the immune system and explains the difference in frequency between infections in adults and children.

The immune system is a complicated structure/organ made up of many parts that have, with time, evolved and become increasingly sophisticated. Different aspects of the immune system are discussed below.

2. THE IMMUNE SYSTEM

2.1 Haematopoietic stem cells

- Multipotent cells capable of giving rise to entire haematopoietic system
- Capable of self-renewal
- Characterized by presence of CD34 surface antigen
- CD34 does not identify stem cells alone, but also more committed progenitor cells
- Present at 1% in the bone marrow
- Found at very low frequency in the periphery but can be mobilized into periphery by the use of granulocyte colony-stimulating factor (G-CSF)
- Can be selected, purified and used in bone marrow transplantation

2.2 T- and B-cell development

Both T and B lymphocytes arise from a common lymphoid progenitor cell:

- B-cell development occurs predominantly in the bone marrow
- B-cell development requires a functional pre-B- and B-cell receptor
- VDJ (variable, diversity and joining) immunoglobulin gene rearrangement is necessary for functional receptor complexes to be assembled
- Immature B cells migrate to periphery
- On meeting antigen, B-cell receptors then undergo antigen-mediated somatic hypermutation to develop high-affinity immunoglobulin receptors
- Cells develop into antibody-secreting plasma cells or become memory cells ready for further antigenic encounter
- T-cell development occurs in the thymus
- Early pro-thymocytes express both CD4 **and** CD8 markers (double-positive cells)
- During thymopoiesis cells rearrange the T-cell receptor (TCR) by VDJ recombination as for B cells
- Thymic epithelium expresses self-antigen, allowing elimination of T cells bearing receptors that recognize self
- Single positive CD4+ or CD8+ cells exit the thymus
- T cells recognize antigen presented by professional antigen-presenting cells

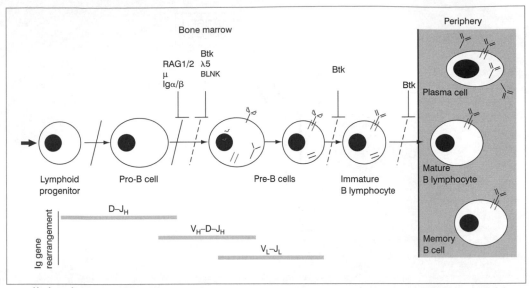

B-cell development

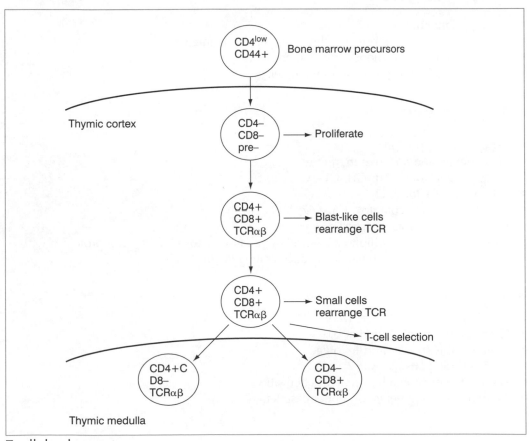

T-cell development

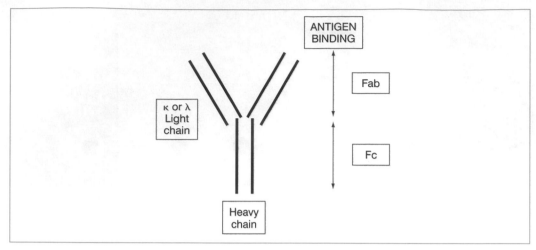

Antibody structure

2.3 Antibody structure

- κ and λ light chains
- Digestion with papain releases the antigen-binding fragment
- Fc region has complement-activating domains
- Fc bound by Fc-receptors on immune cells

2.4 Complement

- 10% of serum proteins
- Links innate and adaptive immunity
- Classical pathway: C1q, C1r, C1s, C4, C2, C3
- Alternative: Factor B, D
- Membrane attack complex: C5, 6, 7, 8, 9
- Upregulating factors: properdin
- Downregulating: C1 inhibitor, C4 binding protein, factor H, factor I, S protein
- Membrane control proteins: decay accelerating factor (DAF)

Nomenclature rules

- Numbered in order of discovery
- Cleavage fragments called a, b, c
- Usually 'a' is smaller and 'b' bigger
- C1 has three parts q, r, s
- A line above the number indicates activation
- Alternative components use upper-case letters

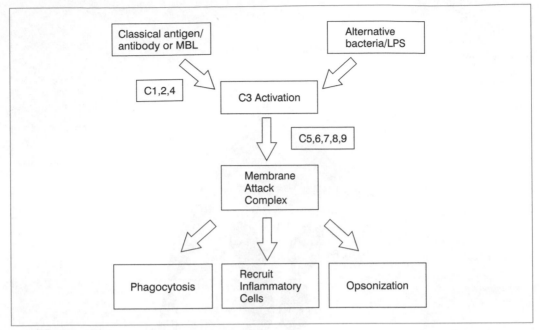

Complement pathway

2.5 Recognition of antigens

Substances that induce an immune response are called *antigens,* The specific region of an antigen that is recognized by an immune receptor is termed an *epitope.* Antibody and antigen binding is non-covalent and is dependent on complementary molecular structures. The strength of this interaction defines antibody *affinity,* and the likelihood of cross-reactivity with similar epitopes on alternative antigens dictates the antibody *specificity.*

T-cell receptors recognize short linear peptides when they are presented in association with MHC (major histocompatibility complex) molecules on the surface of antigen-presenting cells. The α T-cell receptor on *helper* T cells uses the CD4 co-receptor to interact with the MHC class II and peptide complex. *Cytotoxic* T cells use the CD8 co-receptor to stabilize interactions with peptide presented by MHC class I molecules.

Professional antigen-presenting cells (APCs) such as dendritic cells ingest and degrade proteins by endocytosis, and have the intracellular machinery to load short peptide sequences into the groove between the two chains of MHC class II molecules before expressing the complex on their surface.

Most cells employ proteosomes to degrade proteins and traffic selected peptides into the endoplasmic reticulum to be loaded onto class I MHC molecules. The process relies on transporter molecules encoded by the *TAP1* and *TAP2* genes, and mutations of these genes leading to immunodeficiency have been described.

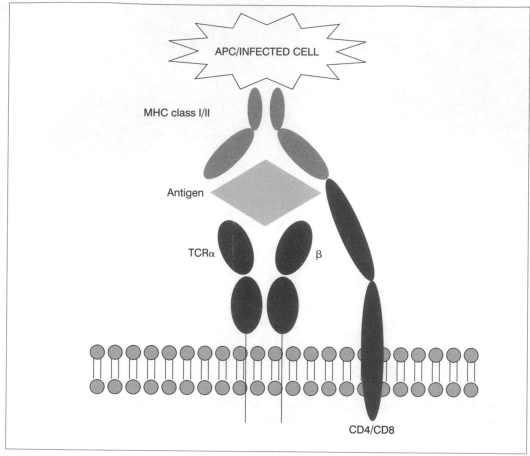

Antigen presentation

A number of polysaccharide and polymerized flagellin antigens carry numerous repeating epitopes that can stimulate B cells without assistance from T cells (*T-independent*). They usually give rise to low-affinity IgM antibodies because of limited class-switching potential, and do not generate memory B cells. Most antigens are *T-dependent* because B cells process and present the antigen to CD4 T cells in association with MHC class II molecules. Once activated, T cells express the CD40 ligand on their surface, which in turn binds CD40 on the B cell, and induces processes of somatic hypermutation and immunoglobulin class-switching. Defects of CD40 ligand result in immunodeficiency associated with increased serum levels of IgM.

2.6 Cytokines

Cytokines are soluble factors that mediate signalling between immune cells. They may act in an autocrine, paracrine or endocrine manner.

Cytokine	Origin	Action
IL-1	Macrophages	Fever, cachexia angiogenesis; activates immune cells
IL-2	T_{H1} cells	Proliferation immune cell activation
IL-4	T_{H2} cells	B-cell class-switching Proliferation
IL-5	T_{H2}	IgA class-switching Proliferation
IL-10	T_{H2} cells, macrophages	Inhibits T_{H1} cells
IL-12	T_{H1} B cells, macrophages	Promotes cytotoxicity
IL-15	Natural killer (NK) cells	NK growth and survival
TNF-α	Macrophages, T cells, B cells, Kupffer cells, astrocytes	Inflammation; Role in rheumatoid arthritis, Crohn's, multiple sclerosis; activates macrophages and other immune cells. Cytotoxic for tumours; sometimes promotes tumour growth; angiogenesis
Interferon-γ	T cells and NK cells	Antiviral

3. INVESTIGATION OF A CHILD WITH PRIMARY IMMUNODEFICIENCY

The usual rules of careful history taking, examination and logical investigations apply.

History

- Recurrent infections at different sites
- Regular courses of antibiotics
- Infections at multiple sites or infections that persist and do not clear easily with antibiotics
- Infection with atypical or unusual organisms
- Prolonged separation of the umbilical cord may be linked to LAD (leucocyte adhesion deficiency)

- Family history of early infant deaths; take careful X-linked history since a number of conditions are X-linked
- Consanguineous family history

Examination

- Failure to thrive and falling off centile charts after 4–6 months (i.e. after protection from maternal immunoglobulin has waned)
- Absence of lymphoid tissue, esp. tonsils and lymph nodes
- Dysmorphism (e.g. Di George syndrome)
- Eczema +/– petechiae in Wiskott–Aldrich syndrome
- Evidence of chronic organ disease (e.g. in lungs or liver)
- Evidence of scar tissue or granuloma formation may be indicative of LAD or CGD (chronic granulomatous disease)
- Gingivitis is associated with LAD
- Ataxic gait and evidence of telangiectasia

Investigations

Need to be directed by accurate history and examination. Initial investigations would include the following:

- Full blood count and differential
- Serum IgG, IgA and IgM (must be compared with age-related normals)
- IgG subclasses
- Antigen-specific antibodies (e.g. diphtheria, tetanus, *Haemophilus influenzae* Hib type b) (reference values for a normal response are available in specialist laboratories)
- Lymphocyte subsets
- T-cell stimulation (response to phytohaemagglutinin (PHA), Candida antigen, tetanus or tuberculin)
- NBT (nitroblue tetrazolium test) (if history suggestive of CGD)
- THC (total haemolytic complement), C3, C4 (if history suggestive of complement defect, i.e recurrent meningitis)
- HIV testing (if clinically appropriate)

(Always check that patient has not received blood products or intravenous immunoglobulin (IVIG) before interpreting immunoglobulin levels — if the patient has received such products, it is necessary to wait approximately 3 months before reassessment.)

Lymphocyte markers

- CD3 — T cell
- CD4 — helper T cell
- CD8 — memory/cytotoxic T cell
- CD19/20 — B cell
- CD14 — monocyte
- CD16/CD56 — NK (natural killer) cell

Normal numbers and percentages of lymphocyte subsets vary with age and with clinical state, i.e. viral infection may lead to a relative CD8 lymphocytosis.

More specialized tests include testing for specific defects, e.g. ADA (adenosine deaminase) metabolites in ADA deficiency or expression of Btk (Bruton's tyrosine kinase) for diagnosis of XLA (X-linked agammaglobulinaemia). These can be carried out in specialist laboratories.

4. IMMUNOGLOBULINS AND B-CELL DEFICIENCIES

- Newborns rely on maternal IgG for 6 months
- Production IgG1 and IgG3 >IgG2 and IgG4
- Adult levels by 7–12 years
- Detect IgM by 1 week of age; adult levels by 12 months
- IgA detectable by 2 weeks; adult levels by 7 years
- Poor response to polysaccharide antigen until >2 years

	IgG	IgM	IgA	IgD	IgE
Size (kDa)	150	950	160	175	190
Cross placenta	Yes	No	No	No	No
Complement	Classical	Classical	Alternative	No	No
Normal levels mg/ml (adult)	13	1.5	3.5	0.03	0.0001

Causes of low immunoglobulins

- **Prematurity**: under 36 weeks' gestation, transfer of maternal antibody is low
- **Excessive losses**: nephrotic syndrome, enteropathy, burns
- **Transient hypogammaglobulinaemia of infancy**: as the name suggests, this is a maturational problem which resolves as patients get older. Protection with Ig may be necessary during this period.
- **Drug-induced**: antimalarials, captopril, carbamazepine, phenytoin, gold salts, sulphasalazine
- **Infections**: HIV, Epstein–Barr virus, congenital cytomegalovirus (CMV), congenital toxoplasmosis
- **Others**: malignancy, systemic lupus erythematosus (SLE)

4.1 X-linked agammaglobulinemia (XLA)

- Primary defect of B cells with <2% CD19+ B cells
- Defect in B-cell development with arrest at the pre-B-cell stage
- Mutations of the Bruton tyrosine kinase (Btk), on the X chromosome (Xq22) a molecule involved in B-cell signalling

- *Streptococcus pneumonia* and *H. influenzae* infections of the upper and lower respiratory tract, sinuses and middle ear
- Particular susceptibility to Mycoplasma infections and CNS infection with enteroviruses
- Severe cases present before the age of two, milder cases may not diagnosed until school age
- Poor or no responses to vaccines and low levels of isohaemagglutinins are found
- In some atypical forms there a small number of circulating B cells and some make Ig
- Patients respond well to IVIG therapy

4.2 Autosomal recessive congenital agammaglobulinaemia

- Other defects giving rise to abnormal B-cell development have been found
- These include components of the pre-B-cell receptor which are essential for B-cell development: μ heavy chain, λ surrogate light chain, Igα accessory molecule

4.3 IgA deficiency

- Produced and secreted at mucosal surfaces
- Two subclasses
- Serum IgA produced by B cells in lymph nodes
- Activates alternative complement pathway
- Most common form of primary immunodeficiency
- 1:600–1:300 incidence of deficiency; usually asymptomatic
- Increased risk of atopy, infections of lungs, gastrointestinal tract
- Association with IgG2 deficiency
- Associations: autoimmunity, ulcerative colitis, Crohn's, coeliac disease, malignancy
- 40% have antibodies to IgA; risk of transfusion/IVIG anaphylaxis

4.4 Common variable immunodeficiency (CVID)

- Catch-all term to describe heterogeneous group of poorly characterized immunodeficiencies
- History of recurrent infections, often of the respiratory tract and involving a range of pathogens
- A subgroup of patients have granulomatous disease affecting GI tract, lungs and skin; normally responsive to steroids
- Autoimmune diseases occur in over half the patients and there is an increased risk of malignancy
- May be reduced T-cell numbers, though the majority of patients have normal numbers of B cells
- Diagnosis is usually made in patients older than 2 years with reduced serum immunoglobulins, absent isohaemagglutinins and poor vaccine responses

The patients with persistently low immunoglobulin levels benefit from supplemental IVIG infusions. Prophylactic antibiotics given to those with recurrent infection despite IVIG. Severe cases may require bone marrow transplantation.

5. SEVERE COMBINED IMMUNODEFICIENCY (SCID)

- SCID arises from severe defects in both cellular and humoral immunity
- Same phenotype arises from different molecular defects
- Both X-linked and autosomal recessive forms of SCID exist
- Characterized by recurrent infections, often severe involving opportunistic pathogens
- Overall prognosis for SCID without effective management is very poor
- Only curative option is bone marrow transplantation; but for certain types of SCID other treatments such as gene therapy (presently for X-SCID) and enzyme replacement therapy (for ADA SCID) are available (see below)

Incidence

- Rare
- Estimated at 1:50,000 to 1:500,000 for all forms of SCID
- Males affected more than females because of X-linked inheritance in one specific type of SCID

Clinical manifestations

- Mean age of presentation is approximately 6–7 months
- **Respiratory complications**: interstitial pneumonitis due to *Pneumocystis carinii* (PCP), respiratory syncytial virus (RSV), cytomegalovirus (CMV), adenovirus, influenza and parainfluenza infections. Bacterial and fungal pneumonias are also described
- **Diarrhoea and failure to thrive**: there may be a viral aetiology (rotavirus, adenovirus) but in many cases no cause is defined. Failure to thrive as a result of diarrhoea or recurrent infection is seen in nearly all patients.
- **Skin rash:** may be due to a viral infection but an erythrodermic macular rash is often indicative of maternal T-cell engraftment or Omenn's syndrome

Immunological phenotype

- SCID is characterized by both humoral and cellular defects
- Abnormality in T-cell development with variable defects in B- and NK-cell development
- IgG present early on due to maternal transfer, but IgM and IgA production impaired
- SCID is categorized by the pattern of T/B/NK-cell development and this can be indicative of the underlying molecular defect

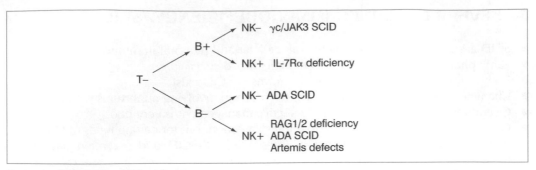

Pattern of T/B/NK-cell development

Exceptions to the above scheme include:

- **Maternal engraftment**: maternal T cells are present but these are non-functional CD8+ cells
- **Omenn's syndrome (OS)**: characteristic immunological profile with activated non-functional CD8+ cells, lack of B cells, increased IgE and eosinophilia
- **Atypical variants**: for many of the defined forms there have been reports of less severe phenotypes where there may be small but not normal numbers of T/B or NK cells present

Genetic diagnosis

- The molecular basis of the known SCID types is shown in the table on p. 363
- Diagnosis is made on the basis of pedigree, immunological phenotype and genetic analysis

Management

- Prophylactic – septrin for prevention of PCP, immunoglobulin replacement, aciclovir for antiviral prophylaxis and itraconazole/fluconazole for antifungal prophylaxis
- Supportive — nutrition, skin care, genetic counselling for family
- Specific treatment of infectious complications

Bone marrow transplantation (BMT) (see section 5.4)

- BMT is the only treatment option for the majority of SCID cases
- Best results are available following a genotypically matched donor transplant (>90% success rates). In most SCID cases such transplants can be undertaken without prior chemotherapy conditioning.
- If no genotypically identical donor is present, BMT from a matched family donor, volunteer unrelated donor or parental haploidentical donor can be undertaken. Results following such procedures are less good, with haplotransplants having the worst outcome.

Gene therapy

- Gene therapy has been used to treat X-linked SCID
- Also being developed for other SCID forms

PEG-ADA (for treatment of ADA-SCID)

- Exogenous enzyme replacement therapy using a bovine form of ADA conjugated to polyethylene glycol (PEG-ADA or Pegademase) has been used in patients who lack a good bone marrow donor
- PEG-ADA can be used indefinitely, or to stabilize the condition until a donor for BMT can be found
- Side-effects such as autoimmune haemolytic anaemia and thrombocytosis have been reported

5.1 Routine vaccination in the immunosuppressed

- All live vaccines are contraindicated in SCID and only poor responses obtained to killed vaccines
- Oral polio should not be given to patients with significant immune deficiency, or to the siblings of such patients; a killed intramuscular preparation may be given.
- BCG contraindicated in all primary immunodeficiencies; chemotherapy patients; patients on significant steroids or immunosuppressants
- HIV patients in UK should not be given BCG; other live vaccines given if asymptomatic
- No specific contraindications for complement deficiencies

5.2 Combined immunodeficiency (CID)

- CID refers to a genetically undefined group of immunodeficiencies in which there are variable defects in T- and B-cell function
- CID patients present at a later stage with less severe infections
- Over time, immune function deteriorates leading to recurrent infection and resulting in chronic damage especially to liver and lungs
- Principles of management are the same as for SCID
- BMT is less successful in CID due to underlying chronic organ damage and increased age at time of transplant

5.3 HIV (human immunodeficiency virus) infection

- HIV infection is an important differential in the diagnosis of a child with immunodeficiency
- Presentation is often similar to that of children with SCID, e.g. PCP infection is common
- Characteristic immunological profile is reversal of the CD4/CD8 ratio, but for infants the T-cell profile may be normal
- Some patients also have hypergammaglobulinaemia

5.4 Bone marrow/haematopoietic stem-cell transplantation (BMT/HSCT)

BMT/HSCT offers curative option for haematological malignancies/congenital immunodeficiencies/haemoglobinopathies/inherited metabolic defects and recently for autoimmune conditions. Bone marrow is a rich source of haematopoetic stem cells (HSC); also contains mature T, B and NK cells. HSC can also be harvested by leucapheresis after giving the donor a course of G-CSF.

Autologous: used for treatment of malignancies especially solid tumours and autoimmune conditions. HSC collected from the patient, usually before intensive chemotherapy/radiotherapy for malignancy and then re-infused to rescue the haematopoetic system.

Allogeneic: from another person who is ideally HLA-matched. Parents are usually haploidentical. Indications in childhood include relapsed leukaemias, primary immune deficiencies, haematological disorders (Fanconi, thalassaemia, sickle) or metabolic conditions (adrenoleucodystropy, Hurler's syndrome, osteopetrosis).

Umbilical cord blood: is also rich in HSC and can be used for transplants. Is associated with less graft vs. host disease (GvHD) (see below) and faster immune reconstitution. However, the number of cells that can be obtained from a cord collection limits the applicability of this source.

Recipients usually require **pre-conditioning** with chemotherapy/radiotherapy to remove the existing immune cells (unless non-functional as in X-SCID).

Cytotoxic agents can have significant side-effects: cyclophosphamide (haemorrhagic cystitis, infertility), busulphan (pulmonary fibrosis).

T cells in the graft may cause **graft versus host disease** (GvHD) and this may be managed by T-cell depleting grafts and/or immunosuppression using cyclosporin and steroids.

GvHD is graded I–IV on the basis of skin rash, liver impairment and gastrointestinal involvement.

T cells also mediate a **graft versus leukaemia** effect which helps eradicate tumour cells.

Early post-transplant complications

Graft rejection or failure; infection (bacterial, CMV, EBV, adenovirus, fungal); GvHD; veno-occlusive disease.

Late complications

Incomplete immune reconstitution; chronic GvHD; growth retardation and endocrine problems; cognitive impairment in some patients.

Disorder	Chromosomal location	Gene	Function/defect	Diagnostic tests other than direct mutation analysis
X-linked severe combined immunodeficiency	Xq13	**Common γ chain (γ$_c$)**	Component of IL (interleukin) 2,4,7,9,15 cytokine receptors; T- and NK-cell development, T- and B-cell function	γ$_c$ Expression by FACS (flow cytometric) analysis
Adenosine deaminase (ADA) deficiency	20q12–13	**Adenosine deaminase**	Enzyme in purine salvage pathway; accumulation of toxic metabolites	Red cell ADA levels and metabolites
Recombinase activating gene (*RAG1/2*) deficiency Omenn's syndrome	11p13	***RAG1* and *RAG2***	Defective DNA recombination affecting immunoglobulin and T-cell receptor gene rearrangements	
Artemis gene defect	10p	**Artemis**	Defective DNA recombination affecting immunoglobulin and T-cell receptor gene rearrangements	
T-cell receptor deficiencies	11q23	***CD3γ/CD3ξ***	T-cell receptor function and signalling	CD3 fluorescence intensity; mutation analysis
Zap70 deficiency	2q12	**ZAP-70**	T-cell function — selection of CD8+ cells during thymocyte development	ZAP—70 expression
JAK3 deficiency	19p13	**JAK3**	IL-2,4,7,9,15 receptor signalling, T- and NK-cell development, T- and B-cell function	JAK3 expression/ signalling
IL-7 receptor deficiency	5p13	**IL-7 receptor-α**	Essential role in T-cell development and function	IL-7 receptor α expression

Major types of SCID and their genetic defect

6. MISCELLANEOUS IMMUNODEFICIENCY SYNDROMES

6.1 Wiskott-Aldrich syndrome (WAS)

- X-linked inheritance pattern
- Approximately 1:1,000,000 live male births
- Classical clinical features include thrombocytopenia, combined immunodeficiency and eczema
- Patients are susceptible to lymphoproliferative disease in later life
- Autoimmune features with peripheral and large-vessel vasculitis are seen in older patients
- Considerable clinical heterogeneity with some patients having thrombocytopenia alone
- Arises from mutations in the *WASP* (Wiskott–Aldrich syndrome protein) gene
- *WASP* expressed in all haematopoietic tissues
- *WASP* involved in organization of cytoskeleton and defects affect immune-cell motility

Thrombocytopenia is the most consistent clinical feature and patients also have small fragmented platelets (<70,000 platelets/mm^3) and a reduced mean platelet volume

Immune defects include decreased IgM levels, decrease in T-cell numbers and function with time and impaired responses to polysaccharide antigens. Extent of eczema is variable.

Diagnosis
Is made on clinical phenotype, platelet count morphology, X-linked pedigree and mutation analysis of the *WASP* gene.

Management
Is orientated to the different clinical problems:

- Topical care of eczema
- Thrombocytopenia sometimes responds to high-dose immunoglobulin (2 g/kg) and steroids
- In most cases splenectomy is successful in improving platelet count
- Immune defect is treated by prophylactic antibiotics, IVIG and aggressive management of active infection
- Only curative option is BMT which can be difficult if a fully matched donor is unavailable
- BMT >5 years is associated with worse prognosis

6.2 Di George syndrome

- Now usually diagnosed in infants with cardiac malformations undergoing genetic analysis for detection of micro deletions of chromosome 22q11.2
- Defects of the fourth branchial arch and third and fourth pharyngeal pouches

- Aortic arch and conotruncal anomalies (truncus arteriosus, tetralogy of Fallot, interrupted aortic arch or aberrant right subclavian) are associated with significant neonatal mortality
- Parathyroid hypoplasia may lead to hypocalcaemic tetany, and thymic hypoplasia may lead to profound cellular immunodeficiency (less than 500/mm^3 CD3 T cells)
- Dysmorphic features include lateral displacement of the inner canthi, short philtrum, micrognathia and ear abnormalities. Learning difficulties are common.
- Increased likelihood of autoimmune phenomena in older children
- Usually confirmed by the detection of the 22q11.2 deletion by fluorescent *in-situ* hybridization
- Attempts to correct T-cell deficiency by thymic transplantation have been unsuccessful

Management
Includes use of irradiated blood products prior to surgery and then management of specific syndromic problems. Management of immunodeficiency is dependent on the severity of immune compromise and varies from prophylactic antibiotics to bone marrow transplantation.

6.3 CD40 ligand deficiency (X-linked hyper-IgM syndrome)

- Presents before the age of 2 years with a history of recurrent infections, usually of the sinuses or middle ear
- Increased susceptibility to PCP, viral infections and mycobacterial organisms
- Cryptosporidium infection often leads to chronic diarrhoea and sclerosing cholangitis
- Liver disease is the major cause of death in older patients
- Predisposition to haematological malignancy and autoimmune diseases
- Maps to Xq26.3–7 and results from mutations in the gene for CD40 ligand — resulting in defects in Ig class-switching
- Associated with anaemia and neutropenia but T- and B-cell numbers are often normal
- Serum levels of IgM are usually elevated but can be normal, with reduced IgG and IgA levels
- Diagnosis by Ig profile, flow cytometric analysis for the absence of CD40 ligand on T cells and by genetic analysis
- Treat with regular IVIG infusions and antibiotic prophylaxis. Patients are screened, treated for Cryptosporidium infection and regularly monitored for liver disease (including cholangiography and liver biopsy in some cases).
- Bone marrow transplantation offers the possibility of cure, but in the absence of matched donors carries high risks of morbidity and mortality

6.4 X-linked lymphoproliferative syndrome (XLP)

Also known as Duncan's syndrome. Affected boys are well until contract EBV infection when they can exhibit a variety of clinical manifestations:

- Fulminant infectious mononucleosis (FIM) (58%)
- Lymphoma (31%)
- Dysgammaglobulinaemia (30%)
- Aplastic anaemia (3%)
- Phenotypes can exist together or evolve from one to another
- EBV is not always the trigger for these dysregulatory phenomena and a significant number of boys are EBV-negative
- FIM has the poorest outcome with greater than 90% mortality. Major cause of death is hepatic necrosis.
- Diagnosis difficult due to clinical variability
- No specific immunological defect in affected boys prior to the onset of severe symptoms
- After infection, a variety of immunological defects seen including reversed CD4/CD8 ratio and dysgammaglobulinaemia
- Gene identified as *SAP* which plays a critical role in regulation of T-cell stimulation
- Identification of mutations in *SAP* can provide unambiguous diagnosis

Treatment

- Is difficult
- In affected boys identified by family history, prophylactic IVIG and antibiotics do not provide protection from severe EBV infection
- BMT offers only curative option but is difficult to perform if child is in acute phase

6.5 Purine nucleoside phosphorylase (PNP) deficiency

- Autosomal recessive inheritance
- Lack of expression of PNP and defect in purine salvage pathway
- Triad of immune deficiency, neurological manifestations and autoimmune phenomena
- Two-thirds have neurological problems ranging from spasticity to global developmental delay
- One-third develop autoimmune disease including AIHA (autoimmune haemolytic anaemia) and ITP (immune thrombocytopenia)
- Infective complications are the most common presenting complaint. Infections as for other forms of SCID/CID but presentation generally at a later age than most SCID types
- BMT offers only cure. Increased risks associated with non-HLA identical transplant
- BMT reported anecdotally to correct/halt neurological deterioration, although other reports contradict this

6.6 Ataxia telangiectasia

- Early onset of progressive neurological impairment: cerebellar ataxia and choreoathetosis
- Oculocutaneous telangiectasia in aged 2 years and above
- Immunodeficiency, leading to recurrent sinopulmonary infection

- Increased risk of developing lymphoid malignancies
- Associations include growth retardation, diabetes and liver dysfunction
- *ATM* (ataxia telangiectasia mutated) gene maps to chromosome 11q22–23
- Usually clinical diagnosis supported by genetic analysis
- IgA levels are reduced and serum alpha-fetoprotein raised
- Cultured cells exhibit increased radiation-induced chromosomal breakage

6.7 Chronic mucocutaneous candidiasis (CMC)

- Presents in childhood with extensive Candida infections of the skin, nails and mucous membranes
- May be associated endocrine abnormalities such as hypoparathyroidism and Addison's disease
- Pathogenesis of this disease is poorly understood
- The mainstay of therapy is prophylactic, systemic antifungal therapy

7. DEFECTS OF NEUTROPHILS

Neutrophil immunodeficiency may arise because of reduced numbers of circulating neutrophils, a failure of neutrophil precursor maturation or defective neutrophil function.

7.1 Congenital neutropenia

- Recurrent bacterial infections (often *Staphylococcus aureus*) in the first year of life leading to abscesses, cellulitis and meningitis
- There is a failure of myeloid-cell maturation, but the condition responds to treatment with G-CSF
- There are a variety of underlying molecular defects, including stem-cell receptor defects, and some patients may later develop myelodysplastic syndromes

7.2 Schwachman–Diamond syndrome

- Combination of pancreatic exocrine insufficiency, skeletal abnormalities and recurrent infections of lungs, bones and skin
- Most patients have neutropenia, and up to 25% may develop pancytopenia
- The risk of myelodysplasia and leukaemia are increased
- BMT may be curative

7.3 Cyclical neutropenia

- Patients recurrently become neutropenic for between 3 and 6 days, and may develop stomatitis, mouth ulcers or bacterial infections
- There is usually a 21-day cyclical pattern, but this can range between 14 and 36 days

- The condition is autosomal dominant and has been linked to mutations in the elastase gene, *ELA2*

7.4 Leucocyte-adhesion deficiency

History of delayed umbilical separation, periodontitis, recurrent orogenital infections. Pathogens include *S. aureus*, Aspergillus, Candida and Gram-negative enteric bacteria.

- Type 1: autosomal recessive defect of d_2-integrin adhesion molecules (CD18) on neutrophils, resulting in defective aggregation and a paradoxical leucocytosis. There is no expression of CD18 on neutrophils and early death occurs without BMT in the most severe forms. CD18 is expressed in milder forms and patients can survive to adulthood.
- Type 2: defective carbohydrate fucosylation. Associated dysmorphic features and growth and developmental retardation.

7.5 Chronic granulomatous disease

X-linked form of CGD accounts for 2/3 of cases and usually presents earlier and with more severe disease than patients with autosomal recessive forms.

- Failure to thrive, severe bacterial infections, abscesses or osteomyelitis within the first year of life are common
- Pneumonia and lymphadenitis due to *S. aureus* or Aspergillus are the most common infections
- Granulomas may result in intrathoracic, gastrointestinal or urinary obstruction
- X-linked CGD is due to mutations in the gene for the phagocyte oxidase cytochrome glycoprotein *gp91phox*
- Defects of *p47phox* account for the majority of recessive cases, and mutations of *p22phox* and *p67phox* are uncommon
- These mutations result in defects of NADPH oxidase and the generation of hydrogen peroxide resulting in defective intracellular killing of pathogens
- Diagnosis is usually made by the demonstration of impaired neutrophil respiratory burst by the nitroblue tetrazolium test (NBT) or by flow cytometric analysis of hydrogen peroxide production using fluorescent detector dyes. Immunoblot analysis or flow cytometry using antibodies to the various NADPH oxidase subunits may help to define the particular subtype of CGD.
- Treatment usually involves antibiotic prophylaxis and the use of steroids to treat granulomatous disease. Aggressive use of antifungal agents and granulocyte infusions along with interferon-gamma may be required to manage severe fungal infections. BMT has been used successfully in those who have a matched sibling donor.

7.6 Chédiak–Higashi syndrome

- Rare autosomal recessive disorder of lysosomal granule-containing cells of the immune and nervous systems caused by mutations of the *LYST* gene.
- Features include peripheral neuropathy, albinism, giant inclusions in hair
- Ocular albinism may result in severe visual defects
- Diagnosis by identification of giant lysosomal granules in neutrophils on peripheral blood film and clinical features of albinism
- Neutrophils respond poorly to infections and patients may develop T-cell and monocytic infiltration of tissues (so-called accelerated phase) which is often fatal
- BMT is the treatment of choice. If a matched donor is available this should be undertaken prior to the onset of the accelerated phase

7.7 *Rac* deficiency

Rare inhibitory mutation of *Rac2* causing neutrophil immunodeficiency, clinically similar to LAD, with abnormal neutrophil chemotaxis and superoxide production.

8. DEFECTS OF THE INTERFERON-γ/INTERLEUKIN-12 AXIS

- Intracellular pathogens normally trigger IL-12 production by antigen-presenting cells, and this in turn binds specific receptors on T cells to induce IFN-γ production which enhances phagocyte-mediated killing through tumour-necrosis factor (TNF) release
- Defects of the interferon-γ receptor, interleukin-12 or interleukin-12 receptor leads to increased susceptibility to intracellular organisms such as Mycobacteria and Salmonella
- Inheritance of autosomal recessive cases of IFN-γ receptor defects occurs in consanguineous Maltese populations
- Infants may present with disseminated BCG and atypical mycobacterial infection and are usually unable to form granulomas
- Milder cases may respond to high-dose infusions of IFN-γ

Disorder	Chromosomal location	Gene	Function/defect	Diagnostic tests
X-linked chronic granulomatous disease	Xp21	*gp91phox*	Component of phagocyte NADPH oxidase–phagocytic respiratory burst	Nitroblue tetrazolium test *gp91phox* by immunoblotting; mutation analysis
X-linked agammaglobulinaemia	Xq22	**Bruton's tyrosine kinase (*Btk*)**	Intracellular signalling pathways essential for pre-B-cell maturation	*Btk* by immunoblotting or FACS analysis and mutation analysis
X-linked hyper-IgM syndrome (CD40 ligand deficiency)	Xq26	**CD40 ligand (CD154)**	Isotype switching, T-cell function	CD154 expression on activated T cells by FACS analysis mutation analysis
Wiskott–Aldrich syndrome	Xp11	*WASP*	Cytoskeletal architecture formation, immune-cell motility and trafficking	*WASP* expression by immunoblotting mutation analysis
X-linked lymphoproliferative syndrome	Xq25	*SAP*	Regulation of T-cell responses to EBV and other viral infections	Mutation analysis *SAP* expression — under development
Properdin deficiency	Xp21	**properdin**	Terminal complement component	Properdin levels
Leucocyte-adhesion deficiency type 1	21q22	CD11/CD18	Defective leucocyte adhesion and migration	CD11/CD18 expression by FACS analysis; mutation analysis
Chronic granulomatous disease	7q11 1q25 16p24	*p47phox* *p67phox* *p22phox*	Defective respiratory burst and phagocytic intracellular killing	*p47phox, p67phox, p22phox,* expression by immunoblotting; mutation analysis
Chédiak–Higashi syndrome	1q42	*LYST*	Abnormalities in microtubule-mediated lysosomal protein trafficking	Giant inclusions in granulocytes; mutation analysis
MHC class II deficiency	16p13 19p12 1q21 13q13	*CIITA (MHC2TA)* *RFXANK* *RFX5* *RFXAP*	Defective transcriptional regulation of MHC II molecule expression	HLA-DR expression; mutation analysis
Autoimmune lymphoproliferative syndrome (ALPS)	10q24	*APT1* (Fas)	Defective apoptosis of lymphocytes	Fas expression; apoptosis assays; mutation analysis
Ataxia telangiectasia	11q22	*ATM*	Cell-cycle control and DNA damage responses	DNA radiation sensitivity; mutation analysis
Inherited mycobacterial susceptibility	6q23 5q31 19p13	**Interferon γ-receptor IL-12 p40 IL-12 receptor β1**	Defective IFN-γ production and signalling function	Interferon-γ receptor expression; IL-12 expression; IL-12 receptor expression; mutation analysis

Major types of non-SCID immunodeficiencies and their genetic defects

9. COMPLEMENT DEFICIENCY STATES

Component	Deficiency
C1q,r,s C4, C2	Infection (pneumococcal) SLE, glomerulonephritis
C5,6,7,8	Infection (*Neisseria*)
Mannose-binding lectin	Recurrent infections
Factor D	Infection (meningococcal)
Properdin	Infection (meningococcal)
C1 inhibitor	Hereditary angioedema
DAF, protectin	Paroxysmal nocturnal haemaglobinuria
C3 receptor	Infections

10. HYPERSENSITIVITY REACTIONS

Type	Type 1	Type 2	Type 3	Type 4
Immune mediator	IgE	IgG, IgM	IgG	T cells
Antigen	Soluble	Cell surface	Soluble	Soluble or cellular
Mechanism	Mast-cell degranulation	Altered signalling; complement activation	Immune Complexes	TH1(IL2, IFNγ) TH2 (IL4, IL5) Cytotoxic T cells
Clinical conditions	Asthma; Food allergy; Disease of hayfever Anaphylaxis	Haemolytic Arthus reaction Newborn penicillin allergy	Serum sickness dermatitis Erythema nodosum	Contact conditions Tuberculin Chronic asthma

11. IMMUNOSUPPRESSANTS AND IMMUNE-MODULATING AGENTS

- T-cell immunosuppressants

Drug	Indications	Major side-effects
Prednisolone	Prevent rejection Prevent GvHD Immunosuppression for many indications	Hypertension, thin skin, truncal obesity, proximal myopathy
Cyclosporin	Prevent rejection Prevent GVHD Suppress autoimmune disease	Nephrotoxicity, hirsutism, hypertension
Tacrolimus	Prevent rejection	Nephrotoxicity, neurotoxic cardiomyopathy
Mycophenolate mofetil (MMF)	Prevent rejection	Leucopenia, marrow suppression
Azathioprine	Prevent rejection Suppress autoimmune disease	Marrow suppression, hepatotoxic

- Clinically used monoclonal antibodies/fusion proteins

Drug	Target	Indication
Rituximab	CD20 on B cells	B-cell lymphoma Lymphoproliferative disease
Infliximab	TNF-α	Rheumatoid arthritis, juvenile idiopathic arthritis, Crohn's
Etanercept	TNF-α receptor	Juvenile idiopathic arthritis; rheumatoid arthritis,
Anti-thymocyte globulin (ATG)	T cells	T-cell depletion
OKT3	T cells	T-cell depletion
Campath	CD52 on human T and B cells	T-cell depletion in BMT and for certain lymphomas

- Interferons

Drug	Possible indications	Side-effects/comments
IFN-α	Myeloma Renal carcinoma Melanoma	Flu-like illness, fever Myelosuppression Depression
IFN-2α	Hepatitis C	Given with ribavirin
IFN-β	Multiple sclerosis	Fever, flu-like illness
IFN-γ	Mycobacterial infection Chronic granulomatous disease	Fever, flu-like illness

12. FURTHER READING

Basic and Clinical Immunology:. Vergani D and Peakman M, Churchill Livingstone, 2000.

Immunologic Disorders in Children and Infants: Steihm ER (ed), 4th edition. WB Saunders, 1995.

Naturally occurring primary deficiencies of the immune system. Fischer A, Cavazzana-Calvo M, De Saint Basile G, *et al. Annual Review of Immunology*; **15**:93–124 1997.

Primary Immunodeficiency Diseases: Ochs M, Smith C and Puck J, Oxford University Press, 1999.

Severe combined immunodeficiency — molecular pathogenesis and diagnosis. *Archives of Diseases in Childhood*; **84**(2):169–73 2001.

Chapter 11

Infectious Diseases

Nigel Klein and Katy Fidler

CONTENTS

Infectious Diseases

1. NOTIFICATION OF INFECTIOUS DISEASES

Doctors in England and Wales have a statutory duty to notify the local authority, usually the CCDC (Consultant in Communicable Disease Control), of cases of certain infections: this is done via the notification book in each hospital.

Notifications of infectious diseases, some of which are microbiologically confirmed, prompt local investigation and action to control the diseases.

Notifiable diseases

Acute encephalitis	Measles	Malaria
Meningitis	Mumps	Yellow fever
– meningococcal	Rubella	Typhoid fever
– pneumococcal	Whooping cough	Paratyphoid fever
– haemophilus influenzae	Viral hepatitis	Relapsing fever
– viral	– hepatitis A	Leptospirosis
– other specified	– hepatitis B	Viral haemorrhagic fever
– unspecified	– hepatitis C	Typhus fever
Meningococcal septicaemia	– other	Plague
(without meningitis)	Smallpox	Rabies
Tetanus	Acute poliomyelitis	Dysentery
Tuberculosis		Food poisoning
Scarlet fever		
Ophthalmia neonatorum		
Anthrax		
Cholera		
Diphtheria		

---

2. PATHOGENESIS OF INFECTION

The course and outcome of any infectious disease is a function of the interaction between the pathogen and host.

The pathogens

Human infections are caused by bacteria, viruses, fungi and parasites. However, despite the vast array of potential pathogens, only a minority have the capacity to cause infection in a human host. Many factors determine an individual organism's ability to initiate disease, but successful organisms have three essential characteristics: the ability to invade a host; to travel to an environment within the host which is conducive to their propagation; and to survive the host's defence mechanisms. Increasing understanding of the molecular mechanisms underlying these pathogenic events, should enable the development of new treatment strategies.

377

Bacterial properties important in the pathogenesis of infections

Bacterial characteristic	Function
Pili	Aid adhesion to host targets
Capsular polysaccharide	Inhibit phagocytosis
Enzyme production	Inactivate antibody, degrade host tissue
Toxin production	Lyse circulating cells
Antigen variation	Evade host defences

The host

The essential elements of all components of the immune system are present at birth. Initially, however, the baby's circulating immunoglobulin is derived predominantly from the mother. It is only after encountering a wide range of potential pathogens that defences fully mature to provide adequate protection in later life. Meanwhile, these children are particularly susceptible to infections.

The importance of acquiring a fully competent host defence system is illustrated clinically by the problems encountered in immunodefective individuals, e.g. primary immunodeficiencies, acquired immunodeficiency syndrome (AIDS) and those receiving chemotherapy and radiotherapy. These patients suffer not only from severe and persistent infections due to common organisms, but are also vulnerable to a range of unusual or opportunistic pathogens. The role played by each component of the host defence system can be deduced from the nature of infections associated with specific immunological defects, many of which present in childhood.

Immune deficiency and susceptibility to infection

Immune defect	Infectious susceptibility	
Antibody	Bacteria	*Staphylococcus, Streptococcus* spp., *Haemophilus influenzae, Moraxella (Branhamella) catarrhalis*
	Viruses	Enteroviruses
	Protozoa	Giardia
Cellular immunity	Bacteria	*Mycobacteria, Listeria* spp.
	Viruses	Cytomegalovirus (CMV), herpesvirus, measles, respiratory syncytial virus (RSV), adenovirus
	Fungi	*Candida, Aspergillus* spp.
	Protozoa	*Pneumocystis* spp.
Neutrophils	Bacteria	Gram +ve, Gram −ve
	Fungi	*Aspergillus, Candida* spp.
Complement	Bacteria	*Neisseria, Staphylococcus* spp.

3. FEVER WITH FOCUS

3.1 CNS infections (see also Chapter 15, *Neurology*)

Meningitis and encephalitis

Common viral causes include:

- enteroviruses (coxsackieviruses-A and -B and echovirus)
- herpes simplex virus (HSV)-1 and -2
- Epstein–Barr virus (EBV)
- varicella zoster
- measles
- mumps

Rare causes include:

- adenoviruses, rubella, arenaviruses (e.g. Japanese B encephalitis), rabies.

Most of these cause a meningoencephalitis. Herpes simplex virus causes a predominantly encephalitic illness.

The peak incidence of viral encephalitis is in the first 6 months of life with up to 1–2 cases/1,000 children. In about 50% of cases a mild lymphocellular pleocytosis is seen.

Aciclovir dramatically reduces mortality if given early in HSV disease.

Bacterial meningitis

- *Neisseria meningitidis* is the commonest cause of community-acquired bacterial meningitis in the UK, with most cases being *N. meningitidis B* since the introduction of the conjugate meningococcal C vaccine.
- *Streptococcus pneumoniae* is the second most common cause.
- The incidence of Hib meningitis has dropped from around 2,500 cases per year to less than 40 per year because of vaccination.
- A rare, but serious form, of bacterial meningitis is caused by *Mycobacterium tuberculosis*. This organism can affect patients of all ages and should be considered in any atypical presentation of meningitis, particularly in patients presenting with an insidious illness.

Neonatal meningitis
In the neonatal period, the group B streptococcus is the prominent meningeal pathogen, followed by Gram-negative bacilli, *S. pneumoniae* and *Listeria monocytogenes*.

Diagnosis of bacterial meningitis
If meningitis is suspected, the diagnosis should be confirmed by lumbar puncture and cerebrospinal fluid (CSF) examination.

- Specific contraindications to LP include:
  - signs of raised intracranial pressure with changing level of consciousness, focal neurological signs or severe mental impairment;
  - cardiovascular compromise with impaired peripheral perfusion or hypotension;
  - respiratory compromise with tachypnoea, an abnormal breathing pattern or hypoxia;
  - thrombocytopenia or a coagulopathy;
  - a lumbar puncture should also be avoided if it will result in a significant delay in treatment.

Very high white cell counts of more than $1,000/mm^3$ can be seen in bacterial meningitis. There is a broad correlation between a predominance of polymorphonuclear leucocytes in the CSF and bacterial meningitis. However, lymphocytes may predominate in early or partially treated bacterial meningitis, in tuberculous meningitis and in neonates.

In bacterial meningitis, the CSF glucose level is usually low with a CSF/blood ratio of less than 0.5, and the protein level is frequently raised to >0.4 g/l. Numerous studies have now shown that, even after the administration of intravenous antibiotics, the diagnostic cellular and biochemical changes in the CSF may persist for at least 48 hours.

Treatment – Antibiotics for bacterial meningitis
In infants up to 3 months of age a combination of ampicillin and cefotaxime is a logical choice: cefotaxime provides cover for both neonatal and infant pathogens, and ampicillin is effective against *L. monocytogenes*.

Penicillin-resistant meningococci are emerging worldwide, as are chloramphenicol-resistant strains, but these have not yet resulted in treatment failures. Fortunately, almost all strains in the UK remain sensitive to the third-generation cephalosporins. At the moment, the routine use of vancomycin for community-acquired meningitis is not justified in the UK.

- If the cause of meningoencephalitis is unclear it is usual to start empirical treatment with cefotaxime/ceftriaxone **and** aciclovir **and** erythromycin to cover bacteria, HSV and Mycoplasma, respectively.

Treatment – The role of corticosteroids
Several studies of patients with Hib meningitis have demonstrated some improvement in morbidity (deafness or neurological deficit) if corticosteroids were given either before antibiotic administration or at the same time. Data supporting the use of steroids in pneumococcal and meningococcal meningitis is lacking.

Complications

- Convulsions occur in 20–30% of children, usually within 72 h of presentation.
- Subdural collections of fluid are common, particularly during infancy. They are usually sterile and rarely require aspiration.
- The commonest long-term complication of meningitis is sensorineural deafness. The overall rate of deafness following meningitis is less than 5%. Hearing impairment is higher in cases of pneumococcal meningitis than in meningococcal infections.

Prevention

Conjugate vaccines against Hib and group C *N. meningitidis* are now routinely given in the UK as part of the primary course of immunization at 2, 3 and 4 months of age.

3.2 Respiratory infections See Chapter 17, *Respiratory*

3.3 Bone and joint infections

Bacterial infections of bones (osteomyelitis) and of joints (septic arthritis) should be suspected in infants of children who present with:

- fever
- unexplained limp and/or abnormal posture/gait and/or reluctance to use the limb
- musculoskeletal pain, especially in the presence of local bone or joint tenderness, swelling, erythema and complete or partial limitation of movement
- osteomyelitis and septic arthritis may occur separately or together and may affect one or many joints, often depending on the organism and host immunity

Osteomyelitis

- Most common in those under 1–year-old or 3–10 years of age
- More frequent in boys than girls
- Often preceded by trauma in the affected extremity

Acute haematogenous osteomyelitis:
- presents as an acute bacteraemic illness with fever and localized bone symptoms in less than a week

Subacute haematogenous osteomyelitis:
- insidious onset, over 1–4 weeks, with fewer systemic features and more pronounced local bone signs

Chronic osteomyelitis
- lasts for months, often due to an infection that has spread from a contiguous site, e.g. a fracture

Organisms

S. aureus is the most common organism causing osteomyelitis in the normal host. Don't forget *M. tuberculosis*.

Organisms involved in acute haematogenous osteomyelitis

Age	Expected organism	Comments
Neonate (0–2 months)	Group B Streptococcus *S. aureus* *Escherichia coli*	Usually affects femur or humerus Multifocal in 20–40%, Usually associated with septic arthritis
Infant (2–24 months)	*S. aureus*, *S. pneumoniae* Hib Group B Streptococcus	Single long-bone metaphysis affected, usually femur
Child	*S. aureus* Streptococci *E. coli* Salmonella	As for infant
Sickle-cell anaemia	Salmonella *S. aureus* Gram-negative bacilli *S. pneumoniae*	Diaphysis rather than metaphysis affected

Diagnosis

- Increased white cell count with neutrophilia, increased erythrocyte sedimentation rate (ESR) and C-reactive protein (CRP)
- Blood cultures
- Needle aspiration of periosteal space or bone or arthrocentesis if associated septic arthritis
- Tuberculin skin test if tuberculosis is suspected
- Characteristic X-ray changes occur after 10–14 days with periosteal elevation and radiolucent metaphyseal lesions
- Technetium bone scan is positive within 24–48 h of infection

Differential diagnosis

Malignant and benign bone tumours, e.g. Ewing's sarcoma, osteosarcomas, leukaemia with bony infiltrates and bone infarcts, e.g. sickle-cell disease.

Treatment

- 4–6 weeks of antibiotics depending on the organism. The commonest cause is *S. aureus* and should be treated with an anti-staphylococcal penicillin. Some authorities also add fusidic acid. Aim to get an accurate diagnosis from bone culture at debridement, blood cultures or joint fluid cultures.
- Surgery is required if dead or necrotic bone is present.
- Associated septic arthritis (especially the hip) may need incision and drainage.

Complications
Serious damage to the growth plate causing differential limb length and limp (if leg involved)

Septic arthritis

- Serious pyogenic infection of the joint space
- Slightly more common than osteomyelitis
- Most common in children less than 3–years-old and sexually active young women
- Usually monoarticular, except in neonates when often multifocal

Clinical presentation
Similar to haematogenous osteomyelitis. Neonates often present with crying when changing their nappy due to movement of the hip joint.

Organism

- Depends on age and immune status of the child
- Infectious arthritis may be due to viral, fungal (very rare in immunologically normal hosts) or bacterial agents
- Septic arthritis implies pyogenic arthritis secondary to bacterial infections, including *M. tuberculosis*
- Organisms are similar to those in osteomyelitis with *S. aureus* being the most common. Group A streptococci are also often implicated
- *N. meningitidis* may present with acute or occasionally chronic arthritis
- *N. gonorrhoeae* is not uncommon in sexually active teenagers who have polyarticular septic arthritis
- *Borrelia burgdorferi* (Lyme disease) may cause an intermittent, migrating polyarticular arthritis
- *Brucella* spp. may cause chronic septic arthritis

Differential diagnosis

- viral infections such as rubella, mumps, parvovirus B19 and hepatitis B
- post-infectious, reactive and immune-complex arthritidies
- connective tissue diseases
- 'irritable hip' – a transient synovitis of the hip in children <5-years-old following an upper respiratory tract infection; there is mild fever and limp with minimal systemic features, a normal ESR and white cell count and an almost full range of movement of the affected limb

Diagnosis
Clinical

- Ultrasound scan and aspiration of joint fluid for Gram staining and microbiological culture
- Look for associated osteomyelitis

Treatment

- Antibiotic treatment depending on the organism for at least 2 weeks
- Open surgical drainage is indicated for recurrent joint effusions and for **any** case of septic arthritis of the **hip** at the time of presentation

Septic arthritis of the hip in a child is an emergency. Immediate open drainage reduces the intra-articular pressure and avoids aseptic necrosis of the femoral head. The femoral metaphysis can be drilled during this procedure if osteomyelitis is suspected.

3.4 Gastrointestinal infections See Chapter 7, *Gastroenterology and Nutrition*

3.5 Urogenital infections See Chapter 14, *Nephrology*

4. FEVER WITH NO FOCUS/PROLONGED FEVER

4.1 Bacteraemia/septicaemia

Definitions

- **SIRS** (systemic inflammatory response syndrome) is defined by the presence of two or more abnormalities in temperature, heart rate, respiratory rate and white blood count. SIRS can follow any severe insult including infection, trauma, major surgery, burns or pancreatitis.

- **Sepsis** is used to describe SIRS in the context of infection
- **Severe sepsis** is used to describe a state characterized by hypoperfusion, hypotension and organ dysfunction.
- **Septic shock** is restricted to patients with persistent hypotension despite adequate fluid resuscitation, and/or hypoperfusion even following adequate inotrope or pressor support.

Microbial aetiology of sepsis

- The most common organisms in childhood are:
  - *Streptococcus pneumoniae*
  - *N. meningitidis*
  - Hib (drastically reduced in countries with a vaccination programme)
- Rarer causes of sepsis in healthy children include:
  - *S. aureus*
  - group A Streptococcus
  - *Salmonella* spp.
these may be associated with wound and skin infections or a history of diarrhoea, respectively.

- In neonates the usual causes of sepsis are:
  - group B Streptococcus
  - *E. coli* and other Gram-negative bacteria
  - *L. monocytogenes*
- In immunocompromised patients:
  - Gram-negative organisms, such as *Pseudomonas aeruginosa*
  - fungi
- In patients with indwelling catheters:
  - coagulase-negative Staphylococci
  - Enterococci

Some viruses including herpesviruses, enteroviruses and adenoviruses can produce diseases that may be indistinguishable clinically from bacterial sepsis, particularly in neonates and infants.

Pathophysiology of sepsis

Lipopolysaccharides from Gram-negative bacteria and a variety of other microbial products have the capacity to stimulate the production of mediators from many cells within the human host.

Tumour-necrosis factor, interleukin-1 and interleukin-6 are just a few of the many inflammatory mediators reported to be present at high levels in patients with sepsis. Recently, a family of receptors has been identified capable of transducing cellular signals in response to bacteria. These are known as human Toll-like receptors (hTLR).

It is the cytokines and inflammatory mediators which are produced in response to microbial stimuli that stimulate neutrophils, endothelial cells and monocytes and influence the function of vital organs, including the heart, liver, brain and kidneys.

The net effect of excessive inflammatory activity is to cause the constellation of pathophysiological events seen in patients with sepsis and septic shock.

Treatment

Successful treatment involves the administration of appropriate antibiotics, intensive care with particular emphasis on volume replacement and inotropic and respiratory support. A number of adjuvant therapies have been investigated, but, at present, none are used routinely.

4.2 Kawasaki's disease

- In 1967, Tomisaku Kawasaki described 50 Japanese children with an illness characterized by fever, rash, conjunctival injection, erythema and swelling of the hands and feet and cervical lymphadenopathy.
- Kawasaki's disease (KD) is associated with the development of systemic vasculitis (multisystem disease affecting medium-sized muscular arteries) complicated by coronary and peripheral arterial aneurysms, and myocardial infarction in some patients.
- It is the commonest cause of acquired heart disease in children in the UK and the USA.
- KD is commonest in Japan, where more than 125,000 cases have been reported. The disease is also commoner in Japanese and other Oriental children living abroad.
- Children aged between 6 months and 5 years are most susceptible, with peak incidence in children aged 9–11 months. Seasonal variation in the disease incidence has been reported, with the peak occurrence during the winter and spring months.
- Slight male predominance (1.6:1)

Diagnosis of KD

- There is no diagnostic test for KD, therefore diagnosis is based on clinical criteria.
- The differential diagnosis includes toxic-shock syndrome (streptococcal and staphylococcal), staphylococcal scalded-skin syndrome, scarlet fever, and infection with enterovirus, adenovirus, measles, parvovirus, Epstein–Barr virus, cytomegalovirus, *Mycoplasma pneumoniae*, rickettsiae and leptospirosis.

Diagnostic criteria

- fever of 5 days' duration plus four of the five following criteria;
  - conjunctival injection
  - lymphadenopathy
  - rash
  - changes in lips or oral mucosa
  - changes in extremities
- **or:** the presence of fever and coronary artery aneurysms (CAA) with three additional criteria are required for the diagnosis of 'complete' cases.
- 'Incomplete' cases comprise those with fewer than the prerequisite number of criteria. Irritability is an important sign – which, although virtually universally present, is not included as one of the diagnostic criteria.
- Other relatively common clinical findings in KD include arthritis, aseptic meningitis, pneumonitis, uveitis, gastroenteritis, meatitis and dysuria as well as otitis. Relatively uncommon abnormalities include hydrops of the gallbladder, gastrointestinal ischaemia, jaundice, petechial rash, febrile convulsions and encephalopathy or ataxia. Cardiac complications other than coronary arterial abnormalities include cardiac tamponade, cardiac failure, myocarditis, endocardial disease and pericarditis.
- Acute-phase proteins, neutrophils and the ESR are usually elevated. Thrombocytosis occurs towards the end of the second week of the illness and therefore may not be

helpful diagnostically. Liver function may be deranged. Sterile pyuria is occasionally observed, and also CSF pleocytosis (predominantly lymphocytes) representing aseptic meningitis.

Treatment of KD

Treatment of KD is aimed at reducing inflammation and preventing the occurrence of CAA and arterial thrombosis. Aspirin and intravenous immunoglobulin are considered to be the best form of treatment.

- An echocardiogram is performed at 10–14 days, 6 weeks, 6 months and longer if an abnormality is detected.

Cardiac complications of KD

- 20–40% of untreated KD patients develop coronary artery abnormalities.
- 50% of these lesions regress within 5 years, and regression occurs within 2 years in most cases of mild CAA (3–4 mm).

In 1993, a report from the British Paediatric Surveillance Unit (BPSU) indicated a mortality rate of 3.7% in the UK for Kawasaki's disease. Current mortality rates reported from Japan are much lower at 0.14%.

4.3 Infective endocarditis

- Usually occurs as a complication of congenital or rheumatic heart disease or of prosthetic valves, but it can occur in children without cardiac malformations.
- There is an increased risk with central lines, intravenous drug use.
- Highest risk lesions are those associated with a high-velocity blood flow, e.g. ventricular septal defects (VSD), left-sided valvular lesions and systemic–pulmonary arterial communications. Uncommon with atrial septal defects (ASD).
- Vegetations occur at the site of endocardial erosion from turbulent flow.

Organisms

Most common

- Native valve:
    - *Streptococcus viridans* group (*S. mutans*, *S. sanguis*, *S. mitis*)
    - *S. aureus*
    - enterococcus (e.g. *S. faecalis*, *S. bovis*)
- Prosthetic valves:
    - *S. epidermidis*
    - *S. aureus*
    - *S. viridans*

Uncommon organisms

- *S. pneumoniae, H. influenzae, Coxiella burnetii* (Q fever), *Chlamydia psittaci, Chlamydia trachomatis* and *Chlamydia pneumoniae, Legionella* spp., fungi and the HACEK organisms (*Haemophilus* spp. (*H. parainfluenzae, H. aphrophilus, H. paraphrophilus*), *Actinobacillus actinomycetemcomitans, Cardiobacterium hominis, Eikenella corrodens*, and *Kingella kingae*)

Clinical presentation

- Acute: with acute fever and septicaemia
- Non-acute: more common – prolonged fever, with none or non-specific symptoms, e.g. fatigue, myalgia, arthralgia, weight loss.
- New or changes in known murmurs, splenomegaly, neurological manifestations, e.g. emboli, cerebral abscesses (usually *S. aureus*), mycotic aneurysms and haemorrhage.
- Cardiac failure from valve destruction.
- The classic skin lesions occur late in the disease and are now rarely seen, e.g. Osler's nodes (tender nodules in pads of the fingers and toes), Janeway lesions (painless haemorrhagic lesions on soles and palms) and splinter haemorrhages (linear lesions below nails). These are caused by circulating antigen–antibody complexes.

Investigations

- At least 3 separate blood cultures from different sites and different times over 2 days, cultured on enriched media for >7 days
- Look for raised white cell count, high ESR, microscopic haematuria
- Echocardiography

Treatment

- Broad-spectrum i.v. antibiotics, e.g. penicillin and gentamicin or vancomycin and gentamicin (depending on most likely organism), at high bactericidal levels should be started immediately as delay causes progressive endocardial damage.
- Treatment duration is usually 4–6 weeks, but may be shorter for fully sensitive organisms.
- Surgical intervention may be required

Prevention

- Antibiotic prophylaxis prior to and after various procedures, e.g. dental extraction in high-risk patients.
- Proper dental care and oral hygiene

4.4 Toxic-shock syndrome

- Syndrome of high fever, conjunctivitis, diarrhoea, vomiting, confusion, myalgia, pharyngitis and rash with rapid progression to severe, intractable shock in some cases.

- Due to exotoxins produced by *S. aureus*, e.g. staphylococcal enterotoxin B or C (SEB, SEC) or toxic-shock syndrome toxin-1 (TSST-1) or group A Streptococcus, e.g. streptococcal pyrogenic exotoxin A (SPEA).
- In staphylococcal toxic shock the focus of infection is often minor, e.g. skin abrasion.
- Classically occurred in the past in females using tampons.
- In streptococcal toxic shock the focus is usually severe and deep-seated, e.g. fasciitis and myositis.
- Superantigen-mediated, i.e. causes massive, non-MHC-restricted, T-cell response.

Diagnostic criteria

- Fever >38.8°C
- Diffuse macular erythroderma
- Desquamation 1–2 weeks after onset, especially on palms and soles
- Hypotension
- Involvement of 3+ organs – gastrointestinal tract, renal, hepatic, muscle, central nervous system (CNS); mucositis, disseminated intravascular coagulation (DIC)

Diagnosis

- Clinical
- Identification of toxin or antibodies to toxin

Treatment

- Supportive
- Intravenous antibiotics
- Intravenous immunoglobulin

4.5 Brucellosis

- *Brucella* species (e.g. *B. abortus*, *B. melitensis*) are non-motile Gram-negative bacilli
- Zoonotic disease, transmitted to humans by ingestion of unpasteurized milk or direct inoculation to abraded skin
- Incubation period 1–4 weeks
- Disease often mild in children

Acute brucellosis

- Fever, night-sweats, headaches, malaise, anorexia, weight loss, myalgia, abdominal pain, arthritis, lymphadenopathy, hepatosplenomegaly
- Complications include meningitis, endocarditis, osteomyelitis

Chronic brucellosis

- Fevers, malaise, depression, splenomegaly

Diagnosis

- Culture of blood, bone marrow or other tissue, paired serology

Treatment

- Co-trimoxazole, high dose, 4–6 weeks

4.6 Lyme disease

- Caused by spirochete *Borrelia burgdorferi*, transmitted by Ixodes ticks
- Incubation from tick bite to erythema migrans is 3–31 days

Clinical manifestations

3 stages:
- Early localized: distinctive rash – erythema migrans – red macule/papule at site of tick bite, which expands over days/weeks to large annular erythematous lesion with partial clearing, approximately 15 cm in diameter. Associated with fever, malaise, headache, neck stiffness.
- Early disseminated: 3–5 weeks' post-bite – multiple erythema migrans, cranial nerve palsies especially VIIth, meningitis, conjunctivitis, arthralgia, myalgia, headache, malaise, rarely carditis.
- Late disease: recurrent arthritis, pauciarticular, large joints, neuropathy, encephalopathy.

Diagnosis

- Clinical
- Culture of biopsy specimen
- Serology and immunoblotting to detect production of antibodies to *B. burgdorferi*, polymerase chain reaction (PCR) amplification

Treatment

- Doxycycline for child >12 years (avoid sun exposure), or amoxyl if <12 years for 14–21 days if early disease, 21–28 days if disseminated or late disease
- Intravenous ceftriaxone or i.v. penicillin if meningitis, encephalitis, carditis or recurrent arthritis

4.7 Listeriosis

- Caused by *Listeria monocytogenes*, a Gram-positive bacillus.
- Variable incubation of 3–70 days.
- Isolated from a range of raw foods, including vegetables and uncooked meats, as well as processed foods and soft cheeses and meat-based patés.

- The majority of cases are believed to be foodborne. Some cases due to direct contact with animals. Mother to fetus transmission *in utero* or during birth or via person-to-person spread between infants shortly after delivery.
- Unborn infants, neonates, immunocompromised individuals, pregnant women and the elderly are at high risk.

Clinical manifestations

- Influenza-like illness or meningoencephalitis/septicaemia; spontaneous abortion.
- Maternal infections can be asymptomatic.

Treatment

- Ampicillin

4.8 Leptospirosis

- Caused by *Leptospira* spp., e.g. *L. weilii*, which are spirochaetes.
- Many wild and domestic animals, e.g. rats, dogs and livestock, harbour and excrete *Leptospira* spp. in their urine.
- Transmission is by direct contact of mucosal surfaces or abraded skin with urine or carcasses of infected animals; or indirect contact, e.g. swimming in water contaminated by infected urine.
- Incubation period is 1–2 weeks.

Clinical manifestations

- Infection is usually symptomatic with 2 presentations: icteric and anicteric.
- Usually abrupt onset with fevers, rigors, headaches, myalgia, malaise and conjunctival injection.
- 90% will be anicteric; however, 10% will be severely unwell with jaundice, renal dysfunction and CNS disease such as aseptic meningitis (Weil's disease). This may be followed by a second phase of illness, thus giving the biphasic course.

Diagnosis

- Special culture of blood and CSF in the first 10 days of illness and urine after 1 week.
- PCR is available in a few laboratories

Treatment

- Penicillin i.v., doxycycline (if child is >12–years-old)

4.9 Cat-scratch disease

- Caused by *Bartonella henselae* – a Gram-negative bacterium

- Organism transmitted between cats by the cat flea, then transmitted to humans by a cat scratch or bite
- More than 90% have a history of contact with cats (usually kittens)

Clinical manifestations

- Fever and mild systemic symptoms occur in 30% of patients.
- A skin papule is often found at the site of presumed bacterial inoculation.
- Predominant sign is regional lymphadenopathy, involving the nodes that drain the site of inoculation.
- In up to 30% of cases the lymph node will suppurate spontaneously.

Complications

Include:
- Encephalitis, aseptic meningitis, neuroretinitis, hepatosplenic microabscesses and chronic systemic disease

Diagnosis

- Serology is best
- PCR is available in some laboratories
- Special staining of the lymph node may show the causative organism

Treatment

- Most disease is self-limiting so treatment is usually only symptomatic.
- For those who are severely unwell, antibiotics such as ciprofloxacin, rifampicin and gentamicin may be used.

5. MYCOBACTERIAL INFECTIONS

5.1 Tuberculosis (TB)

- Disease caused by infection with *Mycobacterium tuberculosis*, an acid-fast bacillus.
- Incubation period, i.e. infection to development of positive tuberculin skin test, is 2–12 weeks (usually 3–4 weeks).
- Incidence is increasing again in the UK (especially in immigrant patients and those with HIV).
- Host (immune status, age, nutrition) and bacterial (numbers, virulence) factors determine whether infection progresses to disease. Defects in interferon-gamma and interleukin-12 pathways predispose to infection.
- Children usually have primary TB, adults both new infections and reactivation disease.
- Children are rarely infectious.
- Children are usually infected by an adult with 'open' pulmonary TB, therefore notification and contact tracing are essential.

- Only approximately 30% of healthy people closely exposed to TB will become infected, of whom only 5–10% will go on to develop TB disease. Young children exposed to TB are more likely to develop disease than healthy adults.
- Risk of disease is highest in the first 6 months after infection.

TB exposure:	Patient exposed to person with contagious pulmonary TB Clinical examination and chest X-ray and Mantoux-negative Some will have early infection, not yet apparent
TB infection:	Positive Mantoux test Asymptomatic with normal clinical examination Chest X-ray normal Treat with chemoprophylaxis
TB disease:	Positive Mantoux test Clinical symptoms/signs of TB, and/or Chest X-ray signs consistent with TB Treat with chemotherapy

Pathogenesis

- Majority acquire infection via respiratory route, occasionally ingested.
- Organisms multiply in periphery of the lung and spread to regional lymph nodes, which may cause hilar lymphadenopathy.
- Pulmonary macrophages ingest bacteria and mount a cellular immune response.
- In the majority of children, this primary pulmonary infection is controlled by the immune system over 6–10 weeks. Healing of the pulmonary foci occurs, which later calcifies (Ghon focus). Any surviving bacilli remain dormant, but may reactivate later in life and cause 'open' TB.

Clinical symptoms/signs

TB infection – usually asymptomatic, may get fever, malaise, cough or hypersensitivity reactions – erythema nodosum or phlyctenular conjunctivitis.

Complications = disease

- Progressive primary pulmonary TB – foci of infection not controlled but enlarge to involve whole middle and/or lower lobes, often with cavitation (look for immunodeficiency) – fever, cough, dyspnoea, malaise, weight loss
- Dissemination to other organs (especially in children <4 years of age):
  - miliary TB – acutely unwell, fever, weight loss, hepatosplenomegaly, choroidal tubercles in retina, miliary picture on chest X-ray
  - TB meningitis (see section 3.1)
  - TB pericarditis – fever, chest pain, signs of constrictive pericarditis
  - bone and joint infection
  - urogenital infection (v. rare in childhood)

- GI tract – abdominal pain, malabsorption, obstruction, perforation, fistula, haemorrhage, 'doughy' abdomen (usually ingested rather than disseminated)

Congenital TB (see section 10)

Neonatal contact of mother with TB

Infant is at high risk of acquiring TB. Evaluate mother and child (with clinical examination and chest X-ray).

- If mother is 'smear positive' or has an abnormal chest X-ray, separate neonate and mother until both on adequate medication and mother non-contagious.
- If congenital TB excluded, give 3 months' prophylactic isoniazid.
- At 3 months Mantoux test – if this is negative and a repeat chest X-ray is negative – give BCG and stop chemoprophylaxis. If it is positive reassess for TB disease – if no disease continue isoniazid for another 3 months. If disease is present then treat.

Diagnosis

Tuberculin tests: intradermal test of delayed hypersensitivity to tuberculin purified-protein derivative (PPD).

- Heaf test – used for mass screening, if positive refer to TB clinic. Positive is grade 2–4 if no previous BCG, grade 3 or 4 if previous BCG received.
- Mantoux test – dose in UK is 0.1 ml of 1:1,000, i.e. 10 tuberculin units (use 1:10,000 if risk of hypersensitivity, e.g. erythema nodosum or phlyctenular conjunctivitis). Measure induration, **not** erythema, at 48–72 h. Interpretation difficult but positive if:
  - >15 mm induration in anyone (equivalent to Heaf 3–4)
  - >5–14 mm induration (equivalent to Heaf 2) if not had BCG and at high risk, e.g. found at contact or new immigrant screening
  - **NB:** A negative Mantoux test does **not** exclude diagnosis – may be negative if: incorrectly inserted; anergy, e.g. from overwhelming disseminated TB; viral infections, e.g. HIV, measles, influenza, young age.

Diagnosis

Microbiological

- Ziehl–Neelsen stain for acid-fast bacilli (AFB), and culture for 4–8 weeks (culture is required as it will give type and sensitivities) of sputum, gastric washings, bronchoalveolar lavage (BAL) fluid, CSF, biopsy specimens.
- All have low yield in children as lower numbers of bacteria.

Other

- Histology: caseating granuloma and AFBs
- PCR: poor sensitivity and specificity at present
- Chest X-ray: typical changes of hilar lymphadenopathy +/– parenchymal changes

Treatment

Chemoprophylaxis

- For those with TB *infection* (i.e. +ve Mantoux/Heaf test, well child, normal chest X-ray) to prevent progression to disease
- Close contacts of smear-positive TB if they are a young child, HIV positive, immunosuppressed as may not develop positive Mantoux
  - isoniazid for 6 months (+ pyridoxine for breast-fed infants and malnourished)
  - **or** isoniazid and rifampicin for 3 months
  - No need to repeat chest X-ray at end of treatment if good compliance and child asymptomatic

Chemotherapy

For those with signs of *disease*

It is now recommended, due to the increase in isoniazid resistance (now 6% in London, UK), that four drugs are used in the initial 2 months instead of three. The fourth drug (usually ethambutol/streptomycin) can be **omitted** if there is a **low** risk of isoniazid resistance, i.e. previously untreated, Caucasian, proven or suspected HIV-negative patients, or those who have had **no** contact with a TB patient with drug resistance.

- Pulmonary and non-pulmonary disease (except meningitis) – isoniazid and rifampicin for 6 months with pyrazinamide and a fourth drug for the first 2 months.
- Meningitis – 12 months' total therapy with isoniazid and rifampicin with pyrazinamide and a fourth drug for the first 2 months.
- Multidrug-resistant TB – seek expert advice.
- **NB:** Directly observed therapy (DOT) recommended if any chance of non-compliance.
- Corticosteroids should be used for 6–8 weeks if TB meningitis, pericarditis, miliary TB and endobronchial disease with obstruction, but only **with** anti-TB therapy.

Prevention

- Improve social conditions and general health.
- BCG vaccination (live attenuated strain of *M. bovis*) gives approximately 50% protection. In UK, BCG given at birth to high-risk groups and at 12–14 years of age to tuberculin test-negative children.

Complications of BCG vaccination

Include subcutaneous abscess, suppurative lymphadenitis and disseminated disease in severely immunocompromised children.

5.2 Atypical mycobacteria

- Caused by non-tuberculous mycobacteria (NTM), e.g. *M. avium* complex (MAC), *M. scrofulaceum, M. kansasii*
- Ubiquitous organisms – found in soil, food, water and animals

- Found worldwide
- Acquired via ingestion, inoculation, inhalation of organism
- Many people exposed, but only a small number have infection or disease
- May cause disseminated disease in immunodeficient patients, e.g. HIV-positive

Clinical presentations

- Lymphadenitis (usually cervical), pulmonary infections, cutaneous infections

Diagnosis

- Isolation and identification by culture (PCR in some labs)
- May have weakly positive Mantoux test (with no signs of TB)

Treatment

- For NTM lymphadenitis: surgical excision alone
- If incomplete excision, or other site involved, need at least 2 drugs, choice depends on sensitivities, for 3–6 months

NB. For differential diagnosis of persistent cervical lymphadenopathy see section 11.2.

6. FUNGAL INFECTIONS

- Many fungi are ubiquitous, growing in soil, decaying vegetation and in animals.
- Infection acquired by inhalation, ingestion and inoculation from direct contact.
- Often produce spores.
- Superficial infections are common.
- Invasive disease occurs almost exclusively in immunocompromised people, mainly those with neutrophil defects or neutropenia. Consider if neutropenic patient not responding to antibacterial therapy after 48 h of illness.

6.1 Cutaneous fungal infections

Tinea versicolour or pityriasis versicolour

- Caused by *Malassezia furfur* (*Pityrosporum orbiculare*)
- Oval, macular lesions on neck, upper chest, back, arms; may be hypo- or hyperpigmented
- Diagnosis by microscopy of skin scrapings
- Treatment with topical antifungals and salicylic acid preparations

Ringworm (dermatophytoses)

These are caused by filamentous fungi belonging to 3 main genera – *Trichophyton*, *Microsporum* and *Epidermophyton*, diagnosed by skin scrapings.

Tinea capitis (ringworm of scalp)

- Causes patchy dandruff–like scaling with hair loss, discrete pustules or kerion – boggy, inflammatory mass +/– fever and local lymphadenopathy
- Treat with oral antifungals, e.g. griseofulvin, terbinafine. Topical agents not effective

Tinea corporis (ringworm of body)

- Usually dry, erythematous annular lesion with central clearing, on face, trunk and limbs
- Treat with topical antifungals for 4 weeks, if no response use oral antifungals

Tinea cruris (Jock itch!)

- Infection of groin and upper thighs causing itchy erythematous, scaly skin
- Treat as tinea corporis

Tinea Pedis (athlete's foot)

- Infection in interdigital spaces, may involve all of foot. Fungi are common in damp areas, e.g. swimming pools. Treat as tinea corporis

6.2 Candidiasis (thrush, monilliasis)

- Usually caused by *Candida albicans*
- Present on skin, in the mouth, GI tract and vagina of healthy individuals
- Person-to-person transmission occurs
- Use of antibiotics may promote overgrowth of yeasts

Clinical manifestations

Mild mucocutaneous infection:

- Oral thrush and/or nappy-area dermatitis common in infants
- Vulvovaginal candidiasis in adolescents
- Intertriginous lesions, e.g. in neck, groin, axilla

Chronic mucocutaneous candidiasis:

- Associated with endocrine disease and progressive T-cell immunodeficiencies

Invasive disease:

- Disseminated disease to almost any organ, especially in very low birthweight newborns and those who are immunocompromised

Diagnosis

- Microscopy showing pseudohyphae or germ-tube formation (*C. albicans* only)
- Culture

Treatment

- For minor mucocutaneous disease – use oral nystatin or topical nystatin/clotrimazole/miconazole
- For severe or chronic mucocutaneous disease – use an oral azole, e.g. fluconazole
- For invasive disease – treat as for Aspergillus infection (see below)

6.3 Aspergillosis

- Caused by *Aspergillus fumigatus*, *A. niger*, *A. flavus* and, rarely, others
- No person-to-person transmission

Clinical manifestations

- Allergic bronchopulmonary aspergillosis – episodic wheezing, low-grade fever, brown sputum, eosinophilia, transient pulmonary infiltrates. Usually in children with cystic fibrosis or asthma. Treat with steroids.
- Sinusitis and otomycosis of external ear canal – usually benign in immunocompetent patients.
- Aspergilloma – fungal balls that grow in pre-existing cavities or bronchogenic cysts – non-invasive.
- Invasive aspergillosis – extremely serious:
  - may cause peripheral patchy bronchopneumonia with clinical manifestations of acute pneumonia;
  - often disseminates to brain, heart, liver, spleen, eye, bone and other organs.

Diagnosis

- High clinical index of suspicion
- Microscopy shows branched and septate hyphae, culture

Treatment

- For invasive disease treat with amphotericin B in high dose +/– 2nd antifungal, e.g. flucytosine or an azole depending on culture results.
- Surgically excise localized lesion.

7. VIRAL INFECTIONS

7.1 Human immunodeficiency virus (HIV)

- Human immunodeficiency virus (HIV) is a retrovirus, i.e. it contains the enzyme reverse transcriptase, which allows its viral RNA to be incorporated into host-cell DNA.
- 2 main types are known: HIV-1 (widespread) and HIV-2 (West Africa).

- Mainly infects CD4 helper T cells, causing reduction of these cells and acquired immunodeficiency.
- As of March 2002, there were 820 HIV-infected children in the UK.

Transmission

- Vertical (most common mode of transmission in children):
  - prenatal
  - intrapartum (most common)
  - postnatally via breast milk
- Blood or blood products, e.g.:
  - haemophiliacs, unsterile needle use
- Via mucous membranes, e.g.:
  - sexual intercourse, **NB** sexual abuse

Diagnosis

- Virus detection by PCR (rapid, sensitive, specific) or viral culture
- Detection of IgG antibody to viral envelope proteins (gp120 and subunits)

Diagnosis of HIV infection if:

- HIV antibody-positive after 18 months old if born to an infected mother, or at any age if mother is not infected – on 2 occasions
- PCR or virus culture-positive on 2 separate specimens taken at different times

Babies of HIV-positive mother:

- Start zidovudine (AZT, azidothymidine) orally for baby within 12 h of birth:
  - 24–48 h: HIV PCR (50% true-positive by 1 week, 90% by 2 weeks) urine for CMV, may need hepatitis screen, may have signs of drug withdrawal
  - 6 weeks: repeat HIV PCR, stop AZT, start septrin prophylaxis
  - 3–4 months: repeat HIV PCR
- If all 3 PCRs are negative then >95% chance baby is **not** infected, Stop septrin. Follow-up until HIV antibody (vertically acquired from mother) is negative. NB. Still HIV Affected, i.e. many issues re infection in family

Follow-up of HIV-positive babies/children:

- Every 3–6 months depending on health
- History and examination for signs of persistent or unusual infections and growth/puberty
- Psychological and social support, issues re awareness of diagnosis
- FBC, T-cell subsets/CD4 count, HIV viral load
- Hepatitis B, C viruses, CMV, Toxoplasma status if indicated
- Immunization information
- Decisions re *Pneumocystis carinii* prophylaxis (PCP) and highly active antiretroviral treatment (HAART)

Clinical manifestations

These include AIDS-defining and non-defining illnesses.

Clinical categories for children <13 years with human immunodeficiency virus (HIV) infection

Category N	Not Symptomatic	Children who have no signs or symptoms considered to be the result of HIV infection, or those who have only one of the conditions listed in Category A
Category A	Mildly Symptomatic	Children with two or more of: lymphadenopathy; hepatomegaly; splenomegaly; dermatitis; parotitis; recurrent or persistent upper respiratory infection, sinusitis or otitis media
Category B	Moderately Symptomatic	Anaemia, neutropenia or thrombocytopenia; single episode of bacterial meningitis, pneumonia, or sepsis; persistent oropharyngeal candidiasis; cardiomyopathy; diarrhoea; hepatitis; recurrent HSV stomatitis; herpes zoster (shingles); leiomyosarcoma; lymphoid interstitial pneumonia (LIP); nephropathy; nocardiosis; persistent fever (lasting >1 month); toxoplasmosis; disseminated varicella
Category C	Severely Symptomatic (AIDS-defining)	1. Serious bacterial infections, multiple or recurrent 2. Opportunistic infections: candidiasis (oesophageal or pulmonary), coccidioidomycosis, cryptococcosis, cryptosporidiosis or isosporiasis with diarrhoea persisting >1 month; CMV disease with onset of symptoms at age >1 month; HSV bronchitis, pneumonitis, or oesophagitis; histoplasmosis; *M. tuberculosis*, disseminated or extrapulmonary; *M. avium* complex or *M. kansasii*, disseminated; *P. carinii* pneumonia; progressive multifocal leucoencephalopathy; toxoplasmosis of the brain 3. Encephalopathy 4. Wasting syndrome 5. Malignancy, e.g. Kaposi's sarcoma, lymphoma

- 1997 – 20% of vertically infected children developed AIDS in infancy, most common AIDS-defining illness was PCP.
- 2001 – improved antenatal detection and prophylaxis, therefore less AIDS-defining illnesses in infancy.
- Approximately 5% of children with HIV develop AIDS per year.

Recurrent bacterial infections

- Due to poor CD4 (T-helper cell) function, there is B-cell dysregulation despite often high immunoglobulin levels.
- Recurrent serious bacterial infections, such as pneumonia, meningitis, septicaemia and osteomyelitis, may occur. Most common organisms are *S. pneumoniae*, *H. influenzae*, coliforms and Salmonella.
- Treatment depends on clinical condition. Antibiotics should be broad-spectrum, e.g. oral augmentin, cefaclor or i.v. cefuroxime and an aminoglycoside.

Failure to thrive

This is frequently multifactorial, e.g.:

- reduced nutrient and fluid intake – psychosocial, oral and oesophageal thrush
- increased nutrient and fluid requirement with chronic disease
- increased fluid loss with diarrhoea – look for gut pathogens, microsporidiosis, cryptosporidiosis, Giardia, atypical Mycobacteria and viruses.
- **Treatment**: improve immune function with HAART; paromomycin may help in treating Cryptosporidium; fluconazole for thrush; dietary supplements.

Lymphocytic interstitial pneumonitis (LIP)

- Caused by diffuse infiltration of pulmonary interstitium with CD8 (cytotoxic) lymphocytes and plasma cells
- Often chest X-ray diagnosis
- May cause progressive cough, hypoxaemia and clubbing
- Is associated with parotitis
- Superimposed bacterial infections and bronchiectasis may occur
- May have element of reversible bronchoconstriction
- **Treatment**: symptomatic; highly active antiretroviral therapy (HAART) may help; if severe use oral prednisolone

HIV encephalopathy

- May present with regression of milestones, behavioural difficulties, acquired microcephaly, motor signs, e.g. spastic diplegia, ataxia, pseudobulbar palsy
- Exclude CNS infections and lymphoma
- **Treatment**: supportive only, or HAART

Thrombocytopenia

- Not associated with other indicators of disease progression
- **Treatment**: only if symptomatic or platelet count persistently <20,000/mm^3. Options include intravenous immunoglobulin, steroids, HAART, or last-resort splenectomy (not recommended as it further increases the risk of sepsis).

Opportunistic infections

Protozoa

- *P. carinii* pneumonia (PCP) +/– CMV pneumonitis:
  - most common at 3–6 months of age; presents with persistent non-productive cough, hypoxaemia, dyspnoea, minimal chest signs
  - chest X-ray shows bilateral perihilar 'butterfly' shadowing; diagnosis by bronchoalveolar lavage; ensure no concurrent CMV infection
  - **Treatment**: supportive, may need to be treated in paediatric intensive care unit. High-dose co-trimoxazole (septrin) for 21 days. Steroids if severe disease. Gancyclovir i.v. if concurrent CMV disease. Once stable, commence HAART. Prophylactic low-dose septrin following treatment.
- Cerebral toxoplasmosis
  - rare in childhood HIV infection compared to adults; may present with focal signs +/– fits
  - CT shows multiple intraparenchymal ring-enhancing lesions. Positive toxoplasmosis serology
  - **Treatment**: 6 weeks of pyrimethamine and sulfadiazine with folinic acid and HAART
- Cryptosporidosis
  - *Cryptosporidium parvum* causes severe secretory diarrhoea, abdominal pain and sometimes sclerosing cholangitis
  - Diagnosis by stool microscopy +/– small-bowel biopsy
  - **Treatment**: supportive, paromomycin

Fungi

- *Candida albicans* – oropharyngeal, oesophageal, vulvovaginal, disseminated (rare)
  - **Treatment**: chronic antifungal therapy, e.g. fluconazole, i.v. amphotericin B if severe
- *Cryptococcus neoformans* – meningitis (insidious onset), pneumonia
  - Diagnosis by CSF examination (Indian ink stain, antigen, culture), serum culture, antigen
  - **Treatment**: fluconazole

Viruses

- CMV – retinitis, colitis, pneumonitis, hepatitis, pancreatitis
  - diagnosis by serum PCR, immunofluorescence in relevant sample and characteristic retinal changes if present; differentiate disease from carriage
  - **Treatment**: i.v. ancyclovir; HAART may help
- Herpes simplex virus (HSV)
  - types 1 and 2 – extensive oral ulceration
  - **Treatment**: i.v. aciclovir, oral prophylaxis if recurrent and severe; ART may help
- Measles, varicella zoster virus (VZV), RSV, adenovirus – all may cause severe disease in HIV-infected children, especially pneumonitis

TB and atypical TB

- Increased risk of TB and atypical TB, especially disseminated *M. avium* complex
- See section 5

Tumours

- Kaposi's sarcoma – tumour of vascular endothelial cells, associated with human herpesvirus-8 (HHV–8); involves skin, gut, lung and lymphatics
  - **Treatment**: HAART, local radiotherapy, chemotherapy if disseminated
- Lymphoma – non-Hodgkin's B-cell primary CNS lymphoma
  - focal neurological signs +/– fits; CT shows single lesion
  - definitive diagnosis by brain biopsy
  - **Treatment**: radio/chemotherapy; poor prognosis

HIV treatment

Highly active antiretroviral therapy (HARRT).

- When to start treatment in children differs in each country.
- In UK, start if AIDS-defining illness, many B-category symptoms, rapidly increasing viral load or decreasing CD4 count.
- Usually give 3 drugs to reduce resistance occurring.
- Many regimes being evaluated involve protease inhibitors, nucleoside reverse transcriptase inhibitors and non-nucleoside reverse transcriptase inhibitors. Liaise with tertiary centre.
- Monitor for efficacy (viral load and CD4 count) and side-effects.

PCP prophylaxis

- Life-long if ever had PCP
- For first 12 months of life if vertically infected
- If CD4 count persistently <15%

CMV prophylaxis

- Life-long if ever had CMV retinitis

Reduction of vertical transmission

With breast feeding and no intervention vertical transmission rate is 14–39%.

- Interventions:
  - no breast feeding (where safe alternative is possible) transmission rate is 15%
  - + antiretrovirals to mother and baby, e.g. ACTG 076 trial – reduces rate to 5%
  - + elective Caesarean section – reduces transmission to 1% (or less if very low maternal viral load)
- In order to allow intervention, women need to be diagnosed before giving birth. National targets and objectives were set in 1999 that involve the offer and recommendation of an HIV test to all pregnant women throughout UK. By 2001 80% of maternity units in the UK offered this service, with an uptake of approximately 70%.
- NB. If vaginal delivery – avoid invasive fetal procedures, e.g. fetal blood sampling.

Major side-effects of antiretroviral drugs used in children

Drug	Side-effect
Nucleoside reverse transcriptase inhibitors	
AZT – zidovudine	Nausea, bone marrow suppression, myopathy
DDI – didanosine	Peripheral neuropathy, pancreatitis
D4T – stavudine	Peripheral neuropathy, pancreatitis, elevation of LFTs
3TC – lamivudine	Rare – peripheral neuropathy, pancreatitis
Abacavir	Life-threatening hypersensitivity reactions – usually present as rash and fever
Non-nucleoside reverse transcriptase inhibitors	
Efavirenz	Rash, +/– Stevens–Johnson syndrome
Nevirapine	Rash, hepatitis
Protease inhibitors	
Ritonavir	GI side-effects common in first 4 weeks, paraesthesia
Indinavir	GI disturbances, rashes
Nelfinavir	Diarrhoea

NB. PI's and D4T are associated with lipodystrophy

7.2 Hepatitis (see Chapter 7, *Gastroenterology and Nutrition*)

7.3 Epstein–Barr virus (EBV)

This causes infectious mononucleosis (glandular fever). EBV infects pharyngeal epithelial cells and then B lymphocytes. These disseminate and proliferate until checked by activated T cells.

- **Transmission**: saliva, aerosol
- **Incubation**: 30–50 days
- **Clinical presentation**:
  - fever, sore throat, lymphadenopathy, palatal petechiae
  - splenomegaly (50%), hepatomegaly (30%), hepatitis (80%), jaundice (5%), thrombocytopenia, haemolytic anaemia
  - maculopapular rash (5–15%), 90% if given ampicillin
- **Complications**:
  - meningitis, encephalitis, Guillain-Barré, syndrome, myocarditis, splenic rupture, airway obstruction from pharyngotonsillar swelling
  - chronic fatigue-like syndrome
  - disseminated disease with B-cell proliferation in those with T-cell immunodeficiencies

- **Diagnosis**: atypical lymphocytosis, positive Paul-Bunnell (often negative in young children) or Monospot test, serology, heterophile antibodies, PCR
- **Treatment**: supportive, steroids for severe airway obstruction

7.4 Cytomegalovirus (CMV)

- **Transmission**: close contact, blood, organ transplant
- **Clinical presentation**:
  - in normal hosts – often asymptomatic or glandular fever-like picture
  - in immunocompromised patients – severe disease may occur with pneumonitis, retinitis, encephalitis, hepatitis and GI disturbance
  - CMV is the most common congenital infection
- **Diagnosis**: immunofluorescence, intranuclear inclusions, culture, detection of early antigen fluorescence foci (DEAFF) test, serology, PCR
- **Treatment**: symptomatic, i.v. gancyclovir and/or i.v. foscarnet if immunosuppressed

7.5 Herpes simplex virus (HSV)

- **Infection**:
  - 2 types recognized: HSV-1 (usually infects skin and mucous membranes) and HSV-2 (usually genital)
  - primary infections – 85% subclinical
  - recurrent infections – reactivation of latent infection
- **Incubation**: 2–12 days
- **Transmission**: direct contact, very rarely congenital
- **Clinical presentation**:
  - acute herpetic gingivostomatitis – primary infection – acute painful mouth ulcers and fever, most common between 1 and 3 years of age, self-limiting, lasts 4–9 days (may be asymptomatic)
  - recurrent stomatitis – localized vesicular lesions in nasolabial folds, 'cold sores'
  - keratoconjunctivitis and corneal ulcers
  - meningoencephalitis
  - eczema herpeticum – widespread infection of eczematous skin with HSV vesicles – may be very severe
  - genital lesions – usually in sexually active adolescents, NB. child abuse
  - neonatal HSV – usually from vaginal secretions at delivery – high morbidity and mortality
- **Diagnosis**:
  - clinical, electron microscopy of vesicular fluid (very fast), PCR, culture, serology
- **Treatment**:
  - aciclovir – i.v. if severe disease, immunocompromised, neonate or eczema herpeticum
  - oral, topical, eye drops

7.6 Varicella zoster virus (VZV)

This produces chickenpox (varicella) as a primary infection. Shingles (herpes zoster) is caused by reactivation of dormant VZV from dorsal root or cranial ganglia. You can catch chickenpox from contact with chickenpox **or** shingles. You cannot 'catch' shingles.

Chickenpox

- **Incubation**: chickenpox: 11–24 days
- **Transmission**: direct contact, droplet, airborne; infectious from 24 h before rash until all spots have crusted over (approx. 7–8 days)
- **Clinical presentation**: prodrome of fever and malaise for 24 h; rash appears in crops, papular then vesicular and itchy, usually start on trunk; crops appear for 3–4 days and each crusts at 24–48 h
- **Complications**:
  - secondary bacterial infection often with group A Streptococcus
  - thrombocytopenia with haemorrhage into skin
  - pneumonia
  - purpura fulminans
  - post-infectious encephalitis
  - immunocompromised – severe disseminated haemorrhagic disease
- **Diagnosis**: clinical, viral culture
- **Treatment**: supportive; intravenous aciclovir for immunosuppressed or severely unwell patient
- **Prophylaxis**: zoster immunoglobulin (ZIG) if high risk (e.g. immunodeficiency, immunosuppressive treatment). **NB:** If mother develops chickenpox within 5 days' pre- to 2 days' post-delivery give neonate ZIG. If baby develops chickenpox treat with i.v. aciclovir.

Herpes zoster

Increased incidence if immunosuppressed
- **Clinical presentation**:
  - prodrome of pain and tenderness in affected dermatome with fever and malaise; within a few days the same rash as varicella appears in distribution of one (sometimes 2 or 3) unilateral dermatomes
  - if infection of Vth cranial nerve occurs, it may affect the cornea (ophthalmic branch)
  - if VIIth nerve involved, may get paralysis of facial nerve and vesicles in external ear (Ramsey–Hunt syndrome)
- **Complications**: dissemination in immunocompromised; post-herpetic pain rare in children
- **Treatment**: supportive; i.v. aciclovir if severe and immunocompromised
  - **NB:** VZV vaccine now available routinely in the USA, and for at-risk patients in the UK

7.7 Parvovirus B19 (Erythema infectiosum, 'slapped cheek' or Fifth disease)

This virus affects red cell precursors and reticulocytes in the bone marrow.
- **Incubation**: approx. 1 week
- **Transmission**: respiratory secretions, blood; not infectious once rash has appeared
- **Clinical presentation**:
  - very erythematous cheeks, then erythematous macular papular rash on trunk and extremities, which fades with central clearing giving the characteristic lacy or reticular appearance
  - rash lasts 2–30 days
- **Complications**:
  - aplastic crisis in chronic haemolytic diseases, e.g. sickle-cell disease, thalassaemia:
  - aplastic anaemia
  - arthritis, myalgia more common in older children/adults
  - congenital infection with anaemia and hydrops (see section 10)
- **Diagnosis**: clinical, serology
- **Treatment**: supportive

7.8 Roseola infantum (exanthem subitum or HHV-6)

- **Transmission**: respiratory secretions
- **Clinical presentation**: characteristic – sudden onset of high fever (up to 41°C) with absence of clinical localizing signs; may have febrile fits; at day 3–4 fever abruptly stops and macular/papular rash appears which lasts <24 h
- **Treatment**: antipyretics

7.9 Measles

- **Incubation**: 7–14 days
- **Transmission**: respiratory droplets; infectious from 7 days after exposure, i.e. from pre-rash to 5 days after rash starts
- **Clinical presentation**:
  - prodrome: 3–5 days, low fever, cough, coryza, conjunctivitis, Koplik's spots (pathognomonic white spots opposite lower molars)
  - eruptive stage: abrupt rise in temperature to 40°C associated with macular rash, starts behind ears and along hairline, becomes maculopapular and spreads sequentially to face, upper arms, chest, abdomen, back, legs; lasts approx. 4 days
- **Complications**:
  - otitis media, laryngitis, bronchitis
  - interstitial pneumonitis, secondary bacterial bronchopneumonia, myocarditis
  - encephalomyelitis: mainly post-infectious, demyelinating
  - subacute sclerosing panencephalitis (see Chapter 15, *Neurology*)
- **Diagnosis**: clinical, viral culture, immunofluorescence, serology

- **Treatment**: symptomatic; human pooled immunoglobulin <5 days of exposure to high-risk patients only
- **Prophylaxis**: immunization – measles, mumps, rubella (MMR)

7.10 Mumps

- **Incubation**: 14–21 days
- **Transmission**: respiratory droplets, infectious 24 h pre- to 3 days' post-parotid swelling
- **Clinical presentation**: mild prodrome of fever, anorexia, headache; painful bilateral (may be unilateral) salivary +/– submandibular gland swelling
- **Complications**: due to viraemia early in the infection:
  - meningoencephalitis clinically 10% (subclinically 65%):
    - infectious – symptoms same time as parotitis
    - postinfectious – symptoms approx. 10 days' post-parotitis
  - orchitis/epididymitis:
    - rare in childhood, 14–35% in adolescents/adults
    - occurs within 8 days of parotitis, abrupt onset of fever and tender, swollen testes
    - approx. 30–40% of affected testes atrophy; may cause subfertility
  - pancreatitis, nephritis, myocarditis, arthritis, deafness, thyroiditis
- **Diagnosis**: viral culture, serology
- **Treatment**: supportive
- **Prophylaxis**: vaccination (MMR) to ensure 'herd immunity'

7.11 Rubella (German or 3–day measles)

- **Incubation**: 14–21 days
- **Transmission**: respiratory droplets; transplacental
- **Clinical presentation**:
  - mild coryza, palatal petechiae
  - characteristic tender, retroauricular, posterior cervical and suboccipital adenopathy 24 h before rash appears, lasting one week
  - rash begins on face, spreading quickly to trunk.
- **Complications**: arthritis, encephalitis, congenital rubella syndrome (see section 10)
- **Diagnosis**: clinical, serology
- **Treatment**: supportive
- **Prophylaxis**: although a mild illness, vaccination of all children prevents childbearing women contacting rubella

7.12 Adenovirus

- **Transmission**: respiratory droplets, contact, fomites, very contagious, strict infection control policy
- **Incubation**: 2–14 days
- **Clinical presentation**:
  - upper respiratory tract infection (URTI)

- conjunctivitis +/– pharyngitis
- gastroenteritis – more common in <4-year-olds
- **Complications**: severe pneumonia (more common in infants); disseminated disease in immunocompromised patients
- **Diagnosis**: viral culture, serology, PCR
- **Treatment**: supportive

7.13 Enteroviruses

These include:
- Polioviruses: types 1–3 (see Chapter 15, *Neurology*)
- Coxsackieviruses: A and B
- Echoviruses

Coxsackie- and echoviruses

- **Transmission**: faecal/oral and respiratory droplets, usually during summer and autumn
- **Clinical presentation**:
    - non-specific febrile illness: abrupt onset of fever and malaise +/– headache and myalgia, lasts 3–4 days
    - respiratory manifestations: pharyngitis, tonsillitis, nasopharyngitis, lasts 3–6 days
    - GI manifestations: diarrhoea, vomiting, abdominal pain
    - skin manifestations: 'hand, foot and mouth' – usually coxsackievirus A16 and enterovirus 71; intraoral ulcerative lesions, vesicular lesions on hands and feet 3–7 mm; rash clears within 1 week
    - pericarditis and myocarditis: usually coxsackie B viruses
    - neurological manifestations: aseptic meningitis (esp. coxsackievirus B5), encephalitis (esp. echovirus 9), cerebellar ataxia and Guillain–Barré, syndrome
- **Diagnosis**: viral culture, PCR
- **Treatment**: supportive
- **Prophylaxis**: Nil for coxsactic and echo viruses. Polio vaccine for prevention of polio. The WHO are aiming for worldwide eradication.

7.14 Molluscum

- **Incubation**: 2–8 weeks
- **Transmission**: direct contact with infected person or fomites or autoinoculation
- **Clinical presentation**: discrete, pearly papules 1–5 mm, face, neck, axillae and thighs
- **Diagnosis**: clinical, microscopy
- **Treatment**:
    - self-limiting but may last months–years
    - need to treat in immunodeficient patients as it will become widespread, e.g. with liquid nitrogen

8. PARASITIC INFECTIONS

8.1 Toxoplasmosis

- Caused by *Toxoplasma gondii*
- Worldwide distribution and infects most warm-blooded animals.
- Cat is the definitive host and excretes oocysts in stools.
- Intermediate hosts include sheep, pigs and cattle who have viable cysts in their tissues.
- Human infection is by eating undercooked meat containing cysts or ingestion of oocysts from soil; may also be acquired from blood transfusion or bone marrow transplantation.
- Congenital infection (see section 10)

Clinical manifestations

- Often asymptomatic, or non-specific fever, malaise, myalgia, sore throat.
- May also have lymphadenopathy or mononucleosis-like illness.
- Complications rarely include myocarditis, pericarditis and pneumonitis, encephalitis.
- Isolated ocular toxoplasmosis is usually a result of reactivation of congenital infection, but may be acquired.
- Immunodeficient patients may have more serious/disseminated disease.

Diagnosis

- By serology (PCR in special cases)
- Isolation of *T. gondii* is difficult
- Atypical lymphocytosis, eosinophilia and inversion of CD4:CD8 ratio

Treatment

- Supportive if mild
- Pyrimethamine (and folinic acid) and sulfadiazine if symptomatic

8.2 Head lice (Pediculosis capitis)

- Caused by lice – *Pediculus humanus capitis*
- Itching is the most common complaint
- Adult lice or eggs (nits) may be seen in the hair
- Very common in school-aged children

Transmission

- Occurs by direct contact with hair of infested individuals

Diagnosis

- Clinical, can confirm by microscopy

Treatment

- 2 applications, 1 week apart, of a parasiticidal lotion, left on overnight, e.g. permethrin and malathion. Resistance is developing, so if the treatment fails try another insecticide for the next course. Many people use mechanical means of lice control, e.g. 'nit comb'. **Remember** to treat whole family (+/– school class at same time).

Malaria (see section 9.1)

Leishmaniasis (see section 9.8)

Schistosomiasis (see section 9.9)

Pneumocystis (see section 7.1)

9. TROPICAL INFECTIONS

Always obtain a travel history as imported infections in returning travellers, those from abroad holidaying in the UK and recent immigrants are part of the differential diagnosis of fever.

In the last decade, 100 people of all ages have died in the UK from malaria contracted in malarious areas. Only one of these people was taking full doses of what would currently be considered an adequate antimalarial. Of these 100 cases, 94 were contracted in Africa and six in the countries of South Asia. Four African countries accounted for 67% of all the fatal cases (Kenya 25%, Nigeria 17%, the Gambia 14% and Ghana 11%).

9.1 Malaria

- Caused by *Plasmodium* spp., *P. vivax*, *P. malariae*, *P. ovale* and *P. falciparum* invading erythrocytes.
- Endemic in tropical world, especially sub-Saharan Africa and parts of SE Asia.
- Transmitted by bite of the female Anopheles mosquito.
- Congenital infection and blood transfusion-acquired infection may also occur.
- *P. vivax* and *P. ovale* have hepatic stages and may cause relapses of infection.
- Recrudescence of *P. falciparum* and *P. malariae* occurs from persistent low levels of parasitaemia.
- *P. falciparum* malaria is the most severe and potentially fatal disease.

Clinical manifestations

Appear 8–15 days after infection with high fevers with chills, rigors and sweats, which classically occur in cyclical pattern depending on the type of Plasmodium.

- Headaches, abdominal pain, arthralgia, diarrhoea and vomiting are common.
- Pallor and jaundice occur secondary to haemolysis.
- Hepatosplenomegaly is more common in chronic infections.
- Nephrotic syndrome may occur with *P. malariae*, due to immune-complex deposition in the kidney.
- *P. falciparum* may present as a febrile illness with no localizing signs, or as one of the following clinical syndromes:
  - cerebral malaria – with confusion, fits, decreased level of consciousness, coma (NB. do blood sugar (BM))
  - severe anaemia with signs of haemolysis
  - hypoglycaemia from disease (metabolic requirements of parasites) and also quinine treatment
  - pulmonary oedema (rare in children)
  - renal failure with acute tubular necrosis, or 'blackwater fever' due to haemaglobinuria resulting from severe, acute intravascular haemolysis (rare in children)

Diagnosis

- Thick blood films allow detection of parasites, thin film allows species identification and determination of parasitaemia (% of erythrocytes harbouring parasites)
- Need at least 3 negative films at 12–24-h intervals to be confident of negative result if there is a high index of clinical suspicion
- New tests being evaluated include PCR and malarial ribosomal RNA
- NB. in hyperendemic areas, a low-level parasitaemia is common and malaria is not necessarily the cause of the symptoms.

Treatment

- Look for and treat hypoglycaemia

Chemotherapy is based on infecting species, possible drug resistance and disease severity

P. falciparum malaria

- In the UK, we assume that all cases of *P. falciparum* malaria are chloroquine-resistant and treat with quinine, orally if possible, or i.v. if severely unwell for 7 days total (monitor glucose and ECG if i.v. regimen used). 1 dose of pyrimethamine–sulfadoxine (Fansidar) is given on the last day of quinine therapy.
- Exchange transfusion may be warranted if parasitaemia exceeds 10%.
- Monitor sequential blood smears.

P. malariae malaria

- Treat with chloroquine (if no resistance).

P. vivax and **P. ovale** malaria

- Treat with chloroquine then primaquine to eradicate the liver stage and prevent relapses. Check patient is not glucose 6–phosphate dehydrogenase (G6PD)-deficient before giving primaquine.

Prophylaxis

- From dusk to dawn (night-biters) use protective clothing, mosquito repellents, bed nets impregnated with insecticide.
- Prescribe chemoprophylaxis from 1 week prior to departure until 4 weeks after return:
  - chloroquine-sensitive area – chloroquine once a week **or** proguanil daily;
  - chloroquine-resistant areas – mefloquine once a week **or** doxycycline daily **or** chloroquine and proguanil (not optimal protection, therefore use only if others not appropriate or low-risk area).

9.2 Enteric (typhoid/paratyphoid) fever

- Caused by *Salmonella typhi, S. paratyphi* – Gram-negative bacilli in family Enterobacteriacae.
- *S. typhi* found only in humans, transmitted by faecal–oral route.
- Onset of illness is gradual with fever, headache, malaise, constipation (initially), diarrhoea (2nd week), abdominal pain, hepato/splenomegaly, rose spots. Infants may present with Gram-negative septicaemia. Within a week, fever becomes unremitting, delirium and disorientation may occur. The paradoxical relationship between high fever and low pulse rate is uncommon in children.

Complications

- Intestinal perforation 0.5–3%, severe haemorrhage in 1–10% of children
- Focal infections, e.g. meningitis, osteomyelitis, endocarditis, pyelonephritis more common in the immunocompromised host
- Osteomyelitis and septic arthritis in children with haemoglobinopathies
- Chronic carriage – local multiplication in the wall of the gallbladder produces large numbers of Salmonellae, which are then discharged into the intestine and may cause chronic carriage and shedding (in 5% adults, much less in children)

Diagnosis

- Perform bacterial cultures on blood, stool, bone marrow or rose spot aspirate.
- Microscopy of stool reveals many leucocytes, mainly mononuclear.
- Blood leucocyte count is at the low end of normal.

Treatment

Drug choice and route of administration depend on susceptibility of organism, host response and site of infection – includes:

- Ampicillin, ceftriaxone, cefotaxime, chloramphenicol; in view of resistance, a fluoroquinolone is now frequently used as first-line therapy for 14 days
- For osteomyelitis – as above for 4–6 weeks
- For meningitis – ceftriaxone or cefotaxime for 4 weeks
- To eradicate carriage – high-dose ampicillin or amoxicillin or cholecystectomy

Prophylaxis

Personal hygiene and proper sanitation for food processing and sewage disposal. Vaccine available, but only 17–66% effective depending on type.

9.3 Dengue fever

- Caused by an arbovirus (i.e. arthropod borne). 570 arboviruses have been identified with more than 30 being human pathogens.
- Dengue fever is caused by the genus *Flavivirus* (which also cause Japanese encephalitis and yellow fever).
- Transmitted by the mosquito *Aedes aegypti* – a day-biting mosquito.
- Dengue fever is now endemic in SE Asia, central and south America and the Caribbean.

Clinical manifestations

- Include fever for 1–7 days, frontal or retro-orbital headaches, back pain, myalgia and arthralgia ('breakbone' fever), nausea and vomiting.
- 1–2 days after defervescence a generalized morbilliform rash occurs lasting 1–5 days. As this rash fades the fluctuating temperature reappears, producing the biphasic temperature curve.

Complications

- Dengue haemorrhagic fever – rare in childhood, since it occurs with 2nd exposure to Dengue

Diagnosis

- PCR, serology, isolation of virus (**NB:** prior yellow-fever vaccination will give positive dengue IgG)

Treatment

- None is specific, supportive only

9.4 Viral haemorrhagic fevers

- Many different viruses found in different parts of world, so accurate travel history necessary, e.g. Lassa fever caused by lassa virus (an arenavirus) or Ebola haemorrhagic fever caused by Ebola virus.
- These diseases range from mild infections to severe acute febrile illnesses with cardiovascular collapse. Fever, headaches, myalgia, conjunctival suffusion and abdominal pain are early symptoms. Mucosal bleeding occurs with vascular damage and thrombocytopenia and may cause life-threatening haemorrhage. Shock develops 7–9 days after the onset of illness.
- Elevated alanine aminotransferase (ALT) is a poor prognostic factor in Lassa fever. Transmission is by inhalation or broken skin contact with the urine or saliva of infected rodents.

Diagnosis

- Serology

Treatment

- Intravenous ribavirin for Lassa fever, especially in the first week of illness reduces mortality.

Prevention

- Strict isolation of patient and contacts
- For suspected cases – examine a malarial film only (labelled 'Very high risk' for laboratory staff awareness). If negative, ie diagnosis is NOT malaria then contact local microbiologist/public health laboratory service urgently re transfer of the patient to the designated unit.

9.5 Giardia

- Caused by *Giardia lamblia*, a protozoan that produces infectious cysts
- Faecal–oral transmission
- Infection limited to small intestine and/or biliary tract
- Worldwide distribution, some animals and humans infected, may infect water supply

Clinical manifestations

- Very varied
- Acute watery diarrhoea with abdominal pain, or foul-smelling stools and flatulence with abdominal distension and anorexia

Diagnosis

- Stool microscopy, rarely by duodenal biopsy

Treatment

- Metronidazole

9.6 Amoebiasis

- Caused by *Entamoeba histolytica*, a protozoan, excreted as cysts or trophozoites in stool of infected patients
- Faecal–oral transmission of cysts
- Worldwide distribution, with infection rates as high as 20–50% in the tropics

Clinical manifestations

- Intestinal disease – asymptomatic or mild symptoms, e.g. abdominal distension, flatulence, constipation, loose stools
- Acute amoebic colitis (dysentery) – abdominal cramps, tenesmus, diarrhoea with blood and mucus – complications include toxic megacolon, fulminant colitis, ulceration and rarely perforation

Extraintestinal disease

- Liver abscess – acute fever, abdominal pain and liver tenderness, or subacute with weight loss and vague abdominal symptoms; rupture of the abscess into the abdomen or chest may occur
- Rarely, abscesses in the lung, pericardium, brain and genitourinary tract

Diagnosis

- Microscopy of stool, biopsy specimens and aspirates, serology if extraintestinal disease

Treatment

- To eliminate the tissue-invading trophozoites as well as cysts
- Metronidazole and a second luminal amoebicide, e.g. paromomycin

9.7 Hookworm

- Caused by *Ancylostoma duodenale* and *Necator americanus*
- Prominent in rural, tropical areas where soil may be contaminated with human faeces
- Humans are the major reservoir
- Infection is by infectious larvae penetrating the skin, usually soles of feet

Clinical manifestations

- May be asymptomatic
- May get pruritis and papulovesicular rash for 1–2 weeks after initial infection
- Pneumonitis associated with migrating larvae in this phase is uncommon and usually mild

Diagnosis

- Stool microscopy

Treatment

- Antihelminthic drug e.g. mebendazole. (NB. Also treat any associated iron deficient anaemia.)

9.8 Leishmaniasis

- *Leishmania* species are obligate intracellular parasites of monocytes/macrophages
- Variety of hosts including canines and rodents
- Vector is the sandfly
- Incubation period is usually days–months, but may even be years
- 3 major clinical syndromes:
  - cutaneous leishmaniasis – shallow ulcer at site of sandfly bite; lesions commonly on exposed skin, i.e. face and extremities; may have satellite lesions and regional lymphadenopathy
  - mucosal leishmaniasis – initial cutaneous infection disseminates to midline facial structures, e.g. oral and nasopharyngeal mucosa
  - visceral leishmaniasis (kala-azar) – parasites spread throughout the reticular endothelial system and are concentrated in the liver, spleen and bone marrow. Present with fevers, weight loss, splenomegaly (may be massive), hepatomegaly, lymphadenopathy, anaemia, leucopenia, thrombocytopenia and hypergammaglobulinaemia.

Diagnosis

- Microscopic identification of intracellular leishmanial organisms from skin or splenic biopsy, or bone marrow
- PCR and serology may be helpful

Treatment

- Sodium stiboglutonate or amphotericin B

9.9 Schistosomiasis

- Caused by the trematodes (flukes) *Schistosoma mansoni, S. japonicum, S. haematobium* and others
- Humans are principal host, snail is intermediate host
- Eggs are excreted in urine or stool into fresh water, hatch and infect snails; after further development, cercariae emerge and penetrate human skin

Clinical manifestations

- Usually infection is asymptomatic
- May have initial transient pruritic, papular rash
- May have acute infection – Katayama fever: 4–8 weeks after infection an acute illness with fever, malaise, cough, rash, abdominal pain, diarrhoea, arthralgia, lymphadenopathy and eosinophilia
- Chronic infection with *S. mansoni* and *S. japonicum* may cause diarrhoea, tender hepatomegaly, chronic fibrosis, hepatosplenomegaly and portal hypertension
- Chronic infection with *S. haematobium* may cause dysuria, terminal microscopic haematuria, gross haematuria, frequency and obstructive uropathy
- Haematogenous spread to the lungs, liver and central nervous system may occur

Diagnosis

- Identification of the eggs in stool/urine, respectively
- Bladder biopsy
- Serology

Treatment

- Praziquantel

9.10 Travellers' diarrhoea

- Travellers' diarrhoea (TD) is a syndrome characterized by a twofold or greater increase in the frequency of unformed bowel movements.
- Food and waterborne diseases are the number one cause of illness in travellers.
- Traveller's diarrhoea can be caused by viruses, bacteria or parasites, which can contaminate food or water.
- The most important determinant of risk is the destination of the traveller.
- Attack rates of 20–50% are commonly reported.

Clinical manifestations

- Diarrhoea, abdominal cramps, nausea, bloating, urgency, and malaise; sometimes vomiting also occurs.
- Nature of stool may indicate particular organism.
- TD usually lasts from 3 to 7 days, but is rarely life-threatening.

Enteric bacterial pathogens

- Enterotoxigenic *E. coli* (ETEC) are among the most common causative agents; ETEC produce a watery diarrhoea associated with cramps and a low-grade or no fever.
- Salmonella gastroenteritis is usually caused by non-typhoidal *Salmonella* spp.; which cause dysentery characterized by small-volume stools containing bloody mucus.
- Shigella bacillary dysentery is seen in up to 20% of travellers to developing countries.

- *Campylobacter jejuni* causes a small percentage of the reported cases of TD, some with bloody diarrhoea.
- *Vibrio parahaemolyticus* is associated with the ingestion of raw or poorly cooked seafood.

Less common bacterial pathogens include other diarrhoeagenic *E. coli*, *Yersinia enterocolitica*, *Vibrio cholerae* 01 and 0139, non–01 *V. cholerae*, *Vibrio fluvialis* and possibly *Aeromonas hydrophila* and *Plesiomonas shigelloides*.

Viral enteric pathogens

- For example, rotaviruses and Norwalk-like virus may cause TD.

Parasitic enteric pathogens

- These include *Giardia intestinalis*, *Entamoeba histolytica*, *Cryptosporidium parvum* and *Cyclospora cayetanensis*. The likelihood of a parasitic aetiology is higher when diarrhoeal illness is prolonged. *E. histolytica* should be considered when the patient has dysentery or invasive diarrhoea (bloody stools).

Treatment

- Antimotility agents should NOT be used in children. Occasionally in adolescents, like adults, they may be used to provide prompt symptomatic but temporary relief of uncomplicated TD. However, they should **not** be used by people with high fever or with blood in their stools.
- Oral rehydration solutions (ORS) and plenty of fluids should be drunk to prevent dehydration.
- Antibiotics should be reserved for: those with severe diarrhoea that does not resolve within several days; if there is blood or mucus, or both, in the stools; if fever occurs with shaking chills.

Prevention

- Treatment of water:
  - boiling for at least five minutes is the most reliable method to make water safe to drink;
  - chemical disinfection can be achieved with either iodine or chlorine, with iodine providing greater disinfection in a wider set of circumstances.
- Food:
  - any raw food can be contaminated, particularly in areas of poor sanitation;
  - foods of particular concern include salads, uncooked vegetables and fruit, unpasteurized milk and milk products, raw meat and shellfish;
  - some fish are not guaranteed to be safe even when cooked because of the presence of toxins in their flesh. Tropical reef fish, red snapper, amber jack, grouper and sea bass can occasionally be toxic at unpredictable times if they are caught on tropical reefs.

10. CONGENITAL INFECTIONS (See Chapter 13, Neonatology)

Congenital infections are acquired *in utero*, usually transplacentally, during maternal infection.

Manifestations are most severe if acquired in the first trimester.

Suspect if:

● small for gestational age
● microcephaly or hydrocephalus
● ocular defects
● hepatosplenomegaly
● thrombocytopenia
● developmental delay/fits

10.1 Diseases

CMV, congenital rubella syndrome, toxoplasmosis

Approximately two-thirds of pregnancies complicated by rubella during the first 8 weeks' gestation will result in fetal death or severe abnormality. There is a 40% risk of toxoplasmosis transmission. In CMV and toxoplasmosis, only approximately 10% of infected infants are clinically affected at birth, although symptoms will often become apparent during childhood.

Characteristic features of CMV, rubella and toxoplasmosis infection

Abnormality	Rubella	CMV	Toxoplasmosis
Neurological:			
Sensorineural hearing loss	+++	++	+
Microcephaly	+	++	+
Hydrocephalus	–	–	++
Calcification	–	++ (periventricular)	++ (widespread)
Eyes:			
Micro-ophthalmia	+	–	+
Cataracts	+++	–	+
Chorioretinitis	+	++	+++
Growth retardation:	++	+++	+
Hepatosplenomegaly	+++	+++	++
Petechiae ('blueberry muffin' rash)	++	++	+
Cardiac malformations	++	–	–
Pneumonitis	+	++	+
bony involvement	++	–	

Parvovirus B19

- Women who become infected with parvovirus B19 during first 20 weeks of pregnancy have a 9% fetal loss.
- Hydrops fetalis occurs in approximately 3% if the mother is infected between 9 and 20 weeks.

Congenital varicella

Infection during the 1st or 2nd trimester may rarely cause congenital varicella syndrome (0.5–2%).

- Skin scarring, limb malformation/shortening, cataracts, chorioretinitis, micro-ophthalmia, microcephaly, hydrocephalus

Herpes simplex

Vast majority of infants are infected peripartum, only 5% transplacentally.

- Cutaneous scars or vesicles
- Choreoretinitis, keratoconjunctivitis, micro-ophthalmia
- Microcephaly, intracranial calcifications
- Hepatosplenomegaly
- Developmental delay

Syphilis

High transmission rate, 40% mortality untreated.

- 'Snuffles', congenital nephrotic syndrome, chorioretinitis, glaucoma
- Osteochondritis, periostitis
- Hepatosplenomegaly, lymphadenopathy
- Rash – maculopapular, desquamative, bullous, condylomas

Mycobacterium tuberculosis

- Very rare, high mortality
- Presents as disseminated disease with fevers and often respiratory distress
- Needs Mantoux testing, chest X-ray, lumbar puncture, quadruple therapy + steroids if meningitis confirmed

Diagnosis:

- 'TORCH screen' – **T**oxoplasmosis, '**O**ther', **R**ubella, **C**MV and **H**erpes-specific IgM in neonates <3-weeks-old implies congenital infection
- Better to screen for specific infection depending on clinical findings in neonate and mother
- **NB**: Look at specific antibody responses in mother's booking-visit blood samples and post-delivery blood samples to see rise/fall in titres depending on time of infection acquisition

- PCR
- Ophthalmological examination – characteristic retinal changes

Treatment

- Prevention through vaccination is the only way to reduce the risk of congenital rubella.
- Spiramycin may be used for toxoplasmosis in pregnancy to reduce transmission to the fetus. Affected infants are treated with pyrimethamine and sulphadiazine after birth.
- Gancyclovir may be used in cases of congenital CMV, aciclovir for herpes simplex, penicillin for syphilis.
- Highly active antiretroviral therapy (HAART) for HIV infection.
- Anti-TB treatment.

11. MISCELLANEOUS

11.1 Differential diagnosis of prolonged fever

Systemic bacterial disease:	Viral:
Salmonellosis	CMV
Mycobacterial infection	Hepatitis viruses
Brucellosis	HIV
Leptospirosis	EBV
Spirochaete infections	Human herpesvirus-6

Focal bacterial infections:	Parasitic infections:	Other infections
Abscesses	Malaria	Chlamydia
Sinusitis	Toxoplasmosis	Rickettsia
Osteomyelitis	Leishmaniasis	Fungi
Endocarditis		
Urinary sepsis		

Non infectious diseases:	
Collagen vascular diseases: Systemic Lupus erythematosus (SLE), Juvenile Inflammatory Arthritis (JIA)	Inflammatory bowel disease
	Malignancies
	Drugs
Familial Mediterranean fever	Haemophagocytic lymphohistiocytosis
Kawasaki's disease	Autonomic/CNS abnormalities
Sarcoidosis	

11.2 Differential diagnosis of cervical lymphadenopathy

Differential diagnosis of cervical lymphadenopathy

- Cervical abscess
- Tuberculosis (usually atypical)
- Cat-scratch fever (caused by Gram-negative organism *Bartonella henselae*)
- Mumps
- Malignancy
- Infectious mononucleosis
- Toxoplasmosis
- Brucellosis
- Salivary stone

11.3 Infections commonly associated with atypical lymphocytosis

- EBV
- CMV
- Toxoplasmosis
- Mumps
- Tuberculosis
- Malaria

11.4 Diseases associated with eosinophilia

An increase above $0.4 \times 10^9/l$ is seen with:

- Allergic disease, e.g. asthma, eczema
- Parasitic disease, e.g. hookworm, amoebiasis, ascariasis, tapeworm infestation, filariasis, schistosomiasis
- Recovery from acute infection
- Skin disease, e.g. psoriasis, pemphigus
- Hodgkin's disease
- Polyarteritis nodosa
- Drug sensitivity
- Hyper-eosinophilia syndrome
- Eosinophilic leukaemia (very rare)

11.5 Causes of hydrops fetalis

10–15% 'immune' aetiology.

- Fetal anaemia due to anti-D, anti-Kell and anti-C antibodies.

85–90% non-immune cause

- Human parvovirus B19 infection (most common), CMV, toxoplasmosis, syphilis, leptospirosis
- Aneuploidy
- Cardiac cause, e.g. supraventricular tachycardia and congenital complete heart block
- Primary hydrothorax

- Cystic hygroma
- Twin–twin transfusion syndrome
- Massive transplacental haemorrhage
- Fetal akinesia and muscular dystrophy

11.6 Oxazolidinones: a new class of antibiotics

Linezolid

- Active against methicillin-resistant *Staphylococcus aureus* (MRSA) and vancomycin-resistant enterococci
- Does not have good activity against Gram-negative organisms
- Reserve for those with infections resistant to other antibacterial agents
- Side-effects include myelosuppression – monitor blood count weekly

11.7 Erythema multiforme (EM)

- Characteristic target lesions; also macules, papules, wheals, vesicles and bullae
- Systemic symptoms common – fever, malaise, arthralgia
- Stevens–Johnson syndrome – severe EM with mucosal bullae in mouth, anogenital region and conjunctiva

Causes

- Idiopathic (>50%)
- Herpes simplex
- Mycoplasma
- Viruses – coxsackieviruses, echoviruses
- Drugs – sulphonamides, penicillins, barbiturates

Treatment

- Treat underlying cause; supportive; steroids in severe EM (early)

11.8 Erythema nodosum

Inflammatory disease of skin and subcutaneous tissues characterized by tender, red nodules predominantly pretibial (also arms and other areas)
- Streptococcal URTI
- Sarcoid
- Primary tuberculosis
- Ulcerative colitis
- Drugs (sulphonamides, contraceptive pills, bromides)
- Other – leprosy, histoplasmosis, psittacosis, lymphogranuloma venereum (LGV), coccidiomycosis

Treatment

- Penicillin (up to 12 months) for Group A streptococcal infection (GAS)
- Steroids: systemic most effective

11.9 Anthrax

- Caused by the Gram-positive organism *Bacillus anthracis*.
- Wild and domestic animals in Asia, Africa and parts of Europe carry the bacterium.
- The bacterium can exist as a spore, which allows the bacterium to survive in the environment (e.g. in the soil).

Cutaneous anthrax (95% of cases)

- Caught by direct contact with the skin or tissues of infected animals. A lesion appears on the skin, often on the head, forearms or hands, and develops into a characteristic ulcer with a necrotic centre. It is rarely painful. Untreated, the infection can spread to cause bacteraemia, which can be fatal in 5–20% of cases.

Inhalation anthrax

- Much less common. Caused by breathing in anthrax spores. Symptoms begin with a flu-like illness, followed by respiratory difficulties and shock after 2–6 days. High fatality rate.

Intestinal anthrax

- Very rare form of food poisoning, which results in severe gut disease, fever and septicaemia. Mortality of up to 50%.
- Vaccine – available for very high-risk groups only.
- Post-exposure prophylaxis with antibiotics can be very effective in preventing disease, providing it is given early enough.

Treatment

- High-dose penicillin and doxycycline or ciprofloxacin.

11.10 Botulism

- Botulism is caused by a botulinum toxin, produced by the bacterium *Clostridium botulinum*.
- The bacterium is anaerobic and common in the soil in the form of spores.
- Foodborne botulism occurs when the spores of *C. botulinum* have germinated and the bacteria have reproduced in an environment (usually food) outside the body and produced toxin. The toxin is consumed when the food is eaten.
- The toxin is destroyed by normal cooking processes.

Clinical manifestations

Botulism is a neuroparalytic disorder that can be classified into 3 categories:

- Foodborne:
  - onset of symptoms is usually abrupt, within 12–36 h of exposure;
  - symmetrical, descending, flaccid paralysis occurs, typically involving the bulbar musculature initially;
  - sometimes diarrhoea and vomiting occur;
  - most cases recover, but the recovery period can be many months; the disease can be fatal in 5–10% of cases.
- Infant botulism:
  - extremely rare, but occurs when spores are ingested that germinate, multiply and release toxin in the intestine;
  - incubation period is much longer, 3–30 days;
  - presents with 'floppy infant' with poor feeding, weak cry, generalized hypotonia.
- Wound botulism:
  - same symptoms as other forms, but occurs when the organisms get into an open wound and are able to reproduce in an 'anaerobic' environment.

Diagnosis

- Enriched selective media are used to culture *C. botulinum* from stools and food.
- A toxin neutralization assay can identify botulinum toxin in serum, stool or food.
- Electromyography has characteristic appearances.

Treatment

- Supportive care, especially respiratory (e.g. ventilation) and nutritional
- Antitoxin
- Concerns about the effectiveness and side-effects of the vaccine against botulism; not widely used
- Immunity to botulism toxin does not develop, even with severe disease

Prevention

Education regarding food preparation

Therapeutics

Botulinum A toxin, in small doses, is used therapeutically to prevent excessive muscular activity, e.g. in torticollis, cerebral palsy and recently in cosmetics to reduce wrinkles!

11.11 Bovine spongiform encephalopathy (BSE) and new variant Creutzfeldt–Jakob disease (nv-CJD)

- Transmissible spongiform encephalopathies (TSEs) are caused by proteinaceous infectious particles or prions. These are abnormal isoforms of a cell-surface glycoprotein designated PrP.
- Disease is caused when a disease-specific isoform, PrP^{Sc}, interacts with PrP producing conversion to PrP^{Sc}. This protein is not readily digested by proteases and therefore accumulates, causing a rapidly progressive and fatal encephalopathy.
- PrP^{Sc} is very resistant to standard methods of sterilization and disinfection. The genotype of polymorphic codon 129 of the human *PrP* gene appears to influence susceptibility to infection and disease phenotype. 37% of Caucasians are methionine-homozygous (MM), 12 % are valine homozygous (VV) and 51% are heterozygous (MV). Cases of nv-CJD have been found in MM individuals.

Creutzfeldt–Jakob disease (CJD)

The principal human spongiform encephalopathy. Features include a progressive dementia, movement disorder and death in a median of 4 months. The incidence is between 0.5 and 1 case per million. Most cases present between 55 and 75 years. Most cases have no known cause. 15% have a hereditary predisposition to CJD, with recognized mutations of the human *PrP* gene on chromosome 20. A small number of iatrogenic cases have occurred following the use of contaminated growth hormone.

Kuru

A disease of motor incoordination, it was endemic in Papua New Guinea in the 1950s and 1960s. Kuru was a TSE spread by the ritual cannibalism of deceased relatives. Cannibalism ceased in the late 1950s, but there are still a few cases in older adults indicating a long incubation period.

New variant CJD (nv-CJD)

This was first reported with 10 cases in 1996. The source appeared to be due to BSE, acquired following the ingestion of infected cattle. The disease starts as a psychiatric illness followed by ataxia, myoclonus, akinetic mutism and death at about 12 months. There are now more than 100 cases. The incubation period may be very long and therefore the total number of cases is difficult to predict.

12. FURTHER READING

British National Formulary, March 2002.

Chemotherapy and management of tuberculosis in the United Kingdom: recommendations: Joint Tuberculosis Committee of the British Thoracic Society BTS guidelines 1998. *Thorax* **53**, 536–48.

Medicines for children: Hull D, British Paediatric Association 1999.

Nelson Textbook of Paediatrics: Behrman, 14th edition. WB Saunders 1992.

Public Health Laboratory Services (PHLS) and Centres for Disease Control (CDC) websites.

Report of the Committee on Infectious Disease's: Georges P, American Academy of Paediatrics *2000 Red Book*.

Textbook of Paediatric Infectious Diseases: Feigin R and Cherry J, 4th edition. WB Saunders 1998.

Chapter 12

Metabolic Medicine

Mike Champion

CONTENTS

Metabolic Medicine

1. APPROACH TO THE METABOLIC CASE

1.1 Inheritance

Inborn errors of metabolism are individually rare; however, collectively probably have an incidence of 1:3–4,000 births. Autosomal recessive inheritance is commonest. Exceptions include:

- X-linked recessive   Lesch–Nyhan syndrome
  Hunter syndrome
  Ornithine transcarbamylase (OTC) deficiency
  Fabry disease
  Adrenoleukodystrophy
- Autosomal dominant   Porphyrias (some recessive)
- Matrilineal   Mitochondrial DNA mutations

1.2 Presentation

Presentation is notoriously non-specific, therefore clues in history should be sought. The commonest misdiagnosis is sepsis.

Historical clues   Consanguineous parents
Previous sudden infant death (especially late, i.e. >6 months)
Previous multiple miscarriages (? non-viable)
Maternal illness during pregnancy
Acute Fatty Liver of Pregnancy (AFLP) and Haemolysis, Elevated Liver enzymes, Low Platelets (HELLP) syndrome association with carrying fetus with long-chain fat oxidation defect
Increased fetal movements (*in-utero* fits)
Faddy eating (avoidance of foods that provoke feeling unwell)
Previous encephalopathic or tachypnoeic episodes (latter implies acidosis)

Inborn errors of metabolism present at times of metabolic stress:

- Neonatal period
- Weaning (increased oral intake, new challenges, e.g. fructose)

- End of first year (slowing in growth rate, therefore more protein catabolized as less used for growth. May exceed metabolic capacity of defective pathway)
- Intercurrent infections
- Puberty

Neonatal presentation can be divided into three groups for diagnostic purposes:

1. Failure to make or break complex molecules
Usually dysmorphic syndromes at birth due to absence of structural molecules important for embryogenesis (failure to make complex molecules). Many storage disorders appear normal at birth and become progressively more obvious with time as storage accumulates (failure to break down complex molecules).

- Smith–Lemli–Opitz (cholesterol synthesis defect)
- Zellweger syndrome (peroxisomal disorder)

2. Intoxication
Key feature is symptom-free period prior to decompensation, whilst toxic metabolites build up once feeds are established and the neonate no longer relies on the placenta for clearance. Classical presentation is collapse on day 3 of life. Differential diagnosis includes sepsis and duct-dependent cardiac problem.

- Aminoacidopathies: tyrosinaemia, maple syrup urine disease (MSUD)
- Urea cycle defects (UCDs)
- Organic acidaemias (OAs)
- Sugar intolerances: galactosaemia

3. Energy insufficiency
Absence of symptom-free period with immediate onset of symptoms in congenital lactic acidosis. There is a spectrum of severity and some may take longer to decompensate. The group includes conditions that only present if delay in fuel provision, e.g. fat oxidation defects, glycogenoses and gluconeogenesis defects.

- Respiratory chain defects
- Pyruvate metabolism defects (pyruvate dehydrogenase, pyruvate carboxylase)
- Fat oxidation defects   MCAD, LCHAD
- Glycogen storage disease (GSD)   types I, III
- Defects of gluconeogenesis   Fructose bisphosphatase deficiency

1.3 Examination

Clinical examination may reveal few clues in many disorders of intermediary metabolism. Dysmorphic features may suggest certain diagnoses. Odours are usually unhelpful and rarely significant. Eyes should be carefully examined for corneal clouding (mucopolysaccharidoses, cystinosis), cataracts (galactosaemia, peroxisomal), pigmentary retinopathy (fat oxidation, mitochondrial) and cherry-red spot (Tay–Sachs, Niemann–Pick, Sandhoff, G_{M1}). Organomegaly is a key revealing sign. Hepatosplenomegaly is a feature of storage disorders. Massive hepatomegaly in the absence of splenomegaly suggests glycogen storage disease, as glycogen is not stored in the spleen. More prominent splenomegaly is suggestive of Gaucher disease.

1.4 Investigation

Perform investigations at the time of decompensation when diagnostic metabolites are most likely to be present and avoid the need for stress tests at a later date.

Key initial metabolic investigations

- Blood gas (venous, capillary or arterial)
- Glucose
- Lactate
- Ammonia
- Amino acids (blood and urine)
- Organic acids (urine)
- Acylcarnitines
- Ketones (urinary dipstick)

Acid–base status

Anion gap = $Na^+ + K^+ - (Cl^- + HCO_3^-)$
A normal anion gap (10–18 mmol/l) in the presence of a metabolic acidosis signifies bicarbonate loss rather than an excess of acid, e.g. renal or gut. Marked ketosis is unusual in the neonate and therefore is highly suggestive of an underlying metabolic disorder. Urea cycle defects may initially present with a mild respiratory alkalosis, as ammonia acts directly on the brainstem as a respiratory stimulant.

Hypoglycaemia

Hypoglycaemia is defined as a blood glucose concentration of ≤2.6 mmol/l, and should always be confirmed in the laboratory. The key additional investigation is the presence or absence of ketosis. Hypoketotic hypoglycaemia has a limited differential diagnosis that can usually be resolved on history and examination:

- Hyperinsulinism (endogenous or exogenous)
- Fat oxidation defects (e.g. MCAD)
- Mitochondrial disease
- Liver failure

Hyperinsulinism is suggested by a persistently increased glucose demand >10 mg/kg per min

$$\text{Glucose requirement (mg/kg per min)} = \frac{\text{ml/h} \times \% \text{ dextrose}}{6 \times \text{weight (kg)}}$$

Lactate

Lactate is a weak acid which can be used directly as a fuel for the brain and is readily produced during anaerobic respiration. Secondary causes are much more common (hypoxia, sepsis, shock, liver failure, poor sampling, etc.) than primary metabolic causes. Ketosis is usually present in primary metabolic disease, unlike secondary causes, with the exception of pyruvate dehydrogenase (PDH) deficiency, GSD I and fat oxidation defects. The level of lactate is unhelpful in distinguishing the cause, and the lactate:pyruvate ratio usually adds little. A low ratio (<10) may indicate PDH deficiency. Exacerbation when fasted is a feature of gluconeogenesis defects and GSD I compared to GSD III and respiratory chain disorders in which lactate may increase post-prandially.

Ammonia

Hyperammonaemia may result from poor sampling (squeezed sample) and/or delays in processing. The level of ammonia may prove discriminatory as to the cause.

Ammonia concentration (µmol/l)	Differential diagnosis
< 40	Normal
40 – <150	Sick patient, fat oxidation defect, OA, liver failure, UCD
150 – <250	Fat oxidation defect, OA, liver failure, UCD
250 – <450	OA, liver failure, UCD
450 – >2000	Liver failure, UCD, (OA rarely)

OA, organic acidaemia; UCD, urea cycle defect.

Amino acids

Amino acids are measured in both blood and urine. The latter may reflect plasma concentration, or renal threshold, e.g. generalized aminoaciduria of a proximal renal tubulopathy, or the specific transporter defect of cystinuria (**C**ystine, **O**rnithine, **A**rginine, **L**ysine). Plasma amino acids are useful in the work up of a number of metabolic disorders, and are essential in monitoring some metabolic disorders.

- ↑ Leucine, isoleucine and valine   Maple syrup urine disease (MSUD)
- ↑ Glutamine, ↓ arginine (+/− ↑ citrulline) UCDs↑
- ↑ Alanine   Lactic acidosis
- ↑ Glycine   Non-ketotic hyperglycinaemia, OAs

Organic acids

These are measured in urine only and are diagnostic in many organic acidaemias, e.g. increased propionate in propionic acidaemia, increased isovalerate in isovaleric acidaemia, etc., but are also essential in other disorders.

- ↑ Orotic acid   UCDs, mitochondrial, benign hereditary
- ↑ Succinylacetone   Tyrosinaemia type I
- ↑ Dicarboxylic acids   Fat oxidation defects, MCT feeds, mitochondrial

Acylcarnitines

Carnitine conjugates with acyl-CoA intermediates proximal to the block in fat oxidation defects. The chain length of the acylcarnitines formed is diagnostic of where the block lies, e.g. medium-chain (MCAD), very long-chain (VLCAD), etc. Likewise, conjugation with organic acids allows diagnosis of organic acidaemias, e.g. propionylcarnitine. Total and free carnitine levels can be measured at the same time.

Secondary investigations include:

- Neuroimaging   basal ganglia signal change in mitochondrial disorders
- Neurophysiology   mitochondrial, peroxisomal
- Echocardiogaraphy   especially hypertrophic cardiomyopathy mitochondrial, fat oxidation, Pompe's (GSD II)
- ECG   fat oxidation, mitochondrial
- EEG   metabolic encephalopathy, e.g. MSUD, hyperammonaemia

Enzymology

Definitive diagnosis is confirmed on enzymology. Sample requirement depends in which tissues the enzyme is expressed, e.g. galactosaemia (blood), OTC deficiency (liver), mitochondrial (muscle). Genotype has superseded invasive biopsy in some conditions, e.g. GSD I (glucose 6-phosphatase deficiency).

White cell enzymes are often requested in patients with potential neurodegenerative or storage disorders. Laboratories usually undertake different lysosomal assays for different presentations. The neurodegeneration panel includes Tay–Sachs, Sandhoff, Sly mucopolysaccharidosis (MPS VII) and mannosidosis in plasma; G_{M1} gangliosidosis, arylsulphatase A deficiency, Krabbe and fucosidosis in white cells. The organomegaly panel includes Sly (MPS VII), and mannosidosis in plasma, G_{M1} gangliosidosis, Gaucher, Niemann–Pick A and B, mannosidosis, fucosidosis and Wolman in white cells.

1.5 Acute management

- Stop feeds
- Promote anabolism : 10% dextrose (add insulin rather than reduce % dextrose if hyperglycaemic)

NB. High-concentration glucose can exacerbate the lactic acidosis of pyruvate and respiratory chain defects, therefore 5% dextrose used if primary lactic acidosis suspected.

- Correct biochemical disturbance along standard guidelines

  e.g. hypernatraemia, low phosphate, etc.

- Clear toxic metabolites   Dialysis   lactate, organic acids, ammonia, leucine

                                    Drugs   UCDs: phenylbutyrate, sodium benzoate
  OAs: carnitine, glycine

- Supplement enzyme cofactors   e.g. biotin, thiamine, riboflavin

- Specific treatment   dietary restriction
  drugs e.g. NTBC in tyrosinaemia
  enzyme replacement therapy in Gaucher, Fabry, Pompe
  transplantation (liver, bone marrow)
  hepatocyte transfer (future)
  gene therapy (future)

- Genetic counselling (+/– future prenatal)

- Screen siblings if indicated

In defects of intermediary metabolism, during intercurrent infections, feeds are stopped to reduce metabolic load and glucose polymer drinks substituted to avoid catabolism. Failure to tolerate the emergency regime requires admission for intravenous therapy.

2. DISORDERS OF AMINO ACID METABOLISM

2.1 Phenylketonuria (PKU)

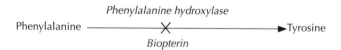

This is the commonest inborn error of metabolism in the UK with an incidence of 1:10,000; carrier rate 1:50. Untreated classical PKU (phenylalanine >1,000 µmol/l) presents with developmental delay in the first year. Characteristic features include mental retardation, behavioural problems, decreased pigmentation and eczema. There is considerable variation in phenotype and genotype. 1–2% of cases result from biopterin defects, the essential cofactor for phenylalanine hydroxylase and neurotransmitter synthesis.

Diagnosis

Detection of a raised phenylalanine level on neonatal screening; confirmed on plasma amino acids and exclusion of biopterin defects.

Management

Phenylalanine is an essential amino acid and therefore cannot be totally excluded from the diet. The developing brain is most vulnerable to the deleterious effects of high phenylalanine; however, evidence is increasing that diet should be continued for life.

- Phenylalanine restriction (given as exchanges of natural protein titrated against phenylalanine levels monitored on home fingerprick blood tests)
- Amino acid supplement (no phenylalanine)
- Special PKU products (minimal or no phenylalanine)
- Free foods (negligible phenylalanine)
- Neurotransmitter replacement in biopterin defects (+/– folinic acid)

2.2 Tyrosinaemia (type 1)

Tyrosinaemia type 1 results from a block in the catabolism of tyrosine-producing by-products which damage the liver and kidney.

Clinical features of tyrosinaemia

- Early onset (severe) liver disease with coagulopathy, proximal renal tubulopathy
- Late onset: failure to thrive and rickets (secondary to renal Fanconi)
- Development of hepatocellular carcinoma in late childhood/adolescence

Diagnosis

Tyrosine is raised in plasma and the presence of succinylacetone in urine is pathognomonic. Coagulation is almost always deranged even in the minimally symptomatic patient and should be actively sought in a patient with renal tubulopathy. Confirm on liver enzymology (fumarylacetoacetase).

Management

A low phenylalanine and low tyrosine diet supplemented with a tyrosine and phenylalanine-free amino acid supplement has been the mainstay of management; improving both liver and renal function but failing to prevent the development of hepatocarcinoma. NTBC has revolutionized the management, by blocking the catabolic pathway proximal to the production of the damaging metabolites. NTBC is a derivative of the bottle-brush plant

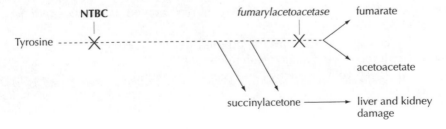

437

originally developed as a weedkiller. Dietary restriction remains but it is hoped that the risk of tumours is greatly reduced. Liver transplantation is reserved for patients failing to respond to NTBC, or who develop tumours or progressive cirrhotic liver disease. Tumour surveillance includes interval hepatic MRI and monitoring of α-fetoprotein.

2.3 Maple syrup urine disease (MSUD)

MSUD results from a block in the degradation of the branch-chain amino acids (BCAAs) leucine, isoleucine and valine. MSUD also belongs to the family of organic acidaemias.

Clinical features

The severe neonatal form presents as a classic intoxication with encephalopathy and seizures. The neonate has a sweet odour, hence the name. Intermittent forms may present at a later age, patients appearing entirely symptom-free between bouts. Cerebral oedema is a well-recognized complication during acute episodes.

Diagnosis

- Elevated BCAAs plus alloisoleucine
- Elevated branch-chain oxo-acids on urinary organic acids
- Enzymology on fibroblasts

Management

Long-term management centres on controlling leucine levels with a low-protein diet supplemented with a BCAA-free amino acid supplement. Valine and isoleucine may require additional supplementation as levels may fall too low whilst controlling leucine. The enzyme cofactor thiamine is given in the hope of improving residual enzyme activity.

2.4 Homocystinuria

Homocystinuria may result from a number of metabolic defects. Classical homocystinuria (cystathione-β-synthase deficiency) presents with the typical dysmorphology similar to Marfan's. Differences include lower IQ, stiff joints, direction of lens dislocation and malar flush.

Clinical features of homocystinuria

- Marfanoid habitus (span greater than height), high arched palate, arachnodactyly
- Restricted joint movements
- Ectopia lentis (classically downward, but may be sideways!)
- Developmental delay/retardation (variable severity)
- Thrombosis (deep vein thrombosis and pulmonary embolus commonest)
- Osteoporosis

Diagnosis

Measurement of total plasma homocysteine is becoming the method of choice superseding free homocystine plasma levels. In classical homocystinuria, the plasma methionine is elevated. Definitive diagnosis is based on enzymology in fibroblasts.

Management

Treatment aims to reduce plasma total homocysteine. Protein restriction is used in patients diagnosed on screening, but is particularly difficult to institute in the cases who present later. 50% of patients respond to cofactor supplementation (pyridoxine). Folate should also be supplemented as depletion affects response. Betaine is effective at lowering homocysteine by remethylation and is particularly useful in the pyridoxine non-responsive patient.

2.5 Non-ketotic hyperglycinaemia (NKH)

Defective glycine cleavage produces this early-onset convulsive disorder. Glycine is a neurotransmitter; excitatory centrally and inhibitory peripherally. In the absence of birth asphyxia, metabolic causes of neonatal seizures include NKH, pyridoxine-dependent seizures, biotinidase deficiency and sulphite oxidase deficiency.

Clinical features of non-ketotic hyperglycinaemia

- Increased fetal movements (*in-utero* seizures)
- Hiccups, hypotonia
- Progressive apnoeas/encephalopathy
- Seizures
- Marked developmental delay/psychomotor retardation

Diagnosis

The first clue is usually an elevated glycine on urinary or plasma amino acids. The diagnosis is confirmed by measuring simultaneously the CSF:plasma glycine ratio (>0.09). Enzymology is traditionally assessed in the liver, but a new assay using lymphocytes is available.

Management

Glycine is reduced with sodium benzoate but has little effect on neurological outcome. Dextromethorphan (partial *N*-methyl-D-aspartate (NMDA)) receptor antagonist) helps block the central action of glycine and has helped reduce fits in some patients compared to conventional anticonvulsants. Prognosis remains poor for development. Newer NMDA receptor blockers are currently under investigation. Prenatal testing is available.

3. ORGANIC ACIDAEMIAS

Defects in the catabolism of amino acids result in the accumulation of organic acids which are detected in urine. Propionic acidaemia (PA) and methylmalonic aciduria (MMA) result from blocks in BCAA degradation, isovaleric acidaemia from a block in leucine catabolism and glutaric aciduria type 1 (GA-I) from a block in lysine and tryptophan metabolism.

3.1 Propionic, methylmalonic and isovaleric acidaemias

Clinical features of acidaemia

- Acute neonatal encephalopathy (intoxication), or chronic intermittent forms
- Dehydration
- Marked acidosis ($\uparrow$ anion gap), ketosis
- Neutropenia +/– thrombocytopenia (acute marrow suppression)
- Progressive extrapyramidal syndrome (MMA, PA) basal ganglia necrosis
- Renal insufficiency (MMA)
- Pancreatitis
- Acute-onset cardiomyopathy (PA, MMA)

Diagnosis

Marked acidosis with ketosis is a key feature. Lactate and ammonia are invariably raised. Blood glucose may be low, normal or raised. Propionate is partly produced by gut organisms, therefore decompensation in PA and MMA may be precipitated by constipation. Neutropenia is another useful clue to the diagnosis. The key metabolites are detected on urinary organic acids, and enzyme deficiency confirmed on enzymology.

Management

Long-term management is based on dietary protein restriction. Carnitine supplementation helps eliminate organic acids via conjugation and renal excretion. Glycine is used similarly in isovaleric acidaemia (IVA). Some forms of MMA are vitamin B_{12} responsive. Metronidazole is used in MMA and PA to alter the gut flora to reduce propionate production and help avoid constipation. Liver transplantation is gaining acceptance as a definitive treatment in PA in view of the high risk of subsequent neurological decompensation, however the procedure may not eliminate the risk of neurological deterioration in MMA.

3.2 Glutaric aciduria type 1 (GA-1)

Prior to decompensation precipitated by an intercurrent infection, usually towards the end of the first year, there may be little clue as to the underlying disorder except macrocephaly.

Diagnosis

The diagnosis must be actively sought in children with large heads and no other explanation, aiming to prevent metabolic decompensation and subsequent severe neurology.

GA-1 may mimic non-accidental injury with encephalopathy and bilateral subdurals. Diagnosis is made on urinary organic acid metabolites. A minority of cases are non-excretors, therefore fibroblasts are required for definitive enzymology in cases that have a strongly suggestive clinical picture but negative organic acids.

Clinical features of glutaric aciduria type 1

- Macrocephaly
- Normal development prior to catastrophic decompensation (usually <1 year)
- Choreoathetosis and dystonia (basal ganglia involvement)
- MRI features: bifrontotemporal atrophy, subdurals, basal ganglia decreased signal

Management

In the absence of screening, the diagnosis is usually only made post-decompensation. In prospectively treated siblings, protein restriction in conjunction with aggressive treatment of infections and hyperalimentation have improved the prognosis, however there is a broad spectrum of phenotypes and some children still decompensate in spite of treatment.

4. UREA CYCLE DEFECTS

The urea cycle is the pathway by which waste nitrogen is converted to urea for disposal. Urea cycle defects (UCDs) are inherited in an autosomal recessive manner except ornithine transcarbamylase (OTC) deficiency which is X-linked recessive. Girls may present symptomatically if during lyonization enough good genes are switched off in the liver.

Clinical features of urea cycle defects

- Vomiting (may be a cause of cyclical vomiting)
- Encephalopathy (intoxication following symptom-free period in neonate)
- Tachypnoea (ammonia is a respiratory stimulant acting centrally)
- Progressive spastic diplegia and developmental delay (arginase deficiency)
- Arginase deficiency rarely presents with classical hyperammonaemia

Diagnosis

UCDs are suggested by the presence of a respiratory alkalosis in the child with encephalopathy. Indication of the exact level of the enzyme block depends on plasma amino acids and urinary organic acids for the presence or absence of orotic acid. Orotic aciduria indicates a block at the level of OTC or beyond. Final confirmation of the diagnosis requires enzymology.

Urea cycle defect	Enzyme deficiency	Amino acids	Orotic acid
NAGS deficiency	*N*-acetyl glutamate synthase	Glu ↑, Arg ↓ Cit ↓	**Normal**
CPS deficiency	Carbamyl phosphate synthase	Glu ↑, Arg ↓ Cit ↓	**Normal**
OTC deficiency	Ornithine transcarbamylase	Glu ↑, Arg ↓ Cit ↓	↑↑↑
Citrullinaemia	Argininosuccinic synthase	Glu ↑, Arg ↓ **Cit ↑↑↑**	↑
Argininosuccinic aciduria	Argininosuccinic lyase	Glu ↑, Arg ↓ Cit ↑ **Argininosuccinate ↑**	↑
Argininaemia	Arginase	Glu ↑, **Arg ↑↑↑**	↑

Glu, glutamine; Arg, arginine; Cit, citrulline.

Management

Treatment follows the basic principles as detailed at the beginning of this chapter. Elimination of ammonia is accelerated by dialysis, earlier reduction in ammonia improving long-term neurological outcome. Sodium benzoate and sodium phenylbutyrate conjugate with glycine and glutamine, respectively, to produce water-soluble products that can be excreted by the kidney, therefore bypassing the urea cycle and reducing the nitrogen load on the liver. Arginine becomes an essential amino acid in UCDs (except argininaemia) and is supplemented. Long-term protein is restricted and medicines adjusted according to growth, amino acids and ammonia.

Liver transplantation has been used successfully in patients with brittle control, however numbers are small and follow-up limited.

5. FAT OXIDATION DISORDERS

The fat oxidation defects form a large group of conditions which commonly present with hepatic, cardiac or muscle symptoms. Fatty acids are a major fuel source in the fasted state and are oxidized by most tissues except the brain, which is reliant on hepatic fatty acid β-oxidation for ketone production. Fatty acids are the preferred substrate for cardiac muscle, and during prolonged exercise a vital energy source for skeletal muscle.

5.1 Medium-chain acyl-CoA dehydrogenase (MCAD) deficiency

MCAD is the commonest fat oxidation disorder with an incidence of 1 in 10,000 in the UK (as common as PKU). Peak presentation occurs in autumn and winter precipitated by inter-current infections.

Clinical features of MCAD deficiency

- Encephalopathy
- Reye-like syndrome: hepatomegaly, deranged liver function
- Hypoketotic hypoglycaemia
- Mean age at presentation 15 months, commonest precipitant is diarrhoea
- Sudden infant death (consider in older infant >6 months)
- Common *G985* mutation

Diagnosis

Detection requires a strong clinical suspicion to ensure appropriate investigations are done at the time. The presence or absence of ketosis should be sought in all cases of hypoglycaemia. Plasma-free fatty acids are raised, whilst ketone formation is impaired. Urinary organic acids reveal a characteristic dicarboxylic aciduria in the acute state, but may be normal between episodes. Acylcarnitines detect an elevated octanoyl carnitine, and genotyping is used for confirmation. The *G985* common mutation accounts for >90% alleles so far detected in the UK cases. It is thus a useful tool to assess at-risk siblings. Neonatal screening occurs in the US, Germany, Australia and others, but at present is not part of the UK screening programme.

Management

Prevention is better than cure. Mortality is 25% on first presentation, and 33% of survivors have neurological sequelae. Once the diagnosis is known, further decompensations can be avoided by employing an emergency regime of glucose polymer drinks during intercurrent illnesses or admission for a 10% dextrose infusion if not tolerated. In the at-risk neonate born to a family with a previously affected sibling, feeds should be frequent with intervals no longer than 3 hours, and top-up feeds established if needed whilst acylcarnitine results are awaited. Neonatal deaths have been reported.

5.2 Long-chain defects

The long-chain fat oxidation defects, very long-chain (VLCAD) and long-chain hydroxy acyl-CoA dehydrogenase (LCHAD) are more severe, presenting at an earlier age and requiring meticulous dietary management to ensure normoglycaemia and reduce long-term complications. Liver dysfunction may occur in the carrier mother during pregnancy: acute fatty liver of pregnancy (AFLP) or haemolysis, elevated liver enzymes and low platelets (HELLP).

Clinical features of long-chain defects

- Hypoketotic hypoglycaemia
- Myopathy
- Hypertrophic cardiomyopathy
- Pigmentary retinopathy (LCHAD)
- Peripheral neuropathy (LCHAD)
- Maternal hepatic symptoms in pregnancy

Diagnosis

Characteristic dicarboxylic aciduria is noted in acute episodes on urinary organic acids. Creatine kinase (CK) may rise acutely and frank rhabdomyolysis can occur. Acylcarnitines form the mainstay of diagnosis with confirmation on fibroblast flux studies. There is a common LCHAD mutation. Urine and blood samples from infants born to mothers with AFLP or HELLP should be screened post-delivery.

Management

Long-chain fat intake is severely restricted and the diet supplemented with medium-chain fat and essential fatty acids. Normoglycaemia is maintained with frequent bolus feeds during the day, and overnight nasogastric or gastrostomy feeds in infancy. Uncooked cornstarch (UCCS) can be introduced from 2 years of age to smooth and prolong glycaemic control. An emergency regime is used during intercurrent infections, and admission for i.v. therapy if not tolerated. Carnitine supplementation is used to correct acute depletion, secondary to increased excretion of carnitine–fatty acid conjugates in the urine.

6. MITOCHONDRIAL CYTOPATHIES

Mitochondria are ubiquitous organelles that are the power stations of the cell producing ATP to drive cellular functions. The respiratory chain, the site of oxidative phosphorylation, is embedded in the inner mitochondrial membrane and consists of five complexes. Electrons are donated from reduced cofactors and passed along the chain, ultimately reducing oxygen to water, whilst the energy so produced pumps hydrogen ions from the mitochondrial matrix into the intermembrane space. Discharge of this electrochemical gradient through complex V (ATP synthase) generates ATP.

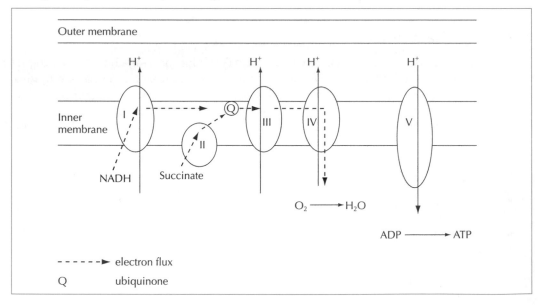

6.1 Mitochondrial genetics

Mitochondria are unique in containing their own DNA (mtDNA) contained within a circular double-stranded molecule. mtDNA is inherited solely from the maternal egg, the sperm's mitochondria being left outside within the tail at fertilization. Inheritance of mtDNA mutations is therefore matrilineal; only being handed on by females. However, the mitochondrion is not self-sufficient but relies on nuclear genes for many essential proteins, including respiratory chain subunits. All complex II's subunits are encoded within the nucleus. If a nuclear gene is at fault then normal mendelian inheritance applies. Autosomal recessive inheritance is probably the commonest mode of inheritance for paediatric practice.

Mitochondria also contain more than one copy of mtDNA, and each cell may contain many mitochondria. It is possible to have mutant mtDNA and wild-type present in the same cell (heteroplasmy). The accumulation of mutant mtDNA will result in symptoms when a threshold is breached. Due to heteroplasmy, symptoms may be patchy within and between organ systems. In rapidly dividing cells such as the bone marrow and gut, wild-type cells may have a reproduction advantage and therefore symptoms in these organ systems may improve compared to the progressive brain and muscle involvement. Unless a nuclear defect is identified, prenatal diagnosis is not available.

6.2 Clinical features

As mitochondria are ubiquitous, any organ system can be involved at any time with any inheritance. High-energy demand tissues are more commonly involved, particularly brain, muscle, kidney, liver, but any system can be involved. 33% of paediatric patients present in the neonatal period, and 80% in the first 2 years. Many syndromes have been described; however, these were initially reported in adults and are associated with mtDNA mutations which are less common in children (e.g. mitochondrial encephalomyopathy with lactic acidosis and stroke-like episodes (MELAS), myoclonic epilepsy-ragged red fibres (MERRF) and Kearns–Sayre syndrome). Syndromes may also be incomplete.

- CNS   Leigh's syndrome, hypotonia, deafness, epilepsy, stroke-like episodes
- Muscle   myopathy, fatigue
- Heart   hypertrophic cardiomyopathy, heart block
- Kidney   proximal tubulopathy
- Liver   failure, cirrhosis
- Gut   diarrhoea, malabsorption, pancreatic insufficiency, failure to thrive
- Eye   external ophthalmoplegia, pigmentary retinopathy
- Bone marrow refractory anaemia
- Endocrine   short stature, diabetes, endocrinopathies

Investigation

mtDNA studies are preferred if a classic mitochondrial syndrome is identified. Usually mitochondrial disease is suspected when there is multiorgan involvement in apparently unrelated organs: 'illegitimate associations'. Peripheral lactate may be persistently elevated. Further organ involvement may be sought prior to muscle biopsy for histochemistry (staining for complex II and IV), and respiratory chain enzymology (complexes I–IV).

- CNS   MRI, brainstem auditory evoked potentials (BSAEPs), CSF lactate
- Heart   echocardiography, ECG
- Kidney   proximal tubular proteins, tubular resorption of phosphate

445

- Liver   biopsy, enzymology
- Eye   fundoscopy, electroretinogram (ERG), visual evoked responses (VERs)
- Marrow   full blood count (FBC), aspirate
- Endocrine   electrolytes

Management
Management remains supportive. A variety of antioxidants and respiratory-chain pick-me-ups have been described with success in only a handful of cases, e.g. ubiquinone, riboflavin. Dichloroacetate resolves the raised lactate but does not appear to improve outcome.

7. DISORDERS OF CARBOHYDRATE METABOLISM

7.1 Glycogen storage disease

Glucose is stored in the liver and muscles as glycogen. Glycogen storage disorders (GSDs) result from defects of glycogen breakdown. Hepatic forms present with hepatomegaly and hypoglycaemia, the muscle forms with weakness and fatigue.

GSD Ia (glucose 6-phosphatase deficiency) von Gierke's disease

The enzyme deficiency fails to remove the phosphate from glucose 6-phosphate, therefore export of glucose from the liver from glycogenolysis and gluconeogenesis is blocked. Fasting tolerance is therefore limited to approximately 4 hours. Infants usually present at around 3 months when feeds are spread further apart. Massive hepatomegaly in the absence of splenomegaly is strongly suggestive of a hepatic GSD, as glycogen is not stored in the spleen (unlike the material in lysosomal storage disorders). Nephromegaly is common. Abnormal fat distribution results in 'doll-like' faces and thin limbs. Bruising is a feature of poor control. Long-term complications include renal insufficiency, liver adenomas with potential for malignant change, gout, osteopenia and polycystic ovaries.

Investigations show raised plasma lactate levels, hyperuricaemia and hyperlipidaemia. Lactate level falls on glucose loading. Genotyping has superseded liver enzymology for confirmation.

Treatment consists of frequent feeds during the day with continuous feeds overnight. From age 2, uncooked corn starch (UCCS) is introduced as a slow-release form of glucose, prolonging the gap between feeds. Allopurinol controls the uric acid level in the blood. Liver transplantation is reserved for patients with malignant change in an adenoma or failure to respond to dietary treatment.

GSD Ib (glucose 6-phosphate translocase deficiency)

The translocase deficiency shares the above phenotype plus the addition of neutrophil dysfunction with associated recurrent skin sepsis, large mouth ulcers and inflammatory bowel disease. Management is as above with the addition of prophylactic septrin for severe recurrent mouth ulcers, or granulocyte colony-stimulating factor (GCSF) in resistant cases.

GSD II (Pompe's disease)

GSD II, acid maltase deficiency, is really a lysosomal storage disorder with accumulation of glycogen in lysosomes. The infantile form presents with severe hypotonia, weakness, hyporeflexia and a large tongue. ECG reveals giant QRS complexes. Vacuolated lymphocytes are seen on the blood film. Confirmatory enzymology is performed on fibroblasts. Death is usual within the first year; however, enzyme replacement therapy trials have shown encouraging results. Milder forms with mainly myopathy exist.

GSD III (debrancher enzyme)

Type IIIa affects liver and muscle, whereas type IIIb is purely hepatic. Type III may be clinically indistinguishable from type I, however fasting tolerance is longer as gluconeogenesis is not blocked, and glycogen can be pruned to near the branch points. Nephromegaly is not a feature. Myopathy is notable and may be progressive in type IIIa. Cardiomyopathy is a rare complication. Adenomas, liver fibrosis and cirrhosis are rare.

Lactate level rises, unlike type I, on glucose loading. The diagnosis may be confirmed on white cell enzymology. Dietary management is similar but not as intensive as type I. A high protein diet has been suggested for the type IIIa.

GSD IV (branching enzyme)

This form is very rare and presents with hepatomegaly and progressive liver disease. The diagnosis is usually made on liver histology and enzymology. Liver transplantation is the treatment for progressive disease.

GSD VI (liver phosphorylase deficiency) and GSD IX (phosphorylase-b-kinase deficiency)

Hypoglycaemia is rarely a problem. Hepatomegaly may be an incidental finding. GSD IX enzymology is assayed in red cells but may be normal in the isolated liver form. Treatment consists of uncooked corn starch one to two times a day to aid growth. Inheritance is X-linked or recessive depending on subgroup.

Muscle GSDs

GSD V (muscle phosphorylase deficiency) McArdle's disease
GSD VII (phosphofructokinase deficiency)

Weakness and fatigue with post-exercise stiffness are the presenting features. Serum creatine kinase (CK) is usually elevated along with uric acid. On exercise, lactate fails to rise with excessive increases in uric acid and ammonia. After a brief rest, exercise can be restarted ('second-wind') as fatty acids slowly become available as an alternative fuel. Protein in the diet may be beneficial. Glucose is of benefit in McArdle's disease as glycoloysis is still intact. Extreme exercise should be avoided but regular gentle exercise is probably of benefit.

7.2 Galactosaemia

Clinical features of galactosaemia

- Neonatal onset — jaundice, hepatomegaly, coagulopathy and oil-drop cataracts, usually at the end of the first week
- Later presentation with failure to thrive, proximal tubulopathy and rickets at a few months
- Association with *Escherichia coli* sepsis

Diagnosis

Diagnosis is based on the clinical picture, presence of reducing substances in the urine and enzymology for galactose 1-phosphate uridyltransferase (Gal 1-Put) in red cells. If the child has already received a transfusion, the parents should be screened for carrier-level activity instead. Even in the absence of obvious major liver involvement, the clotting is nearly always slightly prolonged. Galactosaemia should be considered in all cases of severe early-onset jaundice.

Management

This consists of a strict lactose/galactose-free diet for life. Milk is replaced with a soya-based formula. Long-term complications, in spite of good control, include developmental delay, particularly involving speech, feeding problems and infertility in girls.

7.3 Hereditary fructose intolerance

The key to diagnosis is the linking of symptoms to the exposure to fructose which usually occurs at weaning.

Clinical features of hereditary fructose intolerance

- Acute: vomiting and symptomatic hypoglycaemia
- Chronic exposure: failure to thrive, hepatomegaly, ascites, jaundice and proximal renal tubulopathy
- Milder cases: learn to avoid sugary foods
- Exacerbations may occur following exposure to fructose contained in medicines

Diagnosis

Lactic acidosis and hyperuricaemia are common features. Confirmation of exposure to fructose, and measurement of aldolase b activity in liver. Genotyping is used when liver biopsy is contraindicated due to coagulopathy.

Management

Lifelong avoidance of fructose.

8. HYPERLIPIDAEMIAS

Cholesterol and triglycerides are transported in the circulation bound to lipoproteins.

The four major classes are:

- Chylomicrons: carry dietary lipids, mainly triglycerides, from the gut to the liver. Lipoprotein lipase releases free fatty acids from chylomicrons in the portal circulation
- VLDL (very low-density lipoprotein): carries predominantly triglycerides and some cholesterol synthesized in the liver to the peripheries. Lipoprotein lipase releases the free fatty acids leaving IDL (intermediate-density lipoprotein).
- LDL (low-density lipoprotein): transports cholesterol and some triglyceride from the liver to the peripheries. Direct uptake by cells via the LDL receptor.
- HDL (high-density lipoprotein): carries cholesterol from the peripheries to the liver. Inverse association with ischaemic heart disease ('good cholesterol').

8.1 Hypertriglyceridaemias

- Defective chylomicron removal: lipoprotein lipase deficiency, ApoC-II deficiency
- Overproduction of VLDL: familial hypertriglyceridaemia

Hypertriglyceridaemias are rare. Clinical features include colic, hepatosplenomegaly, eruptive xanthomas and creamy plasma. Complications include abdominal pain and pancreatitis, but rarely develop in patients until the level exceeds 20 mmol/l. Secondary causes of elevated triglycerides include obesity, chronic renal failure, diabetes mellitus and liver disease. Treatment comprises a very low-fat diet supplemented with essential fatty acids. Drugs used to lower triglycerides include fibric acid derivatives, niacin or the statins. Fibrate drugs reduce hepatic triglyceride synthesis and enhance peripheral triglyceride clearance, statins reduce triglycerides probably by reducing VLDL synthesis.

8.2 Hypercholesterolaemias

- Defective LDL removal: familial hypercholesterolaemia
- Familial combined hyperlipidaemia

Familial hypercholesterolaemia (FH) is a monogenic disorder with a heterozygote incidence of 1:500, and homozygote 1:1 million. It is the commonest hyperlipidaemia, resulting from LDL-receptor gene mutations. Patients are picked up through premature ischaemic heart disease, or through screening for hypercholesterolaemia following diagnosis in a relative. Family history is an important risk factor for ischaemic heart disease, particularly at a young age and especially in females. In homozygotes, xanthomas may appear in the first decade, and angina before the age of 20.

In children, diet and exercise are the mainstay of treatment, supplemented with binding resins, e.g. cholestyramine and colestipol. These bind cholesterol and bile acids in the gut increasing their loss in the faeces. They are preferred in paediatrics as they are not system-ically absorbed. The new cholesterol-lowering margarines containing plant sterols are a more palatable alternative, reducing cholesterol absorption in the gut, but are extremely expensive at present. Smoking is strongly discouraged. Increasingly, statins are being used in the over-tens as more safety data becomes available. However, theoretical concerns remain over their safety in this age group, particularly with regard to puberty. Statins are ter-atogenic. Liver function and CK are regularly monitored for adverse-effects. Their mecha-nism of action is the competitive inhibition of HMG-CoA reductase, the rate-limiting step of cholesterol synthesis. Liver transplantation, or plasma apheresis, is the treatment of choice for homozygotes.

9. PEROXISOMAL DISORDERS

Peroxisomes harbour many vital cellular functions, including the synthesis of plasmalogens, (essential constituents of cell walls), cholesterol and bile acids, and the β-oxidation of very long-chain fatty acids and breakdown of phytanic acid (vitamin A) and glyoxylate. Disorders are biochemically characterized by the number of functions impaired:

- Multiple enzymes affected: Zellweger syndrome (ZS), neonatal adrenoleukodystrophy (NALD), infantile refsum disease (IRD)
- Several enzymes involved: rhizomelic chondrodysplasia punctata (RCDP)
- Single enzyme block: X-linked adrenoleukodystrophy (ALD), Refsum's disease, hyperoxaluria

Inheritance is autosomal recessive with the exception of ALD. The first-line investigation is very long-chain fatty acids which are elevated in ZS and ALD, but normal in RCDP. In this group plasmalogens are the first screen. Further investigation requires fibroblast studies.

9.1 Zellweger syndrome

Zellweger syndrome (ZS) is the classic peroxisomal biogenesis disorder with distinctive dys-morphic features. There is clinical overlap with NALD and IRD, which are milder with better prognosis.

Clinical features of Zellweger syndrome

- Dysmorphic faces: prominent forehead, hypertelorism, large fontanelle
- Severe neurological involvement including hypotonia, seizures and psychomotor retardation
- Sensorineural deafness
- Ocular abnormalities: retinopathy, cataracts
- Hepatomegaly and liver dysfunction
- Calcific stippling (especially knees and shoulders)
- Failure to thrive

Diagnosis

Loss of all peroxisomal functions: raised very long-chain fatty acids (VLCFAs), phytanate, bile acid intermediates and decreased plasmalogens. Confirmatory enzymology on fibroblasts.

Treatment

Management is supportive. Docosahexaenoic acid supplementation has been tried, but no clear benefit has been demonstrated. Death usually occurs within the first year.

9.2 X-linked adrenoleukodystrophy (XALD)

The paediatric cerebral form presents with severe neurological degeneration usually between 5 and 10 years, progressing to a vegetative state and death within a few years. Brothers in the same family may present at different ages.

Clinical features of XALD

- School failure, behaviour problems
- Visual impairment
- Quadriplegia
- Seizures (late sign)
- Adrenal insufficiency

Adrenal involvement may precede or follow neurological symptoms by years. Some only develop neurological symptoms, and others just adrenal insufficiency. All males developing adrenal failure should have VLCFAs measured to ensure the diagnosis is not missed. Neurological symptoms may occur for the first time in adults (adrenomyeloneuropathy — AMN) resembling a cord syndrome with spastic gait and bladder involvement. Female carriers may develop multiple sclerosis-like symptoms in adulthood.

Diagnosis

Elevated VLCFAs, blunted synacthen response or frank hypoglycaemia. Neuroimaging shows bilateral, predominantly posterior, white-matter involvement. The differential diagnosis for neurodegeneration in the school-age child includes:

- Subacute sclerosing panencephalitis (SSPE)
- Batten's disease
- Wilson's disease
- Niemann–Pick C disease.

Management

Lorenzo oil (oleic and erucic acid) normalizes VLCFAs, but fails to prevent progression. Bone marrow transplantation is the mainstay of therapy in patients prior to neurodegeneration, i.e. prospectively diagnosed siblings, and those diagnosed having presented with adrenal insufficiency or other problems. Serial psychometry and neuro imaging are used to detect the first signs of neurological deterioration: the stimulus for transplantation. Adrenal function should be closely monitored, and steroid replacement therapy given once indicated.

10. MUCOPOLYSACCHARIDOSES (MPS)

Mucopolysaccharides (glycosaminoglycans — GAGs) are structural molecules integral to connective tissues such as cartilage. Degradation occurs within lysosomes, requiring specific enzymes. Patients with mucopolysaccharidoses appear normal at birth and usually present with developmental delay in the first year. The features of storage become more obvious with time.

10.1 Classification

Type	Disorder	Inheritance	Corneal clouding	Skeleton	Hepato-splenomegaly	Mental retardation
I	Hurler	AR	+	+++	+++	+++
II	Hunter	X-linked	–	+++	+++	+++
III	Sanfillipo	AR	+	+	+	+++
IV	Morquio	AR	+	+++	+	–
VI	Maroteaux–Lamy	AR	+	+++	+++	–
VII	Sly	AR	+	+++	+++	+++

Hurler is the classical MPS with storage affecting the body and CNS. Sanfillipo predominantly affects the CNS and Morquio and Maroteaux–Lamy the body. Atlantoaxial instability is common in the latter two, often necessitating prophylactic cervical spinal fusion in the first 2–3 years. Hunter syndrome is phenotypically similar to Hurler, however there is no corneal clouding and scapular nodules are seen.

10.2 Hurler syndrome

Hurler syndrome typifies the MPS group and their associated clinical problems. The enzyme deficiency is α-iduronidase shared with Scheie disease, the milder variant.

Clinical features of Hurler syndrome

- Coarse faces, macroglossia, hirsuitism, corneal clouding
- Airway/ENT problems, secretory otitis media
- Dysostosis multiplex
- Cardiomyopathy, valvular disease
- Hepatosplenomegaly
- Hernias: umbilical, inguinal, femoral
- Stiff joints
- Developmental delay and retardation

Diagnosis

Urinary screen for GAGs (raised dermatan and heparan sulphate). Enzymology confirmed on white cells.

Management

Treatment depends on early recognition to allow early bone marrow transplantation, which significantly modifies the phenotype. Enzyme-replacement clinical trials are currently underway. Supportive care is the mainstay of untransplanted patients, with particular regard to the chest and airway requiring 3-monthly sleep studies.

11. SPHINGOLIPIDOSES

Sphingolipids are complex membrane lipids. They are all derived from ceramide and divide into three groups: cerebrosides, sphingomyelins and gangliosides. Lysosomal hydrolases break down these molecules; deficiencies result in progressive storage and disease. Typical features include psychomotor retardation, neurological degeneration including epilepsy, ataxia and spasticity, with or without hepatosplenomegaly.

11.1 Tay–Sachs disease

Clinical features of Tay–Sachs disease

- Developmental regression within first year
- Macrocephaly
- Hyperacusis
- Cherry-red spot
- Spastic quadriplegia
- Death within 2–4 years
- No hepatosplenomegaly compared to Sandhoff's

Diagnosis

Vacuolated lymphocytes present on the blood film is a further clue. Hexosaminidase A deficiency is confirmed on white cell enzymology.

Management

Currently, management is supportive. However, research into substrate-deprivation therapy, thereby avoiding accumulation in the first place, is under investigation.

11.2 Gaucher disease

Glucocerebrosidase deficiency results in the accumulation of cerebroside in visceral organs +/– the brain depending on the type.

Clinical features of Gaucher disease

- Type 1
  - Non-neuropathic (commonest)
  - Splenomegaly > hepatomegaly
  - Anaemia, bleeding tendency
  - Skeletal pain, deformities, osteopenia
  - Abdominal pain (splenic infarcts)

- Type 2
  - Acute neuropathic
  - Severe CNS involvement (especially bulbar), rapidly progressive
  - Convergent squinting and horizontal gaze palsy
  - Hepatosplenomegaly

- Type 3
  - Sub-acute neuropathic
  - Convergent squint and horizontal gaze palsy (early sign)
  - Splenomegaly > hepatomegaly
  - Slow neurological deterioration

Diagnosis

Elevated angiotensin-converting enzyme (ACE) and acid phosphatase are markers for the disease. Bone marrow aspiration may reveal Gaucher cells (crumpled tissue-paper cytoplasm). White cell enzymes for glucocerebrosidase give the definitive diagnosis. The enzyme chitotriosidase is markedly elevated and may be used to follow disease activity.

Management

Enzyme replacement therapy is effective in visceral disease in types 1 and 3. Bone marrow transplant has been used in the past, and may have benefit for cerebral involvement in type 3. Splenectomy has been used to correct thrombocytopenia and anaemia and relieve mechanical problems, but may accelerate disease elsewhere. There is no effective treatment for type 2.

11.3 Niemann–Pick disease

Niemann–Pick is the eponymous name for the sphingomyelinoses, however types A and B are biochemically and genetically distinct from C and D.

Type 1 (sphingomyelinase deficiency)

Clinical features of type 1

- Type A (infantile)
  - Feeding difficulties
  - Hepatomegaly > splenomegaly
  - Cherry-red spot
  - Lung infiltrates
  - Neurological decline, deaf, blind, spasticity
  - Death within 3 years

- Type B (visceral involvement)
  - Milder course, no neurological involvement
  - Hepatosplenomegaly
  - Pulmonary infiltrates
  - Ataxia
  - Hypercholesterolaemia

Diagnosis
Bone marrow aspirate for Niemann–Pick cells. White cell enzymes. Genotyping may help distinguish between the two types prior to the onset of neurological signs.

Management
Supportive.

Type 2 (lysosomal cholesterol-export defect, secondary sphingomyelin accumulation)

Clinical features of type 2

- Type C
  - Conjugated hyperbilirubinaemia (earliest sign)
  - Hepatosplenomegaly
  - Neurological deterioration (variable age of onset)
  - Dystonia
  - Cherry-red spot
  - Vertical ophthalmoplegia

- Type D (Nova Scotia variant)
  - As above, single mutation (founder effect)

Diagnosis

Niemann–Pick cells on bone marrow aspirate; however, white cell enzymes show normal or mildly decreased sphingomyelinase deficiency. Definitive diagnosis requires cholesterol studies on fibroblasts.

Management

Supportive. Prognosis is guided by age of onset.

11.4 Fabry disease

α-Galactosidase deficiency results in the storage of glycolipids in blood vessel walls, heart, kidney and autonomic spinal ganglia. It is X-linked recessive. Increasingly, female carriers with symptoms are being recognized.

Clinical features of Fabry disease

- Severe pain in extremities (acroparaesthesia)
- Angiokeratoma (bathing-trunk area)
- Corneal opacities
- Cardiac disease
- Cerebrovascular disease
- Nephropathy
- Normal intelligence

Diagnosis

Maltese crosses (birefringent lipid deposits) on urinary microscopy. White cell enzymes.

Management

Analgesia, dialysis and renal transplantation are the established therapies. Enzyme replacement therapy has now been licensed for the treatment of Fabry disease in adults, with clinical trials in children underway.

12. MISCELLANEOUS

12.1 Porphyria

Porphyrias are a group of disorders of haem biosynthesis, which may be classified as acute (neuropsychiatric), cutaneous or mixed. Symptoms in children are extremely rare. Inheritance is autosomal dominant except congenital δ-aminolaevulinc acid dehydratase deficiency, erythropoietic porphyria and hepatoerythropoietic porphyria.

Clinical features of porphyria

- Acute (acute intermittent porphyria, aminolaevulinic acid dehydratase)
  - Abdominal pain, vomiting
  - Polyneuropathy (muscular weakness)
  - Neuropsychiatric disturbance
  - Postural hypotension/hypertension

- Cutaneous (erythropoietic protoporphyria, porphyria cutanea tarda, congenital erthropoietic porphyria, hepatoerythropoietic porphyria)
  - Photosensitive skin lesions
  - Liver damage

- Mixed (variegate porphyria, hereditary coproporphyria)

Diagnosis

- Acute attacks   Raised urinary aminolaevulinic acid and porphobilinogen during attacks (fresh urine)
  Faecal porphyrin analysis to distinguish type
- Cutaneous forms   Total plasma porphyrins (raised if active lesions)
  Total faecal porphyrins
  Erythrocyte porphyrins

Management

Cutaneous forms are managed by avoidance of precipitants, especially sunlight, and good skin care. Acute attacks are managed with glucose and haem arginate, reducing synthesis of aminolaevulinic acid by negative feedback. Many drugs precipitate attacks, therefore only those known to be safe should be used during an attack.

Drugs used:

- Pain   opiates
- Psychosis   chlorpromazine
- Tachycardia, hypertension   β-blockers
- Seizures   gabapentin, vigabatrin

12.2 Smith–Lemli–Opitz syndrome

Smith–Lemli–Opitz (SLO) is the commonest sterol biosynthesis defect; a group of disorders characterized by limb defects, major organ dysplasia and skin abnormalities.

Clinical features of Smith–Lemli–Opitz syndrome

- Dysmorphic faces: microcephaly, narrow frontal area, upturned nose, ptosis
- Genital anomalies
- Syndactyly 2nd and 3rd toes
- Mental retardation
- Renal anomalies
- Failure to thrive

Diagnosis

SLO is due to a block in the penultimate step of cholesterol biosynthesis, therefore cholesterol is low with a raised 7-dehydrocholesterol level, the immediate precursor.

Management

At present, management is supportive; however, trials are underway evaluating statins to block the build-up of precursors. Cholesterol supplementation has not shown convincing benefit.

12.3 Congenital disorders of glycosylation (CDG)

This group of disorders result from defects in the synthesis of the carbohydrate moiety of glycoproteins. Group I contains defects of the oligosaccharide chain synthesis and transfer to the protein, and group II defects in the further processing of the protein-bound oligosaccharide chain. The two commonest disorders are CDG Ia (phosphomannomutase deficiency), and CDG Ib (phosphomannose isomerase deficiency)

CDG are multiorgan disorders affecting particularly the brain, except CDG Ib which is mainly a hepatogastrointestinal disorder. CDG Ia has typical dysmorphology.

Clinical features of CDG 1a

- Dysmorphic features – inverted nipples, fat pads
- Muscular hypotonia
- Failure to thrive
- Cerebellar hypoplasia

Diagnosis

Transferrin isoelectric focusing is used to screen for CDG syndromes. Enzymology is performed on white cells and fibroblasts.

Management

CDG Ib is effectively managed with mannose supplementation. The other types are treated symptomatically.

12.4 Lesch–Nyhan syndrome

This is an X-linked disorder of purine metabolism due to hypoxanthine guanine phosphoribosyltransferase (HGPRT) deficiency.

Clinical features of Lesch–Nyhan syndrome

- Self-mutilation
- Gout
- Motor retardation

Diagnosis

Elevated urate and hypoxanthine in urine.

Management

A low-purine diet, allopurinol and liberal fluids are used to reduce renal complications.

12.5 Menkes syndrome

An X-linked membrane copper-transporter defect. Copper uptake by cells is normal, however export from the cell is blocked and the copper-requiring enzymes do not receive the necessary copper for normal function.

Clinical features of Menkes syndrome

- Hypothermia
- Epilepsy
- Hypotonia
- Pudgy cheeks
- Pili torti
- Retardation
- Connective tissue problems
- Early death

Diagnosis

Low serum copper and caeruloplasmin, although may be normal in the neonatal period. Confirmed on copper-flux studies in fibroblasts, and ultimately genotype.

Management

Daily copper–histidine injections have proven effective in altering the neurological outcome if the diagnosis is made early and treatment not delayed. The connective tissue complications subsequently dominate the clinical picture in treated patients.

13. SCREENING

13.1 Principles of screening

Screening for defined disorders aims to prevent avoidable morbidity and mortality. The sensitivity of a screening test is the rate of true-positives, and specificity the rate of true-negatives. The aim is not to miss any cases with the minimum of false-positives. The necessary requirements for including a condition in a screening programme are:

- Important health problem
- Accepted treatment
- Facilities available for diagnosis and treatment
- Latent or asymptomatic disease
- Suitable test
- Natural history understood
- Agreed case definition
- Early treatment improves prognosis
- Economic
- Case-finding may need to be continuous

The UK National Screening Committee added a further requirement; randomized controlled trial evidence to support introduction of new screens. This is a major obstacle to expanding the current programme as such data does not exist. An application for such a national trial in the UK for MCAD screening following two health-technology, assessment recommendations in 1997, is still awaiting approval.

13.2 UK neonatal screening programme

Neonatal blood spots are collected on day 7 with the aim of commencing treatment by day 21 for hypothyroidism and PKU. Labs still using the Guthrie test for PKU, which relies on phenylalanine-dependent bacterial growth, may give false-negatives if the baby is receiving antibiotics. This information is requested on the card in those regions. The feeding status is also requested to ensure adequate protein intake, but newer techniques are able to detect PKU reliably on day 1 (routine screening day in the US).

Current UK programme:

Universal	Congenital hypothyroidism (thyroid-stimulating hormone (TSH))
	Phenylketonuria (phenylalanine)
Some regions	Haemoglobinopathies (Sickle-cell disease and thalassaemia)
	Cystic fibrosis
	Galactosaemia
	Homocystinuria
	Duchenne muscular dystrophy

Haemoglobinopathies and cystic fibrosis have now been agreed for inclusion in the national screening programme.

Duchenne muscular dystrophy is an example of a condition not fulfilling the criteria (being ultimately incurable); however, the public and professional support for the programme has grown with time. An 'important health problem' has been interpreted on an individual rather than population basis. Potential benefits include 'avoidance of the diagnostic odyssey', with all its associated emotional and financial expense before the correct diagnosis is made, influences on reproductive choice in the parents (at a time before subsequent pregnancies) and the hope that earlier identification may lead to positive interventions to influence outcome and better research.

Newer screening technologies, such as tandem mass spectrometry (TMS), further challenge the established criteria as it is now much easier to diagnose a whole number of not only inborn errors of metabolism, but also liver disease, haemaglobinopathies, etc. Although additional screening costs may be minimal as the current system of blood-spot collection can be utilized, there is a large burden placed on diagnostic and support services dealing with the new caseload. Rarity may no longer preclude screening a whole population when there is an effective treatment available, e.g. biotinidase deficiency cured with biotin supplementation.

14. FURTHER READING

Campbell A, McIntosh N (Editors). *Forfar and Arneil's Textbook of Paediatrics*, 5th edition. Churchill Livingstone 1998 – Chapter 20, Inborn Errors of Metabolism.

Fernandes J, Saudubray J-M, van den Berghe G (Editors). *Inborn Metabolic Diseases: Diagnosis and Treatment*, 3rd edition. Springer-Verlag 2000.

Scriver CR, Beaudet AL, Sly WS, Valle D (Editors). *The Metabolic and Molecular Bases of Inherited Disease*, 8th edition. McGraw Hill 2001.

Chapter 13

Neonatology

Grenville F Fox

CONTENTS

Neonatology

1. EMBRYOLOGY, OBSTETRICS AND FETAL MEDICINE

1.1 Embryology of the cardiovascular system

- The heart develops initially as a tube from yolk sac mesoderm. It begins to beat from about 3 weeks' gestation.
- In the fourth week the primitive heart loops to form four chambers. Septation between the four chambers and the aorta and pulmonary trunk occurs in the fifth week. The septum primum grows down from the upper part of the primitive atrium and then fuses with the endocardial cushions (septum intermedium) in the AV canal.
- Bulbotruncal septation divides the common arterial trunk into the aorta and pulmonary trunk as spiral ridges develop in the caudal end of the heart. Completion of ventricular septation occurs as these fuse with the septum intermedium.
- Blood is pumped caudally from the embryonic heart by six pairs of pharyngeal arch arteries to the paired dorsal aortas. Some of this system regresses and the 3rd arch arteries form the carotid vessels. The right 4th arch artery forms the right subclavian artery with that of the left forming the aortic arch. The left 6th arch artery forms the ductus arteriosus with branch pulmonary arteries forming from the right.

1.2 Embryology and post-natal development of the respiratory system

- Embryonic phase (3–5 weeks' gestation) — the lung bud begins as endodermal outgrowth of foregut. This branches into the surrounding mesoderm to form the main bronchi.
- Pseudoglandular phase (6–16 weeks) — airways branch further to terminal bronchioles (preacinar airways). Cartilage, lymphatics and cilia form. Main pulmonary artery forms from 6th left branchial arch.
- Canalicular phase (17–24 weeks) — airways lengthen, epithelium becomes cuboidal, pulmonary circulation develops. The acinar structures (gas-exchanging units) begin to develop and surfactant production begins by 24 weeks' gestation as type 1 and 2 pneumocytes become distinguishable. Lungs fill with amniotic fluid, which facilitates further lung growth.
- Terminal sac phase (24–40 weeks) — further development of the acinar structures (respiratory bronchioles, alveolar ducts and terminal sacs (alveoli)) occurs and increasing amounts of surfactant are produced. Type 1 pneumocytes eventually cover approximately 95% of the alveolar surface and facilitate gas exchange. The surfactant-producing type 2 cells cover only about 5%. Development of the pulmonary

circulation continues and results in a thicker intra-arteriolar smooth muscle layer by term, which may respond to intrauterine hypoxia by vasoconstriction. This regresses rapidly after birth.

- Post-natal lung development — the number and size of alveoli increases rapidly during the first 2 years (approximately 150 million at term to 400 million by 4 years). The conducting airways also increase in size.
- Diaphragm development — arises as a sheet of mesodermal tissue, the septum transversum. It begins close to the 3rd, 4th and 5th cervical segments and therefore its nerve supply, the phrenic nerve, is derived from this area. The primitive septum transversum migrates caudally to form the pleural space and the two posterolateral canals in which the lung buds develop fuse. Failure to do this results in a Bochdalek hernia. Failure of the retrosternal part of the septum transversum to form causes a Morgagni type of diaphragmatic hernia. The diaphragm is completed as primitive muscle cells migrate from the body wall. If this fails eventration of the diaphragm results.

1.3 Embryology of the gastrointestinal system

- The endodermal lining of the yolk sac forms the primitive gut.
- The midgut lengthens and protrudes into the yolk sac via the vitelline duct. Meckel's diverticulum is the remnant of this.
- The extra-abdominal gut rotates 270° anticlockwise around the mesentery which contains the superior mesenteric artery. Failure to complete this results in malrotation.
- The gut returns to the abdominal cavity by the end of the 12th week. Exomphalos is the result of this not occurring.
- Gastroschisis is a failure of closure of the anterior abdominal wall.

1.4 Embryology of the central nervous system

- The neural plate develops from ectoderm and forms the neural tube by 3 weeks' gestation. The neural groove closes in a cranial to caudal direction by the end of the fourth week.
- Three swellings evolve from the caudal end of the neural tube — the prosencephalon (forebrain) forms the cerebral hemispheres, the mesencephalon forms the midbrain and the rhombencephalon (hind brain) forms the pons, medulla and cerebellum.
- Neuroblasts migrate from the centre of the brain to further develop the cerebral hemispheres.
- Myelination from Schwann cells occurs from 12 weeks' gestation.
- Neural crest cells form the meninges, peripheral nerves, chromaffin cells, melanocytes and adrenal medulla.

1.5 Embryology of the genitourinary system

- The genitourinary systems develop from mesoderm on the posterior abdominal wall and drain into the urogenital sinus of the cloaca.

- The pronephros is the primitive kidney resulting from this and is replaced initially by the mesonephros. The ureteric bud appears at the start of week 5 of embryogenesis as a small branch of the mesonephric duct. The mesonephric (Wolffian) ducts drain urine from primitive tubules into the urogenital sinus. Repeated branching from week 6 onwards gives rise to the calyces, papillary ducts and collecting tubules by week 12.
- Differentiation of the metanephros into nephrons — glomeruli, tubules and loop of Henle occurs from 4 weeks. These structures then join with the lower Wolffian ducts to form the collecting systems. Branching and new nephron induction continues until week 36.
- The metanephros develops from the most caudal part of the mesodermal ridge, but the kidney eventually becomes extrapelvic due to growth of surrounding areas.
- The Y chromosome (*SRY* gene) influences development of primitive gonads to form testes after 6 weeks. Testes 'secrete' Mullerian inhibition factor (MIF) which results in regression of Mullerian structures (uterus, Fallopian tubes and vagina).
- Testosterone influences the development of Wolffian structures (prostate, seminiferous tubules and vas deferens) as well as later masculinization

1.6 Maternal conditions affecting the fetus and newborn

- **Diabetes** — three times risk of congenital malformations (congenital heart disease, sacral agenesis, microcolon, neural tube defects); small for gestational age (SGA) — three times normal rate, due to small-vessel disease; macrosomia due to increased fetal insulin; hypoglycaemia, hypocalcaemia; hypomagnesaemia; surfactant deficiency; transient hypertrophic cardiomyopathy (septal); polycythaemia, jaundice
- **Hypertension** and pre-eclampsia — SGA, polycythaemia, neutropenia, thrombocytopenia, hypoglycaemia
- **Maternal thyroid disease**
  Neonatal thyrotoxicosis can be caused by transplacental thyroid-stimulating antibodies (LATS) with maternal Grave's disease.
  - Rare — only 1:70 mothers with thyrotoxicosis
  - May present with fetal tachycardia or within 1–2 days of birth, but sometimes delayed if mother taking antithyroid drugs
  - Usually causes goitre
  - Only severe cases require treatment with beta-blockers and antithyroid drugs as it resolves spontaneously as antibody levels fall over the first few months

Neonatal hypothyroidism may be caused by maternal antithyroid drugs taken during pregnancy.

Systemic lupus erythematosus (SLE)

Maternal SLE is associated with:

- Increased risk of miscarriage. Recurrent miscarriage is associated with antiphospholipid antibody.
- Increased risk of small for gestational age babies. Risk is higher with maternal hypertension and renal disease.

- Congenital complete heart block — associated with presence of anti-Ro and anti-La antibodies
- Butterfly rash — transient due to transplacental passage of SLE antibodies

Thrombocytopenia

Transplacental passage of maternal antiplatelet antibodies causes neonatal thrombocytopenia. If the mother is also thrombocytopenic the cause is likely to be maternal idiopathic thrombocytopenia (also associated with maternal SLE).

- Platelet count proportional to that of mother's
- Rarely causes very low neonatal platelet counts or symptoms
- Risk of intracranial haemorrhage if platelet count $<50 \times 10^9/l$ (may occur antenatally, therefore Caesarean section not always protective)
- Treatment: intravenous IgG and platelet transfusion

Alloimmune thrombocytopenia occurs following maternal sensitization if mother is PL^{A1} Ag-negative.

- Approximately 3% of White people are PL^{A1} Ag-negative
- First pregnancies may be affected; severity usually more severe in subsequent pregnancies
- Antenatal intracranial haemorrhage is common (20–50%)
- Treatment — washed irradiated maternal platelets or intravenous IgG and random donor platelets

See Chapter 9, *Haematology and Oncology.*

Myasthenia gravis

Babies of mothers with myasthenia gravis have a 10% risk of a transient neonatal form of the disease.

- Usually due to transplacental passage of anti-acetylcholinesterase receptor antibodies but baby may produce own antibodies
- Risk increased if previous baby affected
- Maternal disease severity does not correlate with that of baby; a range of symptoms from mild hypotonia to ventilator dependent respiratory failure may occur
- Diagnosis — antibody assay, EMG and edrophonium or neostigmine test (also used as treatment)
- Babies of mothers with myasthenia gravis should be monitored for several days after birth
- Usually presents soon after birth and resolves by 2 months. Physiotherapy may be required to prevent/relieve contractures
- Congenital myasthenia gravis should be considered if antibodies are absent or if symptoms persist or recur

Fetal alcohol syndrome

Fetal alcohol syndrome. Although more than 3–4 alcohol units per day during pregnancy are thought to be necessary to cause fetal alcohol syndrome, even moderate alcohol intake may reduce birth weight. Features of fetal alcohol syndrome include:

- Small for gestational age
- Dysmorphic face with mid-face hypoplasia — short palpebral fissures, epicanthic folds, flat nasal bridge (resulting in small upturned nose), long philtrum, thin upper lip, micrognathia and ear abnormalities
- Microcephaly with subsequent intellectual impairment
- Congenital heart disease
- Post-natal growth failure

Maternal smoking

- Reduces birth weight by 10% on average
- Increases risk of sudden infant death syndrome (SIDS)

Maternal drugs

Teratogenic drugs include:

- Phenytoin (fetal hydantoin syndrome) — dysmorphic face (broad nasal bridge, hypertelorism, ptosis, ear abnormalities)
- Valproate — neural tube defects, fused metopic suture, mid-face hypoplasia, congenital heart disease, hypospadias, talipes, global developmental delay
- Retinoids (isotretinoin) and large doses of vitamin A — dysmorphic face (including cleft palate), hydrocephalus, congenital heart disease
- Cocaine — small for gestational age, prune belly and renal tract abnormalities, gut, cardiac, skeletal and eye malformations
- Other teratogenic drugs include — thalidomide (limb defects), lithium, carbamazepine, chloramphenicol, warfarin.

Maternal opiate abuse

- Causes small for gestational age infants
- Results in withdrawal symptoms or neonatal abstinence syndrome — onset usually within 1–2 days of birth but may be delayed until 7–10 days and continue for several months; onset is later and symptoms persist for longer with methadone

Symptoms

W — wakefulness
I — irritability
T — tremors, temperature instability, tachypnoea
H — high-pitched cry, hyperactivity, hypertonia
D — diarrhoea, disorganized suck
R — respiratory distress, rhinorrhoea
A — apnoea
W — weight loss
A — autonomic dysfunction
L — lacrimation

Also — seizures, myoclonic jerks, hiccups, sneezing, yawning

- Surfactant deficiency is less common
- SIDS is more common
- Management — monitor using withdrawal score chart. Less than 50% require pharmacological intervention. Indications for this are severe withdrawal symptoms or seizures. Oral morphine is the usual treatment of choice. Methadone, phenobarbital, benzodiazepines and chlorpromazine have also been used.

1.7 Placental physiology, fetal growth and well being

The fertilized ovum divides to form a blastocyst which attaches itself to the inside wall of the uterus. The outer cells of the blastocyst, the trophoblasts, eat their way into the endometrium and these and surrounding endometrial cells form the placenta and membranes. The trophoblasts are therefore the source of nutrition for the early embryo in the first 12 weeks.

In the second and third trimester, maternal blood flows into placental sinuses which surround the placental villi. Active transport of amino acids and other nutrients occurs across the chorionic epithelium into the villi, early in pregnancy, but this becomes less after the first trimester. Oxygen and nutrients diffuse into the fetal blood supply via the villi. Diffusion of oxygen occurs because maternal PO_2 is approximately 7 kPa, compared to 4 kPa in the fetus.

Oestrogen

- Initially produced by the corpus luteum and then in increasing amounts by the placenta as pregnancy progresses
- Causes the uterine smooth muscle to proliferate
- Enhances development of the uterine blood supply
- Changes pelvic musculature and ligaments to facilitate birth
- Causes breast development by increasing proliferation of glandular and fatty tissue

Progesterone

- Limited amounts produced by the corpus luteum in the early part of pregnancy — much larger amounts produced by the placenta after the first trimester
- Causes endometrial cells to store nutrients in first trimester
- Relaxes uterine smooth muscle; decrease in secretion of progesterone in the final few weeks of pregnancy coincides with onset of labour
- Facilitates glandular development of breasts

Human chorionic gonadotrophin (HCG)

- Secreted by trophoblasts
- Prevents degeneration of corpus luteum
- Peak concentration at around 10 weeks, falls rapidly to low levels by 20 weeks' gestation

Human placental lactogen (HPL)

- Secreted by placenta in increasing amounts throughout pregnancy
- Has growth hormone-like effect on fetus
- Has prolactin-like effect on breasts, facilitating milk production

Oxytocin

- Produced by the hypothalamic–posterior pituitary axis
- Release is stimulated by irritation of the cervix
- Oxytocin causes contraction of uterine smooth muscle
- Causes milk secretion — stimulation via the hypothalamus

Prolactin

- Produced by the hypothalamic–anterior pituitary axis
- Production is inhibited during pregnancy by high levels of oestrogen and progesterone produced by the placenta; the sudden decrease in these after delivery of the placenta increases prolactin release
- Prolactin causes secretion of milk from the breasts
- Hypothalamic production of a prolactin inhibitory factor increases if the breasts are engorged with milk and decreases as the baby breast feeds
- Prolactin inhibits follicle-stimulating hormone (FSH) immediately post-partum, thereby preventing ovulation

Identifying fetal compromise

- Kick charts
- Symphysis–fundal height — to estimate fetal size/growth
- Ultrasound scan measurement — to estimate fetal size/growth
- Amniotic fluid volume (see below)
- Umbilical artery Doppler studies — reflect placental blood flow
- Fetal Doppler's — reflect hypoxia if abnormal
- Biophysical profile — fetal movement, posture and tone, breathing, amniotic fluid volume and cardiotacograph (CTG) assessed

1.8 Amniotic fluid, oligohydramnios and polyhydramnios

- Amniotic fluid is produced by the amnion, fetal urine and fetal lung secretions
- Diagnosed on ultrasound scan if clinically suspected
- Deepest pool of amniotic fluid normally 3–8 cm. The amniotic fluid index (AFI) is the sum of the depth of the deepest pool in each quadrant
- Oligohydramnios (decreased AFI) may be due to:
  - Placental insufficiency (intrauterine growth retardation (IUGR) usually also present)
  - Fetal urinary tract abnormalities
  - Prolonged rupture of membranes (PROM)
- Polyhydramnios (increased AFI) may be due to:
  - Maternal diabetes
  - Karyotype abnormalities
  - Twin to twin transfusion syndrome (sometimes called polyhydramnios–oligohydramnios sequence)
  - Neuromuscular disorders
    - Congenital myotonic dystrophy
    - Spinal muscular atrophy (SMA type 1 or 0) (Type 0 is antenatal presentation of SMA)
    - Congenital myopathies
    - Moebius syndrome
- Oesophageal atresia
- Congenital diaphragmatic hernia
- Idiopathic/unexplained (NB cause more likely to be found in severe cases)

1.9 Hydrops fetalis

Definition — subcutaneous oedema and fluid in at least two of pleural effusions, ascites, pericardial effusion.

Causes
- Immune — usually rhesus disease
- Non-immune:
  - Anaemia:
    - Twin to twin transfusion
    - Fetomaternal haemorrhage
    - Homozygous α-thalassaemia
  - Heart failure:
    - Arrhythmias (SVT, complete heart block)
    - Structural (cardiomyopathy, hypoplastic left and right heart, etc.)
    - High-output (AV malformations, angiomas)
  - Chromosomal abnormalities (Turner's, trisomy 21 and other trisomies)
  - Congenital malformations:
    - Congenital cystic adenomatoid malformation
    - Diaphragmatic hernia
    - Cystic hygroma
    - Chylothorax and pulmonary lymphangiectasia
    - Osteogenesis imperfecta
    - Asphyxiating thoracic dystrophy
  - Infection:
    - Parvovirus B19
    - CMV
    - Toxoplasmosis
    - Syphilis
    - Chagas disease (a South American parasite infection)
  - Congenital nephrotic syndrome
  - Idiopathic — 15–20% cases in recent series

1.10 Fetal circulation, adaptation at birth and PPHN

Fetal haemoglobin (HbF)
- 4 globin chains are $\alpha_2\gamma_2$ (adult is predominantly α2β2).
- The γ-chains have reduced binding to 2,3–DPG (2,3-diphosphoglycerate).
- The reduced 2,3-DPG in HbF causes the oxyhaemoglobin dissociation curve to be shifted to the left — i.e. there is a higher saturation for a given PO_2 or P50 decreases (PO_2 at which half the haemoglobin is saturated). Fetal red blood cells therefore have a higher affinity for oxygen making it easier to unload from the maternal circulation. Delivery of oxygen to the fetal tissues is facilitated by the steep oxyhaemoglobin dissociation curve of HbF, but the lower P50 leads to a decreased rate of tissue unloading to tissues. 2,3-DPG levels rise rapidly in the first few days to meet the increased metabolic requirements that occur after birth. Preterm infants have lower 2,3-DPG levels and therefore have a limited ability for oxygen to be unloaded from red blood cells.
- Approximately 80% of haemoglobin is HbF at term. This falls to <10% by 1 year.

The following also shift the oxyhaemoglobin dissociation curve to the left:

- Alkalosis
- Hypocarbia
- Hypothermia

Circulatory changes at birth

- Functional closure of ductus venosus occurs within hours of birth, with anatomical closure completed within 3 weeks.
- Ductus arteriosus patency is maintained in fetal life by prostaglandins (PGE_2, PGI_2). Functional closure of the ductus arteriosus usually occurs within 15 hours of birth and is facilitated by:
    - Reduced sensitivity of the ductus to prostaglandins and increased breakdown of PGE_2 occurring in the lungs towards the end of pregnancy
    - Increased PO_2 after the onset of breathing
    - Reduced pulmonary vascular resistance.
- Prior to birth only about 10% of cardiac output goes to the lungs as pulmonary vascular resistance is higher than systemic.
- Chemosensitivity of the pulmonary arteriolar bed increases with advancing gestation.
- Increase in PO_2 and lung expansion immediately after birth along with increased release of vasodilator substances (prostaglandins, bradykinin and nitric oxide) lead to a fall in pulmonary vascular resistance after birth.
- Pulmonary artery pressure falls to half pre-birth levels within 24 hours and pulmonary blood flow doubles as a result.
- After birth, left atrial pressure increases due to increased pulmonary blood flow and right atrial pressure falls due to absence of placental blood from the umbilical vein. This results in a functional closure of the foramen ovale within a few minutes of birth. Anatomical closure may take weeks.

Persistent pulmonary hypertension of the newborn (PPHN)

Normal circulatory changes after birth are delayed due to either increased muscularization of the pulmonary arterioles or as a response to hypoxia.

Treatment includes ventilation with hyperoxia, induced metabolic alkalosis and the use of pulmonary vasodilators such as nitric oxide.

Nitric oxide (NO)

- Free radical
- Synthesized in endothelial cells from L-arginine by enzyme NO synthase — also known as endothelium-derived relaxing factor (EDRF)
- In vascular smooth muscle — nitric oxide activates guanylate cyclase to increase intracellular cyclic guanosine monophosphate (cGMP). This leads to smooth muscle relaxation and vasodilation by stimulating cGMP-dependent protein kinase which reduces intracellular calcium.

2. PREMATURITY — DEFINITIONS AND STATISTICS

2.1 Mortality:Definitions

- Stillbirth — *in utero* death after 24 weeks' gestation (28 weeks in most other European countries, 20 weeks in USA, 12 weeks in Japan)
- Perinatal mortality rate — stillbirths and deaths within 6 days of birth per 1,000 live and stillbirths (England and Wales perinatal mortality rate 1997 = 8.3)
- Neonatal mortality rate — deaths of liveborn infants <28 days per 1,000 live births (England and Wales neonatal mortality rate 1997 = 3.9) NB this includes infants born at less than 24 weeks' gestation if liveborn

2.2 Incidence and causes/associations of preterm birth

Approximate UK incidences (live births):

- Preterm birth (i.e. prior to 37 completed weeks' gestation)   7%
- Low birth weight (LBW = <2500 g)   7%
- Very low birth weight (VLBW = <1500 g)   1.2%
- Extremely low birth weight (ELBW = <1000 g)   0.5%

All of these incidences are higher in developing countries but lower in some other European countries.

The incidence of preterm birth appears to be increasing both in the UK and in other countries and this is likely to be due to:

- Increase in the number of multiple births due to assisted conception
- Increased obstetric intervention
- Increased use of gestational age assessments (which tends to decrease estimates of gestational age)
- An increase in the registration of live births at very low gestations

The following are associated with an increased risk for spontaneous preterm birth:

- Social/demographic factors:
  - Maternal country of birth Africa or Caribbean
  - Low socioeconomic class
  - Age <20 or >40
- Past obstetric or medical history
  - Previous preterm birth
  - Uterine abnormalities
  - Cervical abnormalities
- Current pregnancy
  - Multiple pregnancy
  - Poor nutrition

- Low pre-pregnancy weight
- Poor pre- and antenatal care
- Anaemia
- Smoking
- Bacteruria
- Genital tract colonization (particularly Group B Streptococcus)
- Cervical dilatation >1 cm
- Preterm prolonged rupture of membranes (PPROM)

2.3 Outcome after preterm birth

The only national study of survival and long-term follow-up after extreme preterm birth published so far is the EPICure study. This documented outcome after birth between 20 and 25 weeks' gestation in 1289 live births in the UK and Republic of Ireland in 1995.

Survival to discharge from hospital was as follows:

- 22 weeks   1%
- 23 weeks   11%
- 24 weeks   26%
- 25 weeks   44%

Neurodevelopmental follow-up of survivors at 30 months showed:

- no disability   49%
- severe disability   23%
- mild to moderate disability   25%
- died after hospital discharge   2%
- not followed up   1%

Outcome for preterm small for gestational age infants is less well documented, but there is some evidence that outcome is marginally better than that expected in an appropriately grown infant of the same birth weight — i.e. a baby born at 28 weeks weighing 750 g (<3rd centile) would be expected to have the same outcome as a 25-week gestation infant of the same weight (50th centile).

The ethics of resuscitation of extremely preterm infants are controversial and any decisions in individual cases should be made by the most senior paediatrician available at the time, with parents' views taken into consideration when possible. It seems reasonable to actively resuscitate most appropriately grown (i.e. > approximately 500 g) infants greater than 23 weeks' gestation who have reasonable signs of life after birth.

3. RESPIRATORY PROBLEMS

3.1 Surfactant deficiency

Endogenous surfactant is produced by type 2 pneumocytes, which line 5–10% of the alveolar surface. Surfactant-containing osmiophilic granular inclusion bodies cause these to appear different from the thinner and more numerous type 1 pneumocytes, which are responsible for gas exchange.

Composition of endogenous surfactant

Phospholipids — 85%

- Main surface-active components which lower surface tension at air–alveolar interface preventing alveolar collapse
- Dipalmitoylphosphatidylcholine (DPPC) — 45–70% is the major constituent of all exogenous surfactant preparations
- Others phospholipids include:
  - Phosphatidylcholine
  - Phosphatidylglycerol
  - Phosphatidylinositol
  - Phosphatidylethanolamine
  - Phosphatidylserine
  - Sphingomyelin

Neutral lipids — 10%

Apolipoproteins — 5%
Facilitate adsorption, spreading and recycling of surfactant and have immunoregulatory properties.

Surfactant associated proteins:

- A — mainly immune function but also has a role in spreading and recycling of surfactant
  - Has been shown to increase microbial killing by alveolar macrophages
  - Increases resistance to inhibitors of surface activity which occurs in sepsis
- B — major role in adsorption, spreading and recycling of surfactant
  - Case reports suggest that congenital deficiency of surfactant protein B is a lethal, autosomal recessive condition
- C — similar function to surfactant protein B
- D — immune function

Platelet activating factor (PAF) — may increase surfactant secretion

Exogenous surfactants

	Contains	Onset	Mortality	Air leak	CLD/BPD
Synthetic	DPPC Hexadecanol	Hours ↓	↓	↓	
Tyloxapol Animal Surf. proteins B+C	Lipids (inc. DPPC)	Minutes ↓↓	↓↓	↓↓	

Estimated incidence of surfactant deficiency by gestational age (without maternal steroids)

Gestation (completed weeks)	Incidence of surfactant deficiency (%)
26	90
27	85
28	80
29	75
30	70
31	60
32	55
33	40
34	25
35	20
36	12
37	6
38	3
39	2
40	<1–2

Increased incidence of surfactant deficiency in:

- Prematurity
- Male sex
- Sepsis
- Maternal diabetes
- 2nd twin
- Elective Caesarean section
- Strong family history

478

Surfactant deficiency decreased:

- Female sex
- PROM
- Maternal opiate use
- IUGR
- Antenatal glucocorticoids
- Prophylactic surfactant

Amniotic fluid (or gastric aspirate) lecithin/sphingomyelin (L/S) ratios
<1.5   = immature   — 70% risk of surfactant deficiency
1.5–1.9 = borderline   — 40% risk of surfactant deficiency
2.0–2.5 = mature   — very small risk unless mother diabetic
>2.5   = safe

Management of surfactant deficiency

There is currently no evidence that routine high-frequency oscillation (HFO) is of any long-term benefit in preterm infants with surfactant deficiency, although this mode of ventilation may be used as a 'rescue' in severe cases. Routine paralysis is not used in most neonatal units, although this sedation with opiates and various modes of trigger ventilation may help reduce the incidence of pneumothoraces. Exogenous surfactant considerably reduces mortality and incidence of pneumothoraces and chronic lung disease. Early treatment with surfactant and use of animal rather than synthetic surfactants enhance these outcomes.

3.2 Chronic lung disease — (bronchopulmonary dysplasia (BPD))

Definition — respiratory support with supplementary oxygen +/– mechanical ventilation >28 days with typical chest X-ray changes (see below). In VLBW infants an alternative definition has been suggested — requiring oxygen +/– mechanical ventilation >36 weeks' corrected gestational age and typical chest X-ray changes.

Risk factors for chronic lung disease

- Prematurity
- Prolonged mechanical ventilation with high pressures and high F_iO_2
- Baro- (volume) trauma
- Pulmonary air leak (pneumothoraces or pulmonary interstitial emphysema)
- Gastro-oesophageal reflux
- Patent ductus arteriosus (PDA)
- Pulmonary infection (particularly *Ureaplasma urealyticum*)

Radiological stages

- Stage 1   1st few days   indistinguishable from surfactant deficiency
- Stage 2   2nd week   generalized opacity of lung fields
- Stage 3   2–4 weeks   streaky infiltrates
- Stage 4   >4 weeks   hyperinflation, cysts, areas of collapse/consolidation, cardiomegaly

Management of chronic lung disease

- Ventilatory support as required
- Supplementary oxygen to maintain oxygen saturations 94–96% or PO_2 >7kPa (to reduce risk of pulmonary hypertension and cor pulmonale)
- Good nutrition is of paramount importance; increased alveolar growth accompanies general growth — particularly in the first 1–2 years
- Treatment of underlying exacerbating factors — infection, gastro-oesophageal reflux, fits, cardiac problems, etc.
- Dexamethasone — the only proven benefit is to facilitate weaning off mechanical ventilation but concern has been raised over short- and long-term side-effects, particularly adverse neurodevelopmental outcome
- Inhaled steroids — only proven benefit is to reduce the need for systemic steroids
- Bronchodilators
- Diuretics — only likely to be of benefit in the presence of PDA, cor pulmonale or excessive weight gain
- Respiratory syncytial virus (RSV) prophylaxis with monoclonal antibodies (Palivizumab) has been shown to reduce hospitalization in high risk cases, but use is controversial because of high cost of drug and need for monthly i.m. injections throughout RSV season

Outcome of babies with chronic lung disease

- Most are weaned off supplementary oxygen before discharge home
- Few require home oxygen
- Most babies discharged on home oxygen are weaned off before 1–2 years
- High risk of readmission to hospital with viral respiratory infections in the first 1–2 years of life
- Increased risk of recurrent cough and wheeze in pre-school age group but most outgrow this tendency and have normal exercise tolerance in childhood

3.3 Meconium aspiration syndrome (MAS)

Risk factors

- Term or post-term (incidence much higher >42 weeks)
- Small for gestational age
- Perinatal asphyxia

Rare in preterm, but said to occur with congenital listeriosis (more likely to be pus than meconium). The passage of meconium in fetal distress may be due to increased secretion of motilin. Meconium may be inhaled antenatally or postnatally. Antenatal inhalation is more likely in fetal distress due to abnormal fetal breathing (equivalent to gasping) that occurs with hypoxia and acidosis.

Major effects of MAS on lung function

- Airway blockage
  - Increased airways resistance with ball-valve mechanism and gas trapping
  - High risk of pneumothorax
- Chemical pneumonitis
- Increased risk of infection
  - Although meconium is sterile
  - *E. coli* most common
- Surfactant deficiency
  - Lipid content of meconium displaces surfactant from alveolar surface
  - Persistent pulmonary hypertension of the newborn (PPHN)

CXR changes of MAS include initial patchy infiltration and hyperinflation. Pneumothoraces are common at this stage. A more homogeneous opacification of the lung fields may develop over the next 48 hours as chemical pneumonitis becomes more of a problem. In severe cases, changes similar to chronic lung disease may develop over the next few weeks.

Uncontrolled trials of vigorous airway suction immediately after delivery suggest that it is possible to reduce the incidence of MAS. Intubation for lower airway suction is only needed if meconium can be seen below the vocal cords. Thoracic compression and routine bronchial lavage has no proven benefit. Intermittent positive-pressure ventilation with a relatively long expiratory time to prevent further gas trapping may be required in moderate to severe MAS. Surfactant replacement therapy in these infants with MAS has proven benefit, but large doses may be required. Extracorporeal membrane oxygenation (ECMO) may be used in the most severe cases.

3.4 Pneumonia

Pneumonia may be:

- **Congenital** — onset usually within 6 hours of birth
  - **Bacterial**
    - Streptococci (group B Strep. (GBS))
    - Coliforms (*E. coli*, Klebsiella, Serratia, Shigella, Pseudomonas, etc.)
    - Pneumococci
    - Listeria
  - **Viral**
    - CMV
    - Rubella
    - Herpes simplex
    - Coxsackie
  - **Other**
    - Toxoplasmosis
    - Chlamydia
    - *Ureaplasma ureolyticum*
    - Candida

- **Intrapartum** — onset usually within 48 hours
  - **Bacterial**
    - GBS
    - Coliforms (as above)
    - Haemophilus
    - Staphylococci
    - Pneumococci
    - Listeria
  - **Viral**
    - Herpes simplex
    - Varicella zoster
- **Nosocomial** — onset after 48 hours
  - **Bacterial**
    - Staphylococci
    - Streptococci
    - Pseudomonas
    - Klebsiella
    - Pertussis
  - **Viral**
    - Respiratory syncytial virus (RSV)
    - Adenovirus
    - Influenza viruses
    - Parainfluenza viruses
    - Common cold viruses
  - **Other**
    - *Pneumocystis carinii*

3.5 Pulmonary air leak

Pneumothorax

Occurs in up to 1% of otherwise healthy term infants (usually asymptomatic).

Overdistension of alveoli is more likely to occur in immature lungs because of a decreased number of pores of Kohn, which redistribute pressure between alveoli. Air ruptures through overdistended alveolar walls and moves towards the hilum where it enters the pleural or mediastinal space.

More common in surfactant deficiency, MAS, pneumonia and pulmonary hypoplasia.

Risk reduced by lower ventilator pressures to avoid overdistension, faster rate ventilation with shorter inspiratory times, paralysis of infants fighting the ventilator and surfactant replacement therapy.

Pulmonary interstitial emphysema (PIE)

May occur in up to 25% of VLBW infants, usually confined to those with the worst surfactant deficiency

- PIE may be more common in chorioamnionitis
- Alveolar rupture results in small cysts in the pulmonary interstitium
- Ventilation is difficult and mortality and incidence of chronic lung disease is high

Pneumomediastinum

- May complicate surfactant deficiency or other forms of neonatal lung disease, when it may coexist with pneumothorax or may be iatrogenic following tracheal rupture secondary to intubation
- No symptoms may occur in isolated pneumomediastinum, but respiratory and cardiovascular compromise are more likely to occur if pneumothorax is also present

3.6 Congenital lung problems

Pulmonary hypoplasia

Primary pulmonary hypoplasia is rare but may present with persistent tachypnoea which resolves with lung growth several months after birth.

Secondary pulmonary hypoplasia may be due to:

- Reduced amniotic fluid volume — Potter's syndrome (renal agenesis) or other severe congenital renal abnormalities resulting in markedly decreased urine volume (infantile (autosomal recessive) polycystic kidney disease, severe bilateral renal dysplasia, posterior urethral valves)
- Preterm rupture of membranes — only occurs if membranes ruptured before 26 weeks; 23% of pregnancies with rupture of membranes before 20 weeks are unaffected; outcome with rupture of membranes before 24 weeks is usually poor
- Amniocentesis — mild to moderate respiratory symptoms are more likely to occur in the neonatal period and incidence of respiratory symptoms in the first year of life are increased
- Lung compression — pulmonary hypoplasia is common in small-chest syndromes including asphyxiating thoracic dystrophy and thanatophoric dwarfism, diaphragmatic hernia, congenital cystic adenomatoid malformation and pleural effusions
- Reduced fetal movements — pulmonary hypoplasia occurs in congenital myotonic dystrophy, spinal muscular atrophy and other congenital myopathies

Outcome with pulmonary hypoplasia depends on the severity and the underlying cause.

Congenital diaphragmatic hernia

- Commonest congenital abnormality of the respiratory system — incidence 1 in 2,500–3,500 births.
- Twice as common in males.
- Other congenital malformations common: 30% have karyotype abnormalities and 17% have other lethal abnormalities; 39% have abnormalities in other systems — malrotation occurs in 20%; those with other congenital abnormalities have double the mortality rate.

- 90% are Bochdalek or posterolateral hernias.
- 85–90% are left-sided.
- Bilateral pulmonary hypoplasia occurs — ipsilateral >contralateral.
- Usually diagnosed on routine antenatal ultrasound. May present with polyhydramnios. Those that have a normal routine antenatal ultrasound scan are likely to have a better outcome as the hernia usually occurs later, allowing for reasonable lung growth. *In utero* repair and tracheal plugging has been attempted but with variable outcomes.
- Respiratory distress (usually severe), heart sounds on the right side of the chest, bowel sounds on the left side, a scaphoid abdomen and vomiting may be found at birth. Less severe cases may not present initially but develop increasing respiratory distress over the first 24 hours as the gut becomes more air-filled. Differential diagnosis is congenital cystic adenomatoid malformation (or even pneumothorax).

During resuscitation

- Bag and mask positive-pressure ventilation should be avoided
- Wide-bore nasogastric tube should be placed as soon as possible to deflate gut and to confirm diagnosis, and therefore distinguish between differential diagnoses of congenital cystic adenomatoid malformation or pneumothorax on subsequent CXR
- Consider paralysing baby to avoid air swallowing and to reduce the risk of pneumothorax

Surgical management

- There is some evidence to suggest that stabilizing the baby prior to surgery improves outcome
- Malrotation is corrected if present; the diaphragmatic defect is usually closed with a synthetic patch

Post-operative care

- High-frequency oscillation, nitric oxide or ECMO may be of benefit, but evidence for routine use of these is lacking
- Mortality overall is approximately 50–60%
- Survivors may have problems associated with underlying pulmonary hypoplasia

Congenital cystic adenomatoid malformation (CCAM)

- Rare, abnormal proliferation of bronchial epithelium, containing cystic and adenomatoid portions
- Lower lobes affected more frequently
- May disappear or become smaller spontaneously before or after birth
- Differential diagnosis is congenital diaphragmatic hernia
- Prognosis worse with associated hydrops, preterm birth and with type 3 lesions
- Recurrent infection and malignant change have been described

There are three types:

Type 1 CCAM

- Single or small number of large cyst
- Commonest type (50% cases)
- May cause symptoms by compression or be asymptomatic initially
- Good prognosis after surgery

Type 2 CCAM

- Multiple small cysts
- Usually cause symptoms by compression of surrounding normal lung
- Prognosis variable

Type 3 CCAM

- Airless mass of very small cysts giving the appearance of a solid mass
- Worst prognosis

Congenital lobar emphysema

- Affected lobe is overinflated
- Left upper lobe is affected most commonly (also right middle and upper lobes); rare in lower lobes
- More common in males
- Associated with congenital heart disease in 1:6 cases (usually due to compression of airways by aberrant vessels)
- Unaffected lobes in affected lung are compressed
- Mediastinal shift and compression of the contralateral lung may also occur
- Presents with signs of respiratory distress, wheezing, chest asymmetry and hyperresonance
- CXR shows hyperlucent affected lobe +/– compression of other lobes
- Reduced ventilation and perfusion of the affected lobe is seen on a ventilation/perfusion scan in more severe cases
- Surgical correction of underlying vascular abnormalities or resection of the affected lobe may be required, but symptoms and signs may resolve following bronchoscopy

Chylothorax

- Effusion of lymph into the pleural space due to either:
  - Underlying congenital abnormality of the pulmonary lymphatics
  - Iatrogenic following cardiothoracic surgery
- Diagnosis by antenatal ultrasound scan allows antenatal drainage by insertion of intercostal drains, which may reduce the risk of pulmonary hypoplasia and facilitate resuscitation after birth

- Ventilatory support may be required postnatally, along with intermittent intercostal drainage
- Volume of chyle can be reduced by using a medium-chain triglyceride milk formula or avoiding enteral feeds for up to several weeks as the underlying abnormality resolves with time; protein and lymphocyte depletion may complicate this
- Surgical treatment is needed for the small number of cases that do not resolve spontaneously

3.7 Chest wall abnormalities

Asphyxiating thoracic dystrophy

- Autosomal recessive
- Variable severity
- Short ribs with bell-shaped chest
- May have polydactyly and other skeletal abnormalities also
- Long-term prognosis good in infants who survive >1 year

Ellis van Crefeld syndrome

- Autosomal recessive
- Short ribs, polydactyly, congenital heart disease, cleft lip and palate
- Pulmonary hypoplasia is usually not severe and symptoms improve later

Short-rib polydactyly syndromes

- 4 variants — all autosomal recessive
- Death from severe respiratory insufficiency occurs in the neonatal period

Thanatophoric dysplasia

- Usually sporadic
- Very short limbs — femur X-ray described as 'telephone handle' shape
- Very small, pear-shaped chest
- Death from lung/chest hypoplasia occurs in the neonatal period

Camptomelic dysplasia

- Autosomal recessive
- Very bowed, shortened long bones
- Death from respiratory insufficiency usually occurs in childhood

3.8 Upper airway obstruction

Neonates are obligate nasal breathers.

Choanal atresia

- Incidence 1 in 8,000 (more common in females)
- Occurs due to failure of breakdown of bucconasal membrane
- May be unilateral or bilateral, bony or membranous
- 60% associated with other congenital abnormalities including the CHARGE association: C = colobomata, H = heart defects, A = atresia of choanae, R = retarded growth and development, G = genital hypoplasia in males, E = ear deformities
- Presents at birth with respiratory distress and difficulty passing a nasal catheter. Oral airway insertion relieves respiratory difficulties. Diagnosis confirmed by contrast study or CT scan
- Surgical correction by perforating or drilling the atresia requires post-operative nasal stents

Pierre Robin sequence

- Consists of protruding tongue, small mouth and jaw and cleft palate
- Incidence 1 in 2,000
- Problems include obstructive apnoea, difficulty with intubation and aspiration
- In order to maintain airway patency and prevent obstructive apnoea, prone position should be used initially; if this fails an oral airway should be inserted; intubation may be needed in severe cases which may eventually require tracheostomy
- Glossopexy and other surgical procedures have been attempted with some degree of success
- Gradual resolution of airway problems occurs as partial mandibular catch-up growth occurs during the first few years of life

Laryngomalacia

- Commonest cause of stridor in the first year of life
- Inspiratory stridor increases with supine position, activity, crying and upper respiratory tract infections
- Usually resolves during the second year of life
- Upper airway endoscopy is merited if persistent accessory muscle use occurs, with recurrent apnoea or failure to thrive

Subglottic stenosis

May be congenital but usually acquired.

Risk factors for acquired subglottic stenosis

- Prematurity
- Recurrent reintubation
- Prolonged intubation
- Traumatic intubation
- Inappropriately large or small endotracheal tube
- Black babies (keloid scar formation)
- Oral as opposed to nasal intubation (this is a theoretical but unproven factor)
- Gastro-oesophageal reflux
- Infection

Systemic steroids may facilitate extubation in mild to moderately severe subglottic stenosis. Laser or cryotherapy to granulomatous tissue seen on upper airway endoscopy may also be of benefit in these cases. Severely affected babies require surgery — anterior cricoid split or tracheostomy.

Tracheomalacia

Causes expiratory stridor. Usually caused from extrinsic compression — most commonly due to vascular rings. Also associated with tracheo-oesophageal fistula. Surgical treatment of underlying pathology usually leads to resolution, but tracheostomy and positive-pressure ventilation may be required.

3.9 Extracorporeal membrane oxygenation (ECMO)

A membrane 'lung' is used to rest the lungs and allow them to recover in severe respiratory failure. ECMO may be:

- Venoarterial (VA) — blood removed from right atrium (usually via right internal jugular vein) and returned via a common carotid artery
- Venovenous (VV) — a double-lumen, right atrial cannula is used

Consideration for ECMO should be made in severe neonatal respiratory failure if:

- Lung disease is reversible
- >35 weeks' gestation
- Weight >2 kg
- Cranial ultrasound scan with no intraventricular haemorrhage > grade 1
- No clotting abnormality
- Oxygenation index >40 (see below)

Oxygenation index (OI) is used to quantify the degree of respiratory failure.

$OI = $ (mean airway pressure $\times FiO_2 \times 100) \div PaO_2$ (post-ductal)
NB mean airway pressure is in cmH_2O, FiO_2 is a fraction, PaO_2 is in mmHg

OI >25 indicates severe respiratory failure. OI >40 indicates very severe respiratory failure with a predicted mortality of >80% with conventional treatment — therefore consideration to refer for ECMO is appropriate.

Other measures of the degree of respiratory failure that may be used include:

Alveolar–arterial oxygen difference (A–aDO_2)
$= (716 \times FiO_2) - (PaCO_2/0.8) - PaO_2$

Normal A–aDO_2 = <50 mmHg. If >600 mmHg for successive blood gases over 6 hours = severe respiratory failure with predicted mortality of >80% with conventional treatment

Ventilation index (VI) = PCO_2 × RR × PIP/1,000; where RR is the respiratory rate and PIP is the peak inspiratory pressure

VI >70 indicates severe respiratory failure. VI >90 indicates very severe respiratory failure — suitable for consideration of ECMO.

4. CARDIOVASCULAR PROBLEMS

4.1 Patent ductus arteriosus (PDA)

- Uncommon in term infants after 1–2 days
- Often presents around third day of life in VLBW infants as left to right shunt increases as pulmonary vascular resistance falls; approximately 40% of VLBW infants with surfactant deficiency have clinically significant PDA on day 3 of life
- Clinical signs — systolic or continuous murmur, bounding pulses, wide pulse pressure, active precordium and possibly signs of cardiac failure and reduced lower body perfusion
- A clinically significant PDA in VLBW infants is associated with an increased risk of
  - Pulmonary haemorrhage
  - Chronic lung disease
  - Intraventricular haemorrhage
  - Necrotizing enterocolitis (NEC)
  - Mortality
- Early treatment of PDA with indomethacin has been shown to reduce NEC and chronic lung disease
- Ibuprofen is likely to be equally effective in closing PDA but has less side-effects than indomethacin

4.2 Hypotension

Causes of hypotension in neonates

- Hypovolaemia
  - Antenatal acute blood loss
    - Placental abruption
    - Placenta praevia
    - Maternofetal haemorrhage
    - Twin to twin transfusion (usually not acute)
    - Vasa praevia
  - Postnatal acute blood loss
  - Internal
    - Intracranial haemorrhage
    - Intra-abdominal haemorrhage
    - Intrathoracic/pulmonary haemorrhage
    - Severe bruising
  - External
    - Dislodged vascular lines
- Excessive water loss
  - High urine output
  - High insensible losses — common in extreme prematurity
- 3rd spacing
  - Hydrops
  - Pleural effusions
  - Ascites
  - Post-operative
- Vasodilation
  - Common in preterm infants
  - Sepsis
  - Drug-induced (tolazoline, prostaglandins, prostacyclin)
- Cardiogenic
  - Myocardial dysfunction
    - Perinatal asphyxia
    - Metabolic acidosis
  - Congenital heart disease
    - Hypoplastic left heart
    - Other single-ventricle physiology conditions
  - Arrhythmias
    - Supraventricular tachycardia
    - Complete heart block
  - Reduced venous return
    - Pulmonary air leak
    - Pericardial effusion/tamponade
    - Lung hyperinflation (more common in HFO or with high positive end-expiratory pressure (PEEP))

4.3 Hypertension

Causes of hypertension in neonates

- Vascular
  - Renal artery thrombosis (associated with umbilical artery catheterization (UAC)
  - Aortic thrombosis (associated with UAC)
  - Renal vein thrombosis (more common in infants of diabetic mothers)
  - Renal artery thrombosis
  - Coarctation of aorta
  - Middle aortic syndrome
- Renal
  - Obstructive uropathy
  - Dysplastic kidneys
  - Polycystic disease
  - Renal tumours
- Intracranial hypertension
- Endocrine
  - Congenital adrenal hyperplasia
  - Hyperthyroidism
  - Neuroblastoma
  - Phaeochromocytoma
- Drug-induced
  - Systemic steroids
  - Inotropes
  - Maternal cocaine

4.4 Cyanosis in the newborn

Causes of cyanosis in the newborn

- Congenital cyanotic heart disease
  - Transposition of the great arteries (TGA)
  - Pulmonary atresia
  - Critical pulmonary stenosis
  - Severe tetralogy of Fallot
  - Tricuspid atresia
  - Ebstein's anomaly
  - Truncus arteriosus
  - Total anomalous pulmonary venous drainage (TAPVD)
  - Hypoplastic left heart syndrome
- PPHN
- Respiratory disease
- Methaemoglobinaemia
  - Arterial PO_2 is normal
  - Cause can be:
    - Congenital
      NADH-methaemoglobin reductase deficiency (autosomal recessive)
      Haemoglobin-M (autosomal dominant)
    - Iatrogenic
      Secondary to nitric oxide therapy
      Nitrate or nitrite ingestion
  - Treat with i.v. methylene blue
  - Acrocyanosis and facial bruising also give the appearance of cyanosis

5. GASTROENTEROLOGY AND NUTRITION

5.1 Necrotizing enterocolitis (NEC)

Incidence varies — usually about 10% VLBW infants.

Risk factors

- Prematurity
- Antepartum haemorrhage
- Perinatal asphyxia
- Polycythaemia
- PDA
- PROM

Early enteral feeding has also been suggested as NEC rarely occurs in infants who have not been fed. However, randomized controlled as a risk factor trials suggest that early feeding with small amounts of breast milk is beneficial. The incidence of NEC in preterm infants is

6–10 times higher in those fed formula milk compared to breast milk. There is some evidence that enteral vancomycin prior to initiating milk feeds, reduces the incidence of NEC.

The severity of NEC can be classified using Bell's staging:

Stage 1 — suspected NEC

- General signs — temperature instability, lethargy, apnoea
- Increased gastric aspirates, vomiting, abdominal distension

Stage 2 — confirmed NEC

- Stage 1 signs, plus
- Upper or lower gastrointestinal bleeding
- Intramural gas (pneumatosis intestinalis) or portal vessel gas on abdominal X-ray

Stage 3 — severe NEC

- Stage 1 and 2 signs, plus
- Signs of shock, severe sepsis and/or severe gastrointestinal haemorrhage
- Bowel perforation

Complications

- Perforation occurs in 20–30% of confirmed NEC
- Overwhelming sepsis
- Disseminated intravascular coagulation (DIC)
- Strictures — occur in approximately 20% cases of confirmed NEC
- Recurrent NEC — occurs in <5% cases (consider Hirschsprung's disease)
- Short-bowel syndrome following extensive resection
- Lactose intolerance

Medical management

- Cardiorespiratory support as required
- Stop enteral feeds for 7–14 days (depending on the severity of illness)
- NG tube on free drainage
- i.v. fluids/TPN
- i.v. antibiotics
- Treatment of thrombocytopenia, anaemia, DIC
- Serial abdominal X-rays (to exclude perforation)

Surgical management, may include

- Placement of peritoneal drain
- Early laparotomy — with resection of bowel +/– ileostomy/colostomy; indications for early surgery include perforation or failing medical management
- Late laparotomy +/– bowel resection; most common indication is stricture formation confirmed with contrast X-rays.

5.2 Composition of infant milks

		Breast	Term formula	Preterm formula	Cows' milk
Carbohydrate	g/100 ml	7.4	7.2	8.6	4.6
Protein	g/100 ml	1.1	1.5	2.0	3.4
Fat	g/100 ml	4.2	3.6	4.4	3.9
Sodium	mmol/100 ml	6.4	6.4	14	23
Potassium	mmol/100 ml	15	14	19	40
Calcium	mmol/100 ml	8.5	10.8	18	30
Phosphate	mmol/100 ml	5	10.6	13	32
Calories	per 100 ml	70	65	80	67

NB.   Cows' milk — increased casein:lactalbumin ratio (4:1, whereas breast milk = 2:3)

5.3 Maternal drugs and breast feeding

Drugs contraindicated in breast feeding mothers

- Amiodarone
- Antimetabolites (chemotherapy drugs)
- Atropine
- Chloramphenicol
- Dapsone
- Doxepin
- Ergotamine
- Gold
- Indomethacin
- Iodides
- Lithium
- Oestrogens (decrease lactation)
- Opiates (high dose should be avoided but weaning low dose may facilitate withdrawal in infant)
- Phenindione
- Vitamin D (risk of hypercalcaemia with high dose)

Maternal drugs that should be used with caution/monitoring if breast feeding

- Some antidepressants
- Some antihistamines
- Carbamazepine
- Carbimazole
- Clonidine
- Co-trimoxazole
- Ethambutol

- H$_2$ antagonists
- Isoniazid
- Gentamicin
- Metronidazole (makes milk taste bitter)
- Oral contraceptives
- Phenytoin
- Primidone
- Theophylline
- Thiouracil

If in doubt refer to *British National Formulary* or discuss with pharmacist.

5.4 Congenital abnormalities of the gastrointestinal system

Oesophageal atresia (OA) and tracheo-oesophageal fistula (TOF)

Occurs due to failure of development of primitive foregut. Incidence approximately 1:3,000.

- 85% — blind proximal oesophageal pouch with a distal oesophageal to tracheal fistula
- 10% — oesophageal atresia without fistula
- 5% — proximal +/– distal fistula

Clinical presentation

- Polyhydramnios
- Excessive salivation
- Early respiratory distress
- Abdominal distension
- Vomiting/choking on feeds
- Inability to pass NG tube
- Absence of gas in gut on X-ray if no TOF
- Other anomalies in 30–50%   VACTERL (**V**ertebral, **A**nal, **C**ardiac, **T**OF, **E**ars, **R**enal, **L**imb), rib anomalies, duodenal atresia
- Prematurity common

Management

- Respiratory support as needed.
- Riplogle tube (large-bore, double-lumen suction catheter) on continuous suction is placed in the proximal oesophageal pouch.
- Surgical management includes early division of the fistula and early or delayed oesophageal anastomosis. This depends on the distance between the two ends of atretic oesophagus — for wide gaps, delayed anastomosis to allow growth may improve outcome. Cervical oesophagostomy or colonic transposition may also be used in this situation.

H-type tracheo-oesophageal fistula (tracheo-oesophageal fistula without oesophageal atresia) is much less common and usually not associated with preterm birth or other severe anomalies. It may present in the neonatal period or later with respiratory distress associated with feeding, or recurrent lower respiratory infections.

Duodenal atresia

- Approximately 70% associated with other congenital anomalies (trisomy 21, congenital heart disease, malrotation, etc.)
- Often diagnosed antenatally with ultrasound 'double-bubble' or polyhydramnios
- Usually presents postnatally with bilious vomiting

Malrotation

- Occurs due to incomplete rotation of the midgut in fetal life resulting in intermittent and incomplete duodenal obstruction due to Ladd's bands
- Associated with diaphragmatic hernia, duodenal and other bowel atresias and situs inversus
- Presents with bilious vomiting and some abdominal distension with sudden deterioration in the event of midgut volvulus
- Upper gastrointestinal contrast studies show the duodenal–jejunal flexure on the right of the abdomen with a high caecum

Meconium ileus

- Commonest presentation of cystic fibrosis (CF) in neonates (10–15% cases)
- >90% babies with meconium ileus have CF, therefore need to confirm with genetic testing for all common mutations and serum immune reactive trypsin (IRT)
- May present with antenatal perforation, peritonitis and intra-abdominal calcification or postnatally with intestinal obstruction
- Water-soluble contrast enemas may lead to resolution of meconium ileus
- Important to distinguish between meconium ileus and meconium plug — with meconium plug, symptoms usually resolve after passage of plug and not associated with CF

Anorectal atresia

- May have other features of VACTERL association
- May be high or low with the puborectalis sling differentiating — more likely to be low lesion in females
- Colostomy is needed for all high atresias
- Renal tract ultrasound scan, micturating cystogram (MCUG) +/– cystoscopy needed to exclude rectovaginal, rectourethral or rectovesical fistula or other urinary tract anomaly
- High atresias often have problems with faecal incontinence, whereas those with intermediate/low lesions usually have good outcomes

Hirschsprung's disease

- Occurs due to absence of ganglion cells in either short or long segment of bowel; the rectum and sigmoid colon are most often affected, but cases extending to the upper GI tract have been described
- May present with delayed passage of meconium (>24 hours), bowel obstruction relieved by rectal examination (may be explosive!), enterocolitis or later constipation
- Diagnosis is made by rectal biopsy
- Regular rectal washouts are required prior to temporary colostomy formation (usually reversed at 6 months)

Exomphalos

- Results from failure of the gut to return into the abdominal cavity in the first trimester
- The defect is covered by peritoneum which may be ruptured at birth
- Approximately 75% cases have other congenital anomalies — trisomies, congenital heart disease, Beckwith–Wiedemann syndrome
- Primary or staged surgical closure is required

Gastroschisis

- Rarer than exomphalos and much less likely to be associated with other congenital anomalies
- Aetiology unknown but may be associated with teenage pregnancy
- Bowel is not covered by peritoneum and therefore gets stuck together with adhesions; this leads to functional atresias and severe intestinal motility problems post-surgical repair of the abdominal wall defect
- Prognosis is mostly good

6. NEUROLOGICAL PROBLEMS

6.1 Peri-intraventricular haemorrhage (PIVH)

The germinal matrix or layer occurs in the caudothalamic notch of the floor of the lateral ventricles. It is the site of origin of migrating neuroblasts from the end of the first trimester onwards. By 24–26 weeks' gestation this area has become highly cellular and richly vascularized. This remains so until 34 weeks' gestation by which time it has rapidly involuted. The delicate network of capillaries in the germinal matrix is susceptible to haemorrhage, which is likely to occur with changes in cerebral blood flow. Preterm infants have decreased cerebral blood flow autoregulation which contributes to the pathogenesis. In term infants PIVH may originate from the choroid plexus.

Risk factors for PIVH

- Prematurity (28% at 25 weeks; <5% after 30 weeks)
- Lack of antenatal maternal steroids
- Sick and needing artificial ventilation
- Hypercapnia
- Metabolic acidosis
- Pneumothoraces (due to increased venous pressure or possibly related to surge in blood pressure when drained)
- Abnormal clotting
- Rapid volume infusions (particularly with hypertonic solutions) or increases in blood pressure with inotropes
- Perinatal asphyxia
- Hypotension
- PDA

Timing of PIVH

- 50% in first 24 hours
- 10–20% in second 24 hours
- 10% after first week

Classification of PIVH

Grade 1 — germinal matrix haemorrhage
Grade 2 — intraventricular haemorrhage without ventricular dilatation
Grade 3 — intraventricular haemorrhage with blood distending the lateral ventricle
Grade 4 — echogenic intraparenchymal lesion associated with PIVH; previously this was thought to be extension of bleeding from the lateral ventricles into surrounding periventricular white matter, but is likely to be venous infarction.

Several classification systems have been described. The most widely accepted is that of Papile (above). It may, however, be better to use a more descriptive classification.

Prevention of PIVH
The following have been shown to reduce the incidence of PIVH:

- Antenatal steroids
- Maternal vitamin K
- Indomethacin (but long-term neurodisability not reduced)

The following have been evaluated but have no proven benefit:

- Vitamin E
- Ethamsylate
- Phenobarbital
- Fresh–frozen plasma (FFP)
- Nimodipine

Clinical presentation of PIVH

Grades 1 and 2 PIVH presents silently and are detected by routine ultrasonography. Grade 3 PIVH occasionally presents with shock from blood volume depletion. Grade 4 PIVH may present similarly and occasionally with neurological signs (seizures, hypotonia, bulging fontanelle).

Sequelae of PIVH

1. Death — 59% in one series of large grade 4 PIVH

2. Post-haemorrhagic ventricular dilatation (PHVD) — defined as lateral ventricle measurement >4 mm above 97th centile following PIVH

- 30% develop PHVD — higher risk with more severe lesions
- Spontaneous resolution occurs in approximately 50% of cases of PHVD, rest develop hydrocephalus (i.e. PHVD that requires drainage)
- As a sequel to PIVH, **communicating hydrocephalus** (due to malfunction of arachnoid villi) is more common than **non-communicating** (due to blockage of cerebral aqueduct)
- Early, aggressive intervention with repeated lumbar puncture and/or ventricular taps has not been shown to be of benefit; drainage should probably be considered if the baby is symptomatic, CSF pressure is very high (>12 mmHg or 15.6 cm CSF; normal CSF pressure is 5.25 mmHg or 6.8 cm CSF) or head circumference and/or ventricular measurement on ultrasound scan are increasing rapidly
- Timing of surgical intervention with CSF reservoir or ventriculoperitoneal shunt insertion is controversial
- Drug treatment with acetazolamide with or without diuretics has been shown to be ineffective
- Intraventricular fibrinolytic administration is experimental

3. Adverse neurodevelopment

Cerebral palsy is the commonest adverse neurodevelopmental sequel, but other and global problems may also arise. Approximate risk of adverse outcome is as follows:

- 4% in grades 1 and 2 PIVH if ventricles remain normal size
- 50% in grade 2 with PHVD or grade 3 PIVH
- 75% in PIVH requiring shunt
- 89% with large, grade 4 lesions (difficult to quantify as pathology varied)

6.2 Periventricular leucomalacia (PVL)

PVL is haemorrhagic necrosis in the periventricular white matter which progresses to cystic degeneration and subsequent cerebral atrophy. It is often associated with infection and may be cytokine-mediated. Hypoxia and ischaemia may also play a role. On ultrasound scan, the initial necrosis appears as echogenicity within a few days of the causative insult. This sometimes resolves, but may become a multicystic area after 1–4 weeks. The long-term neurological effects are usually bilateral, although initial ultrasound appearances are often unilateral.

Long-term neurodevelopmental effects of cystic PVL:

- Spastic diplegia or tetraplegia (>90%)
- Learning difficulties
- Seizures (including infantile spasms)
- Blindness

Worse outcomes are associated with subcortical PVL. Transient periventricular echodensities are associated with a risk of spastic diplegia of approximately 5–10% if they persist for more than 7–14 days.

6.3 Neonatal encephalopathy

Neonatal encephalopathy is also known as hypoxic–ischaemic encephalopathy (HIE). The underlying cause is often unclear but may have origin antenatally, peripartum or postnatally, hence the term 'perinatal asphyxia'. Other evidence of organ dysfunction often occurs concurrently, especially if the insult occurs close to the time of birth. Placental insufficiency is a factor in the vast majority of cases.

Pathophysiology of neonatal encephalopathy
Primary and secondary neuronal injury have been described.

Primary neuronal injury results from energy failure due to the inefficiency of anaerobic respiration to produce high-energy phosphocreatine and ATP. Glucose utilization increases and lactic acid accumulates. Energy failure and myocardial dysfunction further exacerbate this leading to ion-pump failure ($Na^+ - K^+$-ATPase) and neuronal death due to cerebral oedema.

Secondary or delayed neuronal injury occurs as there are marked changes in cerebral blood flow with initial hypoperfusion and then reperfusion following resuscitation. This is associated with neutrophil activation and exacerbated by prostaglandins, free radicals and other vasoactive substances. Excitatory amino acid neurotransmitters such as glutamate and *N*-methyl D-aspartate (NMDA) lead to excessive calcium influx and delayed neuronal death. The cellular mechanism for this may be necrosis or apoptosis (programmed cell death).

Clinical presentation
This can be staged according to the scheme suggested by Sarnat and Sarnat.

- Stage 1 — hyperalert, irritable; normal tone and reflexes.; signs of sympathetic overactivity; poor suck; no seizures; symptoms usually resolve <24 hours; good outcome in approximately 99%
- Stage 2 — Lethargic, obtunded, decreased tone and weak suck and Moro reflexes; seizures are common; approximately 75–80% have good outcomes; this is less likely if symptoms persist for >5 days
- Stage 3 — Comatose with respiratory failure; severe hypotonia and absent suck and Moro reflexes; seizures less common but EEG abnormalities common — flat background or burst suppression; over 50% die and majority of survivors have major handicap

Management is largely supportive but brain cooling may offer improved outcomes in the future.

6.4 Neonatal seizures

Causes of seizures in the newborn

- Neonatal encephalopathy
- Cerebral infarction:
  - Usually presents on day 1 or 2
  - Often presents with focal seizures
  - Aetiology uncertain but thrombosis secondary to hypercoagulation tendency is a possibility
  - Outcome good in approximately 50%; other 50% may develop mono- or hemiplegia or long-term seizure disorder
- Intracranial haemorrhage (massive PIVH, subarachnoid or subdural haemorrhage)
- Birth trauma (head injury equivalent)
- Meningitis
- Other sepsis
- Congenital infection
- Neonatal drug withdrawal
- Fifth-day fits (onset day 3–5, unknown cause, resolve spontaneously)
- Hypoglycaemia
- Hypocalcaemia
- Hypo- or hypermagnesaemia
- Inborn errors of metabolism:
  - Non-ketotic hyperglycinaemia
  - Sulphite oxidase deficiency
  - Biotinidase deficiency
  - Maple-syrup urine disease (MSUD)
  - Pyridoxine dependence
  - Urea cycle defects
  - Organic acidaemias (e.g. methylmalonic acidaemia)
- Structural brain abnormalities (migration disorders, etc.)
- Hydrocephalus
- Polycythaemia
- Neonatal myoclonus – not a true seizure, benign and common in preterm infants

Management of neonatal seizures

- Investigate for, and treat underlying condition
- Initial treatment with phenobarbital, followed by midazolam, other benzodiazepines and paraldehyde
- Currently no evidence that suppression of clinical or electrographic seizures improves outcome

6.5 Causes of hypotonia in the newborn

Central causes

- Neonatal encephalopathy
- Intracranial haemorrhage

501

- Infection — generalized sepsis, meningitis, encephalitis
- Chromosomal abnormalities — trisomy 21, 18 or 13
- Structural brain abnormalities — neuronal migration disorders, etc.
- Metabolic disease — amino and organic acidaemias, urea cycle defects, galactosaemia, non-ketotic hyperglycinaemia, peroxisomal disorders, mitochondrial disorders, congenital disorders of glycosylation (CDG), Menkes
- Drugs — opiates, barbiturates, benzodiazepines, etc.
- Prader–Willi syndrome
- Hypothyroidism
- Early kernicterus

Spinal cord lesions

- Trauma to the cervical spinal cord during delivery — usually involves traction and rotation with forceps
- Tumours, cysts and vascular malformations of spinal cord

Neuromuscular disease

- Spinal muscular atrophy
- Congenital myotonic dystrophy
- Congenital myopathies
- Myasthenia gravis

6.6 Retinopathy of prematurity (ROP)

ROP is abnormal retinal vascular development which occurs in preterm infants, usually after oxygen dependence. Neovascularization occurs due to hyperoxia which produces oxygen free-radical-induced changes in the presence of depleted antioxidant levels. Limiting hyperoxia and supplementation with vitamin E decreases the risk of severe ROP.

Preterm infants should be screened by indirect ophthalmological examination at 6 weeks of age and repeat examination should be made every two weeks until vascularization is complete at 40–42 weeks.

Staging of ROP

- Stage 1 — demarcation line between vascular (posterior) and avascular (anterior) zones
- Stage 2 — demarcation line forms a ridge
- Stage 3 — vascular proliferation occurs posterior to the ridge
- Stage 4 — subtotal retinal detachment
- Stage 5 — total retinal detachment

Plus disease occurs at any stage and includes vascular dilatation and tortuosity.
Stages 1 and 2 disease regresses with time and require no treatment. Stage 3 sometimes requires treatment with cryo- or laser therapy. (See also Chapter 16, *Ophthalmology*.)

7. GENITOURINARY PROBLEMS

7.1 Congenital abnormalities of the kidneys and urinary tract

Nephrogenesis (branching and new nephron induction) continues up to 36 weeks' gestation, but glomerular filtration rate (GFR) is still <5% of adult values at this stage. This increases rapidly in the 1st week and then more gradually over the next 2 years to adult values.

The renal function of a neonate is limited by:

- ↓ renal blood flow
- ↓ glomerular filtration rate
- ↓ tubular concentrating and diluting ability
- ↓ tubular excretion
- ↓ urine output

>90% neonates pass urine within 24 hours of birth. The collecting ducts have increased sensitivity to antidiuretic hormone (ADH) after birth and urine concentrating ability increases rapidly.

Preterm infants have immature tubular function leading to a high fractional excretion of sodium and high sodium intake requirements.

Antenatally, congenital renal abnormalities may present with:

- Oligohydramnios (Potter's syndrome if severe)
- Urinary ascites — due to obstructive uropathy
- Other abnormalities seen on antenatal ultrasound scan:
    - Obstructive uropathy — dilated renal tracts
    - Cystic dysplasia/polycystic disease

Obstructive uropathy

Posterior urethral valves

- Mucosal folds in posterior urethra of male infants leading to dilatation of renal tract proximal to obstruction
- Bladder is often hypertrophied
- Diagnosed by micturating cystourogram (MCUG)
- Suprapubic catheter is inserted initially, followed by surgical resection by cystoscopy or vesicostomy, followed by later resection

Pelviureteric junction (PUJ) obstruction

- Usually unilateral
- Diagnosed on antenatal ultrasound scan or presents with abdominal mass
- Gross hydronephrosis is associated with decreased renal function (confirmed with $^{99}Tc^m$ MAG-3 (mertiatide) renogram), nephrectomy is usually required. Ureteroplasty is carried out for milder cases

Mild renal pelvis dilatation

- Should be confirmed on postnatal ultrasound scan and investigated with MCUG to exclude reflux nephropathy, which is a risk for recurrent urinary tract infection and subsequent scarring

Prune-belly syndrome (megacystis-megaureter)

- Lax abdominal musculature, dilated bladder and ureters and undescended testes
- Neurogenic bladder
- Usually due to abnormalities of lumbosacral spine

Ureterocele

- Dilatation of distal ureter leading to obstruction

Urethral stricture

Tumours (Wilms' tumour, neuroblastoma)

7.2 Haematuria in the newborn

Causes of haematuria in the newborn

- UTI
- Obstructive uropathy
- Acute tubular necrosis
- Renal artery or vein thrombosis
- Renal stones
- Trauma
- Tumours
- Cystic dysplasia and other malformations
- Abnormal clotting

7.3 Causes of acute renal failure in neonates

Pre-renal

- Hypotension
- Dehydration
- Indomethacin

Renal

- Cystic dysplasia and infant polycystic kidney disease
- Renal artery/vein thrombosis
- Congenital nephrotic syndrome
- DIC
- Nephrotoxins — gentamicin

Post-renal

- Obstructive nephropathy

7.4 Ambiguous genitalia

See (section 1.5) for embryology of sexual differentiation.

On examination, note the following:

- If gonads are palpable they are nearly always testes
- Length of phallus — if <2.5 cm stretched length in a term baby it is unlikely that the baby can function as a male
- Severity of hypospadias and fusion of labia
- Other dysmorphic features/congenital abnormalities

The parents should be told that the child's sex is uncertain at this stage and that the genitalia are not normally/completely formed. Prompt diagnosis and appropriate management is essential to resolve this and to exclude or treat congenital adrenal hyperplasia (CAH) before electrolyte imbalances occur. Also gonadal tumours may be a risk.

Differential diagnosis

- True hermaphroditism:
  - Testes and ovaries both present (rare)
- Male pseudohermaphroditism:
  - Underdevelopment ($\downarrow$ virilization) of male features
    - Androgen insensitivity (= testicular feminization) — most common
    - Defects in testosterone synthesis

    Some forms of CAH
    Panhypopituitarism (should be suspected if hypoglycaemia also present):
    - Defects in testosterone metabolism (5α-reductase most common)
    - Defects in testicular differentiation (rare)
- Female pseudohermaphroditism
  - Virilization of female:
    - CAH — commonest enzyme deficiency is 21–hydroxylase deficiency ($\uparrow$ 17α-hydroxyprogesterone)
- Chromosomal abnormalities
  - 45X/46XY mosaicism (rare)

Investigations

- Karyotype
- Daily electrolytes until diagnosis established
- Blood pressure monitoring
- Blood sugar monitoring

- Abdominal ultrasound scan
- Serum hormone assay — 17α-hydroxyprogesterone, 11–deoxycortisol, testosterone, oestradiol, progesterone, luteinizing hormone (LH), follicle-stimulating hormone (FSH)
- Urine steroid profile
- Genitogram/MCUG

8. INFECTION

8.1 Bacterial infection

Group B Streptococcus (GBS)

- Up to 20% pregnant women have genital tract colonization with GBS
- 3 serotypes identified
- Neonatal GBS infection may be early (within first few days, usually presenting by 24 hours) or late (after first week, usually at 3–4 weeks)
- Early disease often presents with septicaemia and respiratory distress (pneumonia or PPHN)
- Late disease is usually septicaemia or meningitis — may be vertical or nosocomial transmission; antibiotics given intrapartum or in first few days do not always prevent late GBS disease
- Serotype 3 is more common in late-onset GBS disease or meningitis if this is part of early-onset disease

E. Coli

- Usually causes vertical infections in neonates and is often associated with preterm birth; can also cause nosocomial infection
- K1 capsular antigen is commonest serotype
- Septicaemia and meningitis are commonest presentations if vertically transmitted; UTI and necrotizing enterocolitis (NEC) have been noted in nosocomial *E. coli* sepsis in neonates

Coagulase-negative Staphylococci

- Commonest nosocomial pathogen in neonatal intensive care units
- VLBW infants with indwelling catheters are most at risk
- Often resistant to flucloxacillin

Listeria monocytogenes

- Gram-positive rod
- Outbreaks have been caused by dairy products, coleslaw, paté and undercooked meat
- May present with a flu-like illness in pregnant women and then lead to stillbirth or severe neonatal septicaemia and meningitis
- Early- and late-onset disease have been noted similar to GBS

- Early-onset disease is associated with preterm birth and 'meconium'-stained amniotic fluid (often pus rather than meconium)
- A maculopapular or pustular rash is typical
- Amoxicillin and gentamicin is the antibiotic combination of choice

Other bacterial pathogens in neonates include

- *Haemophilus influenzae*
- *Klebsiella* spp.
- *Pseudomonas* spp.
- Pneumococcus

Risk factors for vertically acquired bacterial sepsis

- Preterm rupture of membranes
- Prolonged rupture of membranes (>12–24 hours)
- Maternal fever (>38°C or other signs of chorioamnionitis — e.g. WCC >15 × 10⁹/l)
- Maternal colonization with GBS
- Fetal tachycardia
- Lack of intrapartum antibiotics in the presence of above risk factors
- Foul-smelling amniotic fluid
- Preterm birth/low birth weight
- Twin pregnancy
- Low Apgar scores

Risk factors for nosocomial sepsis

- Prematurity/low birth weight
- Small for gestational age infants
- Neutropenia
- Indwelling catheters
- TPN
- Surgery

8.2 Congenital viral infection

Cytomegalovirus (CMV)

- Member of Herpersviridae family (DNA virus)
- Transmitted by close personal contact, blood products or breast feeding. May also be sexually transmitted.
- Causes mild symptoms in healthy adults or children
- Up to 1% of pregnancies are affected but symptoms occur in less than 10% of those infected
- Primary infection or reactivation may occur in affected pregnancies
- Symptoms in affected neonates include:
  - IUGR
  - Prematurity

- Hepatosplenomegaly
- Thrombocytopenia
- Anaemia
- Jaundice (raised conjugated and unconjugated bilirubin — often prolonged)
- Pneumonitis
- Microcephaly
- Intracranial calcification
- Choroidoretinitis
- Osteitis
- Long-term neurodevelopmental sequelae are common and include cerebral palsy, learning disability, epilepsy, blindness and deafness

Diagnosis

- Rising specific IgG antibodies in mother or baby
- Specific IgM may be raised for up to 16 weeks after primary infection
- Virus can be isolated from urine or throat swab
- Detection of early-antigen fluorescent foci (DEAFF) is a newer technique used to detect viral antigen from urine and other body fluids
- Ancyclovir has been used with some success in immunosuppressed adults but may be toxic in neonates and is not of proven efficacy

Rubella

First-trimester infection of the fetus results in congenital rubella syndrome. The most common features of this are:

- Congenital heart disease
- Cataracts
- Deafness

IUGR, microcephaly, hepatosplenomegaly, thrombocytopenia, choroidoretinitis, osteitis may also occur similar to congenital CMV infection. Vaccination of children has virtually eradicated congenital rubella in the UK.

Toxoplasmosis

Toxoplasma gondii is a unicellular, protozoan parasite. Cats are the definitive hosts. Infection of humans occurs following ingestion of sporocysts after handling cat faeces or in contaminated vegetables or undercooked meat. Toxoplasmosis is a mild illness in healthy adults.

Congenital infection is more likely with increasing gestation as the placenta provides less of a barrier with age. However, severe infection becomes less likely, falling from 75% in the first trimester to <5% in the third.

Severe congenital toxoplasmosis causes:

- IUGR
- Preterm birth
- Hydrocephalus and sequelae
- Choroidoretinitis
- Intracranial calcification
- Hepatitis
- Pneumonia
- Myocarditis

Babies born with no symptoms may go on to develop choroidoretinitis after months or even years. Serological diagnosis is made by specific IgG and IgM titres. Treatment of affected pregnant women with spiramycin reduces the rate of transmission to the fetus but does not reduce the severity of disease. Affected infants are treated with pyrimethamine and sulfadiazine for up to 1 year.

Parvovirus

Parvovirus is a DNA virus. Serotype B19 causes epidemics of erythema infectiosum ('Slapped cheeks' syndrome or Fifth disease) in winter months. Fetal infection, particularly in the first trimester, leads to severely decreased red cell production and subsequent severe fetal anaemia, resulting in heart failure and non-immune hydrops. Fetal blood can be used to confirm the diagnosis by viral antigen detection with PCR. Fetal blood transfusions may reverse hydrops and improve outcome.

Neonatal HIV

Vertically transmitted HIV is the commonest cause of childhood AIDS. Approximately a third of infections are transmitted across the placenta and two-thirds during birth. Babies of all HIV positive mothers are also seropositive initially as IgG crosses the placenta. Non-infected infants become negative by 9 months. There is no evidence of HIV causing an embryopathy. Babies are usually initially asymptomatic but may present with hepatosplenomegaly and thrombocytopenia in the neonatal period. The following increase the risk of vertical transmission:

- Low maternal CD4 count
- High maternal viral load
- Presence of p24 Ag in mother
- Preterm birth
- Rupture of membranes >4 hours
- Vaginal birth
- No maternal anti-retroviral treatment/poor compliance

Maternal zidovudine (AZT) during 3rd trimester and labour and to baby for 6 weeks post-natally reduces transmission rate from 25.5% to 8.3%. Other measures leading to avoidance of above risk factors have been shown to reduce risk further to well under 5%.

Vaccinations should be given routinely to infants of HIV-positive mothers apart from:

- Give killed (Salk) rather than live (Sabin) polio vaccine
- Give BCG early

Hepatitis B

- Babies of women who are HbsAg-positive or who have active hepatitis B during pregnancy should all receive hepatitis B vaccine in the neonatal period, and at 1 and 6 months.
- Hepatitis B immunoglobulin should be given within 48 hours of birth to all babies of mothers who are HbsAg-positive apart from those with the HbeAb
- Breast feeding is not contraindicated

8.3 Fungal infection

Candida albicans may cause superficial mucocutaneous infection or severe systemic sepsis, particularly in extremely preterm infants. Amphotericin, flucytosine and fluconazole may be used to treat severe fungal infections.

9. NEONATAL JAUNDICE

9.1 Physiological jaundice

Jaundice becomes visible when serum bilirubin (SBR) >80–100 mmol/l and up to 65% term infants become clinically jaundiced. However, only 1.2% become significantly jaundiced requiring treatment (i.e. >340 mmol/l). Physiological jaundice occurs due to:

- Increased haemolysis:
  - Bruising
  - Antibody-induced
  - Relative polycythaemia
  - Life span of RBCs (term — 70 days, preterm 40 days)
- Immature hepatic enzyme systems
- 'Shunt' bilirubin from breakdown of non-RBC haem pigments
- Enterohepatic circulation

Breast fed babies have higher max. SBR and remain jaundiced for longer

9.2 Causes of non-physiological jaundice

Non-physiological jaundice if any of the following are present:

- Onset before 24 hours of age
- 270 mmol/l
- Lasting >14 days (>21 days in preterm)
- Associated with pathological conditions known to cause jaundice

Causes of non-physiological jaundice (unconjugated hyperbilirubinaemia)

- Haemolysis
  - Isoimmunization (Rh, ABO, other)
  - Spherocytosis, etc.
  - G6PD or PK deficiency
  - Sepsis
  - α-Thalassaemia
- Polycythaemia
- Extravasated blood
- Increased enterohepatic circulation
- Endocrine/metabolic
- Rare liver enzyme deficiencies (Crigler–Najjar syndrome, etc.)

Haemolytic disease of the newborn

May be caused by Rhesus D (Rh) incompatibility (mother Rh D-negative, baby Rh D-positive) or by other antibodies (c, E, Kell, Duffy, etc.). Approximately 15% of the UK population are Rh D-negative. Sensitization occurs from previous pregnancy, antepartum haemorrhage, trauma or antenatal procedure.

Prevention of haemolytic disease is by the following:

- Intramuscular anti-D is given following any possible event leading to sensitization in Rh D-negative women
- Maternal serum screening for antibodies at booking with retesting between 28 and 36 weeks for Rh D-negative women with no antibodies
- Referral to a specialist fetal medicine centre for all those with significant levels of antibodies; initially antibody levels are measured but correlate poorly with the degree of fetal anaemia above a certain threshold; once this is reached, further monitoring is by ultrasound scanning to detect signs of hydrops, amniocentesis and spectrophotometric estimation of bilirubin in the amniotic fluid or fetal blood sampling to detect anaemia
- Serial fetal blood transfusions in severe cases
- Preterm delivery

Causes of conjugated hyperbilirubinaemia:

- TPN cholestasis
- Viral hepatitis (hepatitis B, CMV, herpesvirus, rubella, HIV, coxsackievirus, adenovirus)
- Other infection (Toxoplasmosis, syphilis, bacterial)
- Haemolytic disease (due to excessive bilirubin)
- Metabolic (α1-antitrypsin deficiency, CF, galactosaemia, tyrosinaemia, Gaucher's and other storage diseases, Rotor syndrome, Dubin–Johnson syndrome)
- Biliary atresia
- Choledochal cyst
- Bile-duct obstruction from tumours, haemangiomas, etc.

10. MISCELLANEOUS NEONATAL PROBLEMS

10.1 Haemorrhagic disease of the newborn and vitamin K

- Due to relative deficiency of factors II, VII, IX and X and prevented by vitamin K
- Breast milk contains inadequate amounts of vitamin K, therefore the recommendation in UK is to give all babies either a single i.m. injection of vitamin K at birth or an oral dose at birth followed by two further oral doses at 1–2 weeks and 6 weeks in those that are predominantly breast fed.
- May be exacerbated by perinatal asphyxia, liver dysfunction and maternal phenytoin or phenobarbital
- Usually presents between days 2 and 6 with gastrointestinal haemorrhage, umbilical stump bleeding, nose bleeds or intracranial haemorrhage
- Prothrombin time (PT) and activated partial thromboplastin (APTT) are prolonged with normal thrombin time and fibrinogen
- Treat with FFP and i.v. vitamin K +/– blood transfusion
- Late haemorrhagic disease may occur between 8 days and 6 months; intracranial haemorrhage is more common in these cases

10.2 Congenital dislocation of the hip

- Also known as 'developmental dysplasia of the hip'
- 4 times more common in girls; also more common with positive family history, 1st pregnancy and breech delivery
- Clinical examination with Ortolani (abduction) and Barlow (adduction) may miss up to 50% cases; a second examination and ultrasound scan screening have been shown to decrease this
- Approximately one-third of cases resolve with little or no intervention; more severe cases require flexion and abduction with a harness or hip spica device; very few cases require surgery

11. FURTHER READING

A review of the therapeutic efficacy and clinical tolerability of a natural surfactant preparation (Curosurf) in Neonatal Respiratory distress syndrome: Wiseman LR, Bryson HM. *Drugs* **48**(3):386–403, 1994.

Breast milk and neonatal necrotising enterocolitis: Lucas A, Cole TJ, *Lancet* **336** (8730):1519–23, 1990.

Breast milk and subsequent intelligence quotient in children born preterm: Lucas A, Morley R, Cole TJ, Lister G, Leeson-Payne C, *Lancet.* **339**(8788):261–4, 1992.

Current topics in Neonatology: TN Hansen, McIntosh N (eds), Volume 3, pp 43–61, W.B. Saunders, 1999.

Early diet of preterm infants and development of allergic or atopic disease: randomised prospective study: Lucas A, Brooke OG, Morley R, Cole TJ, Bamford MF. *BMJ* **300**(6728):837–40, 1990.

Fetal and Neonatal Physiology: Polin RA, Fox WW (eds), 2nd edition. WB Saunders 1998.

Neonatal drug withdrawal: American Academy of Pediatrics Committee on Drugs. *Pediatrics* **101**(6):1079–88, 1998.

Neonatal respiratory disorders: Greenough A, Robertson NRC, Milner AD (eds). Arnold 1996.

Neurologic and developmental disability after extremely preterm birth: Wood NS, Marlow N, Costeloe K, Gibson AT, Wilkinson AR. EPICure Study Group. [see comments]. *New England Journal of Medicine* **343**(6):378–84, 2000.

Pulmonary problems in the new-born and their sequelae. Yu VYH (ed.). *Balliere's Clinical Paediatrics* 3:1, 1995.

Surfactant replacement therapy for meconium aspiration syndrome: Findlay RD, Taeusch HW, Walther FJ. *Pediatrics* **97**:48–52, 1996.

Textbook of Neonatology: Rennie JM, Roberton NRC (eds), 3rd edition. Chap. 44, pp 1252–71, Churchill Livingstone, 1999.

The EPICure study: outcomes to discharge from hospital for infants born at the threshold of viability: Costeloe K, Hennessy E, Gibson AT, Marlow N, Wilkinson AR. *Pediatrics* **106**(4):659–71, 2000.

UK Collaborative randomised trial of neonatal ECMO: UK Collaborative ECMO Trial Group. *Lancet* **348**:75–82, 1996.

Chapter 14

Nephrology

Christopher J D Reid

CONTENTS

Nephrology

1. EMBRYOLOGY

- At the start of week 5 of embryogenesis, the **ureteric bud** appears
- Small branch of the mesonephric duct
- Evolves into a tubular structure which elongates into the **primitive mesenchyme** of the **nephrogenic ridge**
- Ureteric bud forms the ureter and from week 6 onwards repeated branching gives rise to the calyces, papillary ducts and collecting tubules by week 12
- The branching elements also induce the mesenchyme to develop into nephrons — proximal and distal tubules and glomeruli
- Branching and new nephron induction continues until week 36
- Abnormalities in the signalling between branching ureteric bud elements and the primitive mesenchyme probably underlie important renal malformations including renal dysplasia
- There are on average 600,000 nephrons per kidney; premature birth and low weight for gestational age may both be associated with reduced nephron numbers
- This in turn may underlie the later development of glomerular hyperfiltration, glomerular sclerosis and hypertension and may explain the firmly established inverse association between birth weight and later adult-onset cardiovascular morbidity

2. FETAL AND NEONATAL RENAL FUNCTION

The placenta receives 50% of fetal cardiac output and the fetal kidneys only 5% of cardiac output. By 36 weeks' gestational age nephrogenesis is complete, but GFR <5% of adult value.

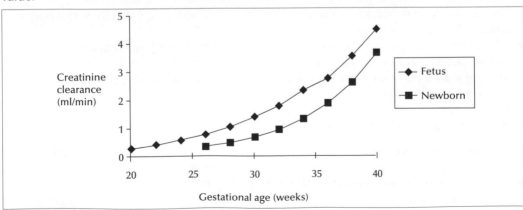

Creatinine clearance (ml/min) in the human fetus and newborn infant

The glomerular filtration rate (GFR) of term infants at birth is approximately 25 ml/min per 1.73 m², increasing by 50–100% during the first week, followed by a more gradual increase to adult values by the second year of life.

The ratio of excreted to filtered sodium, expressed as a percentage. It is calculated as:

$$\frac{\text{Urine Na (mmol/l)}}{\text{Urine creatinine (\mu mol/l)}} \times \frac{\text{Plasma creatinine (\mu mol/l)}}{\text{Plasma Na (mmol/l)}} \times 100\%.$$

- Normal FENa in older children and adults is around 1% and <1% in the sodium- and water-deprived states.
- It is very high in the premature fetus, falling with increasing gestation; and it is significantly lower in the newborn (see figure below), as the kidney adapts to the demands of extrauterine life where renal tubular conservation of sodium and water is important.
- Premature neonates still have a relatively high FENa due to immature renal tubular function and require extra sodium supplementation to avoid hyponatraemia.

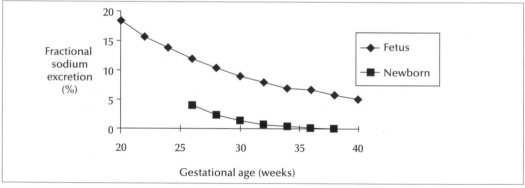

Fractional sodium excretion (%) in the human fetus and newborn infant

- Urine concentrating capacity is low in the premature newborn and leads to susceptibility to dehydration. Fully mature urine concentrating capacity is reached later in the first year of life.
- The plasma bicarbonate concentration at which filtered bicarbonate appears in the urine (bicarbonate threshold) is low in the newborn (19–21 mmol/l), increasing to mature values of 24–26 mmol/l by 4 years. Hence plasma bicarbonate values are lower in infants.

Abnormalities in fetal renal function and morphology are mainly inferred from:

- **Volume of amniotic fluid** — urinary tract obstruction, and/or reduced production of urine by dysplastic kidneys, leads to oligo- or anhydramnios
- **Appearance of kidneys on antenatal ultrasound** — bright echogenicity, lack of corticomedullary differentiation, cyst formation and hydronephrosis are all signs of fetal renal abnormality

Invasive assessment of fetal renal function includes sampling of fetal urine by fine-needle aspiration from the fetal bladder.

- Usually reserved for selected cases of fetal obstructive uropathy, classically caused by **posterior urethral valves** (PUV) in male fetuses
- Analysis of fetal urinary electrolytes and amino acid composition may give further information about fetal renal function and prognosis for postnatal renal function
- Typically, features of poor prognosis for renal function (in addition to oligohydramnios and abnormal ultrasound appearance as detailed above) include high urinary sodium and amino acid levels (implying tubular damage and failure to reabsorb these)
- Severe oligohydramnios may lead to pulmonary hypoplasia; this is the major determinant of whether newborns with congenital renal abnormalities live or die in the immediate postnatal period

3. COMMON UROLOGICAL ABNORMALITIES

3.1 Hydronephrosis

This is dilation of the pelvicalyceal system. Main causes are:

- Vesicoureteric reflux (VUR) — see section 12.1
- Pelviureteric junction (PUJ) obstruction:
    - Usually detected on antenatal ultrasound (US) scan
    - Occasionally detected during investigation of UTI or abdominal pain
    - Main aspects of assessment are:
        - Ultrasound: degree of renal pelvic dilatation measured in the anteroposterior diameter: 5–10 mm, mild; 11–15 mm, moderate; >15 mm, severe
        - MAG-3 renogram: findings that suggest significant obstruction are (a) poor drainage despite furosemide (frusemide) given during scan, and (b) impaired function, e.g. <40% on hydronephrotic side
        - Surgical correction is by pyeloplasty; usual when MAG-3 indicates obstruction, and/or US shows progressive increase in hydronephrosis: when dilatation >30 mm, surgery likely
- Vesicoureteric junction obstruction
    - As for PUJ obstruction, but much less common
    - US shows renal pelvic and ureteric dilatation
    - Interventions include stenting the VUJ (temporary measure); and surgical reimplantation

3.2 Duplex kidney

- Often detected on antenatal US, or during investigation of UTI
- Two ureters drain from two separate pelvicalyceal systems; ureters sometimes join before common entry into bladder, but more commonly have separate entries, with upper-pole ureter inserting below lower-pole ureter

- Common complications associated with duplex systems are:
  - Obstructed hydronephrotic upper moiety and ureter, often poorly functioning, associated with bladder ureterocele
    - Dilatation and swelling of submucosal portion of ureter just proximal to stenotic ureteric orifice; can be seen on bladder US, and as filling defect on MCUG
  - Ectopically inserted upper-pole ureter, entering urethra or vagina; clue to this from history is true continual incontinence with no dry periods at all
  - VUR into lower-pole ureter, sometimes causing infection and scarring of this pole

3.3 Multicystic dysplastic kidney

- Irregular cysts of variable size from small to several centimetres; no normal parenchyma
- Dysplastic atretic ureter
- No function on 99Tc^m MAG-3 or 99Tc^m DMSA (dimercaptosuccinic acid) scan
- 20–40% incidence of VUR into contralateral normal kidney

3.4 Polycystic kidneys — see section 15.1

3.5 Horseshoe kidney

- Two renal segments fused across midline at lower poles in 95%, upper in 5%
- Isthmus usually lies low, at level of 4th lumbar vertebra immediately below origin of inferior mesenteric artery
- Associations include Turner's syndrome, Laurence–Moon–Biedl syndrome
- Usually asymptomatic, but increased incidence of PUJ obstruction and VUR, so may develop UTI

3.6 Hypospadias

- Opening of urethral meatus on ventral surface of penis, at any point from glans to base of penis or even perineum
- Meatus may be stenotic and require meatotomy as initial intervention
- Foreskin is absent ventrally; it is used in surgical reconstruction of deficient urethra and so circumcision should not be performed
- Chordee is the associated ventral curvature of penis, seen especially during erection, and this requires surgical correction also; due to fibrous tissue distal to meatus along ventral surface of penis

3.7 Bladder extrophy and epispadias

- Commoner in males

- Bladder mucosa exposed, and with exposure and infection becomes friable; bladder muscle becomes fibrotic and non-compliant
- Anus anteriorly displaced
- Males: penis has epispadias (dorsal opening urethra) and dorsal groove on glans, with dorsal chordee and upturning; scrotum shallow and testes often undescended
- Girls: female epispadias with bifid clitoris, widely separated labia
- Pubic bones separated
- Requires surgical reconstruction; long-term urinary incontinence common

4. PHYSIOLOGY

4.1 Glomerular filtration rate (GFR)

GFR is determined by:

- The transcapillary hydrostatic pressure gradient across the glomerular capillary bed (ΔP), favouring glomerular filtration
- The transcapillary oncotic pressure gradient ($\Delta \pi$), countering glomerular filtration
- Permeability coefficient of the glomerular capillary wall, k

Hence GFR = $k(\Delta P - \Delta \pi)$

GFR is expressed as a function of body surface area. Absolute values for GFR in ml/min are corrected for surface area (SA) by the formula:

Corrected GFR (ml/min per 1.73 m^2) = absolute GFR (ml/min) $\times$ 1.73/SA

1.73 m^2 is the surface area of an average adult male. Normal mature GFR values are 80–120 ml/min per 1.73 m^2 and are reached during the second year of life.

GFR can be:

1. **Estimated by a calculated value** using the Schwartz formula:

   $$\frac{\text{Height (cm)} \times 49}{\text{Plasma creatinine (μmol/l)}} = \text{ml/min per 1.73 m}^2$$

This method will tend to overestimate GFR in malnourished children with poor muscle mass.

2. **Measured** by single-injection plasma disappearance curve, using inulin or a radioisotope such as chromium-labelled EDTA (ethylenediaminetetra-acetic acid). Following an intravenous injection of a known amount of one of these substances, a series of timed blood samples are taken over 3–5 hours and the slope of the curve generated by the falling

plasma levels of the substance gives the GFR. This technique does **not** require any urine collection, thus making it suitable for routine clinical use.

NB. Creatinine clearance, based on a timed urine collection and paired plasma sample using the formula:

$$\frac{\text{Urine creatinine (µmol/l)} \times \text{urine flow rate (ml/min)}}{\text{Plasma creatinine (µmol/l)}},$$

overestimates the true GFR since creatinine is secreted by the tubules.

4.2 Renal tubular physiology

The renal tubules play a fundamental role in:

- maintaining extracellular fluid volume
- maintaining electrolyte and acid–base homeostasis

These processes are energy-demanding and render tubular cells most vulnerable to ischaemic damage and acute tubular necrosis (ATN). The proximal tubule (PT) and Loop of Henle (LoH) are the sites of major reabsorption of most of the glomerular filtrate.

The distal tubule (DT) and collecting duct (CD) is where 'fine tuning' of the final composition of the urine occurs.

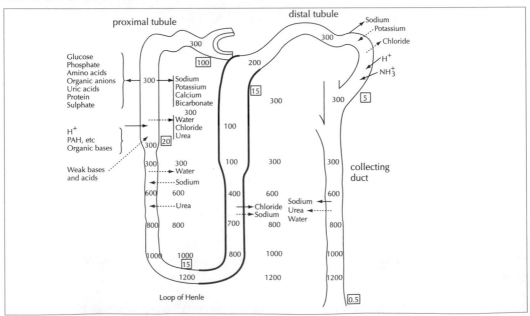

Diagram of tubular function, showing sites of active (solid arrows) and passive (broken arrows) transport. The boxed numbers indicate the percentage of glomerular filtrate remaining in the tubule, and the non-boxed numbers the osmolality of the tubular fluid under conditions of antidiuresis

Proximal tubule

The primary active transport system is the Na^+–K^+–ATPase enzyme, reabsorbing 50% of filtered Na. Secondary transport involves coupling to the Na^+–H^+ antiporter, which accounts for 90% of **bicarbonate** reabsorption with some Cl.

In addition:

- **Glucose** is completely reabsorbed unless the plasma level is high, when glycosuria will occur
- **Amino acids** are completely reabsorbed, though premature and term neonates commonly show a transient aminoaciduria
- **Phosphate** is 80–90% reabsorbed under the influence of parathyroid hormone (PTH), which reduces reabsorption and enhances excretion of phosphate
- **Calcium** is 95% reabsorbed — 60% in PT; 20% in LoH; 10% in DT; 5% in CD
- A variety of organic solutes, including creatinine and urate, and some drugs, including trimethoprim and most diuretics, are secreted in the PT

Loop of Henle

- A further 40% of filtered Na is reabsorbed via the Na–K–2Cl co-transporter in the thick ascending limb of the LoH
- The medullary concentration gradient is generated here as this segment is impermeable to water
- Loop diuretics block Cl binding sites on the co-transporter
- There is an inborn defect in Cl reabsorption at this same site in Bartter's syndrome — (see section 7.2, *Loop of Henle*)

Distal tubule

- A further 5% of filtered Na is reabsorbed here, via a Na–Cl co-transporter
- Thiazide diuretics compete for these Cl-binding sites; and may have a powerful effect if combined with loop diuretics which increase NaCl and water to the DT
- Aldosterone-sensitive channels (also present in the collecting duct) are involved in regulating K secretion. K secretion is proportional to:
  - Distal tubular urine flow rate
  - Distal tubular Na delivery: so natriuresis is associated with increased K secretion and hypokalaemia (e.g. Bartter's syndrome; loop diuretics)
  - Aldosterone level: so conditions of elevated aldosterone are associated with hypokalaemia
  - $[pH]^{-1}$

Collecting duct

- A final 2% of filtered Na is reabsorbed via aldosterone-sensitive Na channels, in exchange for K
- Spironolactone binds to and blocks the aldosterone receptor, explaining its diuretic and K-sparing actions
- H^+ secreted into urine by H^+–TPase

- Antidiuretic hormone (ADH) opens water channels (aquaporins) to increase water reabsorption

4.3 Renin–angiotensin–aldosterone system

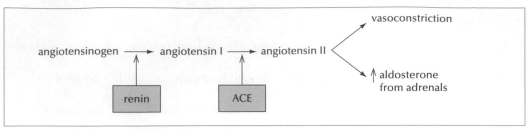

(ACE, acetycholinesterase)

- Renin is released from the juxtaglomerular apparatus in response to decreased perfusion to the kidney, leading to increased angiotensin II levels (causing vasoconstriction); and increased aldosterone release causing enhanced distal tubular sodium and water conservation and hence ECF (extracellular fluid) volume expansion
- Abnormal renin release resulting in hypertension is associated with most forms of secondary renal hypertension, e.g. reflux nephropathy, renal artery stenosis

There are syndromes of **low-renin hypertension**, including:

- **Conn's syndrome** (primary hyperaldosteronism: high aldosterone leading to ECF volume expansion, hypertension, hypokalaemia and renin suppression)
- **Liddle's syndrome** (constitutive **activation** of amiloride-sensitive distal tubular epithelial sodium channel: ECF volume expansion leading to renin and aldosterone suppression and hypokalaemia)

Pseudohypoaldosteronism is constitutive **inactivation** of the amiloride-sensitive distal tubular epithelial sodium channel, leading to excessive loss of salt and water with ECF volume depletion and hyperkalaemia; renin and aldosterone levels are high secondary to the ECF volume depletion. There are transient and permanent forms.

4.4 Erythropoietin (EPO) system

- EPO is released by renal peritubular cells and stimulates marrow erythropoiesis
- Deficiency of EPO in renal disease is a major cause of the associated anaemia
- Recombinant human EPO is available for treatment and prevention of anaemia in renal failure

4.5 Vitamin D metabolism

- Vitamin D_3 (cholecalciferol) is mainly available from the action of UV light on its precursor in the skin

- In the liver it is hydroxylated to 25(OH)-D_3
- Renal 1α-hydroxylase then leads to the production of 1,25(OH)$_2$-D_3, or calcitriol, the most biologically active vitamin D metabolite, in the kidney
- Hypocalcaemia leads to enhanced 1α-hydroxylase activity both directly and indirectly by stimulating PTH secretion, which also stimulates the enzyme; other stimuli for increased 1α-hydroxylase activity include low serum PO_4 and growth hormone.
- Deficiency of renal production of calcitriol underlies the rickets of renal failure

5. INVESTIGATIONS

5.1 Urinalysis

Dipstick testing of urine is routinely used to detect blood, protein, glucose and to measure pH. Multistix® can, in addition, detect **leucocyte esterase** (a marker of the presence of polymorphs) and **nitrite** (produced by the bacterial reduction of nitrate). If the urine appears clear to the naked eye and all panels on a Multistix® are negative, urine infection is almost certainly excluded.

NB. Urinary haemoglobin and myoglobin (from rhabdomyolysis) produce a false-positive dipstick test for blood; microscopy of urine will not, however, reveal RBCs.

5.2 Urine microscopy

A routine investigation for urinary tract infection (UTI) and in patients with dipstick haematuria. The finding of organisms and white blood cells on microscopy is strong supporting evidence for the presence of a UTI before a culture result is available. Apart from infection, the major causes of haematuria in children are glomerular, rather than lower urinary tract. Glomerular RBCs appear deformed or dysmorphic when examined by an experienced microscopist, helping to localize the site of haematuria to the kidneys.

Urinary casts usually signify renal pathology:

- Red cell casts   isolated renal haematuria; or glomerulonephritis
- Tubular cell casts   acute tubular necrosis
- WBC casts   pyelonephritis; Acute tubular necrosis (ATN)

5.3 Haematuria

The main causes are:

- UTI:
  - Other infections including TB and schistosomiasis
- Glomerulonephritis:
  - Often with proteinuria and urinary casts

- Isolated haematuria with no other evidence of clinical renal disease may be the presenting feature of several important glomerulonephritides, including:
  - Alport's syndrome
  - IgA nephropathy
- Trauma — usually a history
- Stones — usually painful
- Tumour
- Cystic kidney disease
- Bleeding disorders
- Vascular disorders, including renal vein thrombosis (especially neonates) and arteritis
- Sickle cell disease
- False-positive (see section 5.1, *Urinalysis*)
- Factitious Munchausen syndrome; Munchausen syndrome by proxy

Other causes of red urine include beetroot consumption, haemoglobinuria and rifampicin.

5.4 Proteinuria

This is usually detected on dipstick testing. The minimum detectable concentration is 10–15 mg/dl, so in a patient producing a large volume of dilute urine the sticks may be negative even though the total amount of protein excreted per day may be significant.

In normal afebrile children, urine protein excretion should not exceed 60 mg/m^2 per 24 hours. Collection of an accurate 24-hour urine collection is difficult in small children. Assessment of proteinuria may be made on a spot early morning urine sample by measuring the urinary protein (mg/l) to creatinine (mmol/l) ratio. The mean value in normal children is 0.3 mg/mmol (range 0.02–1.0).

Orthostatic proteinuria is detectable when the patient has been in the upright position for several hours, but not when the patient is recumbent. It is important to assess protein excretion when recumbent and when upright, since orthostatic proteinuria is a benign condition with a good prognosis and does not warrant investigations such as renal biopsy.

5.5 Renal imaging

Ultrasound

This is a readily available, non-invasive investigation that is operator-dependent for its interpretation. It is standard for antenatal investigation and in almost all renal conditions. It gives good information about:

- Size, shape, symmetry and position of kidneys
- Hydronephrosis, ureteric dilatation
- Bladder distension, bladder emptying post-void, bladder wall thickness
- Stones, though small ureteric stones may not be seen
- Cystic disease, including autosomal dominant and recessive
- Tumours, including renal and adrenal tumours

- Gross cortical scarring
- Vascular perfusion using a Doppler technique

US may not detect minor degrees of scarring. It is not sensitive or specific to detect vesicoureteric reflux (VUR). Doppler US may reveal renal artery stenosis, but there is a significant false-negative rate.

Micturating cystourethrogram

To look for VUR; and the appearance of the bladder outline; and the urethra, specifically posterior urethral valves in males.

Nuclear medicine isotope scans

$^{99}Tc^m$ DMSA

- A **static** scan, i.e. isotope filtered and retained in renal parenchyma
- Divided function and detecting cortical scars
- Main use is in investigation of UTI; and investigating hypertension
- Some perfusion defects seen if DMSA scan done during acute UTI may resolve; defects present 3 months after acute infection are permanent

$^{99}Tc^m$ DTPA (diethylenetriaminepenta-acetic acid), $^{99}Tc^m$ MAG-3 (mertiatide)

- **Dynamic** scans, i.e. isotope filtered and then excreted from kidney down ureters to bladder
- Divided function and assessing drainage and obstruction; main use is in investigating upper tract dilatation seen on US; and for follow-up of surgery for obstructed kidneys or ureters
- **Indirect radioisotope reflux study** is a convenient way of assessing the presence of VUR in children old enough to co-operate with the scan — in practice >3-years-old. It avoids the need for a urethral catheter and has a lower radiation dose than MCUG.

Intravenous urography

Little used now, since the combination of US and isotope scans provides the required information in most cases and avoids the risk of anaphylaxis and radiation dose involved with intravenous urography (IVU). Has a role in:

- Emergency evaluation of painful haematuria, if US uninformative, when IVU may reveal a ureteric stone
- Determining ureteric anatomy, course and insertion if ectopic ureter suspected

Renal arteriography

Used to diagnose renal artery stenosis. Approach is via femoral artery; usually requires general anaesthesia in children. Therapeutic approaches include balloon angioplasty of stenoses and embolization of intrarenal AV aneurysms.

5.6 Renal biopsy

In general, the main indications for renal biopsy are to;

- Make a diagnosis
- Guide therapy and to assess response to therapy
- Assist in giving a prognosis

The commonest reasons for renal biopsy in children are:

- Steroid-resistant nephrotic syndrome
- Haematuria and/or proteinuria
- Unexplained acute nephritis/acute renal failure
- Assessment of renal transplant

6. ACID–BASE, FLUID AND ELECTROLYTES

6.1 Metabolic acidosis

A primary decrease in plasma bicarbonate and decrease in plasma pH, due to:

- **Bicarbonate loss**, e.g.:
  - gastrointestinal loss in severe diarrhoea
  - renal loss in proximal (type 2) renal tubular acidosis (RTA)
- **Reduced hydrogen ion excretion**, e.g.:
  - distal (type 1) RTA
  - acute and chronic renal failure
- **Increased hydrogen ion load**, e.g.:
  - ↑ **endogenous** load
    - **inborn errors of metabolism**, e.g. maple-syrup urine disease; propionic acidaemia
    - **lactic acidosis**, e.g. cardiovascular shock
    - **ketoacidosis**, e.g. diabetic ketoacidosis (DKA)
  - ↑ **exogenous** load, e.g. salicylate poisoning

Anion gap

- A classification of metabolic acidosis involves assessing the **anion gap**: the 'gap' between anions and cations made up by **unmeasured** anions, e.g. ketoacids; lactic acid
- Measured as $[Na]-[HCO_3 + Cl]$; thus **normal** anion gap: $[140]-[25 + 100] = 15$
- Acidosis may be **normal** anion gap, when Cl⁻ will be raised, i.e. hyperchloraemic
- May be **increased** anion gap, when Cl⁻ will be normal, i.e. normochloraemic

Examples:

- Normal anion gap, hyperchloraemic, acidosis: e.g. RTA
    Na, 140; Cl, 110; HCO_3, 15 → AG = 15
- Increased anion gap, normochloraemic, acidosis: e.g. DKA
    Na, 140; Cl, 100; HCO_3, 15 → AG = 25

6.2 Metabolic alkalosis

A primary increase in plasma bicarbonate and increase in plasma pH, due to:

- **Chloride depletion**, the commonest cause in childhood, leading to **low urinary** Cl and **Cl-responsive** alkalosis, i.e. as soon as Cl is made available (e.g. as intravenous saline) it is retained by the kidney at the expense of HCO_3, correcting the alkalosis (also see *Pseudo-Bartter's syndrome*, section 7.2) e.g.:
    - Gastrointestinal loss, for example pyloric stenosis, congenital chloride diarrhoea
    - Furosemide (frusemide) therapy
    - Cystic fibrosis
- **Stimulation of H^+** secretion by the kidney, with **normal urinary** Cl^- and **Cl-unresponsive** alkalosis, e.g.:
    - Bartter's syndrome
    - Cushing's syndrome
    - Hyperaldosteronism
- **Excess intake of base**, e.g. excess ingestion of antacid medicine (rare in childhood)

6.3 Body fluid compartments and regulation

Total body water (TBW)

TBW represents 85% of body weight (Bwt) of premature infants; 80% in term infants; and 65% in children. TBW in children is distributed between intracellular (ICF) and extracellular (ECF) fluid compartments as follows:

TBW (%BWt)	ICF (%BWt)	ECF (%BWt)	
		Interstitial	Intravascular
65	40	20	5

Osmotic equilibrium, cell volume regulation

- The major fluid compartments are separated by semipermeable membranes, which are freely permeable to H_2O. Osmotic equilibrium is maintained between the ICF and ECF compartments by the shift of H_2O from lower to higher osmolality compartments.
- ECF osmolality can be **calculated** as: [(Na + K) × 2] + glucose + urea.
- A rise in ECF osmolality, e.g. in diabetic ketoacidosis (DKA), will lead to shift of H_2O out of the ICF compartment and thus a reduction in ICF volume, i.e. cell shrinkage. Cell shrinkage stimulates the intracellular accumulation of organic osmolytes which

increase ICF osmolality and lead to shift of H_2O back into the cell, restoring cell volume.

- Treatment of DKA may then lead to the **rapid reduction of ECF osmolality**, but the ICF organic osmolytes are degraded **slowly.** Thus an **osmotic gradient** may be created during DKA treatment, favouring movement of H_2O into the cells, causing **cerebral oedema.**

Osmoregulation

A small (3–4%) increase in ECF osmolality stimulates hypothalamic osmoreceptors to cause posterior pituitary ADH release, leading to water retention and return of osmolality to normal. Increases in ECF osmolality also stimulate thirst and water drinking. Significant (>10%) ECF depletion, even if iso-osmolar, will cause carotid and atrial baroreceptors to stimulate ADH release.

6.4 Electrolyte disturbances

Hyponatraemia

Normal plasma Na is 135–145 mmol/l. Hyponatraemia usually defined as plasma Na <130 mmol/l. The causes are:

Gain of H_2O in excess of Na

- **Excess water intake**: increased volume of appropriately hypotonic urine
  - Iatrogenic: excess hypotonic oral or intravenous fluid
  - Psychogenic polydipsia
- **Acute renal failure**: oedema and hypervolaemia, oliguria with urine Na >20 mmol/l
- **Syndrome of inappropriate ADH (secretion) (SIADH)**: inappropriately raised urine osmolality, i.e. not maximally dilute; increased body weight; decreased plasma urea and creatinine; absence of overt renal, liver, or cardiac disease
  - Meningitis; CNS tumour
  - Pneumonia
  - Intermittent positive-pressure ventilation
  - Drugs, e.g. carbamazepine, barbiturates

- **Treatment**
  - Treatment is principally water restriction; for severe hyponatraemia (<120 mmol/l) with neurological symptoms, correction of plasma Na to 125–130 mmol/l over 4 hours is usually safe and effective in correcting symptoms.

Loss of Na in excess of H_2O

- **Renal losses**: dehydration, but inappropriately high urine volume and urine Na content (>20 mmol/l); urine isotonic with plasma
  - Loop diuretics
  - Recovery phase of ATN
  - Tubulopathies (see section 7.1, *Proximal tubulopathies*)
  - Salt-wasting CAH; adrenal insufficiency — **NB. hyperkalaemia**

- **Extrarenal losses**: dehydration, appropriate oliguria and Na conservation with low urine Na (usually <10 mmol/l); urine hypertonic
  - GIT losses — gastroenteritis
  - Skin losses — severe sweating, cystic fibrosis
- **Treatment** involves rehydration and calculation of Na deficit as (140 — plasma Na) × 0.65 × body weight (kg); avoid over-rapid correction of hyponatraemia (risk of cerebellopontine myelinolysis)

Hypernatraemia

Usually defined as plasma Na >150 mmol/l. There is a shift of H_2O from the ICF to ECF compartments, so that in hypernatraemic dehydration, ECF volume is not markedly reduced and thus typical signs of dehydration are less obvious. The causes are:

1. Loss of H_2O in excess of Na
- **Renal losses**: inappropriately high urine output, inappropriately low urine osmolality:
  - Reduced renal concentrating ability, e.g. premature neonates
  - Diabetes insipidus (pituitary and nephrogenic (see section 7.4)
  - Osmotic diuresis, e.g. DKA
- **Extrarenal losses**: appropriate oliguria and high urine osmolality
  - GIT losses
  - Increased insensible H_2O loss, e.g. pyrexia and hyperventilation
- **Inadequate free-water intake**:
  - Breast-fed neonate with inadequate maternal milk flow

- **Treatment**
  - Safest and best given with standard oral rehydration solution
  - If intravenous treatment is essential, **slow** (48–72 hour; or 10–15 mmol/l per 24 hour) correction of hypernatraemia with frequent measurement of plasma electrolytes is safest; a suggested fluid is (1 litre dextrose 5% + NaCl 25 mmol + KCl 20 mmol)

2. Gain of Na in excess of H_2O

- Increased volume of urine with high Na content
  - Iatrogenic: excess hypertonic intravenous fluid, e.g. $NaHCO_3$, hypertonic saline
  - Incorrect reconstitution of infant formula
  - Accidental or deliberate (e.g. Munchausen-by-proxy, salt poisoning)

- **Treatment**
  - Recognition and removal of underlying cause; access to water while kidneys excrete excess salt load

Hypokalaemia

Normal plasma K is 3.4–4.8 mmol/l. The main causes of hypokalaemia are:

- **Inadequate provision of K** with prolonged intravenous fluid administration

- **Extrarenal losses**
  - GIT losses
- **Renal losses**
  - High plasma renin levels
    - Diuretic use — loop and thiazide diuretics
    - Osmotic diuresis, e.g. DKA (hypokalaemia becomes evident when metabolic acidosis and insulin deficiency are corrected)
    - Fanconi's syndrome
    - Bartter's syndrome
    - Gitelman syndrome
      Distal (type 1) RTA
  - **Low plasma renin levels**
    - Conn's syndrome
    - Liddle's syndrome
    - Cushing's syndrome
- **Shift from ECF to ICF compartment**
  - Correction of metabolic acidosis
  - Insulin treatment
  - High-dose or prolonged salbutamol treatment for asthma

Hyperkalaemia

The main causes are:
- **Excess administration** in intravenous fluid
- **Renal failure** — acute and chronic
- **Shift from ICF to ECF**
  - Metabolic acidosis
  - Rhabdomyolysis; acute tumour lysis (both often associated with acute impairment in renal function which compounds the hyperkalaemia)
- **Hypoadrenal states**
  - Salt-wasting congenital adrenal hyperplasia
  - Adrenal insufficiency
  - Pseudohypoaldosteronism (see section 4.3)
- **Potassium-sparing diuretics**, e.g. spironolactone

- **Treatment**
  - Exclusion of K from diet and i.v. fluids
  - Cardiac monitor: peaked T waves → prolonged PR interval → widened QRS → ventricular tachycardia → terminal ventricular fibrillation
  - Calcium gluconate to stabilize myocardium
  - Shift K from ECF to ICF:
    - Correct metabolic acidosis if present, e.g. in acute renal failure
    - Salbutamol: nebulized or short i.v. infusion
    - Insulin and dextrose: NB. Extreme caution in young children as risk of hypoglycaemia.

- Remove K$^+$ from body
  - Calcium resonium
  - Dialysis

Calcium and hypocalcaemia

- **Calcium** is 40% protein-bound (of which 98% bound to albumin), 48% ionized and 12% complexed to anions like PO$_4$, citrate
- Normal values are 2.1–2.6 mmol/l for **total Ca** and 1.14–1.30 for **ionized (Io) Ca**
  - Albumin-corrected Ca = measured total plasma Ca + [(40–albumin) × 0.02]
    e.g. total Ca = 1.98; albumin = 26; corrected Ca = 1.98 + [(40–26) × 0.02] = 2.26
- Degree of protein binding of plasma Ca proportional to plasma pH

Beware in correcting acidosis in renal failure, where total and ionized Ca often already low:

- Acute rise in pH with NaHCO$_3$ Rx $\rightarrow$ $\uparrow$ protein-bound Ca $\rightarrow$ $\downarrow$ Io Ca, which may cause tetany
- Monitoring of Io Ca useful in intensive care patients, where changes in acid–base and albumin levels make interpretation of total plasma Ca difficult

Hypocalcaemia

The main symptoms are tetany, paraesthesias, muscle cramps, stridor, seizures. The main causes are:

- **Calcitriol** (1,25(OH)$_2$-D$_3$) deficiency
  - Dietary deficiency of vitamin D
  - Malabsorption of vitamin D — fat malabsorption syndromes
  - Renal failure (acute and chronic): 1α-hydroxylase deficiency
  - Liver disease: 25–hydroxylase deficiency
- **Hypoparathyroidism**
  - Transient neonatal
  - Di George syndrome — 22q11.2 deletion
  - Post-parathyroidectomy
- **Pseudohypoparathyroidism**
  - Autosomal dominant; end-organ resistance to raised levels of PTH
  - Abnormal phenotype with short stature, obesity, intellectual delay, round face, short neck, shortened 4th and 5th metacarpals
- **Acute alkalosis** (respiratory or metabolic) or acute correction of acidosis in setting of already reduced Ca
- **Hyperphosphataemia**
  - Renal failure (acute or chronic)
  - Rhabdomyolysis; tumour lysis syndrome
- **Deposition of Ca**
  - Acute pancreatitis

- **Treatment**
  - Intravenous 10% calcium gluconate, 0.2 ml (0.045 mmol)/kg, diluted 1:5 with D-glucose 5%, over 10–15 minutes with ECG monitoring; followed by i.v. infusion
  - Oral Ca supplements
  - Vitamin D, or the analogue alfacalcidol (1α-OH-cholecalciferol) for nutritional deficiency, hypoparathyroidism and renal failure

Hypercalcaemia

The main symptoms are constipation, nausea, lethargy and confusion, headache, muscle weakness and polyuria and dehydration. The main causes are:

- **Vitamin D therapy**
  - Renal failure
  - Dietary vitamin D deficiency
- **Primary hyperparathyroidism**
  - Neonatal
  - Part of multiple endocrine neoplasia syndromes I and II
- **William's syndrome**
  - Heterozygous deletions of chromosomal sub-band 7q11.23 leading to an elastin gene defect in >90% (detected by FISH)
  - Hypercalcaemia rarely persists beyond 1-year-old
- **Familial hypocalciuric hypercalcaemia**
  - Inactivation of Ca-sensing receptor gene in parathyroid cells and renal tubules → plasma PTH level inappropriately high, urine Ca inappropriately low
- **↑ Macrophage production of 1,25(OH)$_2$-D$_3$**
  - Sarcoidosis
  - Subcutaneous fat necrosis
    - Prolonged or obstructed labour
- **Malignant disease**

- **Treatment**
  - Intravenous hydration plus loop diuretic
  - Correction/removal or specific treatment of underlying cause, e.g. steroids for sarcoidosis
  - Rarely, bisphosphonates

Phosphate and hypophosphataemia

Phosphate is excreted from the kidney under the influence of parathyroid hormone (increases excretion), and calcitriol (decreases excretion). In hypophosphataemia, calculation of the tubular reabsorption of phosphate(TRP) is useful:

TRP = 1–Fractional excretion PO$_4$

i.e. TRP = $\dfrac{1-\text{urine PO}_4 \text{ (mmol/l)}}{[\text{urine creatinine (µmol/l)}]} \times \dfrac{\text{plasma creatinine } [(\text{µmol/l})]}{\text{plasma PO}_4 \text{ (mmol/l)}} \times 100\%$

Normally, TRP >85%. If the TRP is <85%, in the presence of low plasma PO_4 and normal PTH level, then this implies abnormal tubular leakage of PO_4.

Hypophosphataemia

- With appropriately high TRP, i.e. low urinary PO_4:
  - Dietary PO_4 restriction
  - Increased uptake into bone: the 'hungry bone syndrome' seen after parathyroidectomy for prolonged hyperparathyroidism, or after renal transplantation with preceding hyperparathyroidism of chronic renal failure (CRF); also see hypocalcaemia
  - Additional cause refeeding the malnourished child as required for cell turnover
- With inappropriately low TRP, i.e. high urinary PO_4:
  - Hypophosphataemic rickets — see section 7.1
  - Fanconi syndrome — see section 7.1

Hyperphosphataemia

- With high urinary PO_4:
  - Tumour lysis syndrome, rhabdomyolysis: also see oliguria, hyperkalaemia
- With low urinary PO_4:
  - Chronic renal failure
  - Hypoparathyroidism; pseudo-hypoparathyroidism

Magnesium and hypomagnesaemia

Most filtered Mg is reabsorbed in the distal proximal tubule and Loop of Henle. As with Ca, Mg transport and NaCl transport are associated. Factors enhancing Mg reabsorption include hypocalcaemia and raised PTH levels. Hypomagnesaemia is often found in patients with hypocalcaemia and hypokalaemia, and to correct these the magnesium deficiency must also first be corrected. The main causes of hypomagnesaemia are:

- Poor dietary intake
- Reduced gut absorption
- Increased urinary losses:
  - Recovery from ATN
  - Post-transplant diuresis
  - Drug-induced:
    - loop and thiazide diuretics
    - amphotericin B
    - cisplatinum
  - Gitelman syndrome — see section 7.3

7. RENAL TUBULOPATHIES

7.1 Proximal tubulopathies

Cystinuria

- Defect in reabsorption and hence excessive excretion of the dibasic amino acids cystine, ornithine, arginine and lysine
- Not to be confused with **cystinosis** — see below
- Autosomal recessive; two separate cystinuria genes — on 2p and 19q
- Cystine is poorly soluble in normal urine pH; increased solubility in alkaline urine
- Clinical manifestation is recurrent urinary stone formation
- Stones are extremely hard and densely radio-opaque
- Diagnosis based on stone analysis or high cystine level in timed urine collection
- Treatment based on high fluid intake ($\geq$1.5 l/m^2 per day) and alkalinization of urine with oral potassium citrate
- If stones still form, oral D-penicillamine leads to formation of highly soluble mixed disulphides with cystine moieties

X-linked hypophosphataemic rickets

- Also known as vitamin D-resistant rickets
- Mutation in *PEX* gene on X chromosome
- Isolated defect in PO$_4$ reabsorption leading to:
  - Inappropriately low tubular reabsorption of PO$_4$ (TRP) — typically <85% — with a normal PTH and calcitriol level
  - Hypophosphataemia
- Earliest sign is $\uparrow$ alkaline phosphatase (ALP) (by 3–4 months)
- Plasma PO$_4$ may be normal until 6–9 months of age
- By 12 months, have delayed growth, hypophosphataemia; $\uparrow$ ALP; and radiological signs of rickets
- Other features include delayed dentition and recurrent dental abscesses
- Treatment based on calcitriol or alfacalcidol and phosphate supplements
- Complications of this Rx include hypercalcaemia and nephrocalcinosis
- Recent evidence that addition of growth hormone treatment may improve growth and biochemical disturbance

Proximal (type 2) renal tubular acidosis (RTA)

- Failure to reabsorb filtered HCO$_3^-$
- Renal bicarbonate threshold is low i.e. HCO$_3^-$ is present in the urine at levels of plasma HCO$_3$ lower than normal
- Distal tubular H$^+$ excretion is intact so acid urine can be produced
- Normal acidification of urine in response to ammonium chloride load
- Normal increase in urine *P*CO$_2$ in response to 3 mmol/kg oral bicarbonate load

- Ability to excrete acid from distal tubule and the fact that calcium salts are more soluble in acid urine, is the likely reason that nephrocalcinosis is not a feature of proximal RTA
- May occur as an isolated defect or as part of Fanconi's syndrome — see below
- Symptoms include failure to thrive, vomiting, short stature
- Rx requires large doses of alkali (5–15 mmol/kg per day)

Fanconi's syndrome

- Diffuse proximal tubular dysfunction, leading to excess urinary loss of:
    - Glucose — glycosuria with normal blood glucose
    - Phosphate — hypophosphataemia, low TRP, rickets
    - Amino acids — no obvious clinical consequence
    - HCO_3^- — leading to proximal RTA
    - K^+ — causing hypokalaemia
    - Na^+, Cl^- and water — leading to polyuria and polydipsia, chronic ECF volume depletion, failure to thrive
    - Tubular proteinuria — loss of low MW proteins including retinol binding protein (RBP) and N-acetyl glucosaminidase (NAG)
- Usual clinical features include polyuria and polydipsia, chronic ECF volume depletion, failure to thrive, constipation, rickets, with features of any underlying condition in addition

Main causes of Fanconi's syndrome

- Metabolic disorders
    - Cystinosis
    - Tyrosinaemia
    - Lowe's syndrome (oculocerebrorenal syndrome)
    - Galactosaemia
    - Wilson's disease

- Heavy-metal toxicity
    - Lead; mercury; cadmium

- Idiopathic

Cystinosis

Autosomal recessive defect in transport of cystine out of lysosomes. Gene localized to chromosome 17p.

- Predominant early clinical features are of:
    - Fanconi's syndrome
    - Photophobia due to eye involvement with corneal cystine crystals
    - Hypothyroidism

- Late features include:
  - Renal failure around 8–10 years of age, if untreated
  - Pancreatic involvement with diabetes mellitus
  - Liver involvement with hepatomegaly
  - Gonadal involvement with reduced fertility
  - Neurological deterioration and cerebral atrophy

- Diagnosis based on:
  - Cystine crystals in cornea seen by slit lamp
  - Peripheral blood white cell cystine level
  - Antenatal diagnosis available for families with positive history

Treatment
This should be:

- **Supportive** — PO_4, NaCl, K^+ and $NaHCO_3$ supplements and high fluid intake; alfacalcidol; thyroxine
- **Specific** — cysteamine, which increases cystine transport out of the lysosome; commencing treatment in early infancy appears to delay onset of renal failure
- **Other** — indomethacin reduces the GFR and hence the severe polyuria and secondary polydipsia and electrolyte wasting

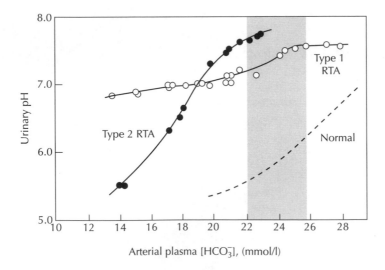

Renal tubular acidosis — graphical representation

In normal subjects, urine pH falls as plasma HCO_3^- decreases through the normal range from 26 to 22 mmol/l. In proximal RTA, the curve has a similar shape but is shifted to the left, such that acid urine is not produced until plasma HCO_3^- has fallen abnormally low, e.g. 16 mmol/l. In distal RTA, acid urine cannot be produced regardless of how low the plasma HCO_3^- falls.

Renal tubular acidosis — classification

	Type 1 (distal)	Type 2 (proximal)
Defect	Impaired excretion of H$^+$	Failure to reabsorb filtered HCO$_3^-$; bicarbonate threshold is low
Urine pH	>5.8 i.e. never 'acid'	Variable; may be <5.3
Plasma K	Usually $\downarrow$	Normal or $\downarrow$
Causes	Primary isolated RTA Nephrocalcinosis Obstructive uropathy Amphotericin; cyclosporin	Primary isolated RTA Transient infantile Fanconi's syndrome
Clinical features	Nephrocalcinosis; failure to thrive; episodes of severe hypokalaemia	Vomiting; failure to thrive; short stature
Response to NH$_4$Cl load	Failure to acidify urine	Production of acid urine
Response to NaHCO$_3$ load	No $\uparrow$ in urine-blood PCO$_2$ gradient	Normal $\uparrow$ in urine–blood PCO$_2$ gradient
Treatment	1–2 mmol/kg per day of NaHCO$_3$	5–15 mmol/kg per day of NaHCO$_3^-$; large doses needed to overcome low renal threshold

- Blood PCO$_2$ is measured with blood gas analyser, urine PCO$_2$ with a dedicated PCO$_2$ meter.

7.2 Loop of Henle

Bartter's syndrome

- This is caused by an inborn defect, autosomal recessive, in the Na$^+$–K$^+$–2Cl$^-$ co-transporter in the thick ascending limb of the LoH, leading to NaCl and water wasting.
- Symptoms are polyuria, polydipsia, episodes of dehydration, failure to thrive, constipation; there may be maternal polyhydramnios with an affected fetus.
- The resultant ECF volume contraction causes 2° renin secretion and raised aldosterone levels, with avid Na$^+$ and water reabsorption in the distal tubule and reciprocal K$^+$ and H$^+$ secretion into the urine. (Note that the blood pressure is normal; the hyper-reninaemia is a compensatory response to maintain normal BP in the presence of chronic ECF volume depletion.) There is also increased renal prostaglandin PGE$_2$ production.
- The above changes produce the characteristic biochemical disturbance of hypochloraemic–hypokalaemic alkalosis.
- Crucial to the diagnosis is the finding of **inappropriately high** levels of urinary Cl$^-$ and Na$^+$ — usually >20 mmol/l; urine Ca^{2+} is normal or high (cf Gitelman syndrome — see below)
- Therapy involves K$^+$ supplementation combined with prostaglandin synthetase inhibitors, usually indomethacin

Pseudo-Bartter's syndrome

The same plasma biochemistry, hypochloraemic–hypokalaemic alkalosis, but **appropriately low** levels of urine Cl^- and Na^+: <10 mmol/l

---

Main causes of Pseudo-Bartter's syndrome

- Cystic fibrosis — sweat loss of NaCl and water
- Congenital chloride diarrhoea — gut loss
- Laxative abuse — gut loss
- Cyclical vomiting

NB. All the changes of Bartter's syndrome, including the high urine electrolyte levels, may be produced by loop diuretics, which block the same site in the thick ascending limb of LoH.

7.3 Distal tubule

Gitelman syndrome

- This condition is considered a variant of Bartter's syndrome
- There is an inborn defect, autosomal recessive, in the DT Na–Cl co-transporter
- Often asymptomatic, with transient episodes of weakness and tetany with abdominal pain and vomiting
- Patients have hypokalaemic metabolic alkalosis, raised renin and aldosterone and **hypomagnesaemia** with increased urinary magnesium wasting and **hypo**calciuria, a feature which helps distinguish it from classical Bartter's syndrome (normal or high urinary Ca^{2+} — see above)
- Biochemical changes resemble those produced by thiazide diuretics, which inhibit this DT co-transporter

7.4 Collecting duct

Nephrogenic diabetes insipidus (NDI)

- Resistance to action of high circulating levels of ADH
- Is associated with ADH-receptor gene mutations (X-linked NDI) and aquaporin (water channel) gene mutations (autosomal recessive NDI)
- High volumes of inappropriately dilute urine with tendency to hypernatraemic dehydration

Liddle's syndrome

Pseudohypoaldosteronism

8. NEPHROTIC SYNDROME

A triad of oedema, proteinuria and hypoalbuminaemia. It is almost always idiopathic in childhood. It is best classified by response to steroid treatment; steroid–sensitive nephrotic syndrome (SSNS; 85–90% cases) or resistant (SRNS; 10–15% cases), since this is the best predictor of outcome.

8.1 Definitions

- **Steroid resistant**: no remission after 4 weeks of prednisolone 60 mg/m^2 per day
- **Remission**: negative urinalysis on first morning urine for three consecutive mornings
- **Relapse**: 3$^+$ proteinuria on three or more consecutive first-morning urines
- **Frequently relapsing**: ≥2 relapses within 6 months of diagnosis; or ≥4 relapses per year

8.2 Clinical features

	SSNS	SRNS
Age at onset	Toddler, pre-school	<1yr; >8 yrs
Sustained hypertension	No	Often
Microscopic haematuria	Mild, intermittent	Persistent
Renal function	Normal	Often reduced
Long-term prognosis	Excellent, even if frequently relapsing	Poor — significant risk of long-term hypertension and renal failure
Usual histology	Usually not biopsied; from historical data known to be minimal changes	Focal segmental glomerulosclerosis (FSGS)

8.3 Complications

Infection

- Typically with *Streptococcus pneumoniae*:
  - Pneumonia
  - Primary pneumococcal peritonitis
- Increased risk due to:
  - Tissue oedema and pleural and peritoneal fluid
  - Loss of immunoglobulin in urine
  - Immunosuppression with steroid treatment

Thrombosis

- Increased risk due to:
  - Loss of antithrombin III and protein S and C in urine
  - Increased production of procoagulant factors by liver
  - Increased haematocrit secondary to reduced oncotic pressure
  - Swelling of legs, ascites and relative immobility
  - Steroid therapy

Hypovolaemia

- Reduced plasma oncotic pressure leads to shift of plasma water from intravascular space to interstitial space
- Symptoms include oliguria, abdominal pain, anorexia, postural hypotension
- Signs include cool peripheries, poor capillary refill, tachycardia
- Poor renal perfusion activates the renin–angiotensin–aldosterone system and **urine Na** will therefore be very low, usually <10 mmol/l
- Occasionally acute tubular necrosis develops secondary to hypovolaemia

Drug toxicity

Most morbidity arises from side-effects of steroid treatment. Other drugs successfully used to enable control without steroids, or on much lower dose of steroids, include:

Cyclosporin A

- Taken twice daily long-term, e.g. 12–18 months' initial trial
- High relapse rate when weaned/stopped
- Hirsutism; gum hyperplasia; nephrotoxicity — need to monitor plasma cyclosporin A levels, GFR

Tacrolimus (FK506)

- nephrotoxicity

Cyclophosphamide

- 2 mg/kg × 12 weeks; or 3 mg/kg × 8 weeks
- Hair thinning; bone marrow suppression
- Significant effect on fertility is very unlikely at this dose (equivalent to 168 mg/kg). Doses of >350 mg/kg are associated with significant reduction in fertility in males. Females are not as vulnerable to this effect.

Mustine

- Given as two courses, each of four consecutive daily doses i.v.

Levamisole

- Need to monitor FBC for bone marrow suppression

8.4 Treatment

Initial presentation

Most commonly used prednisolone regimen in UK is:

- Prednisolone 60 mg/m^2 per day × 4 weeks; then reduce to 40 mg/m^2 alternate days × 4 weeks; then stop.

However, there is good evidence from controlled trials that **longer duration** of initial prednisolone treatment is associated with fewer relapses and lower total prednisolone dose over the first 2 years. Example of 6-month initial course:

- 60 mg/m^2 per day × 4 weeks; then 40 mg/m^2 alternate days × 4 weeks; 30 mg/m^2 alt days × 4 weeks; 20 mg/m^2 alt days × 4 weeks; 10 mg/m^2 alt days × 4 weeks; 5 mg/m^2 alt days × 4 weeks; then stop

Relapse

Most commonly used prednisolone regimen is prednisolone 60 mg/m^2 per day until in remission; then 40 mg/m^2 alternate days for three doses; and reduce alternate day dose by 10 mg/m^2 every three doses until 10 mg/m^2 alt days; then 5 mg/m^2 alt days for three doses; then stop.

Steroid-resistant nephrotic syndrome

- Patient should be referred to specialist renal unit for assessment including renal biopsy
- Usually resistant to other drug treatments also, so full remission not achieved
- Aim is to reduce proteinuria so that patient no longer nephrotic
- Commonest treatment is alternate day prednisolone combined with cyclosporin long-term; enalapril often used to treat **hypertension**, with the added benefit of antiproteinuric effect
- Significant chance of hypertension and progression to renal failure
- If histology is FSGS, associated with 20–40% chance of recurrence in transplant

8.5 Congenital nephrotic syndrome (CNS)

Onset in first 3 months of life; large placenta usually 40% birth weight. Almost always resistant to drug treatment; clinically severe with high morbidity from protein malnutrition, sepsis.

Main causes (in decreasing order of frequency)

- Finnish-type CNS
- Diffuse mesangial sclerosis
- Denys–Drash syndrome

- FSGS
- Secondary CNS

— most severe; autosomal recessive; gene on
  chromosome 19
— less severe; also autosomal recessive
— includes pseudohermaphroditism and Wilms'
  tumour

— congenital syphilis

Treatment

Intense supportive care with 20% albumin infusion, nutritional support and early **unilateral nephrectomy** (to reduce urinary protein loss) combined with anticholinesterase (ACE) inhibitors and indomethacin (to reduce GFR and thus protein loss, of remaining kidney).

Eventual progression to renal failure occurs, when remaining kidney is removed and the child undergoes dialysis and transplantation.

9. GLOMERULONEPHRITIS (GN)

9.1 General clinical features

Inflammation of the glomeruli leading to various clinical features, or **renal syndromes**, which may include:

- Haematuria and/or proteinuria
- Nephrotic syndrome
- Acute nephritic syndrome with reduced renal function, oliguria and hypertension
- Rapidly progressive crescentic GN: rapid-onset severe renal failure and hypertension, usually associated with the histological lesion called a **crescent**

These renal syndromes are not specific to particular conditions and the same condition may present with different renal syndromes in different patients.

- Chronic GN may lead to scarring of the **tubulointerstitial** areas of the kidney, with progressive renal impairment
- The main causes of GN and the associated changes in serum complement, include:

Normal complement	Reduced complement
Primary renal disease	**Primary renal disease**
• FSGS • IgA nephropathy	• Acute post-streptococcal GN $\downarrow C_3$, normal C_4 • Mesangiocapillary GN (MCGN) $\downarrow C_3$ and C_4
Systemic disease	**Systemic disease**
• Henoch–Schönlein nephritis	• SLE $\downarrow C_3$ and C_4 • 'shunt nephritis' $\downarrow C_3$ and C_4

9.2 Acute post-streptococcal GN

Onset of reddish-brown ('Coca Cola coloured') urine 10–14 days after streptococcal throat or skin infection.

- May have any of the **renal syndromes** described above
- Deposition of immune complexes and complement in glomeruli

Investigations

- Throat swab
- Antistreptolysin O (ASO) titre; anti-DNAase B
- Typically, $\downarrow C_3$, normal C_4
- Biopsy if significant renal involvement (see diffuse proliferative GN, with crescents in severe cases)

Treatment

Is mainly supportive, with an excellent prognosis for recovery; in very severe cases with renal failure, steroids have been used.

NB. Always check C_3 and C_4 3 months after acute illness — should normalize; if still $\downarrow$, may be another diagnosis, e.g. SLE, MCGN, which has much worse prognosis.

9.3 Henoch–Schönlein nephritis

- 70% children with Henoch–Schönlein purpura (HSP) will have some degree of renal involvement, usually just microscopic haematuria ± proteinuria
- They may have any of the **renal syndromes** described above
- May have a relapsing course
- Refer to specialist renal unit if nephrotic, or nephritic, or sustained hypertension as these patients may require biopsy

- Prognosis difficult to be certain about, but initial clinical severity and histological score on **biopsy** guide prognosis
- Treatment of severe cases includes steroids, azathioprine; and for very severe crescentic nephritis with renal failure, methylprednisolone combined with cyclophosphamide and plasma exchange has been used (histologically identical to IgA nephropathy — see section 9.4)
- Follow-up should continue for as long as there continues to be any abnormality on urinalysis
- Accounts for 5–8% children in endstage renal failure (ESRF)

9.4 IgA nephropathy

- Presents with incidental finding of persistent **microscopic haematuria**; or with an episode of **macroscopic haematuria** which is typically associated with concurrent upper respiratory infection — these episodes may be recurrent
- Again, may have any of the **renal syndromes** described above
- Prognosis for childhood presentation quite good, though 10–15% will develop proteinuria, hypertension ± renal failure during long-term follow-up
- Treatment as for HSP nephritis; ACE inhibitors used for long-term control of hypertension and to minimize proteinuria

9.5 Systemic lupus erythematosus (SLE) nephritis

- Again, may present with various renal syndromes
- Histologically variable; and the condition may change its clinical and histological features and severity over time
- Patients may also manifest the antiphospholipid/anticardiolipin antibody syndrome, with thrombotic complications affecting the renal vasculature

9.6 'Shunt' nephritis

- Classically associated with infected ventriculoatrial shunts, these are now rarely used so the condition is rare
- Histologically similar to nephritis of subacute bacterial endocarditis

10. ACUTE RENAL FAILURE (ARF)

An acute disturbance in fluid and electrolyte homeostasis, typically associated with oliguria (<300 ml/m^2 per day) and retention of urea, potassium, phosphate, H$^+$ and creatinine. It is rare in childhood compared with the incidence in the elderly. The main cause of severe ARF in otherwise normal children is haemolytic–uraemic syndrome (HUS).

10.1 Classification of ARF

Pre-renal failure, with reduced renal perfusion

- In early stages, kidney reacts appropriately producing small volume of urine with very low Na and high concentration of urea; may be reversible at this stage with fluid therapy (± inotropic support)
- If uncorrected, progresses to established **acute tubular necrosis (ATN)**

Main causes

- ECF volume deficiency
  - Haemorrhage; diarrhoea; burns; DKA; septic shock with '3rd space' fluid loss
- Cardiac ('pump') failure
  - Congenital heart disease (CHD), e.g. severe coarctation, hypoplastic left heart; aortic
    cross-clamping and bypass for correction of CHD; myocarditis

Intrinsic renal failure

ATN due to:

- Uncorrected pre-renal failure as above
- Toxins
  - Gentamicin; X-ray contrast; myoglobinuria
  - **NB**. Gentamicin toxicity most common in neonates and may cause **non-oliguric** renal failure
- Acute glomerulonephritis
- Vascular
  - Small-vessel occlusion — HUS
  - Bilateral renal vein thrombosis (RVT) — neonates
  - Acute renal cortical necrosis — neonatal birth asphyxia
- Tubulointerstitial nephritis
  - Drugs — NSAIDs; furosemide (frusemide); penicillin; cephalosporins

Post-renal (obstructive) renal failure

- Posterior urethral valves is main lesion, but not **acute** renal failure
- Neuropathic bladder (may be **acute** in transverse myelitis, spinal trauma or tumour)
- Stones (bilateral pelviureteric junction or ureteral; or bladder stone)
- Urethral prolapse of bladder ureterocele

10.2 Differentiating pre-renal oliguria from intrinsic renal failure/ATN

Clinical assessment of circulation in oliguric child is crucial:

- Low BP, poor capillary refill and cool peripheries suggest pre-renal cause: may respond to fluid challenge
- Normal/raised BP, raised jugular vein pressure (JVP), good peripheral perfusion, gallop rhythm suggests intravascular volume overload and thus not pre-renal; fluid challenge contraindicated (though challenge with loop diuretic may improve urine output)
- Urine biochemical indices may help

Urine indices	Pre-renal failure	Intrinsic renal failure
Osmolality	>500	<300
Urine Na	<10	>40
Urine:plasma urea ratio	>10:1	<7:1
Fractional excretion of Na	<1%	>1%

10.3 Initial assessment of acute renal failure (ARF)

History

This may give clues to diagnosis, e.g.:

- Sore throat and fever 10 days' earlier suggests post-streptococcal GN
- Bloody diarrhoea and progressive pallor suggests HUS
- Drug history may reveal use of NSAIDs (increasingly used for childhood fever, earache, etc.)

Examination

This aims to:

- Assess circulation
- Look for clues to diagnosis, e.g. drug rash suggests interstitial nephritis; large palpable bladder suggests acute obstructive nephropathy

Initial investigations

Blood

- Electrolytes, chloride, urea, creatinine, phosphate, calcium, magnesium, urate, liver function tests, venous or capillary blood gas
- Full blood count, blood film (RBC fragments in HUS)

Urine

- Urinalysis for blood, protein, glucose (a clue to interstitial nephritis)
- Urine microscopy for casts
- Urine Na, urea, creatinine, osmolality — see table above

Ultrasound of urinary tract

- With most causes of acute renal failure, kidneys appear normal or increased in size and echogenicity (if kidneys appear small with poor corticomedullary differentiation, renal failure is **chronic**)
- Rules out or confirms obstruction of urinary tract; stones
- Can detect clot in RVT

Renal biopsy
If diagnosis not clear from above assessment.

10.4 Initial management of child with ARF

- Early liaison with paediatric renal unit
- Fluid therapy determined by clinical assessment and urine indices, as above
  - Pre-renal failure: fluid challenge with normal saline
  - Intrinsic renal failure:
    - if clinically euvolaemic, give fluid as insensible loss (300 ml/m² per day) + urine output
    - if clinically overloaded, challenge with loop diuretic and restrict to insensible losses
- If hypertensive due to ECF volume overload:
  - Challenge with loop diuretic
  - Nifedipine or hydralazine as simple vasodilating hypotensives
- If hyperkalaemic, treat as discussed previously

NB. If anaemic (e.g. in HUS) transfusion usually delayed until dialysis access established (i.e. until transferred to renal unit), as hyperkalaemia and fluid overload may be worsened.

10.5 Indications for acute dialysis

- Severe ECF volume overload — severe hypertension; pulmonary oedema; no response to diuretics
- Severe hyperkalaemia, not responding to conservative treatment
- Severe symptomatic uraemia — usually urea >40 mmol/l
- Severe metabolic acidosis not controllable with intravenous bicarbonate
- To remove fluid to 'make space' for nutrition (i.v. or enteral), i.v. drugs — a common reason in intensive care patients
- Removal of toxins: haemodialysis will be most effective for small molecular weight substances that are not highly protein-bound. These include;
  - Drugs, e.g. gentamicin, salicylates, lithium
  - Poisons, e.g. ethanol, ethylene glycol
  - Metabolites from inborn errors of metabolism, e.g. leucine in maple-syrup urine disease, ammonia

10.6 Haemolytic–uraemic syndrome (HUS)

- Commonest cause of acute renal failure in children
- Diarrhoea-associated (D$^+$-HUS) is major type, usually due to *E. coli* 0157, which produces verocytotoxin (also called Shiga toxin)
- Toxin is released in gut and absorbed, causing endothelial damage especially in renal microvasculature, leading to microangiopathic haemolytic anaemia with thrombocytopenia and RBC fragmentation (seen on blood film)
- The microangiopathy leads to patchy focal thrombosis and infarction and renal failure which is often severe and requires dialysis
- Brain (fits, focal neurology), myocardium, pancreas and liver are sometimes affected
- Treatment is supportive; antibiotic treatment of the *E. coli* gastroenteritis increases the incidence and severity of HUS and is thus contraindicated
- Long-term follow-up shows 10–15% will develop hypertension, proteinuria or impaired renal function
- Prevention of HUS with a synthetic Shiga toxin-binding trisaccharide linked to silica beads, taken orally, is undergoing clinical trials in Canada and USA, but early results are disappointing
- Atypical D$^-$-HUS rare but more serious with recurrent episodes, progressive renal impairment and higher incidence of neurological involvement
    - Autosomal recessive forms associated with disturbances of complement regulation
    - Rare complication of bone marrow transplantation

11. CHRONIC RENAL FAILURE, DIALYSIS AND TRANSPLANTATION

11.1 Chronic renal failure

A persistent impairment of renal function, classified according to the GFR as mild (60–80 ml/min per 1.73 m^2), moderate (40–59) and severe (<40). Endstage renal failure, where dialysis or transplantation are needed, is reached once GFR <10 ml/min per 1.73 m^2.

Main causes of chronic renal failure

- Congenital dysplasia +/– obstruction
- Reflux nephropathy
- Chronic glomerulonephritis — FSGS; MCGN
- Genetically inherited disease, e.g. hereditary nephritis: Alport's, nephronophthisis, polycystic kidney disease
- Systemic disease — HSP; SLE

Clinical presentations

- Antenatal diagnosis
- Failure to thrive, poor growth; pubertal delay
- Malaise, anorexia
- Anaemia
- Incidental — blood test; urinalysis
- Hypertension

Main clinical features

Poor growth

- Anorexia, vomiting (uraemia)
- Anaemia, acidosis and renal osteodystrophy — see below
- Reduced effectiveness of growth hormone, probably due to raised levels of insulin-like growth factor (IGF) binding protein and hence less free IGF; levels of growth hormone are normal
- Recombinant human growth hormone is effective in improving growth in children with CRF and is licensed for this use

Dietary considerations

- Inadequate calorie intake and catabolism worsens acidosis, uraemia and hyperkalaemia in CRF; aggressive nutritional management is crucial to control these and to achieve growth
- Children with CRF often have poor appetite and infants in particular benefit from nasogastric or gastrostomy tube feeding
- Congenital dysplasia +/– obstruction typically causes polyuria, with NaCl and HCO_3^- wasting and these need supplementing along with generous water intake; note that salt and water restriction is **inappropriate** in many children with CRF, until they reach endstage renal failure
- Protein intake should usually be recommended daily intake for age; note that protein restriction is **inappropriate** for children with CRF
- Dietary restriction of PO_4 (dairy produce) combined with use of PO_4 binders (e.g. calcium carbonate) is essential in controlling secondary hyperparathyroidism
- Dietary restriction of K^+ (fresh fruits, potato) also commonly needed

Anaemia

- Dietary iron deficiency
- Reduced RBC survival in uraemia
- EPO deficiency; recombinant human EPO available for treatment

Renal osteodystrophy (two main contributing processes)

- Phosphate retention leads to hypocalcaemia and both $\uparrow PO_4$ and $\downarrow$ Ca stimulate secondary **hyperparathyroidism** (subperiosteal bone resorption). Deficient renal 1α-hydroxylase activity and deficient $1,25(OH)_2$-D_3 also contributes to hypocalcaemia and leads to **rickets**

- Treatment includes control of hyperphosphataemia (see above) and alfacalcidol (1α-OH-cholecalciferol) or calcitriol

Metabolic acidosis

- Contributes to bone disease, since chronic acidosis is significantly buffered by uptake of H^+ into bone in exchange for Ca loss from bone

Hypertension

Depends on the underlying cause of CRF.

- Congenital dysplasia +/− obstruction: patients tend to be polyuric, salt wasting and normotensive
- Chronic GN, polycystic kidney disease, systemic disease: hypertension common; usually secondary to ↑ renin, so ACE inhibitors often effective

11.2 Dialysis

- Once the GFR falls to 10 ml/min per 1.73 m², the child will usually need dialysis, or transplantation, to be maintained safely. The two main types of dialysis, peritoneal dialysis (PD) and haemodialysis (HD), both use a semipermeable membrane to achieve **solute** removal (K^+, urea, PO_4, creatinine, etc.) and **fluid removal**
- Infants and small children are better suited to PD, which is more 'physiological' and avoids abrupt haemodynamic changes

	Peritoneal dialysis	**Haemodialysis**
Semipermeable membrane	Peritoneum	Synthetic membrane
Access	Peritoneal catheter	Central venous catheter or AV fistula in arm
Frequency and duration	Daily (usually overnight) via automated PD machine	3× weekly, 4 hours/session
Where	Home	Hospital
Complications	Peritonitis; catheter blockage or leakage	Catheter sepsis; haemodynamic instability in infants
Advantages	Independence from hospital; schooling uninterrupted; PD machine portable so can travel on holidays	No burden of care for dialysis procedure on family
Disadvantages	Burden of care on family	Missed school; travel to and from hospital; limited holiday options

11.3 Transplantation

The proportion of living related donor (LRD) transplants in paediatric units (~50% of transplants) is higher than the national figure overall — a parent is usually the donor. Transplantation prior to the need for dialysis is usually the aim.

- There are advantages to LRD transplantation:
    - Better long-term survival of the graft kidney: approximate figures are: –90% at 1 year; 75–80% at 5 years; 60% at 10 years
- Surgery is planned, so family life can be organized to deal with it:
    - Increases the chance of achieving transplantation without dialysis
- HLA-matching is based around HLA A, B and DR; on average, a parent and child will be matched for one allele and mismatched for one allele, at each site
- The main immunosuppressive drugs are prednisolone, cyclosporin (Neoral®) and azathioprine
- Children should be immune to TB, measles and chickenpox prior to transplantation — immunization is available for all these infections
- Children need to weigh ≥10 kg for transplantation to be performed

---

Main complications of transplantation

- **Early surgical complications**
    - Bleeding; transplant artery thrombosis; wound infection

- **Rejection**
    - Diagnosed on biopsy; usually treatable with extra immunosuppression

- **Opportunistic infection**
    - Fungal infections; CMV; pneumocystis pneumoniae

- **Drug toxicity**
    - Hypertension; Cushingoid changes; hirsutism and nephrotoxicity from ciclosporin

- **Post-transplantation lymphoproliferative disorder (PTLD)**
    - Lymphoma-like condition, especially associated with primary EBV infection when immunosuppressed

12. URINARY TRACT INFECTION, NEUROPATHIC BLADDER

12.1 Urinary tract infection

- Commonest presenting urinary tract problem — 1% boys and 3% girls
- Boys > girls until 6 months (posterior urethral valves); thereafter girls > boys
- Significance of UTI:
  - Renal scar gives 15–20% risk of hypertension
  - Reflux nephropathy causes 15–20% ESRF
- Age at greatest risk for renal damage, age in which symptoms of UTI least specific, age group most often seen with fever by GPs and age at which proper urine sample hardest to obtain: **infancy**

- Collection of uncontaminated urine sample crucial to accurate diagnosis of UTI, methods include:
  - Adhesive bag: problems with leakage and faecal contamination
  - Absorbent pad also prone to contamination
  - Clean catch
  - Catheter specimen or suprapubic aspirate: suitable if urine sample needed urgently, e.g. septic screen in ill infant

Predisposing factors for UTI

- **Incomplete bladder emptying**:
  - PUV
  - Neuropathic bladder
- **Catheterization or instrumentation of urinary tract**
- **Stones**
- **Vesicoureteric reflux (VUR)**:
  - Familial, behaves as autosomal dominant condition
  - May be graded according to severity on MCUG
  - Management based on long-term, low-dose antibiotic prophylaxis
  - Significant spontaneous resolution rate; less likely in grades IV–V
  - Controlled studies show no benefit for surgery over conservative management for grades I–III
  - Surgery may be indicated where prophylaxis fails to control infection and where there is progressive reflux nephropathy; options are:
    – Reimplantation of ureters
    – Endoscopic injection of synthetic material at ureteric orifice
  - Screening of newborn siblings or offspring of index children or parents should be considered
  - In children who have normal bladder control and no symptoms of detrusor dysfunction and who have been free of infection on prophylaxis, evidence suggests that there is little benefit from continuing prophylaxis beyond 5-years-old

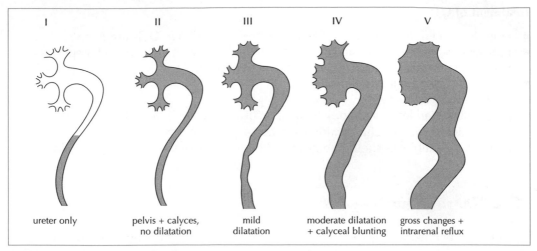

I	II	III	IV	V
ureter only	pelvis + calyces, no dilatation	mild dilatation	moderate dilatation + calyceal blunting	gross changes + intrarenal reflux

Grading of vesicoureteric reflux

Investigation of UTI

Aims

- To identify scarring
- To identify underlying abnormalities likely to cause recurrent infection, e.g. VUR; incomplete emptying

Suggested protocol

- Under 1 year — US + DMSA + MCUG
- Over 1 year — US + DMSA; MCUG if:
    - US or 99Tc^m DMSA abnormal
    - Pyelonephritis clinically
    - Recurrent UTI
    - Family history

Indirect radioisotope reflux study (e.g. 99Tc^m DTPA) (see section 5.5)
May be adequate for initial investigation for VUR in girls, but initial contrast MCUG should always be performed in boys to exclude PUV.

Prevention of UTI

- Non-pharmacological methods:
    - Avoidance of constipation; correct bottom wiping
    - Frequent voiding and high fluid intake; double voiding
    - Lactobacilli in live yoghurt; cranberry juice
    - Clean, intermittent catheterization
- Prophylactic antibiotics

Treatment of UTI

- Empirical antibiotic treat until C&S known; >90% childhood UTIs are *E. coli*
- Intravenous antibiotics for unwell infants and children with clinical pyelonephritis — high fever and rigors, loin pain, vomiting, neutrophilia, ↑ CRP
- Obstructed kidneys may need drainage
- Stones may need removing
- Augmented bladders may improve with mucolytic and bacteriostatic washouts
  - Parvolex washouts; chlorhexidine washouts
- Prophylatic antibiotics should be given until the results of the initial investigations are known.

12.2 Neuropathic bladder

This may be defined as any neurological lesion which leads to major disturbance of the primary functions of the bladder and urethra, which are: (a) to hold a useful volume of urine and to empty fully; (b) bladder emptying to be under voluntary control; and (c) bladder and urethra should not damage the function of the kidneys

Important causes of renal damage

- UTI due to incomplete emptying
- High-pressure vesicoureteric reflux
- Progressive renal scarring

Causes

- Spina bifida; sacral agenesis (maternal diabetes)
- Tumour; trauma
- Transverse myelitis

Types

- Hyper-reflexic; high pressure; detrusor-sphincter dyssynergia
- Atonic — large, chronically distended, poorly emptying

Principles of management

- Videourodynamic assessment of **type** of bladder dysfunction
- Careful assessment of kidney structure, scarring, function, BP
- Improve emptying with clean, intermittent catheterization
- Anticholinergics (oxybutynin) may help reduce unstable contractions
- Augmentation cystoplasty — larger capacity, lower pressure

13. NOCTURNAL ENURESIS

This is a common condition which is benign, but which may cause distress and psychological upset to the child and family. Most children become dry at night 6–9 months after becoming dry by day, which is usually by 3 years. As a simple guide, 10% of 5-year-olds and 5% of 10-year-olds wet the bed ≥1 night per week. It is commoner in boys.

13.1 Definitions

- **Primary nocturnal enuresis** (~80%): never achieved night-time dryness
- **Secondary nocturnal enuresis:** recurrence of bedwetting having been dry ≥ 1 year
- **Initial successful response:** 14 consecutive dry nights within 16 weeks of starting treatment
- **Relapse:** >2 wet nights in 2 weeks
- **Complete success:** no relapse within 2 years of initial success

13.2 Aetiology

- Rarely an organic cause; should be distinguished from true **incontinence**, e.g. due to neuropathic bladder or ectopic ureter, when child is **never** dry
- Genetic component:
  - Commoner where there is a first-degree relative with history of enuresis
  - Concordance in monozygotic twins twice that in dizygotic twins
- No significant excess of major psychological or behavioural disturbance, though family stress, bullying at school, etc. may trigger secondary enuresis and such factors should be sought in the history
- Evidence from studies that:
  - In younger children, bladder capacity is reduced compared with non-enuretic children
  - In older children and adolescents, there is reduction in the normally observed rise in nocturnal ADH levels, and decrease in nocturnal urine volume (hence rationale for DDAVP treatment)

13.3 Assessment

- Careful history is crucial
- Examination should exclude abnormalities of abdomen, spine, lower limb neurology, hypertension
- Investigations should be limited to urinalysis

13.4 Treatment

Sustained and frequent support and encouragement for child *and* parents from an enthusiastic carer (doctor, nurse) is the most essential factor in seeing improvement. Any treatment must involve the child, and success depends on their motivation.

- Star charts; colouring-in charts: simple behavioural therapy that is successful alone in many children; and should be part of the monitoring of all interventions
- Enuresis alarms:
  - Have been used for nearly 100 years
  - Mat on bed attached to bedside buzzer, *or*
  - Small moisture sensor worn between two layers of underwear with vibrator alarm attached to pyjamas (has the advantage of detecting wet underwear rather than waiting to detect a wet bed)
  - May see 85% dry within 4 months, with a low 10% relapse rate
  - More effective than drug therapies in direct comparative trials
  - Should be mainstay of treatment, but enthusiastic and supportive care, and involvement of child (e.g. they should get up and change bedding) is crucial to success
- Drug therapy:
  - **Imipramine:** low long-term success rate; high relapse rate; potentially serious side-effects; rarely used
  - **Desmopressin (DDAVP) (oral or intranasal):** meta-analysis of all published trials showed relatively poor short-term complete response rate, high relapse rate, and poor long-term cure rate; more effective in older children; useful for short-term control for special situations, e.g. school trip
  - **Oxybutynin:** should be restricted to those children with clear history of **detrusor instability** — daytime urgency, frequency, urge incontinence — many of whom also wet the bed

14. HYPERTENSION (HT)

Most significant hypertension in childhood is secondary to an underlying cause. **Essential hypertension** is a diagnosis of exclusion; the typical patient is an obese adolescent with mild hypertension and a family history of hypertension.

What is normal?

- BP rises throughout childhood, related to age and height
- Depends on method and frequency of measurement
- US Task Force on Blood Pressure Control produce centile charts based on 60,000 normal children and teenagers

What is abnormal?

- **Consistently** above the 95th centile for age
- Loss of normal diurnal pattern
- Infants and toddlers may require admission to hospital for BP monitoring to make diagnosis

14.1 Ambulatory blood pressure monitoring (ABPM)

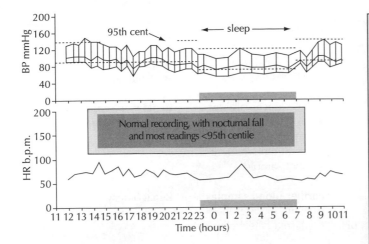

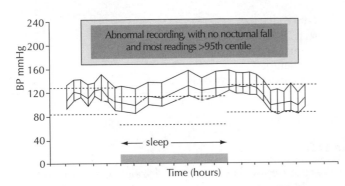

Uses small programmable monitor, oscillometric BP measurement, worn on belt with cuff on arm for 24 hours at home. Monitor downloads to PC for graphical display and statistical analysis

Advantages of ABPM

- Avoids observer error
- More reproducible
- Diagnosis of 'white coat hypertension'

Disadvantages of ABPM

- No normal data for small children
- Poorly tolerated by some young children
- May disturb sleep
- No long-term outcome correlations yet

14.2 Causes of secondary hypertension

Cause	Potentially curable by surgery/intervention
Renal	
Reflux nephropathy	If unilateral only
Polycystic kidney disease	✗
Glomerulonephritis, e.g. FSGS	✗
Renal artery stenosis	✓
Middle aortic syndrome, e.g. NF1; William's syndrome	✓
Coarctation	✓
Endocrine	
Phaeochromocytoma	✓
Cushing's syndrome	✓
Other	Depends on cause

14.3 Evaluation of hypertension by increasing level of invasiveness

Level 1	Level 2	Level 3
Assessment of risk factors • family history; obesity	**Further renal imaging** • 99Tc^m DMSA scan	**Arteriography** • Renal artery stenosis

Consequences of HT
• symptom history
• fundoscopy
• echocardiography
	Urine catecholamines
	• 24 hour total
	• catecholamine:
	  creatinine ratio on
	  spot sample
		Renal vein renin sampling
		IVC catecholamine sampling

Secondary renal causes of HT • urinalysis • urea + electrolytes, creatinine, pH • renal US scan	**Further blood samples** • renin, aldosterone • plasma catecholamines	**Renal biopsy**

	Other imaging
	• [^{131}I]MIBG
	  (metaiodobenzylguanidine)
	  scan for
	  phaeochromocytoma	

14.4 Treatment of hypertension

Short-term treatment of acute HT

- Commonest clinical indication is **acute nephritis** with salt and water retention; simple and well-tolerated combination would be a loop diuretic, e.g. furosemide (frusemide), plus a vasodilating Ca-channel blocker, e.g. nifedipine
- **Phaeochromocytoma** — α- and β-blockers, e.g. phenoxybenzamine and labetalol

Urgent treatment of hypertensive encephalopathy

- Severe hypertension with headache, vomiting, hyper-reflexia, seizures
- Principle of treatment is:
  - **Controllable** reduction with i.v. infusions: labetalol, Na nitroprusside
  - **Gradual** reduction: end-organ damage, e.g. seizures often relieved before **normal** BP seen
  - Risk of treatment is too rapid reduction causing stroke; cortical blindness

Long-term treatment of chronic HT

- Aim to use **single agent** if possible; and select **long-acting** once-daily agent to aid compliance, e.g.
  - β-blocker: atenolol
  - Ca-channel blocker: amlodipine

- ACE inhibitor: enalapril; logical choice for HT secondary to chronic renal disease (e.g. reflux nephropathy; FSGS); also has an antiproteinuric effect; relatively contraindicated in renal artery stenosis

15. INHERITED DISEASES

15.1 Polycystic kidney disease

Autosomal recessive polycystic kidney disease (ARPKD)

- Gene is on chromosome 6
- Tubular dilatation of distal collecting ducts, i.e. not true cysts

Clinical presentation

- Antenatal US: large echobright kidneys; oligohydramnios
- At birth or early infancy:
  - Large palpable renal masses
  - Respiratory distress secondary to pulmonary hypoplasia
- At any time:
  - Signs and symptoms of chronic renal failure
  - Hypertension — often very severe

Median age for onset of endstage renal failure is around 12 years, though may cause severe renal failure in infancy; very variable disease severity even within same family.

Always associated with **congenital hepatic fibrosis** that may vary from subclinical to causing liver disease, which is the dominant clinical feature; complications include ascending cholangitis.

Autosomal dominant polycystic kidney disease (ADPKD)

- At least two gene loci; commonest on chromosome 16 (adjacent to tuberous sclerosis gene)
- True cysts arising from tubules — get larger and more numerous with time and hence cause progressive decline in renal function
- An important cause of hypertension and renal failure in adults, though may present in childhood
- Associated with cerebral aneurysms and subarachnoid haemorrhage

Clinical presentation
(Again, very variable in age and severity)

- Antenatal US: discrete cysts in fetal kidneys (NB. Always scan parents' kidneys)
- Microscopic haematuria

- Hypertension; renal failure
- Incidental finding of renal cysts during abdominal US:
  - First cysts may not appear until patient in twenties; may be unilateral

15.2 Alport's syndrome

- Hereditary nephritis with sensorineural deafness and anterior lenticonus (conical deformity of lens of eye seen with slit lamp)
- X-linked (commonest) and autosomal recessive forms
- Associated with cerebral aneurysms and subarachnoid haemorrhage
  - X-linked: males affected; female carriers all have microscopic haematuria; with Lyonization some females may develop hypertension and renal disease, but milder and later onset
  - Autosomal recessive (chromosome 2): both sexes equally severe
- Basic defect is in production of subunits for type IV collagen (two subunits coded for on X chromosome, two on chromosome 2); type IV collagen located in kidney, eye and inner ear, hence the main clinical features
- Presents with incidental finding of microscopic haematuria, or episode of macroscopic haematuria
- Deafness around 10 years
- Hypertension mid-teens
- Eye signs mid–late teens (not before 12 years of age)
- Average age ESRF develops is 21-years-old

15.3 Nephronophthisis

- Autosomal recessive condition; gene (called *NPHP1*) on chromosome 2
- Produces polyuria (concentrating defect), growth delay and often severe anaemia
- Urinalysis typically 'bland', sometimes a trace of glucose
- Progresses to endstage renal failure towards the end of the first decade
- Sometimes associated with tapetoretinal degeneration: Senior–Löken syndrome

16. NEPHROCALCINOSIS AND NEPHROLITHIASIS

16.1 Nephrocalcinosis

Diffuse speckling calcification seen on US scan or plain X-ray.

Main causes of nephrocalcinosis

- Distal RTA
- Ex-prem neonates:
  - Furosemide   Hypercalciuria
  - Steroids   Hypercalciuria

- Vitamin D Rx for hypophosphataemic rickets:
  - Enhances tubular reabsorption Ca^{2+}
- Oxalosis:
  - Autosomal recessive disorder of liver enzymes
  - Excess oxalate production and urinary excretion
  - Calcium oxalate precipitates, nephrocalcinosis and obstructing stones form, renal failure ensues
  - Systemic oxalosis — joints, heart, blood vessels
  - Rx: liver and kidney transplantation

16.2 Nephrolithiasis

Uncommon in paediatrics.

Clinical presentation

- Painful haematuria
- Revealed during investigation into UTI

Important to undertake metabolic analysis of timed urine collection, or stone itself if possible, since several metabolic diseases cause stones which may be recurrent.

Type	Cause	Radio-opaque
Mg–ammonium–phosphate	Proteus UTI; urinary stasis	+/–
Calcium phosphate	RTA; hypercalciuria	+
Calcium oxalate	Oxalosis	+
Cystine	Cystinuria	+
Uric acid	Lesch–Nyhan; tumour lysis	–
Xanthine	Xanthinuria	–

17. FURTHER READING

Clinical Paediatric Nephrology: Postlethwaite RJ (ed.), 3rd edition. Oxford University Press, 2002
Pediatric Nephrology: Barratt, Avner, Harmon (eds), 4th edition. Lippincott, Williams and Wilkins, 2000
Clinical Physiology of Acid–Base and Electrolyte Disorders, Rose B D (ed.), 5th edition. McGraw Hill, 1999.

Chapter 15

Neurology

Neil H Thomas

CONTENTS

Neurology

1. DEVELOPMENTAL ABNORMALITIES OF THE NERVOUS SYSTEM

1.1 Normal development of the nervous system

The exact details of the normal development of the nervous system are complex, but the important stages can be summarized in the table below:

Stage	Time	Event	Potential disorder
Organ induction: (a) Dorsal	3–7 weeks	Neural tube closure	Anencephaly, spina bifida
(b) Ventral	5–6 weeks	Forebrain, facial development	Holoprosencephaly
Neuronal and glial proliferation	8–16 weeks	Neural proliferation and early cellular differentiation	Microcephaly
Neuronal migration	12–19 weeks	Neuronal migration and formation of corpus callosum	Lissencephaly, pachygyria, agenesis of corpus callosum
Neuronal organization	22 weeks–postnatal	Orientation of cortical structures	Cortical dysplasia
Myelination	24 weeks through early childhood years		Dysmyelination

1.2 Neural tube defects

Spina bifida occulta

Asymptomatic condition characterized by failure of closure of vertebral arch. Occurs in up to 5% of population.

Anencephaly

Failure of closure of the rostral aspect of the neural tube. 75% of affected infants stillborn.

Encephalocele

Protrusion of cerebral tissue through midline cranial defect located in frontal or occipital regions.

Meningocele

Cyst formed by herniation of meninges, usually over dorsum of spine. Neurological disability minimal, risk of bacterial meningitis.

Meningomyelocele

Herniation of meninges, nerve roots and spinal cord through dorsal vertebral defect. Leads to motor and sensory deficits below lesion, including sphincter disturbance. May be associated with other malformations of spinal cord including Arnold–Chiari malformation (downward displacement of cerebellar tonsils through foramen magnum). Hydrocephalus may coexist, secondary to Arnold–Chiari malformation or aqueduct stenosis.

Prevention of neural tube defects

- Clear evidence that preconceptual folate supplementation prevents production of neural tube defects.

Treatment of neural tube defects

- Operative repair of encephalocoele, meningocoele, myelomeningocoele
- Close observation for development of hydrocephalus and operative treatment
- Management of bladder and bowels, possible intermittent bladder drainage
- Orthopaedic management of limb deformities
- Assessment of cognitive abilities
- Treatment of seizures

1.3 Hydrocephalus

Defined as excess fluid within the cranium. Usually refers to increased volume of cerebrospinal fluid (CSF).

Production of CSF

- Secreted by choroid plexus (plasma ultrafiltrate, then modified)
- Flows through lateral ventricles, through third and fourth ventricles into posterior fossa and basal cisterns
- Reabsorbed through arachnoid granulations

Terms such as 'communicating' and 'non-communicating' hydrocephalus are now obsolete.

Main aetiological mechanisms of hydrocephalus

Oversecretion	Choroid plexus papilloma
Obstruction	
	<ul><li>Intraventricular: tumours, malformations, inflammation (post-haemorrhagic)</li><li>Extraventricular: inflammation, tumours, mucopolysaccharidoses</li></ul>
Impaired resorption	Venous sinus compression

Diagnosis

- May be asymptomatic
- Irritability
- Headache
- Vomiting
- Drowsiness
- Increased head circumference
- Tense anterior fontanelle
- Splayed sutures
- Scalp vein distension
- Loss of upward gaze (sunsetting)
- Neck rigidity
- Decreased conscious level
- Cranial nerve palsies

Investigations

- Ultrasonography (when fontanelle open)
- Computed tomography (CT)
- Magnetic resonance imaging (MRI)
- Measurement of CSF pressure by neurosurgical intervention may be indicated

Management

- Decide need for operation by considering symptoms and rate of head growth
- Surgical:
  - Ventriculostomy
  - Shunting (ventriculoperitoneal, ventriculoatrial)

1.4 Disorders of cortical development

Lissencephaly

Brain has very few or no gyri, leaving the surface of the brain smooth. Leads to severe motor and learning disability. Lissencephaly may be associated with facial abnormalities and a deletion on chromosome 17p13.3 in the Miller–Dieker syndrome.

Polymicrogyria

Increased numbers of small gyri, especially in temporoparietal regions.

Periventricular heterotopia

Aggregation of neurones arrested in their primitive positions. May be part of complex brain malformation syndromes.

Pachygyria

Thickened abnormal cortex. Depending on extent, may lead to cerebral palsy picture or to epilepsy.

Agenesis of corpus callosum

Corpus callosum develops between 10th and 12th weeks of embryonic life. Agenesis may be isolated or associated with other malformations. Extent of other malformations determines disability.

1.5 Other nervous system maldevelopments

Dandy–Walker malformation (DWM)

Classical DWM includes:

- Complete or partial agenesis of cerebellar vermis
- Large cystic formation in posterior fossa due to dilatation of fourth ventricle
- Hydrocephalus, which may not develop until adulthood

May be associated with other cerebral malformations. Considered part of a continuum including Dandy–Walker variant (part of vermis present, posterior fossa not enlarged) and megacisterna magna (complete vermis, large retrocerebellar cyst).

Aqueduct stenosis

Cause of hydrocephalus in 11% of cases. Aqueduct may be reduced in size or may be represented by numerous channels within aqueduct location. Can occur in X-linked syndrome.

2. NEONATAL NEUROLOGY

2.1 Neonatal seizures

Seizures are a major neurological problem in the first 28 days of life.

Classification	
Tonic seizures	— Stiffening of trunk and extremities
Multifocal clonic seizures	— Rhythmic clonic movements of different parts of the body and various seizures
Focal clonic seizures	— Repetitive clonic movements of the same part of the body
Subtle seizures	— Episodes of stereotyped bicycling, sucking and swallowing movements
Myoclonic seizures	— Isolated repetitive brief jerks of the body

Causes

- Hypoxic–ischaemic encephalopathy
- Intracranial haemorrhage
- Intracranial infection
- Cerebral malformations
- Metabolic disturbances
- Withdrawal seizures
- Familial neonatal convulsions

2.2 Hypoxic–ischaemic encephalopathy (HIE)

The neonatal brain is highly resistant to hypoxia–ischaemia compared with that of an adult. The degree of hypoxia–ischaemia necessary to damage the neonatal brain usually leads to impairment of other organs.

Hypoxia–ischaemia leads to depletion of brain phosphocreatine and ATP. Lactate increases.

Clinical features

5-minute Apgar score of less than 6, a metabolic acidosis and hypotension are all sugges-tive of asphyxia in term infants.

HIE in term infants

Stage 1 — Hyperalert, tremulousness, poor feeding; seizures infrequent

Stage 2 — Lethargic, obtunded, hypotonic; seizures may occur

Stage 3 — Comatose; seizures within 12–24 hours

Outcome according to severity of HIE

Stage 1 — Largely normal

Stage 2 — 5% die, 25% suffer neurological injury

Stage 3 — 80% die, 20% suffer neurological injury

2.3 Periventricular–intraventricular haemorrhage

Usually a disease of preterm infants. Majority of haemorrhages originate in subependymal germinal matrix.

Potential consequences

- Asymptomatic
- Catastrophic collapse
- Cerebral infarction
- Post-haemorrhagic hydrocephalus

2.4 Periventricular leucomalacia (PVL)

Pathological term to describe bilateral necrosis of periventricular white matter. Gliosis ensues. Leads to interruption of fibres which are responsible for lower limb and optic func-tion, so that PVL is often the underlying pathology to the spastic diplegia and visual impair-ment seen in survivors of preterm birth.

2.5 Brachial plexus injuries

Traction injury to the brachial plexus can follow difficulty in delivery of the shoulders and head during birth. A large baby, narrow birth canal and malpresentation may all contribute. Usually, the nerve roots are stretched but not completely avulsed. Clavicular or humeral fractures may also occur.

Erb's palsy

- C5–C6 lesion
- Affects deltoid, serratus anterior, supraspinatus, infraspinatus, biceps, brachioradialis
- Arm is flaccid, adducted and internally rotated
- Elbow is extended, wrist flexed ('waiter's tip')

Klumpke's paralysis

- C8–T1 lesion
- Affects intrinsic hand muscles so that flexion of wrist and fingers are affected
- Cervical sympathetic involvement may lead to an ipsilateral Horner's syndrome

Management

- Physiotherapy
- Consideration of nerve root surgery

3. DISORDERS OF MOVEMENT

3.1 Cerebral palsy

Cerebral palsy may be defined as a disorder of tone, posture or movement, which is due to a static lesion affecting the developing nervous system. Despite the unchanging nature of the causative lesion, its existence in a developing nervous system means that its manifestations may change over time.

Causes of cerebral palsy

Prenatal insults

- Intrauterine hypoxic–ischaemic injury
- Intrauterine infection
- Toxins
- Chromosomal disorders

Perinatal insults

- Hypoxic–ischaemic injury
- Intracranial haemorrhage
- Bilirubin encephalopathy

Postnatal insults

- Trauma
- Bacterial meningitis
- Viral encephalitis

Epidemiological studies suggest that at least 80% of cases of cerebral palsy are the result of prenatally acquired causes. A minority are the result of intrapartum asphyxia.

Classification
Based on distribution of motor impairment and tone variations.

Spastic (characterized by fixed increase in muscular tone)
- Hemiplegia
- Diplegia
- Quadriplegia

Athetoid (dyskinetic, dystonic)
(athetoid: writhing, involuntary pronation and flexion of distal extremity)
(choreiform: 'dancing' — involuntary rapid semi-purposeful movements of proximal segments of body)

Ataxic
Mixed

Spastic diplegia is most frequently seen as the result of periventricular leucomalacia in preterm infants.

Athetoid cerebral palsy may result from bilirubin encephalopathy or from brief profound anoxic–ischaemic episodes.

Associated clinical features

- Developmental delay
- Tendency to joint contractures
- Epilepsy
- Perceptual difficulties
- Visual and hearing impairment
- Poor growth
- Feeding difficulties

Children with cerebral palsy need the care of a multidisciplinary team.

3.2 Ataxia

Acute cerebellar ataxia may occur following viral infection. Appears to be due to both infectious and post-infectious processes; most commonly follows varicella. Also measles, mumps, herpes simplex virus, Epstein–Barr virus, coxsackievirus and echovirus.

Occult neuroblastoma may also lead to acute ataxia.

A common cause is overdosage of drugs such as carbamazepine, phenytoin, benzodiazepines. Also piperazine, antihistamines.

Other causes

- Posterior fossa tumour
- Migraine

Ataxia–telangiectasia

See section 13.3

Friedreich's ataxia

- Classified as a spinocerebellar degeneration
- Autosomal recessive condition (9cen–*q21*)
- Gene product frataxin
- Involved in modulation of mitochondrial function

Clinical

- Onset of symptoms in first or second decade
- Loss of proprioception
- Increasing impairment of cerebellar function
- Development of pes cavus
- Cardiomyopathy develops
- Deterioration so that patients are usually not ambulant in their twenties or thirties

Treatment

- Currently symptomatic
- Physiotherapy
- Suitable aids and appliances

3.3 Dystonia

Dystonia is a condition in which muscle tone is abnormal without pyramidal involvement. In many dystonias, muscular tone varies with position of limbs. There may be a dystonic component to cerebral palsy of hypoxic–ischaemic origin, but there are a number of clearly defined syndromes in which dystonia is the main feature.

Torsion dystonia (dystonia musculorum deformans)

- Genetically determined
- Autosomal dominant with incomplete penetrance
- Gene maps to *9q34* in Ashkenazim families
- Other unidentified gene responsible in some non-Ashkenazim families

Clinical

- Onset usually after 5 years
- May be focal or generalized
- Dystonia may be task-specific, for example affected children may not be able to walk forwards but can walk backwards normally
- Often gradual spread to other parts of the body
- Wilson's disease should always be excluded

Treatment

- High-dose anticholinergic drugs
- Occasionally L-dopa

Dopa-responsive dystonia

- Described by Segawa
- Idiopathic dystonia
- Symptoms vary throughout the day
- Onset may be in the first 5 years
- Gene map to chromosome 14q
- Symptoms respond dramatically to low-dose L-dopa, which should be continued for life

Other important causes of dystonia

- Wilson's disease
- Juvenile Huntington disease

3.4 Tics and Tourette's syndrome

Tics are involuntary movements affecting specific groups of muscles so that the affected individual appears to have brief purposeless movements or actions. Tics may be motor or vocal.

Simple tics

- Commonly affect children for a few months in mid-childhood
- Up to 25% of children
- Spontaneous resolution

Multiple tics

- Some children are prone to tics of different type
- Different motor tics, vocal tics
- May not remit entirely

Tourette's syndrome

Defined by:

- Multiple motor tics
- One or more vocal tics
- Onset before 21 years of age
- Duration of longer than 1 year

There is probably a continuum between multiple tics and Tourette's syndrome.

Other characteristic features of Tourette's

- Echolalia (compulsive repetition of words or phrases just heard)
- Coprolalia (compulsive swearing)
- Attention-deficit disorder and obsessive–compulsive features are present in 50%

Treatment

- Tics may respond to haloperidol

4. DEVELOPMENTAL DISABILITIES

4.1 Learning disability

The term 'learning disability' is now generally used in preference to the term 'mental retardation'. It covers a wide variety of conditions in which cognitive functioning is depressed below average levels. In the United States, the term 'mental retardation' is retained, with 'learning disability' being used to refer to failure to achieve cognitive potential.

Learning disability tends to be grouped according to severity: moderate learning disability usually refers to IQ 50–70, with severe learning disability being defined as IQ less than 50. The term 'profound learning disability' is sometimes used to refer to IQ less than 20.

The prevalence of learning disability is difficult to estimate. Prevalence of severe learning disability has been estimated at 3–4 per 1,000 but, although moderate learning disability is clearly more common, its exact prevalence remains obscure.

Aetiology

This is easier to determine in severe learning disability. In severe learning disability, the following potential causes are recognized:

- Chromosomal, e.g. trisomy 21
- Genetic, e.g. fragile X

- Congenital anomalies
- Intrauterine insults
- Central nervous system infection
- Unknown (20%)

Moderate learning disability

- Same range of problems as severe learning disability
- Unknown (55%)

Associated problems with learning disability

- Cerebral palsy
- Visual impairment
- Hearing impairment
- Behavioural difficulties

Baseline medical investigations for all children

- Full history and examination
- Karyotype including fragile X
- Thyroid function tests
- Plasma amino acids
- Urine mucopolysaccharide screen
- Plasma creatine kinase (in boys under 5 years)

Other tests may be indicated, depending on clinical features.

4.2 Autism

Autism is a disorder characterized by:

- Disturbance of reciprocal social interaction
- Disturbance of communication (including language, comprehension and expression)
- Disturbance of behaviour, leading to restriction of behavioural range

All the above findings may be seen in learning–disabled individuals.

Associated features in autism

- Learning disability
- Epilepsy
- Visual impairment
- Hearing impairment

Asperger syndrome

Often considered to be on the autistic spectrum. Characterized by autistic features in those individuals of otherwise normal intelligence. Specifically characterized by:

- Impairment in social interaction
- Stereotypic behaviour
- No specific impairment of language

See Chapter 2, *Child Development, Child Psychiatry and Community Paediatrics*

4.3 Attention-deficit hyperactivity disorder (ADHD)

Some children show impulsive, hyperactive behaviour in conjunction with poor concentration and attention. These children are usually of normal intelligence, although functionally they may achieve less than their peers. Medication such as methylphenidate or dexamfetamine may be effective.

See Chapter 2, *Child Development, Child Psychiatry and Community Paediatrics*

4.4 Deficits in attention, motor control and perception (DAMP)

- Often described as 'minimal brain damage' in older literature
- Deficit in motor control and perception often referred to as 'dyspraxia'
- Children have difficulties as described in varying degrees
- Treatment needs to include assessment, and also educational help and physical programme (occupational therapy)

5. EPILEPSY

5.1 Diagnosis

Diagnosis of 'fits, faints and funny turns' is based primarily on clinical assessment of such events with recognition of characteristic patterns, supported by the results of special investigations.

5.2 Definition and classification

Epileptic seizures are clinical events which result from abnormal, excessive electrical discharge from cerebral neurones.

Epilepsy is the tendency to have recurrent, usually unprovoked, epileptic seizures.

The classification of epilepsies can be approached from the viewpoint of the characteristics of individual seizures or by identification of epileptic syndromes.

International classification of epileptic seizures (modified from the International League against Epilepsy Classification)

Partial seizures	Simple partial seizures (no disturbance of consciousness)	with motor signs with somatosensory symptoms with autonomic symptoms with psychic symptoms
	Complex partial seizures (disturbance of consciousness)	
	Partial seizures with secondary generalization	
Generalized seizures	Absence seizures (typical and atypical) – Myoclonic seizures – Clonic seizures – Tonic seizures – Tonic–clonic seizures – Atonic seizures	

Classification of epileptic syndromes

Localization related epilepsies	Idiopathic	Benign childhood epilepsy with centrotemporal spikes ('benign rolandic epilepsy') Childhood epilepsy with occipital paroxysms
	Symptomatic	Temporal lobe epilepsy Frontal lobe epilepsy Parietal lobe epilepsy Occipital lobe epilepsy Epilepsia partialis continua
Generalized epileptic syndromes	Idiopathic	Benign neonatal familial convulsions Benign neonatal convulsions Benign myoclonic epilepsy of infancy Childhood absence epilepsy Juvenile absence epilepsy Juvenile myoclonic epilepsy Epilepsy with grand mal seizures on wakening
	Symptomatic/ cryptogenic	West syndrome (infantile spasms) Lennox–Gastaut syndrome Myoclonic–astatic epilepsy
	Symptomatic	Early myoclonic encephalopathy Ohtahara's syndrome
Epileptic syndromes unclassified as focal or generalized		Neonatal seizures Severe myoclonic epilepsy in infancy Epilepsy with continuous spike-waves in slow-wave sleep Landau–Kleffner syndrome

5.3 Generalized epilepsies

Absence seizures

Typical absence seizures, previously termed 'petit mal epilepsy', is characterized by brief (5–20 seconds) episodes of staring, during which the child is unaware of their surroundings. Associated with 3-Hz spike and wave discharge on EEG. Can be precipitated by hyperventilation. Drugs of choice: sodium valproate, ethosuximide, lamotrigine.

Atypical absences: EEG shows pattern of different frequency.

Myoclonic seizures

Brief, sudden, generalized muscular jerks. Drugs of choice: sodium valproate, benzodiazepines, lamotrigine. May be exacerbated by carbamazepine.

Infantile spasms

Onset in first 12 months — brief sudden muscular contractions resulting in extension or flexion of the body. Attacks occur in runs. Associated with disorganized EEG described as hypsarrhythmia, as well as developmental arrest or regression. May be idiopathic or symptomatic (causes include tuberous sclerosis, perinatal hypoxic–ischaemic injury, inborn errors of metabolism). Treatment of choice: corticosteroids (or ACTH) or vigabatrin.

Juvenile myoclonic

Onset in adolescence — myoclonic seizures on waking, generalized tonic-clonic seizures from sleep at night. Treatment of choice: sodium valproate; carbamazepine may exacerbate seizures.

5.4 Partial epilepsies

Benign childhood epilepsy with centrotemporal spikes ('benign rolandic epilepsy')	Characterized by predominantly nocturnal partial seizures with a slight male preponderance. Seizures may affect face or upper limbs; speech arrest may occur. Excellent prognosis for remission.
Complex partial seizures	Characterized by stereotypic behaviour, loss of consciousness and focal EEG abnormalities. Often arise from temporal lobe foci. May respond to carbamazepine or sodium valproate.

5.5 Assessment and treatment of epilepsy

- Clinical assessment of seizure type and frequency
- EEG allows more specific classification of seizure type; if standard EEG is normal and further EEG confirmation is necessary in the face of clear clinical history of epileptic seizures, then sleep or sleep-deprived EEG may document abnormalities
- Imaging (MRI) is indicated in partial seizures and generalized seizures resistant to treatment

Management

- Explanation of potential risks and benefits of different therapies
- Medication — start, depending on frequency and number of seizures
- Maintenance of seizure freedom with medication for perhaps 2 years
- Subsequent withdrawal of medication
- Some forms of partial epilepsy may be amenable to epilepsy surgery — when seizure disorder is intractable — site of seizure onset can be localized — site is non-eloquent brain
- Other forms of treatment — steroids, ketogenic diet, vagal nerve stimulation

5.6 Anticonvulsant drugs

Drug	Used for seizure types	Dose range	Side-effects	Notes
Carbamazepine	Partial seizures Generalized tonic–clonic seizures	15–25 mg/kg per day	Ataxia, sedation, leucopenia, thrombocytopenia rash	
Sodium valproate	All seizure types	20–40 mg/kg per day	Nausea, vomiting, abdominal pain, tremor, hair loss, thrombocytopenia, liver function abnormalities	
Lamotrigine	All seizure types	With valproate: 5 mg/kg per day Without valproate: 15 mg/kg per day	Rash	Not licensed as monotherapy for under 12-year-olds
Vigabatrin	Partial seizures West's syndrome	50–150 mg/kg per day	Sedation, visual field constriction	
Ethosuximide	Absences	20–50 mg/kg per day	Gastrointestinal disturbance, rash	
Gabapentin	Partial seizures	Up to 45 mg/kg per day	Sedation	
Oxcarbazepine	Partial/generalized seizures	30 mg/kg per day	Sedation, rash	
Topiramate	All seizure types	6–9 mg/kg per day	Sedation, anorexia, paraesthesias	
Clobazam	All seizure types	2 mg/kg per day	Sedation	
Clonazepam	All seizure types		Sedation	
Phenytoin	All seizure types	5 mg/kg per day	Nausea, vomiting, diarrhoea, rash, peripheral neuropathy	Measure level
Phenobarbitone	All seizure types	5–8 mg/kg per day	Sedation	Measure level
Levetiracetam	Partial seizures		Sedation	Not licensed for under 16-year-olds
Tiagabine	Partial seizures		Sedation	Not licensed for under 12-year-olds

5.7 Management of status epilepticus

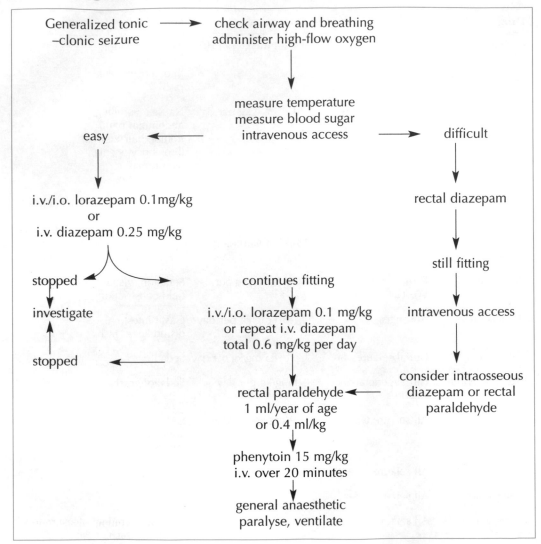

Prognosis

70% of children with epilepsy are seizure-free by their 16th birthday. Remission is less likely in: partial epilepsy, symptomatic epilepsy, some epilepsy syndromes such as juvenile myoclonic epilepsy or epileptic encephalopathies such as Lennox–Gastaut syndrome.

6. NON-EPILEPTIC SEIZURES

6.1 Anoxic seizures

Anoxic (or anoxic–ischaemic) seizures form a group of paroxysmal disorders which are often the main differential diagnosis of epilepsy. Diagnosis is predominantly by clinical assessment. There are two important types seen in childhood: breath-holding attacks and reflex anoxic seizures.

Breath-holding attacks are seen in young children, often in the setting of a tantrum. The thwarted child screams and screams and holds his or her breath, becoming cyanosed and sometimes exhibiting subsequent convulsive movements. It may be possible to encourage the child to take a breath by gently blowing on their face. The tendency to have such episodes abates as children become older.

Reflex anoxic seizures are the clinical manifestation of vagocardiac attacks. The precipitant may be a sudden, unexpected, painful stimulus or occasionally vomiting. Increased sensitivity of the vagus nerve leads to bradycardia, or even brief asystole, leading to pallor and cerebral anoxia–ischaemia. Following collapse, the child may then exhibit convulsive movements. Recovery is spontaneous. Apart from the risk of injury during a collapse, the prognosis is good with few, if any, individuals suffering adverse cerebral effects. The tendency to have such attacks improves with age but is often not completely abolished. Diagnosis can be confirmed by eliciting bradycardia under controlled monitoring conditions by exerting eyeball pressure.

6.2 Psychogenic seizures

A small proportion of children have episodes of collapse, or even epileptiform attacks, which are under conscious or subconscious control. The trigger for these episodes is usually some form of psychological disturbance, which may be deeply hidden.

The nature and setting of the attack is often a clue to the event. The attack itself may include sudden collapse without, for example, pallor or an epileptiform attack during which the child may respond to his/her surroundings. The setting of the attack is often to gain maximum attention for the episode. There is often some form of behavioural trigger to elicit an event.

Prolonged EEG and electrocardiographic monitoring may be helpful in supporting the diagnosis and in helping families accept the nature of the attack.

Management is via psychological or psychiatric treatment.

7. HEADACHES

Headache is a common complaint in childhood. Population studies estimate that up to 35% of children have complained of headache at some time. The commonest cause of headache in Western populations is tension or psychogenic headache.

Classification of headache

Tension or psychogenic headache

Migraine

Vascular disorders	• Subarachnoid haemorrhage • Hypertension • Arteriovenous malformation
Headaches related to raised intra-cranial pressure	• Tumours • Hydrocephalus • Benign intracranial hypertension • Subdural haematomata
Inflammatory disorders	• Meningitis • Vasculitis
Referred pain	• Sinusitis • Optic neuritis • Otitis media
Miscellaneous	• Refractive errors • Carbon monoxide poisoning • Substance abuse

7.1 Tension headaches

- Often occur daily
- Generalized, dull — may involve band-like compression around head
- Worsens over the day
- Worse with stress
- Normal examination
- Anxious or depressed affect
- Depressive features in history

Management

- Reassurance
- Supportive psychotherapy

7.2 Migraine

Defined as: 'Familial disorder characterized by recurrent attacks of headache widely variable in intensity, frequency and duration. Attacks are commonly unilateral and are usually associated with neurological and mood disturbance. All of the above characteristics are not necessarily present in each attack or in each patient.'

Classification of migraine

- Common migraine (no aura)
- Classical migraine (aura preceding onset of headache)
- Complicated migraine (persisting neurological deficit after migraine attack)
- Basilar migraine
- Migraine variance
- Cluster headaches

Treatment

Acute
Analgesics, relaxation, occasionally antiemetics

Prophylaxis
Avoidance of triggers such as cheese, chocolate, yeast extract
Medications such as pizotifen, propranolol

7.3 Other headaches

Post-traumatic headache
Following concussive head injury. May last several months, then resolves. May persist in the setting of depression or ongoing litigation.

Headache due to raised intracranial pressure
Worse in early morning. Worse with coughing and bending.

8. ABNORMALITIES OF HEAD SIZE AND SHAPE

Brain growth is usually the most important determinant of head growth. In full-term infants, the rate of head growth is: 2 cm per month in the first 3 months; in the second 3 months, 1 cm per month; and in the subsequent 6 months, 0.5 cm per month.

8.1 Macrocephaly

Consider:

- Familial macrocephaly
- Hydrocephalus

- Chronic subdural haematomata
- Associated disorders such as tuberous sclerosis or neurofibromatosis
- Metabolic conditions

Investigations depend on rate of growth, deviation from normal and presence of absence of abnormal neurological signs.

Treatment
If necessary, based on underlying pathology.

8.2 Microcephaly

Defined as occipitofrontal head circumference below two standard deviations for age, sex and gestational age.

Consider

- Insults during pregnancy
- Perinatal insults
- Encephalopathies in infancy
- Autosomal recessive microcephaly

Investigations

- Chromosomes
- Antibodies to congenital infections
- Metabolic screen
- MRI scan
- Consider measurement of maternal plasma amino acids to exclude maternal phenylketonuria

8.3 Abnormal head shape

May be associated with specific syndrome, e.g achondroplasia or Down's syndrome. May be the result of craniosynostosis.

Craniosynostosis

Premature closure of one or more cranial sutures. Ultimate skull deformity will depend upon which sutures are involved and the timing of their fusion.

Head shape	Description	Sutures involved	Problems
Scaphocephaly	Elongated narrow skull	Sagittal	Cosmetic
Brachycephaly	Short broad skull	Both coronal	Associated anomalies such as learning disability
Plagiocephaly	Unilateral flattening of skull	Single coronal (occasionally lambdoid)	Cosmetic
Trigonocephaly	Narrow pointed forehead	Metopic	Possible associated forebrain abnormalities
Oxycephaly (acrocephaly)	High pointed head	Coronal, sagittal, lambdoid	Apert's and Crouzon's syndrome (see below)

Apert's syndrome

Acrocephaly, facial underdevelopment, syndactyly, learning disability

Crouzon's syndrome

Acrocephaly, scaphocephaly or brachycephaly, hypertelorism, exophthalmos, increased intracranial pressure, learning disability

9. NEUROMUSCULAR DISORDERS

9.1 The floppy infant

It is important to realize that much of the process leading to a diagnosis in the floppy infant is the clinical assessment of the infant by history and examination. It is this assessment which should direct diagnostic investigations. In an era when specific genetic tests for conditions are increasingly available, a clearer idea of possible diagnoses is even more important.

Causes of hypotonia in infants

General health

- Prematurity
- Intercurrent illness
- Ligamentous laxity

General: neurological

- Chromosomal abnormalities
  e.g. Down's syndrome
- Prader–Willi syndrome
- Hypoxic–ischaemic brain injury
  (especially early basal ganglia injury)
- Metabolic conditions
  - Aminoacidurias
  - Organic acidurias
  - Peroxisomal disorders

Muscle

- Congenital muscular dystrophy
- Congenital myopathies
- Congenital myotonic dystrophy

Spinal

- Cervical cord injury

Anterior horn cell

- Poliomyelitis
- Spinal muscular atrophy

Peripheral nerve

- Peripheral neuropathies

Neuromuscular junction

- Transient myasthenia
- Congenital myasthenic syndrome

9.2 Duchenne muscular dystrophy (DMD)

DMD is easily the commonest neuromuscular condition seen in Western European practice.

- Inherited as X-linked recessive condition
- One-third are new mutations
- Incidence 1 in 3,500 male births
- Female carriers usually asymptomatic, occasionally manifesting carriers

Molecular genetics

- Due to mutations in dystrophin gene
- Gene approximately 2 million base pairs
- DMD patients produce no dystrophin
- Becker muscular dystrophy (allelic, milder form) patients produce abnormal but functional protein
- Dystrophin localized to muscle-cell membrane

Clinical features

- Onset in early years
- Some cases identified presymptomatically by abnormal transaminases measured during intercurrent illness
- Sometimes leads to failure to thrive
- Early delay in motor milestones
- Difficulties in climbing stairs
- Lordosis with waddling gait
- Pseudohypertrophy of calves
- Progressive muscular weakness
- Tendency to joint contractures
- Typically, boys lose ability to walk between 8 and 12 years
- When dependent on wheelchair, boys are prone to develop scoliosis
- Respiratory failure supervenes

Also

- Increased incidence of learning disability
- Cardiomyopathy occurs
- Survival to late teens, early twenties

Diagnosis

- High plasma creatine kinase (greater than 5,000 IU/l)
- Mutations in dystrophin gene
- Muscle biopsy — dystrophic picture with absent dystrophin

Treatment

- No curative treatment
- Physiotherapy
- Appropriate seating
- Management of scoliosis

Becker muscular dystrophy (BMD)

- Allelic disease to DMD
- Milder than DMD
- Patients walk beyond 16 years of age
- Similar clinical pattern to DMD
- Cramps can be problematical
- Prone to cardiomyopathy

Diagnosis

DMD and BMD distinguished clinically and on muscle biopsy findings. Nature of genetic mutation can give pointer as to severity of condition but current routine genetic testing does not distinguish reliably between DMD and BMD; it just identifies a dystrophinopathy.

9.3 Other muscular dystrophies and congenital myopathies

Muscular dystrophies are characterized by dystrophic muscle histopathology: muscle fibre necrosis and regeneration with increased fat and connective tissue. May be progressive or static.

Emery–Dreifuss muscular dystrophy

- Uncommon X-linked muscular dystrophy (Xq28)
- Mild proximal muscular weakness
- Joint contractures
- Cardiac involvement — affected individuals may be prone to sudden cardiac death

Facioscapulohumeral muscular dystrophy

- Autosomal dominant muscular dystrophy (4q35)
- Facial, scapular and humeral wasting and weakness
- Slowly progressive
- Other muscles may be involved
- Variable expression within families

Limb–girdle muscular dystrophies

- Common on a worldwide basis
- May be inherited as autosomal dominant or autosomal recessive traits (at least three separate autosomal dominant and nine autosomal recessive limb-girdle muscular dystrophies identified so far)
- Variations in clinical phenotype
- Many are similar to DMD or BMD

Congenital muscular dystrophies

This is a group of disorders in infants characterized by muscular weakness, hypotonia and joint contractures from birth.

- Muscle biopsy shows typical dystrophic changes
- Different subtypes now being described

Merosin-negative congenital muscular dystrophy

- Characterized by absence of merosin on muscle biopsy
- Clinically hypotonia, weakness, contractures
- Often associated with learning disability
- Functionally, affected children do not achieve independent walking

Merosin-positive congenital muscular dystrophy

- Clinically less severe than merosin-negative congenital muscular dystrophy

Fukuyama congenital muscular dystrophy

- Autosomal recessive (9q31–q33)
- As well as severe weakness, affected individuals have brain malformations

Congenital myopathies

A group of disorders characterized by hypotonia and weakness from birth. Differentiated on clinical and histological features.

- Central cord disease
- Nemaline myopathy
- Myotubular myopathy

Myotonic dystrophy

- Common (incidence 13.5 per 100,000 live births) neuromuscular condition
- Autosomal dominant inheritance (19q13)
- Severity appears to be related to size of triplet repeat (CTG) in gene mutation

Congenital myotonic dystrophy

- Condition often unrecognized in mothers
- Preceding polyhydramnios
- Baby often born unexpectedly 'flat'
- Facial weakness, hypotonia
- Often requires respiratory support
- Joint contractures, especially talipes

Myotonic dystrophy in older children and adults

- Facial weakness initially
- Then weakness affecting temporalis, sternomastoid, distal leg muscles
- Progressive weakness
- Difficulties in relaxing muscular contraction, e.g difficulties in relaxing grip
- Cardiac involvement

Diagnosis

- Gene mutation analysis
- Electromyogram in older children upwards (over 3 to 4 years of age) shows characteristic 'dive bomber' discharges

Myotonia congenita (Thomsen's disease)

- Rare
- Autosomal dominant inheritance
- Characterized by myotonia, cramps
- Muscular hypertrophy is typical

9.4 Anterior horn cell disease

Spinal muscular atrophy (SMA)

The spinal muscular atrophies are a group of heterogeneous conditions which are characterized by the clinical effects of anterior horn cell degeneration. The commonest SMAs in childhood are the autosomal recessive proximal SMAs.

Clinical

- Symmetrical muscle weakness of trunk and limbs, more marked proximally than distally and in legs more than arms
- Tongue fasciculation
- Investigations confirming neurogenic abnormalities

Genetics

- Autosomal recessive
- Gene at chromosome 5q11–13
- Disease caused by mutations of *SMN* gene
- Severity-determining mechanism remains unclear

Childhood-onset proximal SMAs

Severity	Synonyms	Functional abilities
Severe	Type I, acute, Werdnig–Hoffman disease	Unable to sit or walk
Intermediate	Type II	Able to sit, but not walk
Mild	Type III, Kugelberg–Welander disease	Able to walk

Severe SMA

- Incidence 1 in 20,000 live births
- In approximately 30% onset is prenatal
- Symmetrical weakness
- Paralysis of intercostal muscles
- Absent deep tendon reflexes

- Tongue fasciculation
- Death occurs within first 18 months from respiratory failure/infection

Diagnosis

- EMG
- Muscle biopsy
- Genetic analysis

Intermediate SMA

- Autosomal recessive
- Usual onset after 3 months
- Infant learns to sit
- Prone to early scoliosis
- Prognosis depends on degree of respiratory muscle involvement

Mild SMA

- Autosomal recessive
- Able to walk, but proximal weakness evident
- Tendon jerks may not be absent

9.5 Neuropathies

Hereditary motor and sensory neuropathies (HMSN) are the most common degenerative disorders of the peripheral nervous system. Often known by their eponymous title Charcot–Marie–Tooth disease (CMT) or peroneal muscular atrophy.

Previously, X-linked, autosomal recessive and autosomal dominant forms were recognized, but the advent of molecular genetics has identified numerous genetically distinct forms (see table on following page).

Clinically, affected individuals develop slowly progressive distal weakness with areflexia. In the early phases, foot drop is often the main clinical problem. In later stages, which in the common forms may be several decades after onset, hand weakness, joint deformity and distal sensory loss may be problematical.

Hereditary motor and sensory neuropathies (CMT)

Type	Inheritance	Genetic defect	Gene	Neurophysiology	Onset
Type I (Demyelinating)					
CMT 1A	AD	Duplication 17p11.2	*PMP22*	Low motor-nerve conduction velocity	First decade
CMT 1B	AD	1q21–q23	*PO*		
CMT 1C	AD	?	?		
CMT 4	AR	8q (one type)	?		
Type II (Axonal)					
CMT 2A	AD	1p36	?	Normal motor-nerve conduction velocity	Second to third decade
CMT 2B	AR	3q13–q22	?		
Type III (Hypertrophic)					
Déjerine-Sottas	AD	17p11.2	*PMP22*	Low motor-conduction velocity	First year
		1q21–q23	*PO*		
X-linked forms					
CMTX	XL	Xq13	*connexin 32*		

HMSN and Friedreich's ataxia (FA) are sometimes confused. In HMSN there is areflexia and evidence of distal weakness. In Friedreich's ataxia there is much more clear ataxia with evidence of loss of joint position sense. On neurophysiological testing HMSN patients have abnormal motor conduction, whereas FA patients have evidence of a sensory neuropathy.

9.6 Acute neuromuscular disorders

Guillain-Barré syndrome

Acute demyelinating disease of peripheral nerves characterized by progressive weakness.

- Usually follows viral infection or immunization
- Numerous other infections including *Campylobacter jejuni,* gastroenteritis has been implicated

Clinical features

- Sudden onset of weakness, usually affecting lower limbs
- Ascending paralysis
- Usually symmetrical weakness
- Pain often prominent feature
- Sensory involvement in about 50%
- Respiratory muscle weakness may occur

Diagnosis

- High CSF protein
- A marked slowing of motor-neurone conduction velocity
- Conduction block

Course

- Deterioration over the first 10 to 20 days
- Plateau
- Recovery
- Mortality 2–3% in children

Treatment

- Symptomatic
- Respiratory support
- Plasma exchange
- High-dose immunoglobulin

Juvenile dermatomyositis

- Systemic illness affecting primarily skin, muscles and gastrointestinal tract
- Unlike adult dermatomyositis, juvenile dermatomyositis is not associated with malignancy

Clinical

- Age of onset 5–10 years
- May present with fever, muscle pain
- Onset can be insidious
- Increasing muscular weakness, mainly proximal
- Rash involving upper eyelids (heliotrope rash) and periorbital region develops
- Rash on extensor surfaces; calcinosis is a feature
- May have difficulty swallowing
- Children are often miserable in advance of other symptoms

Diagnosis

- Creatine kinase may or may not be raised
- Muscle biopsy may show perifascicular atrophy, but changes can be patchy

Treatment

- Corticosteriods
- Other immunosuppressive treatment such as methotrexate or cyclosporin

9.7 Disorders of neuromuscular junction

Myasthenia gravis

- Commonest disease of neuromuscular junction
- Caused by antibodies directed against postsynaptic acetylcholine receptors

Clinical features

- Onset after 1 year
- Adolescent girls most commonly affected
- Generalized form affects extraocular muscles first
- Then goes on to affect proximal limbs and bulbar muscles
- Variable natural course

Diagnosis

- Edrophonium test
- Electromyography confirming neuromuscular block
- Demonstration of anti–acetylcholine receptor antibodies

Treatment

- Anticholinesterase drugs
- Immunosuppressants
- Thymectomy
- Plasma exchange or immunoglobulin infusion acutely

Other myasthenic syndromes

There are rare congenital myasthenic syndromes which result from specific defects in the process of neuromuscular transmission. Some affect presynaptic mechanisms, others affect postsynaptic components. Some such infants may have joint contractures.

10. CENTRAL NERVOUS SYSTEM INFECTIONS AND PARAINFECTIOUS DISORDERS

10.1 Meningitis

Acute bacterial meningitis remains an important cause of neurological morbidity in childhood. Causative organisms vary depending on the age of the child, and the pattern of infection has been altered by changing immunization patterns.

Age	Organism
Neonatal	Group B Streptococcus *Escherichia coli* *Listeria monocytogenes* *Staphylococcus aureus*
First 2 months	Group B Streptococcus *Escherichia coli* *Haemophilus influenzae* *Streptococcus pneumoniae*
Older infants and young children	*Haemophilus influenzae* *Neisseria meningitidis* *Streptococcus pneumoniae*

Clinical features

In neonates — meningitis is usually part of septicaemic illness. Symptoms and signs may be non-specific: lethargy, poor feeding, respiratory distress. Neck stiffness is rarely seen.

In young infants also, signs may be non-specific and meningeal irritation may be absent.

In older children, signs are more typical: lethargy, headache, photophobia, neck stiffness. Meningococcaemia is associated with a haemorrhagic rash.

Outcome

Neurological sequelae may occur in up to 30% of children: focal neurological deficits, learning disability, hydrocephalus and deafness may all occur. Mortality is improving with earlier diagnosis and treatment.

Diagnosis

Lumbar puncture and cerebrospinal fluid (CSF) analysis is definitive. White cell count is raised with predominance of neutrophils, CSF glucose is reduced and protein is raised. Gram staining of CSF and immunoassays may allow identification of the organism. However, lumbar puncture is contraindicated if signs of raised intracranial pressure are present or if consciousness is impaired. Treatment then needs to be aimed at the most likely organisms. Blood cultures can be taken before starting treatment.

Management

- Antibiotic treatment — agent will depend on age of patient and likely infecting organism
- Watch for subdural effusions and hydrocephalus — measure head circumference
- Evidence re steroid use to prevent neurological sequelae unclear — some evidence to support prevention of deafness in *H. influenzae* meningitis

Viral meningitis may result from a wide variety of viruses: coxsackie virus, echoviruses, mumps, measles, herpes simplex, poliomyelitis, varicella zoster.

- Symptoms similar to bacterial meningitis, but less pronounced
- Specific diagnosis may be suggested by other disease stigmata
- CSF clear with lymphocytosis
- Prognosis of uncomplicated viral meningitis good

Tuberculous meningitis

Generally occurs within 6–8 weeks of primary pulmonary infection or during miliary tuberculosis (TB). Commonest in age range 6 months to 3 years.

Leads to basal arteritis, which may cause hydrocephalus and cranial neuropathies. Symptoms otherwise often non-specific, lethargy, fever, headache.

CSF — high white cell count, predominantly lymphocytes, raised protein level often greater than 2 g/l, low glucose, tuberculous cultures may be positive.

Treatment

- Antituberculous chemotherapy
- Optimal treatment not determined
- Usually triple therapy (isoniazid, rifampicin, pyrazinamide – sometimes four drugs) for 3 months, maintenance treatment with two drugs for 12 months
- The place of corticosteroids is unclear but these are often used in the first few months to reduce inflammation

Mortality and morbidity remain high despite treatment.

10.2 Encephalitis

Numerous viruses may lead to inflammation of the brain: herpesviruses, adenoviruses, arboviruses and enteroviruses for example. The underlying causative agent in undiagnosed encephalitis may remain obscure. It is therefore usual practice to treat with cefotaxime/ceftriaxone, aciclovir and erythromycin/azithromycin until results are available.

Clinical features

Confusion, coma, seizures, motor abnormalities. Infection usually starts to resolve 7–14 days after the onset. However, recovery may be delayed for several months.

Herpes simplex encephalitis

- Most commonly identified cause of encephalitis
- Often focal brain inflammation, located in temporal lobes
- High mortality, high morbidity (50%)
- Specific treatment: aciclovir

Investigations for encephalitis

- CSF examination/cultures
- EEG
- Brain imaging
- Occasionally, brain biopsy

Treatment for encephalitis

- Supportive (fluid management/ventilation if necessary)
- Aciclovir

10.3 Immune-mediated and other infectious disorders

Sydenham's chorea

- Main neurological feature of rheumatic fever
- Chorea results from immune reaction triggered by Group A streptococcal infection
- May be associated with emotional lability
- Probably overlaps with PANDAS (psychiatric and neurological diseases associated with streptococcal infection)
- In about 75%, chorea resolves within 6 months

Subacute sclerosing panencephalitis (SSPE)

SSPE is a slow viral infection, caused by an atypical response to measles infection. Exposure to measles is usually in the first 2 years. Risk of SSPE is higher after contracting natural measles, compared with that after measles immunization. Median interval between measles and SSPE is 8 years.

- Subtle deficits initially
- Increasing memory difficulties
- Worsening disabilities: seizures, motor difficulties, learning disability

Mycoplasma encephalitis

Mycoplasma pneumoniae is the commonest cause of community-acquired pneumonia in adults and commonly leads to infection in the paediatric age range. It may cause encephalitis, predominantly through immune-mediated mechanisms which may respond to steroid administration. The evidence base is small.

Acquired immune deficiency syndrome (AIDS)

Caused by human immunodeficiency virus, an RNA retrovirus which eventually leads to the death of its host cell CD4+T lymphocyte.

Neurological features

- Neurological features of opportunistic infection such as meningitis or encephalitis
- Dementia

11. CEREBROVASCULAR DISEASE

11.1 Arterial occlusion

May result from embolism or thrombosis

Effects of arterial occlusion	
Internal carotid artery	Hemiplegia, hemianopia, aphasia if dominant hemisphere
Middle cerebral artery	Hemiplegia with upper limb predominance, hemianopia, aphasia if dominant hemisphere
Anterior cerebral artery	Hemiplegia affecting predominantly lower limbs
Posterior cerebral artery	Homonymous hemianopia, ataxia, hemiparesis, vertigo

Investigations

- MRI
- MR angiography
- Possible formal angiography
- Carotid Doppler studies
- Echocardiography
- Full blood count, plasma homocysteine
- Clotting studies, especially factor V Leiden, prothrombin 20210A, lipoprotein (a)

The place of deficiencies of antithrombin III, protein C and protein S in the genesis of childhood stroke remains debatable.

11.2 Venous thrombosis

- Less common than arterial occlusion
- Produces a variable clinical picture
  - Intracranial hypertension
  - Seizures
  - Focal neurological signs

Causes

- Sepsis
  - Otitis media
  - Sinusitis
  - Cutaneous infection

- Dehydration
- Coagulopathy

Treatment

- Disputed
- Heparin may be given in the acute phase

12. NEURO-ONCOLOGY

Brain tumours are the second commonest malignancy in children after leukaemia. In infants, supratentorial tumours predominate, whereas in older children, infratentorial tumours are much more common. The trend reverses in children over 8 years of age, with a slight preponderance of supratentorial tumours.

Central nervous system tumours are of varying degrees of malignancy. Those which do metastasize tend to do so within the central nervous system. It is also important to note that a 'benign' tumour situated so that it cannot be removed may have a more serious effect than a 'malignant' tumour differently situated.

General symptoms and signs associated with brain tumours in children may include headache, vomiting, papilloedema, cranial nerve palsies, other focal symptoms such as ataxia.

12.1 Posterior fossa tumours

Cerebellar astrocytoma

Commonest tumour in children; may involve vermis, cerebellar hemispheres or both. Majority are cystic, slow growing.

Treatment
Surgical. Occasionally more malignant tumours require radiotherapy also.

Medulloblastoma

Common tumour. Highly malignant, rapid growing. Arises from cerebellar vermis. Often leads to hydrocephalus. May metastasize along CSF pathways. Often solid tumours.

Treatment
Surgery and radiotherapy. Trials have sought to clarify the position of chemotherapy.

Outlook has improved: 75% 5-year survival, 50% 10–year survival. Prognosis poorer in young children. Evidence is emerging that specific genetic constitution of tumour is most important in determining outcome.

Ependymoma

6–10% of childhood tumours. Arises from fourth ventricle. May lead to hydrocephalus and may metastasize.

Treatment — surgical resection and radiotherapy
Poor 5-year survival often related to localization of tumour.

	Percentage total tumours in childhood	Spread	Location	Structure	Treatment	5-year survival (%)
Astrocytoma	14–20	Local	Vermis/cerebellar hemispheres	Cystic	Surgery	c 100
Medulloblastoma	14–20	CSF pathways	Vermis	Usually solid	Surgery/radiotherapy/chemotherapy	75
Ependymoma	6–10	CSF pathways	Floor fourth ventricle	May be cystic	Surgery/radiotherapy	40

12.2 Brainstem tumours

Brainstem gliomas, which may vary in their degree of malignancy, form approximately 15% of brain tumours in childhood. Peak incidence 5–9 years of age. Presents with multiple cranial nerve palsies plus long tract signs. Vomiting may be a feature.

Treatment
Radiotherapy

Survival
Poor

12.3 Supratentorial tumours

Cerebral astrocytomas

- Presentation depends on location
- Often leads to seizures

Low-grade astrocytomas (benign): more common in children
High-grade astrocytomas: fortunately, more rare

Ependymoma

30–40% of ependymomas are supratentorial. These are more malignant than their infratentorial counterparts.
They have a tendency to metastasize and thus prognosis is poor.

Optic gliomas

One-third prechiasmatic, two-thirds chiasmatic or post-chiasmatic.
Generally, these tumours are pilocytic astrocytomas. One-quarter occurs in the setting of neurofibromatosis type 1.

Clinical presentation
Pre-chiasmatic lesions may present late with proptosis with associated visual loss. Post-chiasmatic lesions lead to visual loss.

Treatment
Controversial. Often conservative, but surgery and radiotherapy may be indicated.

Craniopharyngioma

Tumour arises from small aggregates of cells which are remnants of Rathke's pouch. Tumour is either suprasellar or suprasellar and intrasellar. Often cystic.

Clinical features

- Endocrine disturbance
  - Delayed growth
  - Hypothyroidism
  - Diabetes insipidus

- Raised intracranial pressure
  - Headache
  - Ataxia

- Local features
  - Visual disturbance (bitemporal hemianopia)
  - Depressed consciousness
  - Vomiting
  - Nystagmus

Investigations

- Skull X-ray may show erosion of dorsum sellae, also calcification
- MRI scan will delineate lesion better
- Also, endocrine investigations and visual field mapping.

Treatment

- Controversial
- Surgery
- Radiotherapy

13. NEUROCUTANEOUS SYNDROMES

Neurocutaneous syndromes form a group of unrelated disorders in which skin and neurological features coexist. Most are genetically determined.

13.1 Neurofibromatosis

Neurofibromatoses are predominantly inherited disorders.

Neurofibromatosis type 1

Gene localized to chromosome 17q11.2

Diagnostic criteria (two or more are necessary for diagnosis)

- Six or more café-au-lait spots >5 mm in diameter in prepubertal patients and >15 mm in post-pubertal patients
- Two or more neurofibromas or one plexiform neurofibroma
- Axillary or inguinal freckling
- Optic glioma
- Two or more iris hamartomas (Lisch nodules)
- Typical osseous lesions such as sphenoid dysplasia
- First-degree relative affected

Neurological manifestations

- Macrocephaly
- Learning disability
- Epilepsy
- Optic gliomas

Neurofibromatosis type 2

Gene localized to chromosome 22q11.2

Diagnostic criteria

- Bilateral VIIIth nerve neurofibromas
- Unilateral VIIIth nerve mass in association with any two of the following: meningioma, neurofibroma, schwannoma, juvenile posterior capsular cataracts
- Unilateral VIIIth nerve tumour or other spinal or brain tumour as above in first-degree relative

13.2 Tuberous sclerosis

Dominantly inherited disorder with variable expression. Characterized by skin and central nervous system abnormalities, although there may be cardiac, renal and bony abnormalities as well. At least two mutant genes on chromosomes 9p34 and 16p.

Clinical features

- Seizures
- Neurodevelopmental impairment
- Cutaneous manifestations:
  - Adenoma sebaceum
  - Periungual fibromata
  - Hypopigmented patches
  - Shagreen patch
- Retinal hamartomas
- Renal angiolipomatas
- Cardiac rhabdomyomata

Brain imaging may reveal cortical tubers, subependymal nodules with calcification

13.3 Other neurocutaneous disorders

Ataxia–telangiectasia

Characterized by conjunctival telangiectasia, progressive cerebellar degeneration and immunological impairment. Multisystem disease with autosomal recessive inheritance. Responsible gene, at least in some families, mapped to chromosome 11q22–23.

Clinical features

- Progressive ataxia
- Scleral telangiectasia
- Abnormalities of cell-mediated and humoral immunity leading to increased sinopulmonary infections and high incidence of reticuloendothelial malignancies in later life

Diagnosis

- Elevated alpha-fetoprotein level
- Reduced IgA
- Reduced IgM
- Inversions and translocations involving chromosomes 7 and 14
- Gene mutation analysis

Sturge–Weber syndrome

Characterized by port-wine stain, facial naevus and ipsilateral leptomeningeal angioma which leads to ischaemic injury to the underlying cerebral cortex leading to focal seizures, hemiparesis and variable degrees of intellectual deficit.

Incontinentia pigmenti

- Rare
- Probably inherited as X-linked dominant
- Characterized by skin lesions — initially erythematous, papular, vesicular or bullous lesions on trunk and limbs, then pustular lesions, then pigmented lesions
- 30–50% of neurological features:
  - Seizures
  - Encephalopathy
- Eye lesions in 30%

Hypomelanosis of Ito

- Also rare
- Sporadic inheritance
- Hypopigmented areas
- CNS involvement common including seizures, hemimegalencephaly

14. NEUROMETABOLIC DISEASES

Disorders of intermediary metabolism are a huge group of heterogeneous conditions which have effects of different nature and severity on the nervous system (see Chapter 12, *Metabolic Medicine*). Inborn errors with predominant neurological involvement include:

14.1 Amino and organic acid disorders

Glutaric aciduria type I

- Inborn error of lysine and tryptophan catabolism
- Leads to extrapyramidal syndrome
- Initially, children may develop normally
- May be hypotonic or irritable
- Chronic subdural haematomata may be present
- Acute neurological deterioration occurs
- Brain imaging shows striatal changes

14.2 Neurotransmitter disorders

Non-ketotic hyperglycinaemia

- Autosomal recessive
- Glycine accumulates in body fluids
- Neuropathology — identifies poor myelination

Clinical

- Poor respiratory effort at birth
- Hypotonia
- Gradual improvement over first week
- Evolution of myoclonic encephalopathy
- Severe seizure disorder and major developmental delay ensues

14.3 Mitochondrial disease

Respiratory chain disorders

Abnormalities of mitochondrial energy production produce a variety of clinical syndromes, many of which have significant neurological features.

Potential clinical features of respiratory chain disorders

- Lactic acidosis
- Failure to thrive
- Progressive external ophthalmoplegia
- Myopathy
- Seizures
- Dementia
- Movement disorders
- Cardiomyopathy
- Retinopathy
- Deafness

Specific syndromes

Kearns–Sayre syndrome	Progressive external ophthalmoplegia, heart block, cerebellar dysfunction
MERRF	Myoclonic epilepsy with ragged red fibres (on muscle biopsy)
MELAS	Mitochondrial myopathy, encephalopathy, lactic acidosis and stroke-like episodes
Leigh disease	Subacute necrotizing encephalopathy — hypotonia, progressive deterioration in neurological abilities
Alpers disease	Grey matter disease; seizures are a prominent feature; liver abnormalities are seen, often late in course of disease

14.4 Abnormalities of copper metabolism

Wilson disease

- Autosomal recessive
- Excessive accumulation of copper in nervous system and liver due to lack of binding globulin (caeruloplasmin)
- Approximately 30% present with neurological symptoms alone, one-third with CNS symptoms after 8 years and one third with a mixture of CNS and hepatic signs
- Leads to movement disorder which may include dystonia, rigidity, chorea and that may also be characterized by intellectual deterioration and behavioural lability
- Diagnosis by biochemical means
- Treatment — copper chelation therapy with penicillamine

Menkes disease (kinky-hair disease)

- Uncommon X-linked disorder
- Low serum copper and caeruloplasmin
- Gene map to chromosome Xq13.3

Clinical

- Onset neonatal period or early infancy
- Hypothermia, poor weight gain
- Hair is sparse, brittle
- Progressive cerebral infarction occurs leading to seizures and neurological impairment
- Diagnosis confirmed by biochemical, genetic means or by hair examination
- Death in first 2 years

14.5 Storage disorders

In these conditions, an enzymatic block leads to accumulation of products of cellular metabolism in the nervous system.

Sphingolipidoses

These are lysosomal diseases involving disorders of sphingolipid metabolism. Sphingolipids are important components of central nervous system membranes.

GM$_2$ gangliosidosis (Tay–Sachs disease)

Neurodegenerative, onset 3–9 months, startles, seizures, blindness

Gaucher disease

Types 2 and 3 have neurological involvement: hypotonia, progressive deterioration, hepatosplenomegaly

Niemann–Pick disease
Types A and C have neurological involvement leading to progressive deterioration.

Fabry disease
Presents with painful hands and feet. May run slow progressive course with renal involvement.

Mucopolysaccharidoses
These are disorders characterized by accumulation of mucopolysaccharides (glycosaminoglycans) in lysosomes. Numerous different types.

Hurler disease (MPS 1H)
Characteristic facies, marked dwarfism, corneal clouding, neurological involvement progressive. Hydrocephalus may ensue.

Sanfilippo disease (MPS III)
Typical mycopolysaccharidosis features may be mild. However, severe neurological involvement with intellectual deterioration and seizures.

14.6 Peroxisomal disorders

Peroxisomes are cellular organelles containing proteins and enzymes. Peroxisomal disorders are characterized by accumulation of metabolites normally degraded by peroxisomal enzymes or by decreased amounts of substances normally synthesized by peroxisomes.

Zellweger syndrome

- Presents in neonatal period
- High forehead, patent fontanelles; severe hypotonia and poor sucking or swallowing
- Very poor subsequent neurological development
- Often associated with cerebral gyral abnormalities

X-linked adrenoleucodystrophy

- Relatively common disease which involves central nervous system and adrenals
- Over half present with CNS features; this group present at 4–8 years with cognitive decline and progressive gait disturbance
- Brain imaging shows leucodystrophy
- Levels of very long chain fatty acids (VLCFAs) are elevated

14.7 Leucodystrophies and other neurodegenerative disorders

Leucodystrophies are degenerative disorders which affect the white matter of the brain through abnormalities of myelin. In some, the metabolic features are known, in others the diagnosis is based on clinical features.

Leucodystrophies

- **With known metabolic defect**
  - Metachromatic leucodystrophy
  - Krabbe leucodystrophy
  - Adrenal leucodystrophy
  - Canavan's disease

- **Without recognized metabolic defect**
  - Pelizaeus–Merzbacher disease
  - Cockayne disease
  - Alexander disease
  - Leucodystrophy with subcortical cysts
  - Leucodystrophy with vanishing white matter

Canavan disease

- *N*-acetylaspartic aciduria
- Autosomal recessive (17p13–ter)
- Leads to spongy degeneration of the subcortical white matter
- Progressive neurological impairment
- Death in first decade

Grey matter disorders

Neuronal ceroid–lipofuscinoses (NCL) (Batten disease)

These disorders are characterized by storage of pigments which are similar to ceroid and lipofuscin. Although originally thought to be related, genetic analysis has shown them to be separate disorders.

The neuronal ceroid–lipofuscinoses

Disease	Onset	Clinical features	Course
Infantile NCL	8–18 months	Myoclonus, ataxia, extrapyramidal features, visual impairment slight	Death in first 5 years
Late infantile NCL	18 months–4 years	Epilepsy, marked ataxia, late visual deficit	Death 5–15 years
Juvenile NCL	4–7 years	Visual failure, later dementia	Death 15–30 years
Adult NCL	Adulthood	Slow cognitive decline, normal vision	Slow

Rett's syndrome

Syndrome of dementia, autistic behaviour and motor stereotypes seen in girls.

Classical clinical features

- Normal perinatal period and normal first year
- Deceleration of head growth from around 9 months
- Loss of neurological skills
- Hand wringing
- Episodic hyperventilation (inability to walk on command)
- Gait apraxia
- May develop scoliosis
- Diagnosis was clinical but now by mutation analysis of *MeCP2* gene (chromosome Xq28)
- Mutation analysis has shown that mutations in this gene lead to severe neonatal encephalopathy in boys

Angelman's syndrome

- Previously known as 'happy puppet' syndrome
- Caused by deletion of chromosome 15q11.2–12, which is maternally inherited
- Deletion includes gene for β3-subunit of GABA receptor

Clinical features

- Severe learning disability
- Ataxia
- Jerky movements
- Seizures
- Often cheerful demeanour

15. HEAD INJURY

It has been estimated that 1 in 10 children suffer a head injury severe enough to impair consciousness. Boys outnumber girls by 2–3 to 1. The overall incidence of head injury is 2–3 per 1,000 population. Around 5% are severe (Glasgow Coma Scale (GCS) 8 or less), 5–10% moderate (GCS 9–12) and 85–90% are minor.

15.1 Mild closed head injury

Clinical features

- Impaired consciousness
- Lethargy
- Crying
- Vomiting
- Ataxia

Symptoms may develop immediately or within 6–8 hours of injury. There is usually complete resolution of symptoms within 24 hours of the injury.

15.2 Severe closed head injury

Characterized by major loss of consciousness which is deeper and persists longer than in milder head injury. The greatest neurological deficit usually occurs immediately after the injury. Injuries may be the result of:

- Primary trauma to brain
- Secondary changes due to inflammation and ischaemia

Paediatric Glasgow Coma Scale

Eye opening (E)	Spontaneous	4
	To speech	3
	To pain	2
	None	1
Best verbal response (V)	Oriented	5
	Words	4
	Inappropriate sounds	3
	Vocalisation	3
	Cries	2
	None	1
Best motor response (M)	Obeys command	6
	Localises pain	5
	Withdraws to pain	4
	Abnormal flexion to pain	3
	Abnormal extension to pain	2
	None	1

Clinical assessment

- Level of consciousness
- Respiratory pattern
- Pupil size and reaction
- Brainstem signs
- Leakage of cerebrospinal fluid
- Focal signs
- Consider potential of cervical spine fracture

Management

- Airway, breathing, circulation
- X-ray cervical spine
- Assess intracranial pressure

- CT scan
- Fluid restriction
- After first 4–5 days — supportive care

Late complications

- Learning disability (global and specific)
- Behavioural disturbance
- Motor deficits
- Post-traumatic epilepsy
- Headaches

15.3 Non-accidental head injury

The incidence of non-accidental head injury is unknown but most estimates almost certainly underdiagnose the problem. Non-accidental head injury may include blunt trauma, sometimes leading to skull fracture, and the so-called 'shaken (or shaken-impact) baby syndrome'.

Clinical features of 'shaken baby syndrome'

- Peak incidence 5 months of age
- History inconsistent with severity of injury
- Baby presents shocked, possibly apnoeic, following apparent sudden spontaneous collapse at home
- Impaired consciousness
- Shocked
- Irregular breathing
- Retinal haemorrhages
- Possible bruising on arms or trunk
- Brain imaging identifies acute and/or chronic intracranial bleeding with brain swelling
- There may be signs of other non-accidental injury

Mechanism

- Unclear
- Cerebral parenchyma may be damaged by blunt trauma
- Recent evidence suggests brainstem injury leading to apnoea and ischaemic injury

Prognosis

- Non-accidental head injury may lead to death
- Prognosis for neurological recovery guarded

16. SPECIFIC NEUROLOGICAL LESIONS

16.1 Cranial nerve lesions

Facial nerve paralysis

Symptoms and signs will depend on location of lesion in the course of the nerve with potential abnormalities of taste, lacrimation and salivation as well as hyperacusis.

Congenital facial paralysis

- May be due to birth trauma or prenatal compression
- May also be non-traumatic due to anomalies of nerve and nerve cell body

Moebius syndrome

- Bilateral facial paralysis with bilateral abducens paralysis
- Other lower cranial nerves may be affected
- Up to one-quarter have learning disability

Acquired facial palsy (Bell's palsy)

- Acute, usually idiopathic, paralysis which is unilateral
- Lower motor neurone VII palsy (whole side of face affected)
- Weakness maximal for 2–4 weeks
- Complete recovery is usual
- Steroids often given, but no evidence to support their use

Other facial paralyses

- Lyme disease
- Otitis media/mastoiditis
- Hypertension

Lower cranial nerve palsies (VII–XII)

Congenital

- Often present in Chiari I and II malformations

16.2 Disorders of eye movement

Acquired ophthalmoplegia

IIIrd nerve palsy

- Common
- Most frequently due to closed head trauma, infections and tumours

IVth nerve palsy

- Traumatic

VIth nerve palsy

- Due to raised intracranial pressure
  - Tumours
  - Benign intracranial hypertension

Congenital ophthalmoplegia

- Can affect all above nerves

Nystagmus

- Involuntary, rhythmical, conjugate, oscillatory movements of the eyes which may occur in any plane
- Results from dysfunction of complex mechanisms that maintain ocular fixation

Type	Cause
Pendular	Congenital
	Acquired — disease of brainstem/cerebellum
Horizontal jerk:	
Vestibular	End-organ
Gaze-evoked	Posterior fossa
Rotary	Vestibular or medullary lesions

Differential diagnosis

- Roving eye movements of blind children
- Opsoclonus

16.3 Unequal pupils

- May be due to physiological anisocoria
- Establish which pupil is abnormal
- Ptosis and large pupil — IIIrd nerve palsy
- Ptosis and constricted pupil — Horner's syndrome
- Extremely important in unconscious patient (much more so than establishment of papilloedema, for example)

17. NEUROLOGICAL INVESTIGATIONS

17.1 Electroencephalography (EEG)

The EEG allows an assessment of changes in cortical function. Electrodes applied to scalp allow the cortical action potential between two electrodes to be amplified and displayed. The quality of the normal EEG will depend upon:

- Age of the patient
- Whether the patient is awake or asleep

Uses

- Investigation of patients with seizures
- Detection of cerebral dysfunction
- Evaluation of depressed consciousness
- Investigation of neurodegenerative disorders

Typical EEG appearances

Epilepsies

- 3 cycles/s (c/s) spike and wave in typical absences ('petit mal')
- 4 c/s spike and wave and poly spike and wave bursts in juvenile myoclonic epilepsy
- Clusters of high-amplitude spike and wave complexes in one or both Rolandic areas in benign focal epilepsy with Rolandic spikes

Epileptic encephalopathies

- High-voltage chaotic slow waves and spike and sharp waves in hypsarrhythmia
- Spike and waves in absence of seizures and loss of language skills in Landau–Kleffner syndrome
- Slow spike-wave discharges at 1.5–2.5 c/s in Lennox–Gastaut syndrome

Undiagnosed neurological illness

- Burst suppression in asphyxia, early myoclonic epilepsy, glycine encephalopathy
- Slowing of background in encephalopathies generally
- Focal slowing may indicate structural lesions such as cerebral abscess
- Focal flattening may indicate subdural haemorrhage or effusion
- Diffuse, moderate-amplitude, fast β activity is the result of some drug intoxications

Suspect cerebral malformation or mental handicap

- High-voltage activity in the α frequency or lower part of β characteristic of lissencephaly or pachygyria

- High-voltage posterior spike and wave accentuated by passive eye closure is a feature of Angelman's syndrome
- Trains of spikes or sharp waves, at first in sleep, with poorly organized background activity develop in Rett's syndrome

Suspect neurodegenerative disorder

- Stereotyped high-voltage polyphasic complexes repeated every few seconds and often associated with transient reduction in tone — subacute sclerosing panencephalitis
- Progressive reduction in EEG amplitude after infancy is typical of infantile neuronal ceroid–lipofuscinosis
- High-voltage posterior complexes induced by slow stroboscopic activation at less than 0.5 c/s is typical of late infantile neuronal ceroid — lipofuscinosis
- β activity of moderate amplitude develops after 2 years in infantile neuroaxonal dystrophy
- Multiple spikes superimposed on lateralized large slow waves suggest progressive neuronal degeneration of childhood, and predict later hepatic involvement

17.2 Evoked potentials

Used to assess the function of auditory, visual and somatosensory pathways.

Auditory brainstem evoked potentials

- Assessment of peripheral hearing in infants and young children

Visual evoked potentials

- Detection of disease in anterior visual pathway

Electroretinogram (ERG)

- Measures response of retina to repeated light flashes
- Used in investigation of low vision and in neurological regression

Somatosensory evoked potentials

- Diagnosis of spinal cord disease
- Intraoperative monitoring

17.3 Peripheral neurophysiology

Measurement of peripheral nerve conduction allows assessment of the function of the motor unit — the anterior horn cell, the peripheral axon and the innervated muscle.

Nerve conduction studies allow measurement of:

- Motor-nerve conduction velocity — reduced in demyelination
- Amplitude of action potential — reduced in axonal neuropathies
- Sensory nerve conduction velocity — reduced in Friedreich's ataxia, for example

Electromyography

- Denervation: Shorter and lower voltage action potentials — later giant potentials

- Myopathic change: Reduced action potentials

17.4 Brain imaging

Computed axial tomography (CT) scanning

Useful in:

- Initial evaluation of coma
- Trauma
- Calcification

Magnetic resonance imaging (MRI) scanning

Useful in:

- Detection of parenchymal lesions, especially white matter lesions
- Posterior fossa lesions

17.5 Lumbar puncture

Useful in diagnosis of:

- Infection
- Demyelinating diseases
- Subarachnoid haemorrhage
- Benign intracranial hypertension (measure pressure)

18. FURTHER READING

Diseases of the Nervous System in Childhood. Clinics in Developmental Medicine: Aicardi J, 2nd edition. MacKeith Press 1998.

Handbook of Neurological Investigations in Childhood: Stephenson, JBP, King MD, Wright 1989.

Neurological Differential Diagnosis: Patten J, 2nd edition. Springer Verlag 1995.

Neurology of the Newborn: Volpe J, 4th edition. WB Saunders 2001.

Chapter 16

Ophthalmology

Majeed H Jawad

CONTENTS

Ophthalmology

1. BASIC ANATOMY OF THE EYE

1.1 Orbits

The orbits are related to the frontal sinus above, the maxillary sinus below and the ethmoid and sphenoid sinuses medially. The orbit houses the eyeball which occupies only one-fifth of the space, fat and muscle accounting for the bulk of the remainder. Other orbital structures include the lacrimal glands, attendant arteries, veins and nerves.

1.2 Extraocular muscles

Six extraocular muscles control the movement of each eye — 4 rectus and 2 oblique muscles.

Muscle	Nerve supply	Primary action	Secondary action
Lateral rectus nerve	VI (abducens)	Abduction	None
Medial rectus	III (oculomotor)	Adduction	None
Superior rectus	III	Elevation	Adduction, intorsion
Inferior rectus	III	Depression	Adduction, extorsion
Superior oblique	IV (trochlear)	Depression	Intorsion, abduction
Inferior oblique	III	Elevation	Extorsion, abduction

NB. Easy way to remember extraocular muscles innervations L6 SO4/3 (where L = lateral rectus, innervated by sixth nerve, SO = superior oblique innervated by fourth nerve, and all the rest innervated by third nerve).

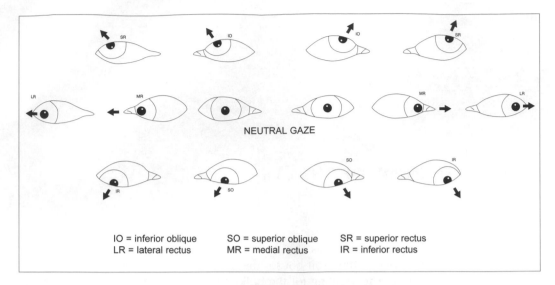

IO = inferior oblique   SO = superior oblique   SR = superior rectus
LR = lateral rectus   MR = medial rectus   IR = inferior rectus

The action of the external ocular muscles with the patient confronting the examiner.

1.3 The globe

The eyelid

Protective cover for the eyeball.

The eyeball

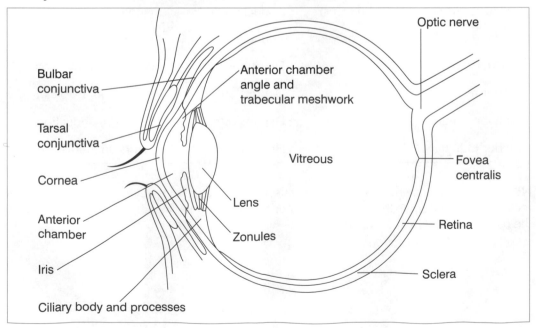

The most important contents are:

Cornea
A transparent avascular tissue inserted into the sclera at the limbus, functioning as a protective membrane and a 'window' through which light rays pass en route to the retina. Sensory innervation is supplied by the first division of the trigeminal nerve. Transparency of the cornea is due to its uniform structure, avascularity and the state of relative dehydration of the corneal tissues which is maintained by the active bicarbonate pump of the endothelium.

Conjunctiva
Thin, transparent mucous membrane that covers the posterior surface of the lids (the palpebral conjunctiva) and the anterior surface of the sclera (the bulbar conjunctiva).

The sclera
The fibrous outer protective coating of the eye. In the infant, the sclera is thin and translucent with a bluish tinge.

Uveal tract
Consists of iris, ciliary body and choroid, each of which has a rich vascular supply and pigment. The choroid's vascular supply provides nutrition for 65% of the outer retinal layers.

Anterior chamber
Fluid-filled space between the cornea and the iris diaphragm. The aqueous fluid is secreted by the ciliary body, reaches the anterior chamber by passing through the pupillary space and drains via the trabecular meshwork in the periphery of the anterior chamber into the venous circulation. The aqueous provides nutrition for the corneal endothelial surface.

Lens
Lies posterior to the iris and anterior to the vitreous humour, suspended by zonular fibres from the ciliary body. Anterior to the lens is the aqueous humour; posterior to it the vitreous. The lens of the newborn infant is more nearly spherical than that of the adult with greater refractive power helping to compensate for the relative shortness of the young eye.

Vitreous
A transparent gelatinous structure that fills the posterior 4/5 of the globe. It is firmly attached to the pars plana anteriorly and has a loose attachment to the retina and optic nerve posteriorly. The vitreous is about 99% water.

The retina
During the first 2–3 months of life, children develop the ability to focus images at any range. The retina contains the sensory receptors: the rods and cones. The fovea centralis is the centre of the macula and it has the greatest concentration of cones, and therefore has the greatest potential for visual acuity. Light falling on the fovea and peripheral retina is converted into nerve impulses by the rods and cones. Nerve fibres emanate from the ganglion cell layer of the retina, coalesce to form the optic nerve and synapse in the lateral geniculate body. Fibres

from the temporal retina travel without crossing at the chiasm to the ipsilateral visual cortex. Nerve fibres from the nasal retina will decussate at the chiasm and are directed toward the contralateral visual cortex. The decussation of nerve fibres causes portions of each retina to image a different part of the visual field.

2. EYELID ABNORMALITIES

2.1 Congenital eyelid abnormalities

Cryptophthalmos

A rare condition. The eyebrow is usually absent and the globe microphthalmic (complete cryptophthalmos) or rudimentary lid and conjunctival sac is present (incomplete cryptophthalmos).

Coloboma

Clefting (defect) of the eyelid. It may occur as an isolated anomaly or in association with other clefting abnormalities or first arch syndromes. Coloboma of the upper lid usually involves the medial side and is full thickness, whilst the lower lid is the lateral side and partial thickness. It may be unilateral or bilateral. The latter can be a sign of Goldenhar's and First Arch syndrome. Management depends on the size of the cleft and the other associated signs. For larger clefts urgent reconstruction of the lid is necessary. Ocular exposure can be controlled with lubricants.

Ablepharon

Congenital absence of the eyelids. An association with ichthyosis is reported.

Ankyloblepharon

Partial or complete fusion of the eyelid margins.

Ectropion

Congenital ectropion is an outward rotation of the eyelid margin present at birth. The condition may occur in the upper or lower lids and is usually associated with other conditions such as ichthyosis which may present as collodion baby at birth. It may also be associated with Down's syndrome.

Management may be initially conservative using lubrication. Surgical intervention is indicated for exposure keratitis and may include skin grafting.

Entropion

Turning inward of the lid margin with lashes rubbing against the conjunctiva.

Epicanthus

Epicanthal folds are folds of skin which extend from the upper eyelid towards the medial canthus. The epicanthus may give rise to a false appearance of strabismus (pseudosquint).

Telecanthus

There is an increased width between the medial canthi with normal interpupillary distance.

Hypertelorism

Increased intralobular distance.

Hypotelorism

Reduced intralobular distance.

Blepharophimosis

Small eyelids.

2.2 Infections and inflammations of the lids

Hordeolum (stye)

A staphylococcal infection of the lid glands, characterized by a localized, red, swollen and acutely tender area at the lid margin. It is a painful abscess of the sebaceous gland at the root of the lashes. They can be treated by removing the lash and draining the abscess. Topical antibiotic may be necessary.

Chalazion (meibomian cysts)

A chronic granulomatous inflammation of the meibomian gland which results from obstruction of the gland duct. Usually occurs away from the lid border as a painless hard nodule. Treatment involves the use of warm compresses to help drainage of the lipid material. Small chalazia may resolve spontaneously, but incision and drainage may be necessary for persistent ones.

2.3 Haemangiomas

Capillary haemangiomas can affect either lids and are usually noticed soon after birth as reddish discolorations of the eyelid which progressively develop into an enlarging mass. Size increases usually up to the age of 2 years or so before involution. Complete resolution may take up to the age of 8 years. If large enough to interfere with the visual axis, intervention with steroids and/or other modalities such as laser therapy may be required.

2.4 Ptosis

Drooping of the upper lid, which may be unilateral or bilateral, congenital or acquired. The essential differentiation is between a simple congenital dystrophy of the levator muscle and other causes of ptosis. If the levator is dystrophic, there will be some lid-lag on downgaze. If the levator is not dystrophic the eyelid remains ptotic in all positions of gaze. The most common cause of ptosis in childhood is simple congenital ptosis, which is due to a dystrophy of the levator palpebrae superioris muscle. It is inherited as autosomal dominant trait with variable penetrance.

Causes of ptosis

- **Congenital ptosis**
    - **Dystrophic**: e.g. simple congenital ptosis
    - **Non-dystrophic**: aponeurotic defect, e.g. neurogenic, mechanical

- **Acquired ptosis**
    - **Aponeumotic** (trauma or oedema)
    - **Lid inflammation** (trauma, oedema)
    - **Neurogenic** (e.g. third nerve palsy, Horner's syndrome and Marcus Gunn's jaw-winking syndrome)
    - **Myogenic** (e.g. progressive external ophthalmoplegia, ocular myopathies and myasthenia gravis
    - **Mechanical** (e.g. lid tumours and lacerations)
    - **Infections** (e.g. encephalitis and botulism)
    - **Syndromes** (e.g. Sturge–Weber syndrome and neurofibromatosis)
    - **Drugs** (e.g. vincristine)

Horner's syndrome

This is caused by sympathetic denervation. May be congenital or acquired.

Features

- Ptosis (partial)
- Miosis (pupil constriction)
- Enophthalmus
- Anhidrosis (ipsilateral)
- Heterochromia iridis (congenital type)
- Normal direct and consensual reflex to light

Congenital may be caused by obstetric trauma, with cervical vertebral anomalies, congenital tumours and infection such as varicella syndrome.

Acquired may be caused by trauma, surgery or tumours such as neuroblastoma.

Marcus Gunn jaw-winking syndrome

This is due to an abnormal synkinesis between the levator and the lateral pterygoid muscle. The affected eyelid is usually ptotic, but elevates when the jaws open and deviates to the contralateral side. To perform the test, look for ptosis when the jaw is closed then ask the child to open his/her mouth wide, this will result in rising of the ptotic upper lid.

Treatment of ptosis

Ptosis of sufficient degree to interfere with vision requires early correction to prevent permanent loss of vision (amblyopia). Surgical treatment such as levator resection. In severe congenital ptosis the eyelid can be suspended from the brow and elevated by the frontalis muscle.

3. LACRIMAL SYSTEM DISORDERS

The lacrimal system function is to produce and remove tears.

Congenital nasolacrimal sac (mucocele or dacryocystocele)

This presents shortly after birth as a bluish mass in the region of the nasolacrimal sac. Fluid becomes trapped within the nasolacrimal sac. Treatment varies from conservative massage to probing within a few days.

Dacryocystitis

This may be caused by bacterial infection of the nasolacrimal sac associated with nasolacrimal duct obstruction. It presents with swelling of the nasolacrimal sac region with cellulitis of the surrounding tissues.

Stenosis or obstruction of the nasolacrimal duct

This may occur in 30% of newborn infants. Signs include mucopurulent discharge or tearing which may start three to five weeks later. Gentle pressure over the nasolacrimal sac expresses tears and mucopurulent material from the sac. Spontaneous resolution is common, but probing of the nasolacrimal duct may be required.

3.1 The watering eye (lacrimation and epiphora)

Lacrimation means excessive secretion of tears, e.g. in crying, whereas epiphora means watering of the eyes, i.e. overflow because of inadequate drainage. The newborn baby does not usually shed tears during crying for the first 4–6 weeks of age.

Causes of epiphora

- Blocked nasolacrimal system
- Congenital glaucoma

631

- Acquired foreign body
- Keratitis and conjunctivitis
- Facial palsy
- Chronic blepharitis
- Migraine
- Contact lens
- Drugs (e.g. maternal heroin addiction)
- Congenital glaucoma (epiphora in conjunction with photophobia may herald congenital glaucoma)
- Non-patent nasolacrimal system

3.2 The dry eye

The child with a dry eye rarely complains that it is dry, but complains of a burning sensation. It is a relatively uncommon problem.

Causes of dry eye

- **Tear mucin-deficiency** — e.g. vitamin A deficiency (xerophthalmia), trachoma, burns and Stevens–Johnson syndrome
- **Tear lipid-layer deficiency**
- **Aqueous tear-deficiency** — keratoconjunctivitis sicca
- **Congenital alacrima**
- **Ectodermal dysplasia** — dry skin, the anhidrotic type — absence of sweat and sebaceous glands, poor hair formation and abnormalities of nails and teeth
- **Familial dysautonomia** — (Reilly–Day syndrome) (autosomal recessive almost exclusively in children of Ashkenazi Jewish origin) emotional lability, paroxysmal hypertension, sweating, cold hands and feet and blotchy skin
- **Sjögren's syndrome** — uncommon in childhood, arthritis, dryness of mouth and other mucous membrane and dry eyes, tendency to bronchitis and pneumonia with pulmonary disease
- **Drug-induced**

Treatment of dry eyes

Treatment is not always satisfactory. Generally avoidance of dry atmosphere (e.g. excessive central heating), active use of sleeping-room humidification and increasing humidity by the use of glasses or goggles. The mainstay of treatment is artificial tears.

4. PROPTOSIS

Is defined as abnormal protrusion of the eyeball. Proptosis (exophthalmos) is most easily appreciated when the examiner looks at patient's eyes from above the top of the head. May be unilateral or bilateral (due to pressure from behind) or false (due to prominent eyeball).

Causes of proptosis

- Infection such as orbital cellulitis and ethmoiditis
- Cavernous sinus thrombosis
- Tumours
  - Neuroblastoma
  - Retinoblastoma
  - Optic nerve glioma
  - Histiocytosis
  - Angioma
  - Rhabdomyosarcoma
- Thyrotoxicosis
- Craniosynostoses
- Dermoid
- Orbital encephalocele
- Mucocele of the paranasal sinus
- Coagulation disorders (haemorrhage) and other orbital and frontal bone osteomyelitis

4.1 Orbital infections

Pre-septal cellulitis

Occurs when the infection is anterior to the orbital septum. Commoner than orbital cellulitis. Causes include eyelid trauma, extraocular infection and upper respiratory tract infection (URTI). Usually unilateral. No associated proptosis. Causative organism varies with age: being streptococcal pneumonia and staphylococcal abscess in the neonatal period and *Haemophilus influenzae* in later infancy.

Treatment: antibiotic and treatment of the underlying condition: e.g. dacryocystitis.

Orbital cellulitis

Uncommon but serious infection, may give rise to ocular and septic intracranial complications. More frequent in children older than 5 years. Over 90% of cases occur secondary to sinusitis, usually of the ethmoid sinus. Type B *Haemophilus influenzae* is the commonest organism during infancy, but other common organisms are *Staphylococcus* spp, causing abscess, and *Streptococcus pneumoniae*.

Presentation: usually with painful red eye and lid Oedema; conjunctival chemosis, injection and axial proptosis with limitation of eye movement. The child is usually pyrexial.

Treatment: admission to a hospital. Investigations (blood culture, computed tomography (CT) scan and sinus X-ray). ENT assessment. Systemic antibiotics initially given intravenously.

4.2 Orbital tumours

The most common primary orbital malignancy in childhood is rhabdomyosarcoma, which usually occurs between the age of 7 and 8 years and presents with progressive unilateral proptosis. Secondary metastases (especially neuroblastoma) present with an abrupt onset of proptosis and ecchymosis which may be bilateral.

Proptosis may be secondary to optic nerve glioma. Dermoid and epidermoid cyst are relatively uncommon. The commonest site of dermoid cyst is lateral brow area.

5. EYE MOVEMENT AND STRABISMUS

5.1 Squint (strabismus)

Definition: misalignment of the visual axis.

Prevalence: approximately 4% of children younger than 6 years of age have strabismus. Some 25% of children with childhood-onset strabismus have either a parent or a sibling with strabismus.

Pseudostrabismus: this is seen in infants with prominent epicanthal folds, closely placed eyes and flat nasal bridges. Observation of symmetrical corneal light reflexes or cover-testing will confirm or exclude the presence of true deviation.

Classification of squint

- Heterophoria (latent squint)
- Concomitant squint (non-paralytic strabismus)
  - Esotropia (convergent squint) — is an inward deviation of the eyes (most common type of squint).
  - Exotropia (divergent squint) — is an outward deviation of the eyes
- Inconcomitant squint (paralytic strabismus)

Causes of strabismus

- **Congenital**
- **Cranial nerve palsy** and developmental abnormalities.
- **Moebius syndrome:** (association of congenital bilateral facial palsy and bilateral abducens palsy). Facial palsies usually spare lower face. May be inherited, usually sporadic.
- **Duane syndrome:** congenital hypoplasia of the VIth nerve nucleus. IIIrd nerve compensates by innervating lateral rectus muscle, resulting in failure of abduction on lateral gaze and globe retraction (palpebral fissure narrows) on adduction. 15–20% bilateral. Usually sporadic. Associations include Goldenhar's syndrome, hemivertebra and Marcus Gunn jaw-winking.

- **Brown's syndrome:** (failure of elevation of the eye, maximal in adduction) Usually congenital developmental anomaly of the superior oblique tendon. Occasionally acquired as a result of trauma or surgery. Present with abnormal head posture, elevations of the chin and turning the head away from the affected eye in order to acquire binocular vision. May resolve spontaneously, but surgery may be indicated especially when deterioration takes place.
- **Congenital ptosis and myasthenia gravis** (rare)
  - **Acquired**
    - **Cranial nerve palsies** — features:
    - third nerve lesion: complete ptosis, diplopia, eye turned 'down and out' (unopposed lateral rectus and superior oblique muscles) and failure of pupil to react to light or accommodation;
    - fourth nerve palsy: diplopia and failure of inferior – lateral gaze (failure of the superior oblique muscle);
    - sixth nerve palsy: diplopia and medial gaze (failure of lateral rectus muscle)
  - **Neuromuscular disease:** myopathy, myasthenia gravis and botulism.
  - **Infections of the orbit or brain:** raised intracranial pressure, e.g. tumour and post-infectious (Miller–Fisher syndrome; a variant of Guillain-Barré syndrome).
  - **Brainstem disorders**

Causes of esotropia (convergent squint)

- Refractory error — hypermetropia
- Cataract
- Lesions of the optic nerve or macular
- High refractive error or asymmetrical refractive errors

Causes of exotropia (divergent)

- Intermittent exotropia is common, and is most evident when child is tired and fixating on a distant object. Constant exotropia may be congenital or caused by poor vision in the outward turning eye.

Heterotropia

This is a constant ocular malalignment. Children with heterotropia suppress the image of one eye to avoid diplopia. Amblyopia will result in the suppressed eye when one eye is used for fixation. Early diagnostic assessment to prevent permanent loss of vision in one eye. A fixed squint is commonly found in cerebral palsy, microcephaly and hydrocephalus. The rapid development of a squint may suggest the possibility of a cerebral tumour.

Amblyopia

Is a term used to describe severe impairment of vision as a result of significant interruption of normal visual development.

Causes of amblyopia

- Strabismus is by far the most common cause
- Anisometropia — refractive state of one eye significantly different from the other eye
- Ametropia — high refractive error in both eyes and then deprivation — as a result of opacity within the visual axis such as cataract. Usually unilateral. Strabismus is the commonest cause.

Treatment

Depends on the cause. If significant refractive error exists, then optical correction must be made early. Intervention rarely effective after 8 years of age. Opacities such as cataract should be treated. If strabismus is present then amblyopia must first be reversed with occlusion therapy prior to surgical treatment.

Assessment of squint

It is important to check that the child can see with each eye first, and that each eye moves to a normal range when tested separately (to exclude paralytic squint). Latent tendency for ocular misalignment under certain conditions, e.g. fatigue, illness and stress.

Facial appearance

Squint may be obvious on general inspection, however broad epicanthic fold can give the appearance of a convergent squint. An abnormal head posture may be a sign of a squint.

Corneal reflections

These should be identical in position in both eyes. Using a penlight held about 30 cm (12 inches) from the eye.

Ocular movements

Should be tested in both horizontal and vertical axis using small fixation object. Limitation of movement in one direction suggests a paralytic squint.

The cover test consists of three parts:

- Cover test
- Uncover test
- Alternate cover test

In all three tests the patient looks intently at a target, which may be in any direction of gaze, distant or near. In each test, each eye is encouraged to take up fixation separately whilst the other is covered.

Cover test

As the examiner observes one eye, a cover is placed in front of the other eye so as to block its view of the target. If the observed eye moves to take up fixation, it clearly is not fixating the target, and manifest deviation (strabismus) is present.

LATENT SQUINT	**MANIFEST SQUINT**

LATENT SQUINT

Normally, both eyes appear to be aligned and centrally fixed

MANIFEST SQUINT

One eye is deviated towards the other

Cover the esotropic eye — there is no movement of either eye

 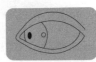

Exophoria

Cover one eye — that eye deviates away from the other eye

 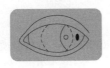

The cover is then removed — the now uncovered eye returns to a central position

The cover is then removed — again, there is no movement of either eye — no proof of tropia

The other eye is now covered — as a result, that eye becomes esotropic and the formerly esotropic eye moves to a central position to take up fixation (Hering's law)

If the cover is removed and no eye movement occurs, this indicates that the eyes have equal visual acuity **or** fixation. This also indicates a relative absence of amblyopia

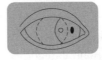

Esophoria

Cover one eye — that eye deviates toward the other eye

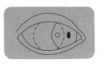

The cover is then removed — the now uncovered eye returns to a central position

If the cover is removed and both eyes move so that the original fixing eye is again centrally fixed and the originally esotropic eye is again esotropic, this indicates that there is amblyopia present

Uncover test

As the cover is removed from the eye following the cover test, the eye emerging from under cover is observed. If the position of the eye changes, interruption of binocular vision has allowed it to deviate, and heterophoria (latent squint) is present.

Alternate cover test

The cover is alternately placed in front of one eye and then the other. This tends to break up the control of heterophoria that may last through a single cover–uncover cycle. This test shows the total deviation of constant squint plus latent squint.

Management of squint

Any squint after the age of 6 months should be referred to an ophthalmologist. A fixed squint should be referred early as it is always abnormal.

The following four approaches are possible:

- Occlusion (occlusion of the good eye encourages the use of squinting eye and the development of fixation)
- Correction of refractory errors: glasses
- Orthoptist involvement as with amblyopia
- Surgery — mainly cosmetic

5.2 Nystagmus

Defined as involuntary rhythmic movement of one or both eyes about one or more axis. Broadly divided into three main categories:

- Nystagmus secondary to a visual deficit
- Nystagmus secondary to intracranial lesions and drug toxicity
- Congenital benign idiopathic nystagmus

Each cycle of nystagmus oscillation may have a slow phase and a fast component, in which case it is called 'jerk nystagmus'. Oscillations without a quick phase are called 'pendular'.

Other classifications

- Physiological
- Congenital (appear before the age of 6 months): blindness, familial and idiopathic

Acquired nystagmus

(Usually after the age of 6 months)

- Spasmus nutans
- Ictal nystagmus (with epilepsy)

- Cerebellar disease
- Spinocerebellar degeneration
- Vestibular
- Drugs: e.g. carbamazepine
- Optic nerve and chiasma tumour (rare)

Spasmus nutans

- Acquired nystagmus characterized by the triad of pendular nystagmus, head nodding and torticollis. The nystagmus is fine, rapid, horizontal and pendular. Signs usually develop within the first 2 years of life, but the components of the triad may develop at various times.

  Often benign and self-limiting resolving in few months but sometimes years. Some children with brain tumours may exhibit signs resembling those of spasmus nutans. Therefore careful assessment and neuroimaging may be required.

Cerebellar nystagmus is the most important to recognize. It is usually horizontal and worsens on looking to the side of the lesion, with the first component directed towards the side of the lesion.

Vestibular nystagmus differs in that the slow phase is directed towards the side of the lesion due to disorders of labyrinth, vestibular system, vestibular nuclei of the brainstem, or cerebellum.

Vertical nystagmus

This is usually due to lesion of the brainstem at the pontomedullary junction (roughly at the foramen magnum), e.g. achondroplasia or Arnold–Chiari malformations.

Clinical test for nystagmus

Ask the child to look at a flashlight or a toy held in front of the eye. Ask the child to follow the object as you move it quickly, first to one side, then to the other, and also up and down.

6. DISEASES OF THE CONJUNCTIVA

6.1 Conjunctivitis

This is the commonest conjunctival disease. May be bacterial, viral, allergic, toxic or part of a systemic disease.

Bacterial conjunctivitis

Neonatal conjunctivitis (previously referred to as ophthalmia neonatorum) — A common problem with an incidence as high as 7–19% of all newborns in the first month of life. Usually bacterial.

Gonococcal conjunctivitis — A hyperacute bacterial conjunctivitis with thick purulent discharge and lid oedema caused by *Neisseria gonorrhoea* (Gram-negative). Incubation period 2–5 days. Requires prompt treatment since untreated can rapidly progress to corneal perforation and potentially blinding. Treatment with systemic antibiotics, usually third-generation cephalosporin for 7 days because of the increasing resistance, together with topical irrigation of the eyes.

Chlamydia trachomatis — Is the most common organism causing ophthalmia neonatarum in the United States. Infection may vary from mild inflammation to severe swelling of the lids and copious purulent discharge. Potentially blinding. Treatment is with tetracycline ointment for 2 months and systemic erythromycin.

Pseudomonas aeruginosa — Usually acquired in the nursery, characterized by the appearance of oedema on day 5 to 18, erythema of the eyelids, and purulent discharge. Progression to endophthalmitis and septic shock can occur. Treatment is with systemic antibiotics. *Pseudomonas aeruginosa* ulcers may frequently affect young children and contact-lens' wearers.

Other bacterial infections in infants and older children
Staphylococcus Haemophilus spp. and *S. pneumococcus* all cause purulent conjunctivitis and need treatment with systemic antibiotics.

Allergic conjunctivitis

Occurs as a hypersensitivity to dust, pollen, animal dander and other airborne allergens, characterized by tearing and itching with conjunctival oedema. Usually seasonal. Topical anti-mast cell stabilizer or topical steroids are helpful. Systemic antihistamines may be required.

Vernal conjunctivitis

Usually occurs later in the prepubertal period. Atopy may be a factor. Extreme itching is the usual complaint with redness, watering of the eye and lid-swelling. It results in cobble-stone appearance of the palpebral conjunctiva. Recommended treatment: topical corticosteroid therapy, a mast-cell inhibitor and cold compress.

Chemical conjunctivitis

Results from irritant substances such as smoke, industrial pollution, sprays, alkalis and acids.

Viral conjunctivitis

Caused by a wide range of viruses, commonly influenzavirus, adenovirus, infectious mononucleosis and with exanthems such as measles. Characterized by a watery discharge and redness of the conjuctiva. May be haemorrhagic. Usually self-limiting and no specific treatment is required unless caused by herpes simplex virus, in which case treatment with topical antiviral agents (aciclovir) as required.

Other causes of conjunctivitis

For example, acute systemic disorders, i.e. Steven–Johnson syndrome and Kawasaki disease. Conjunctivitis is usually non-purulent and self-limiting, but in Steven–Johnson syndrome topical steroids are recommended. There are other systemic signs.

6.2 Other conjunctival disorders

Subconjunctival haemorrhage

May occur spontaneously or secondary to trauma, e.g. physical injury (e.g. non-accidental injury (NAI)), coughing (e.g. pertussis), seizure, post-birth or any activity involving Valsalva type manoeuvres. Pertussis infection is an important cause. They usually resolve spontaneously within 2 weeks and do not require treatment.

Limbal dermoid

May be isolated or part of syndrome, e.g. Goldenhar's syndrome — coronal limbal dermoids appear as yellowish-white, usually rounded elevations sometimes with pigmentation and hair at the apex.

Pigmented lesions

For example, pigmented limbal naevus, conjunctival haemangioma or increased vascularity, e.g. ataxia telangiectasia (usually on the temporal side of the bulbar-conjunctiva), tumours and infiltrates of the conjunctiva, e.g. neurofibromatosis, sarcoidosis.

7. DISEASES OF THE CORNEA

Developmental anomalies

- Sclerocornea present at birth, rare, cornea is white and resembles sclera
- Microcornea corneal diameter is 9 mm or less, may be associated with glaucoma, cataract, iris abnormalities or anterior segment dysgenesis
- Corneal dermoid cyst (limbal dermoid)
- Congenital coloboma

The cornea is also the site of many systemic diseases:

- **Hurler's syndrome** (mucopolysaccharidosis) produces clouding of the cornea
- **Cystinosis** seen in the early months of life (involves the deposition of L-cystine in the cornea)
- **Glaucoma** produces hazy and opaque cornea due to corneal oedema
- **Wilson's disease** produces Kayser–Fleischer ring (it is a greenish/grey ring along the outer margin of the cornea)
- **Infections** may cause corneal opacity, e.g. keratitis (also may be caused by vitamin A deficiency (rare) and injury)

- **Juvenile chronic arthritis** can cause keratopathy
- **Keratoconus** characterized by thinning and bulging of the central cornea which becomes cone-shaped. Descemet's membrane may occasionally rupture with sudden and marked corneal oedema (acute hydrops). Some degree of corneal scarring occurs. Mostly managed conservatively with contact lenses. Occasionally corneal transplant is indicated. Usually sporadic. Associations with atopy, Down's syndrome, Marfan, Ehlers–Danlos syndrome, aniridia and congenital rubella.
- **Corneal inflammations** are associated with viral, bacterial, fungal and allergic diseases. Bacterial infection may cause corneal ulcers and abcess leading to visual impairment and corneal perforation. Herpes simplex infection of the cornea may be transmitted from maternal birth canal or direct contact with active lesion, and is a serious infection. Requires urgent attention and treatment with aciclovir. Herpetic keratis may also require topical steriods.

Deposits

Corneal deposits are not easily visible. Slit-lamp examination is essential. Seen in cystinosis, uric acid crystals (brownish colour), calcium deposits and other rare conditions.

8. DISEASES OF THE SCLERA

Blue sclera although seen in certain normal people. It is more common in osteogenesis imperfecta, and in Ehlers–Danlos syndrome.

Yellow discoloration of the sclera indicates jaundice.

Black patches on the sclera may be due to either naevi or thinning of the sclera which allows the colour of the choroid to show through.

Episcleritis is very rare in infants and children. Inflammation can be either nodular, as in the chickenpox lesion, or diffuse. Episcleritis is associated with subconjunctival injection and may involve the overlying conjunctiva as well. Usually causes mild ache in the eye.

Scleritis is characterized by pain on movement, deep redness and mild proptosis. The vision may be reduced by serous retinal detachment; association with Wegener's granulomatosis.

Episcleritis and scleritis may occur in autoimmune disease, dry eyes and graft-versus-host disease.

9. PHOTOPHOBIA

Definition: light sensitivity in normal lighting conditions which makes the child uncomfortable.

Causes of photophobia

1. **Systemic causes:** meningitis, encephalitis, migraine, vitamin A deficiency and xeroderma pigmentosum.

2. **Drugs:** Atropine eye drops, ethosuximide and para-aminosalicyclic acic (PAS).

3. **Ophthalmic causes:**
- **Corneal:** most causes of true photophobia are of corneal origin, e.g. epithelial disruption, as with a foreign body. The most important cause of corneal photophobia is buphthalmos, which is the hallmark of congenital glaucoma. The corneas are enlarged due to breaks in Descemet's membrane which allows stretching of the cornea in the infantile eye.
- **Iris:** anirida, iritis
- **Uvea:** photophobia may be present in albinism (absent uveal pigment) and uveitis. Juvenile chronic arthritis and spondyloarthropathy account for the majority of paediatric uveitis.

Uveitis is classified according to location, clinical characteristics of the inflammatory pathology with further differentiation based on primary site such as iritis, choroiditis, iridocyclitis or pan-uveitis.

- **Anterior uveitis:** Characterized by triad of symptoms: pain, redness and photophobia. Causes include trauma, infections such as Kawasaki disease, Lyme disease, spondylo-arthropathy and Crohn's disease. In severe inflammation vision is reduced. Slit-lamp examination should be used to assess the extent of the inflammation and in diagnosis.
- **Posterior uveitis:** inflammation of the choroid. The only symptoms are visual. Chorioretinitis may be focal or diffuse, unilateral or bilateral. Causes include toxoplasmosis, CMV infection, sarcoidosis, syphilis, TB and toxocariasis. Signs are usually scarring and pigmentation often with visual impairment. Complications include retinal detachment and glaucoma.
- **Lens diseases:** such as partial cataract.
- **Optic nerve disease:** optic neuritis (although the most important symptom is visual loss).
- **Vitritis**
- **Retinal problems:** retinal dystrophies.

10. CAUSES OF PAINFUL RED EYE

- Trauma — haemorrhage
- Conjunctivitis (bacterial or viral)
- Uveitis
- Iridocyclitis
- Corneal damage: foreign bodies, direct injury, keratitis (e.g. herpes zoster and herpes simplex and other viral infections)
- Glaucoma
- Headache: eye pain but without red eye

11. UVEAL TRACT DISORDERS (IRIS, CILIARY BODIES AND CHOROID)

11.1 Aniridia

Complete absence of the iris. Hereditary and sporadic forms. The usual mode of inheritance is an autosomal dominant trait. Aniridia occurs spontaneously in one-third of cases and they may have a chromosome 11p13 deletion.

Associations of aniridia

- Poor vision
- Cataract — 50–85% by the age of 20 years
- Glaucoma — not present at birth but later in childhood
- Optic nerve hypoplasia
- Ectopia lentis may also occur in conjunction with aniridia

Aniridia with systemic disease

WAGR syndrome: Wilms' tumour, aniridia, genitourinary abnormalities and retardation. Deletion of the short arm of chromosome 11 usually present. High incidence of bilateral Wilms' tumours.

11.2 Albinism

A hereditary error of metabolism within pigment cells. The loss of melanin may be limited to the eye (ocular albinism), or affect the skin and eye (oculocutaneous albinism).

Occular albinism

Usually inherited as X-linked

Features

- Males with photophobia, reduced visual acuity, nystagmus and iris transillumination defects with foveal hypoplasia and scanty retinal pigmentation.

Oculocutaneous albinism

Tyrosinase-negative

- Clinical picture:
Hair steely white, pink skin (sensitive to sunburn), reduced visual acuity, nystagmus – pink/blue eyes. This is associated with one or more of the lesions in the large tyrosinase gene at 11q14–21.

Tyrosinase-positive

- Clinical picture:
Tyrosinase gene is normal. Usually has more pigment and therefore better vision.

Albinism in conjunction with other diseases:

- Chédiak–Higashi syndrome — autosomal recessive, albinism, repeated infections, mild bleeding diathesis, hepatosplenomegaly, peripheral and cranial neuropathy.
- Hermansky–Pudlak syndrome — autosomal recessive, albinism, platelet dysfunction, pulmonary fibrosis and inflammatory bowel disease.

11.3 Brushfield spots

These are silvery-grey spots on the iris. Found in 85% of children with Down's syndrome, and also in 24% of normal people.

11.4 Heterochromia iridis

Difference in iris colour. May be congenital or acquired.

Congenital:

- The involved iris is darker
- Horner's syndrome — ipsilateral hypopigmentation, miosis and ptosis
- Waardenburg's syndrome (autosomal dominant); lateral displacement of the inner canthi, prominent root of the nose, white forelock and sensorineural deafness

Acquired:

- Heterochromia may be result of infiltrative processes such as naevi and melanomatous tumours.

11.5 Coloboma

Congenital defect due to failure of some portion of the eye or ocular adnexa to complete growth resulting in a cleft. They may occur as isolated defects or in association with systemic syndromes.

Usually sporadic, but isolated coloboma may be inherited as a dominant trait.

Iris coloboma

Appears as a keyhole when complete and as a notch when partial, usually affect inferior and nasal part of the iris.

Optic disc coloboma

Appear as a hole of variable size usually in the temporal side of the margin of the disc.

- CHARGE association: **C**oloboma; **H**eart disease; choanal **A**tresia, **R**etarded growth and development; **G**enital hypoplasia; and **E**ar anomalies
- Cat-eye syndrome: Tri- or tetrasomy 22; colobomatous microphthalmia; anal atresia; and preauricular skin tags
- 4P-syndrome (Wolff–Hirschhorn syndrome): severe learning difficulties, characteristic face, fish-like mouth, coloboma, epicanthic fold, hypertelorism and squint, congenital heart disease
- Trisomy 13 (Patau's syndrome): coloboma, cleft lip and palate and severe cardiac abnormalities

Iris abnormalities not related to coloboma

Nodular lesions of the iris may be seen in the neurofibromatosis (Lisch nodules).

11.6 Inflammation of the iris

Iritis/iridocyclitis/uveitis

The incidence of iridocyclitis is approximately 20% in pauciarticular arthritis, more common in females with a ratio of 3:1. This is usually bilateral and asymptomatic and it may precede the arthritis. Common complications include band keratopathy, cataract and secondary glaucoma. Because of the painfree course of iridocyclitis associated with juvenile chronic arthritis, the recommended follow-up is required. Treatment includes: topical corticosteroids and mydriatics.

Half of the patients with mild uveitis have an excellent prognosis, being controlled with topical medication.

Other causes: measles, mumps, chickenpox, Lyme disease, Kawasaki's disease, Reiter's syndrome, Behçet's disease and sarcoidosis. Diagnosis is made through various immunological and serological tests.

12. ABNORMALITIES OF THE PUPIL

Anisocoria

This is inequality of the pupils. May be physiological or due to neurological disorders. In the absence of associated signs, diagnosis can be difficult as to which pupil is abnormal. Examination in light and dark will help to diagnose sympathetic and parasympathetic lesions. In Horner's syndrome the anisocoria is greater in the dark, whereas in a parasympathetic lesion the difference is greatest in the light.

Small pupil

- Horner's syndrome
- Microcoria syndrome: congenital miosis — pupil less than 2 mm in size, when patient look at a distant object
- Uveitis
- Drugs

Large pupil

- Third nerve lesion
- Trauma, aniridia, coloboma, complication of surgery and drugs (mydriatics, e.g. atropine)

Abnormal shaped pupil: coloboma (inferonasal), partial aniridia, hyperplastic pupillary membrane.

Tonic pupil syndrome (Adie's syndrome)

Children may present on school-screening with failed vision or blurred near vision or photophobia. The effect is of a pupil slightly larger than the other pupil. Corneal sensation may be reduced. Patients may be hyporeflexic or areflexic with intact vibration sense.

Leukocoria

White pupillary reflex.

Causes of leukocoria

- Retinoblastoma
- Cataract
- Uveitis
- Retinopathy of prematurity
- *Toxocara* spp.
- Vitreous haemorrhage
- Coloboma

Diagnosis can often be made by direct examination of the eye by ophthalmoscope. Absence of red reflex requires immediate expert attention to determine the cause.

13. CHILDHOOD GLAUCOMA

Definition: damage of the optic nerve with visual field loss caused by, or related to, elevated pressure within the eye. Normal intraocular pressure in infants and young children is less than 20 mmHg.

Congenital glaucoma begins within the first 3 years of life. Juvenile glaucoma between the age of 3 and 30 years.

Classification broadly into:

- primary glaucoma caused by an intrinsic disorder of the aqueous outflow mechanism; and
- secondary glaucoma caused by other ocular diseases or systemic abnormalities.

When the intraocular pressure is raised in young children the cornea usually becomes diffusely oedematous and enlarged. When the corneal diameter increases, splits occur in Descemet's membrane and damage occurs to the corneal endothelial cells. If intraocular pressure is raised in a child under 2 years of age the eye may enlarge. This is referred to as 'buphthalmos' (ox-eye).

Clinical manifestations

Symptoms include the classic triad of epiphora (tearing), photophobia and blepharospasm (eyelid squeezing) secondary to corneal irritation. However, only 30% of affected infants demonstrate the classic symptoms' complex. Epiphora in glaucoma is differentiated from nasolacrimal duct obstruction by the presence of rhinorrhoea. When the nasolacrimal duct is obstructed rhinorrhoea is absent. Other signs include corneal oedema, corneal and ocular enlargement, conjunctival injection and visual impairment.

Primary glaucoma

Is caused by an intrinsic disorder of the aqueous outflow drainage — more than 50% of glaucoma is primary. 1:10,000 births. Usually bilateral.

Associated ocular problems:

- Aniridia
- Sturge–Weber
- Neurofibromatosis
- Hypomelanosis of Ito
- Alagille's syndrome
- Down's syndrome
- Marfan's syndrome
- Rubinstein–Taybi syndrome
- Wolf–Hirschhorn syndrome (4P–)
- Lowe syndrome
- Congenital rubella syndrome

Secondary glaucoma

Associated conditions are inflammatory eye disease (in association with Still's disease), ectopia lentis and complication of surgery for cataract.

Management of glaucoma
If untreated, glaucoma will inevitably lead to visual loss. Amblyopia is a major complication in unilateral glaucoma. The treatment remains surgical in most of the cases but sometimes medical treatment with drugs and laser therapy may help.

- Surgical: to establish more normal anterior chamber angle (goniotomy and trabeculectomy) or to reduce aqueous fluid production (cyclocryotherapy and photocyclocoagulation). Children may need several operations to lower the intraocular pressure. Long-term medical treatment may also be necessary.
- Medical: beta-blockers (e.g. timolol) which act by lowering intraocular pressure. New medication such as BeTopics 0.25% have less systemic side-effects.
- Cyclolaser therapy: cyclophotocoagulation may be successful in reducing intraocular pressure. Repeated applications may be required since relapse is common.

14. LENS DISORDERS

Characteristics to be considered are size, shape, location and transparency. The lens can be affected by developmental problems, humidity and systemic disease.

14.1 Developmental anomalies

The normal lens should fill the entire pupillary area. Aphakia (absent lens) and microphakia (small lens) are rare; the latter can be seen as part of microphthalmia of many of the congenital infections (TORCH).

14.2 Dislocated lens (ectopia lentis)

A subluxed lens is a lens partially displaced from its normal position but remaining within the pupillary space, whereas a dislocated or luxated lens is completely displaced from the pupil implying separation of all or nearly all of the zonular attachments. A reduction in visual acuity is the most common presenting symptom of subluxation or dislocation of lens.

Presentation

Blurred vision.

Associations

Marfan's syndrome: the commonest cause of ectopia lentis (superiorly)

Homocystinuria: the lens usually subluxes inferiorly; other causes include aniridia, trauma, coloboma and glaucoma.

Hereditary lens dislocation: usually bilateral.

Treatment

Visual improvement may be achieved with spectacles. A partial dislocated lens is often complicated by cataract formation, in which case the cataract has to be removed but should be delayed because of the possible complication of retinal detachment. Anterior dislocation of the lens may be treated with pupillary dilatation and manual repositioning of the lens by pressure on the cornea. Complete dislocation of lens may lead to development of glaucoma. Asymptomatic dislocation carries a very good prognosis.

14.3 Cataract

A cataract is a lens opacity. Main presentation is visual impairment. Up to one-third of children with bilateral congenital cataract remain legally blind even after surgery. Congenital cataract is the commonest remedial cause of blindness in the developed world.

Presentation

Absent red reflex, leucocoria, squint, nystagmus and visual impairment.

Causes of a congenital cataract

- Idiopathic
- Intrauterine infection (TORCH)
- Genetic without systemic problems (autosomal dominant, recessive and X-linked inheritance)
- Genetic with systemic problems:
  - Autosomal dominant — hereditary spherocytosis, myotonic dystrophy, incontinentia pigmenti (rare), Marshall syndrome
  - Autosomal recessive (rare) — congenital ichthyosis, Conradi disease, Smith–Lemli–Opitz syndrome, Siemens syndrome
  - X-linked inheritance (rare) — Lowe syndrome
- Chromosomal abnormalities (trisomy 21, 18 and 13) and Turner's syndrome
- Metabolic disorders — galactosaemia, galactokinase deficiency and hypocalcaemia
- Maternal factors, e.g. diabetes mellitus and drugs in pregnancy, e.g. corticosteroids and chlorpromazine

Causes of acquired cataract

- Drugs such as corticosteroids
- Trauma
- Metabolic disorders (e.g. diabetes mellitus, hypothyroidism, hypocalcaemia and pseudohypoparathyroidism)
- Radiotherapy
- Infections — varicella, herpes simplex and *Toxocara canis*
- Atopic dermatitis
- Genetic conditions with later presentations such as Down's syndrome, myotonic dystrophy, nail–patella syndrome, Alport's syndrome, Wilson disease, Laurence–Moon–Biedl syndrome, Cockayne syndrome
- Cataract of prematurity
- The most common chromosomal abnormality associated with cataract is trisomy 21 usually later in life.

Bilateral congenital cataracts: should be removed early because of interference with visual development.

Partial cataracts: need careful assessment of the density and size of the lens opacity before removal, since conservative management is indicated at least until the child's visual status can be adequately assessed. It is important that metabolic disease such as galactosaemia, diabetes, hyperthyroidism and hypocalcaemia are ruled out through appropriate investigation. The most common operation for cataract is lensectomy and anterior vitrectomy in infants. Aphakic spectacles are required following surgery. In older children simple lens aspiration with or without implantation of lens is the preferred procedure.

15. RETINAL DISORDERS

Colobomas: defects of closure of the embryonic fissure of the optic cup. It may occur unilaterally or bilaterally.

Myelinated nerve fibres: myelination may continue beyond the optic disc to include the retinal nerve-fibre layer. It is usually visible as yellow–white, flame-shape patches oriented with the retinal nerve fibres. They may produce clinical signs of leucocoria.

Albinism: albino fundus, usually pale with poor macular development and prominent choroidal vasculature.

Coat's disease: occurs in males, peak 8–10 years of age, is predominantly unilateral. Peripheral retinal telangiectasias and aneurysmal dilatation lead to extensive areas of exudates giving the retina a yellow–white appearance which may produce leukocoria.

Retinitis pigmentosa (RP): a pigmentary retinopathy characterized by night blindness (earliest symptom), progressive loss of peripheral visual field and loss of central vision (final symptom). Symptoms may be present in childhood, but usually do not become apparent until the 2nd or 3rd decade of life.

Early retinal changes shows pigment deposition as seen in the mid-peripheral retina then progressing to more diffuse pigment.

Systemic associations include:

- Abetalipoproteinaemia
- Refsum's disease
- Usher's syndrome
- Laurence–Moon–Biedl syndrome
- Kearns–Sayre syndrome

Retinal detachment

This is a rare condition in childhood. Presentation is usually late and the disease advanced at the time of diagnosis. It often occurs in a developmentally abnormal eye and it may follow blunt trauma. Treatment is surgical.

Hypertensive retinopathy

This is rare in children. In early stages of hypertension no retinal changes are observed. Then the arterioles narrow and become irregular, retinal oedema will follow and then appearance of flame-shaped haemorrhages, cotton-wool spots (retinal nerve-fibre layer infarct) and papilloedema.

Diabetic retinopathy

This is uncommon in children but may occur during or after puberty. Prevalence related to duration and control of the disease.

Non-proliferative diabetic retinopathy characterized by retinal microaneurysms, venous dilatation and retinal haemorrhages and exudate. Proliferative characterized by neovascularization and proliferation of fibrovascular tissue on the retina. Most serious form.

Sickle-cell retinopathy

Proliferative changes: arteriolar occlusions leading to arteriovenous anastomosis. Vitreous haemorrhages and retinal detachment.

Non-proliferative changes: deposits, sunburst lesions and salmon-patch haemorrhages.

Retinopathy of prematurity

This is vasoproliferative retinopathy affecting mainly premature infants. The clinical manifestations range from mild, which is usually transient changes of the peripheral retina, to severe vasoproliferative changes with scarring leading to retinal detachment and blindness.

Classification
Five stages based on the location, extent and severity of disease. The extent of the involvement of retinopathy is described as clock hours of retinal circumference affected.

Babies who at birth are less than 1,500 grams or who are 31 weeks' gestation or less should be screened.

Timing of the first examination:

- Infants born at or earlier than 25 weeks' gestation
- Screening at 6–7 weeks postnatally, then fortnightly until 36 weeks' post-menstrual age.

- Infants born between 26 and 32 weeks' gestational age with screening at 6–7 weeks' postnatally, and at 36 weeks' post-menstrual age (or within a week of this to be discharged from hospital)

Treatment

In selective cases cryotherapy or laser photocoagulation of the peripheral avascular retina has been shown to be effective in Stage 3 disease and reduced progression to blinding disease. Recent advances in *in-vitreo* retinal surgical technique has led to some limited success in treatment of retinal detachment.

Prevention

Retinopathy of prematurity largely depends on prevention of premature birth and its associated problems. Despite improvement of our understanding of the natural history and the associated risk factors, such as high oxygen exposure, prevention remains a major challenge.

Retinal haemorrhages

In young infants, by far the most common cause of retinal haemorrhage is non-accidental injury. The haemorrhages may last for many months. Haemorrhage rarely happens accidentally in children or as a complication of blood disorders such as leukaemia.

Retinoblastoma

Is the most common intraocular malignancy of childhood. Incidence — 1:14,000 to 1:20,000 births. Caused by a mutation in a growth-suppressor gene. Both alleles have to be affected to develop the tumour. The most common age of diagnosis between 1 and 1½ years with 90% before the age of 3 years. Presenting signs: leukocoria 60% and squint 22%. Less than 25% of all cases have a family history of retinoblastoma.

Treatment

Enucleation of the eye remains the most common therapy, and will result in a cure if tumour has not metastasized. Where bilateral tumour is present then the eye with the most extensive tumour with no possibility of useful vision is enucleated and attempts are made to save the eye with less involvement. Focal irradiation is used for solitary tumours less than 15 mm in diameter; systemic chemotherapy is also available to offer shrinkage of intraocular tumours, and cryotherapy and laser for small tumours.

Long-term, follow-up and genetic counselling are required for patients with retinoblastomas.

16. INFECTIONS AND THE RETINA

Congenital infections

- **Toxoplasmosis:** Caused by *Toxoplasma gondii*. Congenital toxoplasmosis. 8% of severely affected neonates will have chorioretinitis. Ophthalmological complications include chorioretinitis which appears as a white elevated mass with surrounding pigmentation on the retina. Infants may present later with leukocoria or squint and visual deterioration occurs and retinal detachment is a complication. Treatment is with pyrimethamine and sulfadine both for 1 year.
- **Rubella:** typical ocular findings include microphthalmia, microcornea, anterior uveitis, cataract, corneal opacification and glaucoma. The retinopathy in rubella is diffuse but does not affect vision.
- **Cytomegalovirus:** ocular manifestation includes microphthalmia, cataracts, keratitis, choroiditis and optic atrophy. Diagnosis confirmed with tests and isolation of the virus from urine, stool or throat of the infected neonate.
- **Herpes simplex:** the eye can be the site of disseminated herpes and the most common ocular involvements are blepharoconjunctivitis with vesicles on the eyelids and keratitis. Choroiditis and inflammation of the vitreous with optic atrophy may also occur, particularly in infants with central nervous system involvement.
- **HIV:** ocular manifestations include retinopathy, usually asymptomatic and characterized by cotton-wool spots, retinal haemorrhage and other microvascular abnormalities.
- **Syphilis:** causes bilateral chorioretinitis or salt-and-pepper fundus appearance.

Acquired infections

- **Toxocariasis**: ocular involvement rare. Caused by *Toxocara canis* larvae infection. The change is usually unilateral. Ocular forms include:
  - Endophthalmitis: present between the age of 2 and 9 years and is most confused with retinoblastoma as the red reflex is absent and a complete retinal detachment is present;
  - Macular lesions: presents slightly later and usually solitary granuloma.

Presentation usually composed of strabismus and leukocoria or failed screening examination at school. Confirmation of infection with ELISA for *Toxocara* spp. with peripheral eosinophilia on blood film.

Treatment: Steroids and to a lesser extent antihelminthic drugs which are not very helpful and do not restore the lost vision.

- **Bacterial endocarditis**
  May give picture of cotton-wool spots; frequently developed in patients with bacterial endocarditis as a result of septic emboli.

17. OPTIC NERVE DISORDERS

17.1 Papilloedema

Defined as swelling of the optic nerve in association with raised intracranial pressure. The vision is usually preserved even with marked swelling of the optic disc. The fundoscopic picture is as follows:

- Earliest sign is blurring of the disc margins, followed by elevated disc
- Dilated capillary plexus and retinal veins
- Absent pulsation of the optic disc
- Swollen nerve-fibre bundles
- Splinter haemorrhages and more markedly elevated disc, nerve-fibre infarcts (cotton-wool spots) and exudates follow
- Further engorgement and tortuosity of the retinal and disc capillaries, and haemorrhages become more widespread

Causes of swollen disc in childhood:

Bilateral

- Papilloedema (raised intracranial pressure, hydrocephalus and benign intracranial hypertension)
- Hypertension
- Optic neuritis
- Bilateral pseudopapilloedema, as in myopia and hypermetropia
- Bilateral tumours (e.g. haemangioma, retinoblastoma and hamartoma)

Unilateral

- Pseudopapilloedema as in myopia and myelinated nerve fibres and hypermetropia
- Tumours: haemangioma, retinoblastoma, optic nerve glioma
- Uveitis
- Ischaemic optic neuropathy
- Unilateral optic neuritis

17.2 Optic atrophy

The optic disc loses its colour and appears sharply demarcated with pale yellow–white disc. Usually leads to reduced visual acuity with subsequent visual field defects.

Presentation

Bilateral optic atrophy presents as blindness in early infancy with roving eye movements and sluggish pupil reaction. Milder degrees of bilateral optic atrophy may cause minor visual defects or squint in childhood. Unilateral cases may present as a squint.

Inheritance

Recessive or dominant trait.

Association with generalized neurological conditions such as Behr's optic atrophy with cerebellar ataxia, hypotonia and learning difficulties.

Leber's optic atrophy occurs in late adolescence, but secondary optic atrophy occurs to papilloedema, optic neuritis, compressive lesions of the optic nerve or chiasm, trauma and hereditary retinal disease or glaucoma.

Causes of optic atrophy

- Prenatal
  - maternal disease
  - pregnancy problems
- Perinatal
  - prematurity
  - asphyxia
- Familial
- Ocular
  - glaucoma
  - retinal dystrophy
- Compressive
  - proptosis
  - space-occupying lesion
- Trauma
- Optic neuritis
- Toxic
  - drugs
  - lead
- Meningitis/encephalitis
- Leukodystrophies

18. METABOLIC DISEASES AND THE EYE

Corneal abnormality

- Mucopolysaccharidoses (except Hunter's)
- Mucolipidosis
- Fabry's disease
- Sialidosis
- Cystinosis
- Tyrosinaemia (type II)

Visual failure

- Juvenile Batten's disease
- Leucodystrophies
- Abetalipoproteinaemia
- Gangliosidoses

Eye movement disorder

- Niemann–Pick disease type C, sialidosis type I (vertical gaze palsy)
- Gaucher's disease type 3 (congenital oculomotor apraxia)
- Sialidosis type II (nystagmus), type I (nystagmus and myoclonus)
- GM2 gangliosidosis type III

Cherry–Red spot

- Tay–Sachs
- Sandhoff
- GM1 gangliosidosis type 1
- Niemann–Pick A, C and D
- Sialidosis type 2
- Farber's disease
- Mucolipidosis I

19. MISCELLANEOUS DISORDERS

Neurofibromatosis (NF1)

- Plexiform neuromas of eyelids — often producing ptosis
- Conjunctival neurofibroma
- Lisch's iris nodules
- Hamartomas (phacomas) of disk and retina
- Fundus pigmentary changes
- Optic gliomas
- Strabismus
- Nystagmus
- Proptosis and exophthalmos

Sturge–Weber syndrome

- Glaucoma: 50% before the age of 2 years (20% after the age of 4)
- Choroidal haemangiomas — 40%

Wilson's disease — Kayser–Fleischer ring

Tuberous sclerosis

- Occurs in 50% of patients, although may not be evident in infancy
- Hamartomas of the retina and optic nerve — most common
- Papilloedema — rare
- Optic atrophy

von Hippel–Lindau syndrome

Retinal angiomatosis — usually in the midperiphery. Often multiple with both eyes involved in more than 50% of cases.

Ataxia-telangiectasia

Telangiectasia of bulbar conjunctivae (by the age of 4–6 years), disorder of conjugate eye movements, convergent squint and nystagmus.

Incontinentia pigmenti

Microphthalmos, corneal opacities, cataract and optic atrophy.

Marfan syndrome

Lens dislocation (usually upward), and iridodonesis (tremulous iris), microphakia, cataract, myopia, glaucoma and retinal detachment.

Down's syndrome

Brushfield's spots, cataract, chronic keratopathy, ectropion, glaucoma, keratoconus, lid eversion, myopia and strabismus.

20. OCULAR TRAUMA

In order to assess the extent of ocular trauma vision should always be assessed first. The severity of the injuries are dictated by the amount of disruption to the anatomy. This varies from minor laceration of the eyelids to severe ocular injuries. Examination will require topical anaesthetic in order to examine the eye comfortably.

Blunt trauma to the eye may cause iritis or anterior uveitis. Patients will complain of dull eye pain and light sensitivity. Other signs of iritis include miosis of the pupil, excessive tearing and ciliary injection. A hyphema is blood in the anterior chamber of the eye. Complications include re-bleeding, glaucoma and iron-staining of the cornea. Dislocation of the lens may take place following blunt trauma.

Retinal haemorrhage may occur as a result of trauma.

Penetrating injuries to the eye may necessitate examination and should be brief and gentle in order to avoid exposure of the intraocular contents. Further examination required in the operating room under anaesthesia. Topical medication should not be used in penetrating injuries.

21. ACQUIRED VISUAL LOSS

History is vital to ensure that visual loss is really acquired rather than present from birth.

- Cortical blindness
- Post-traumatic anoxia
- Hypotension
- Hypoglycaemia
- Migraine
- Occipital epilepsy
- Vitreous haemorrhage
- Retinal disease
- Optic nerve disease
- Optic neuritis
- Ischaemia
- Trauma
- Drugs
- Benign intracranial hypertension and pituitary tumour
- Hysteria

22. VISUAL ASSESSMENT AND REFRACTIVE ERRORS

22.1 Visual assessment

Visual acuity measurement is the most important test for assessment of visual function. The age of the child and the level of development dictates what type of test should be used. Fixation reflex generally used to evaluate vision in young infants. A 3-month-old infant may be expected to steadily fixate and begin to follow pen light, toy or face, and by the age of 6 months a child should be able to follow a fixation target to all fields of gaze, therefore the level of vision can be estimated by the quality of fixation response.

From the age of 2½ to 3 years objective measurement of visual acuity is possible. The vision is tested by using schematic picture or other illiterate eye chart. Each eye should be tested separately. The **E** test, in which the child points in the direction of the letter, is the most widely used to test visual acuity in pre-school children. For older children **Snellen** acuity chart should be used from the age of 5 to 6 years, since this is the 'gold standard' for measurement of visual activity.

22.2 Refractive errors

Errors in the refractive power of the eye may lead to subnormal visual acuity. This may result from variation of curvature of the cornea or lens or variation in the axial length of the eye.

The commonest forms of refractive error are:

- **Myopia** (short-sightedness): this is usually due to an increase in axial length of the eye so objects at distance are blurred. Myopia is inherited as a multifactorial trait, which may also be associated with systemic conditions such as Stickler syndrome. Concave lenses are used to correct myopia in most circumstances.
- **Hypermetropia** (far-sightedness): the optical image formed by the hypermetropic eye is focused behind the retina because the visual axis is short, and therefore convex lenses are used.
- **Astigmatism**: this occurs when the cornea, lens or retinal surface has toric shape rather than spherical one. This produces a blurred retinal image of object at any distance. Astigmatism can be corrected by special lenses.
- **Anisometropia**: this refers to a condition where the eyes have different refractive errors with one worse than the other. It may occur with myopia, astigmatism or absence of the lens or a combination of these refractive errors.

23. OPHTHALMOLOGICAL INVESTIGATIONS

Investigations in ophthalmology

Visual evoked potentials
This test is used to define vision development in infants. This measures the time taken for light stimulus to pass along the visual pathway to the occipital cortex and also the amplitude of the response.

Electroretinography (ERG)
This is an electrical recording of the response of the retina to visual stimulus, e.g. flash of light. This test is useful in the detection of retinitis pigmentosa and intraocular foreign bodies.

Electro-oculography (EOG)
This is based on the standing potential of the eye. The EOG is recorded by placing skin electrodes adjacent to the inner and outer canthi of the eye. It is useful in detecting hereditary macular disease and also retinitis pigmentosa, myopic chorioretinal degeneration and helps in diagnosis of Best's disease.

Ultrasonography
This can be used at times to detect ocular abnormalities which are not usually clinically visualized, such as opacification of the cornea, lens and vitreous.

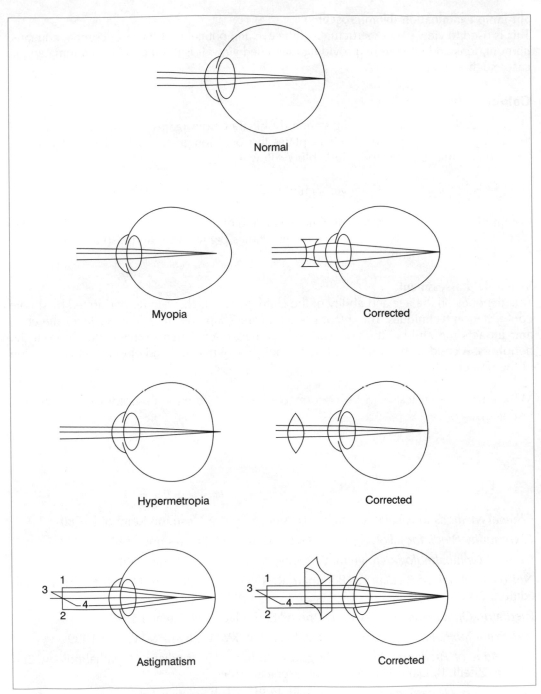

Normal eye and various refractive errors.

Slit-lamp examination (biomicroscopy)

This is used to view various structures of the eye and optical section, e.g., cornea, aqueous, humour, lens and vitreous by providing magnified view. It is often crucial in trauma and in cases such as iritis.

Colour vision

This is usually performed by using standard Ishihara colour plates with some adaptation of the usual testing techniques. Ishihara plates test only red/green colour vision deficiency. Other plates may be used to include blue/yellow testing.

The test is accomplished whenever a child is able to name or trace the test symbol.

Colour vision defect is inherited as X-linked pattern of inheritance but can also be acquired secondary to optic or macula disease, as in retinitis pigmentosa, and also as side-effect of drugs such as rifampicin.

Visual field assessment

This depends on the age and ability of the child. In infants this can be performed by simple confrontation techniques. The infant sits on a carer's lap and the examiner faces the child and attracts the child's attention centrally, using toy or a light moved silently from the periphery. A child with normal fields will readily move his/her head or eyes in the direction of the object or light source.

More formal visual tests can be performed in older children with Goldmann visual field testing.

24. FURTHER READING

Clinical Methods in Paediatric Diagnosis: Athreya, B Van Nostrand Reinhold 1980.

Community Paediatrics: Polnay, L and Hull, D Churchill Livingstone 1985.

General Ophthalmology: Vaughan, D, Taylor, A 11th edition. Lange 1986.

Nelson Textbook of Paediatrics: Behrman, R, Kleigman, R, Jenson, H, WB Saunders, 16th edition, 2000.

Paediatric Ophthalmology: Taylor, D 2nd edition, Blackwell Science 1997.

Pediatric Ophthalmology for Pediatricians: Wright, KW Williams & Wilkins 1999.

Slide Atlas of Paediatric Physical Diagnosis: Volume 19: Paediatric Ophthalmology, 2nd edition. Zitelli, B, Dans, H (eds). Gower Medical, 1992.

Symptoms of Disease in Childhood: David, PJ Blackwell Science 1995.

Chapter 17

Respiratory

Jane C Davies

CONTENTS

Respiratory

1. ANATOMY AND PHYSIOLOGY

1.1 Embryology

In utero development is divided into four stages:

- **Embryonic: up to 5th week**
  - Lung bud grows out from the fetal foregut
  - Single tube branches into two main bronchi

- **Pseudoglandular: 6th–16th week**
  - Airways grow by branching (out to terminal bronchioles)
  - Cartilage and lymphatics appear from 10 weeks onwards
  - Cilia appear
  - Pulmonary circulation develops, arteries arising from the 6th branchial arches

- **Canalicular: 17th–24th week**
  - Conventional architecture of the lung appears
  - Thinning out of distal cells in preparation for gas exchange
  - Further development of arterial circulation, and appearance of venous system
  - Surfactant synthesis begins
  - Lung fills with fluid (lack of fluid at this and later stage (e.g. with renal agenesis) leads to pulmonary hypoplasia)

- **Alveolar sac: 24th–40th week**
  - Formation of the acinus (respiratory bronchioles, alveolar ducts and alveoli)
  - Cell differentiation into type I and II pneumocytes:
    - Type I: >90% of alveolar surface
      Major gas exchanging surface

    - Type II: Produces surfactant which maintains surface tension and prevents alveolar collapse during respiration
      Surfactant-associated proteins: A and D (hydrophilic) involved mainly in innate immunity
      B and C (hydrophobic) important for surface tension

1.2 Fetal and postnatal lung growth

Factors affecting fetal lung growth and development:

- Lack of amniotic fluid
- Glucocorticoids, thyroid hormones, other hormones increase maturation
- Pressure effects (e.g. compression from diaphragmatic hernia, or space-occupying lesion leads to hypoplasia)

Postnatally, lung development and growth continues for 7 years. May be adversely influenced by:

- Ventilation and oxygen toxicity
- Early infection (e.g. adenovirus, respiratory syncytial virus (RSV))

1.3 Changes at birth and persistent fetal circulation

Vaginal delivery compresses the thorax, leading to expulsion of lung fluid and expansion of the lungs with the first breath. The increase in oxygen content leads to closure of the ductus arteriosus (which in fetal life diverts right ventricular blood away from the lungs into the systemic circulation), and the resultant increase in left atrial pressure (from increased pulmonary venous return) closes the foramen ovale. Thus, the right-sided pulmonary and left-sided systemic circulations are effectively separated. Persistent fetal circulation describes the situation where the pulmonary vasculature fails to relax leading to ongoing right to left shunting of (deoxygenated) blood at the ductal and foramen ovale level. Infants are severely hypoxic, mimicking the clinical picture of cyanotic congenital heart disease. Treatment includes ventilation with a high FiO_2, and pulmonary vasodilators such as inhaled nitric oxide or prostacyclin.

1.4 Control of respiration

Inspiration is achieved largely by diaphragmatic effort with additional expansion provided by the intercostal muscles. At rest, expiration is largely passive, although this may become active upon exercise, or in children with respiratory disease. Expiration against a partially closed glottis both prolongs this phase and raises airway pressure leading to increased alveolar gas exchange. This is observed in the common sign of 'grunting' in infants with respiratory distress.

Respiratory drive is provided by both central (medulla) and peripheral (carotid body) chemoreceptors. In normal health high CO_2 leads to increased respiratory drive, although in chronic lung disease sensitivity may be blunted, and there is a dependence on hypoxia for this stimulus.

1.5 Ventilation

Air passes through the trachea, major bronchi and terminal bronchioles (anatomical deadspace) before reaching the sites of active gas exchange, the alveoli. In normal health, alveolar walls are thin (one cell thick) facilitating O_2 and CO_2 exchange. In diseases affecting the alveolus, gas exchange will be impaired, leading to an increase in respiratory rate in response to both a low O_2 and a raised CO_2.

1.6 Perfusion

Perfusion is matched to ventilation via hypoxia-mediated pulmonary vasoconstriction, i.e. vascular constriction leads to diversion of blood flow away from poorly ventilated to well-ventilated areas, decreasing ventilation–perfusion (VQ) mismatch. Pulmonary arterial flow will be increased by vasodilatation in response to both high O_2 and low CO_2, whereas pulmonary vasoconstriction, and thus hypertension, is exacerbated by hypoxia and hypercarbia.

1.7 Lung function testing

Infants

Methods for testing lung function in infancy have been developed and are in use in the research setting, although they are not yet in widespread clinical use. In general, a sedated infant is fitted with a tightly fitted face mask. After either a tidal breath or, with some methodologies, an assisted inspiration, a jacket is rapidly inflated around the infant's chest, leading to forced expiration from which flows and volumes can be measured.

Older children

From the age of between 5 and 7 years, children will usually be able to perform standard lung function tests. The following values can be obtained:

FVC: Forced vital capacity, is the total amount of air exhaled upon forced expiration.

FEV_1: Forced expiratory volume in the first second, gives a measure of large (and medium sized) airway obstruction.

The ratio of these two values gives an indication as to the nature of an abnormality. Restrictive lung diseases such as fibrosis lead to reduction in both parameters, with preservation of the normal ratio (approx. 80%), whilst obstructive diseases (asthma, CF) lead to a greater reduction in FEV_1 and thus a reduced FEV_1:FVC ratio.

FEF_{25-75}: Forced expiratory flow between defined vital capacity (25% being ¾ empty) is a measure of flow at lower lung volumes, is non-effort-dependent, and is thought to be a reasonable representation of small airways function.

RV: Residual volume is the amount of air left in the lungs after maximal expiration. It is increased in diseases such as asthma, as narrowed small airways prevent complete emptying of more distal lung and result in air-trapping.

PEFR: Peak expiratory flow rate. Although useful as a home monitoring device in patients with asthma, it can be quite effort-dependent and can underestimate significant small airways obstruction.

In addition to the above, transfer factor for CO and corrected TLCO (corrected for lung volume) gives an estimate of the lung diffusion capacity. Reduced in diseases where alveolae are abnormal and gas exchange is impaired, and increased in the presence of red blood cells which can absorb CO (e.g. pulmonary haemorrhage or haemosiderosis).

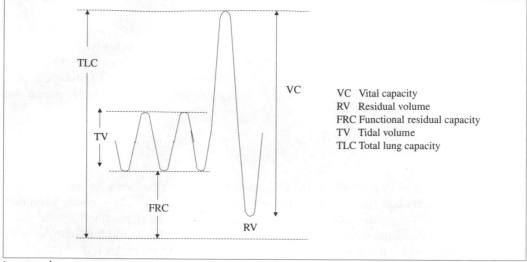

VC Vital capacity
RV Residual volume
FRC Functional residual capacity
TV Tidal volume
TLC Total lung capacity

Lung volumes

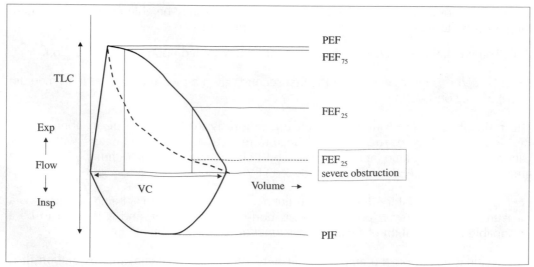

Flow volume loop

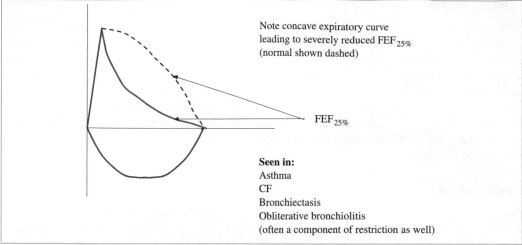

Note concave expiratory curve
leading to severely reduced $FEF_{25\%}$
(normal shown dashed)

$FEF_{25\%}$

Seen in:
Asthma
CF
Bronchiectasis
Obliterative bronchiolitis
(often a component of restriction as well)

Obstructive defect

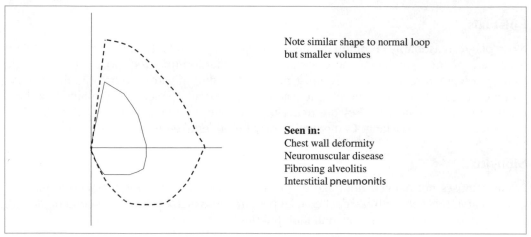

Note similar shape to normal loop
but smaller volumes

Seen in:
Chest wall deformity
Neuromuscular disease
Fibrosing alveolitis
Interstitial pneumonitis

Restrictive defect

2. ENT AND UPPER AIRWAY

2.1 Nose and sinuses

Choanal atresia (CA)

Unilateral or bilateral. Congenital malformation occurring in approximately 1:60–70,000 births. Due to failure of breakdown of bucconasal membrane leading to complete obstruction of the nostril. Bilateral CA presents immediately at birth (neonate obligate nose breather) with severe respiratory compromise and inability to pass nasal catheter. Artificial oral airway life-saving. Surgery required. Associated with other congenital defects, e.g. cardiac.

Allergic rhinitis

Presents as rhinorrhoea, sniffing, altered sense of smell (and taste), +/– itchy eyes and conjunctivitis. May be either seasonal (usually triggered by pollens, grasses, etc.) or related to environmental allergens (e.g. house dust mite, dogs, cats, horses). Often associated with atopic family history, and may be other features in child, e.g. asthma, eczema. Degree of disturbance to a sufferer of severe rhinitis probably underestimated (problems with concentration, poor sleep quality, etc.). Management should include allergen avoidance, topical (nose +/– eyes) administration of corticosteroids or cromoglycate-based agents. In severe cases, oral antihistamines may be required. Children with allergic rhinitis may also have nasal polyps.

Nasal polyps

Occur in atopic children and in cystic fibrosis (CF) (must consider this diagnosis in any child with polyps). Present with runny nose, nasal obstruction, decreased sense of smell, distortion of nasal shape. May respond to topical corticosteroids, but often difficult to treat, necessitating surgical removal. Recurrence post-surgery is unfortunately common.

Epistaxis

Nose bleeds reasonably common in childhood. Usually from Little's area on septum. Often triggered by nose-picking. More common in inflamed/infected nose, (e.g. allergic rhinitis/polyps). If recurrent/severe must rule out bleeding disorder idiopathic thrombocytopenic purpura (ITP), haemophilia, leukaemia, etc.) or anatomical abnormality (e.g. haemangioma, telangiectasia). Pressure under nasal bridge usually adequate to halt bleeding. If severe, may need packing. Cauterization may be undertaken for recurrent episodes.

Sinusitis

Frontal sinuses not aerated until age of 3–5 years, so frontal sinusitis not seen in this age group. Later, presents with headache/facial pain (made worse by coughing/bending down), nasal congestion/discharge, concentration problems.

Associated with CF (almost 100% of patients have opaque sinuses; X-ray therefore not very useful). May also be associated with humoral immunodeficiency, e.g. IgA or IgG subclass deficiency.

Treatment involves decongestants, antibiotics. Surgical drainage required in a minority.

Complications (rare but serious)

- Orbital cellulitis
- Frontal osteomyelitis
- Meningitis/cerebral abscess
- Intracranial (including cavernous sinus) thrombosis

2.2 Cleft lip and palate

Often now diagnosed antenatally on ultrasound scanning. Can be associated with Pierre Robin sequence (micrognathia and glossoptosis), other dysmorphic syndromes (e.g. Stickler's syndrome, Edward's), or occur in isolation, in which case prognosis is usually excellent. Certain antiepileptic medications associated with increased incidence and some evidence of prevention with folic acid (as in spina bifida). Familial cases not uncommon, making a genetic component very likely.

Main problems

Cosmetic: Lip cleft repaired early at approximately 2–3 months of age

Feeding: Special teats for bottles available for some infants
Feeding facilitated by a palatal plate if severe
May be associated oropharyngeal incoordination and aspiration of feeds
Cleft palate surgery usually performed by the age of 1 year
Speech and hearing: often associated with frequent ear infections and glue ear
Large cleft can cause speech difficulties

Airway obstruction: If due to Pierre Robin sequence, some infants require a nasopharyngeal tube to maintain patency of the upper airway.

2.3 Ears

Chronic otitis media (OM)

Chronic otitis media (glue ear) is a major cause of hearing problems and speech delay. Due to accumulation of thick secretions in the middle ear and recurrent acute infections. May be associated with adenoidal hypertrophy; adenoidectomy may improve symptoms. Long-term antibiotics are not very useful.

Insertion of grommets to release fluid and pressure is often performed. Normally extruded spontaneously by about 6–9 months. Studies have suggested that swimming is not harmful to a child with grommets (but should not dive).

Deafness

Types of deafness:

Conductive: Commoner of the two types, detected in up to 3–4% school-children, often mild
Almost always secondary to chronic OM
Preservation of bone conductance with diminished air conductance

Sensorineural: Less common, 0.2–0.3% children
More likely to be severe
Caused by either cochlear or neuronal damage
Equal impairment of both bone and air conductance

671

Causes of sensorineural deafness

- Genetic — associated with dysmorphic syndromes
- Congenital infections (TORCH group)
- Birth asphyxia
- Severe jaundice
- CNS infection
      post-meningitis
      encephalitis
      cerebral abscess
- Aminoglycoside toxicity
- Head injury

Treatment

- Hearing aids may be useful if some preservation of hearing
- Cochlear implants in selected cases
- Multidisciplinary approach

Mastoiditis

Has become rare with the use of antibiotics to treat acute otitis media. Results from breakdown of bony walls of mastoid air cells, secondary to ongoing bacterial middle ear infection. Presents with high fever, toxic, irritability, marked focal tenderness over mastoid process, discharging ear +/– deafness. If early in process may respond to parenteral antibiotics; in more severe cases, surgical intervention may be required.

2.4 Throat

Adenotonsillar hypertrophy and airway obstruction

Adenotonsillar hypertrophy common in childhood, although most cases require no specific treatment and will resolve with age. More severe cases associated with certain disease groups, for example sickle-cell anaemia and HIV.

Symptoms either relate to recurrent infections, or airway obstruction. Obstruction may be obvious to parents (snoring +/– apnoeic pauses, mouth-breathing, halitosis), or may present with right heart failure and cor pulmonale if not recognized until late. Polysomnography may reveal obstructive episodes (increased chest excursion with diminished airflow +/– hypoxia and hypercarbia if severe), although in majority of cases, diagnosis can be made on the history.

Management
Surgical removal in selected cases.

Oropharyngeal incoordination and aspiration

Swallowing is a complex mechanism requiring intact anatomy and neuromuscular co-ordination. Diseases affecting either pathway can lead to saliva and food/drink entering the respiratory tract.

Should be considered as a cause of respiratory symptoms especially in at-risk groups:

- Premature babies: immature swallowing mechanisms
- CNS disease, e.g. cerebral palsy
- Anatomical abnormality: cleft palate/larynx
- Any cause of generalized hypotonia especially with bulbar involvement

Aspiration with intact swallow also seen with severe gastro-oesophageal reflux and tracheo-oesophageal fistula.

Symptoms may be overt (choking and coughing with feeds), but are often absent. Leads to recurrent wheeze and aspiration pneumonias. It is diagnosed on video-fluoroscopy. Management depends on cause, but severe cases may require surgical intervention.

2.5 Larynx

Web

Rare. If complete is obviously incompatible with life. More commonly, results in partial laryngeal obstruction, respiratory distress and stridor. Diagnosed by direct visualization and requires surgical repair.

Cleft

Very rare. Failure of closure of tracheo-oesphageal septum at 35 days of embryonic development. Presents with aspiration, choking, episodes of cyanosis +/– apnoea. May coexist with other abnormalities. Diagnosed by laryngo/bronchoscopy. Requires surgical repair.

Haemangioma

Presents with airway obstruction, cough or stridor. May coexist with cutaneous haemangiomata — examine the child completely. Visible as soft mass on instrumentation of the airway. May bleed copiously if traumatized or biopsy attempted. Topical application of adrenaline may be life-saving in such a situation. Surgical removal similarly often hazardous. May decrease in size in response to local corticosteroid injection.

Papillomatosis

Rare cause of hoarseness if affecting the larynx. May present with stridor or barking cough. Diagnosed on upper airway examination or bronchoscopy.

Notoriously difficult to treat. Some evidence of response to cimetidine. Initial hopes of response to interferon appear unfounded.

2.6 Malacias

Any tubular component of the respiratory tract may be malacic (floppy).

Results in partial or complete collapse on inspiration.

Presentation: Stridor and respiratory distress
Apnoea
Feeding problems
Recurrent croupy episodes
Diagnosis can be confirmed on laryngo/bronchoscopy (although usually possible clinically)
Mild cases (the majority) become less severe with growth
Severe cases may benefit from aortopexy

Causes of stridor

Common
Croup
Laryngo/tracheomalacia
Subglottic stenosis/granuloma (post-intubation)
Vascular ring
Inhaled foreign body (if large and proximally lodged)

Rarer
Epiglottitis (much less common since Hib vaccination)
External tracheal compression
Mediastinal mass, e.g. lymphoma/leukaemia
TB lymphadenopathy
Enlargement of heart/great vessels associated with congenital cardiac malformation
Laryngeal web
Haemangioma, papillomatosis
Vocal cord palsy
Vocal cord dysfunction
Hypocalcaemia

2.7 Sleep disordered breathing

Spectrum of problems, ranging from snoring through to hypoxia/hypercarbia leading to pulmonary hypertension and cor pulmonale. May be related to local (e.g. adenotonsillar hypertrophy) or systemic (e.g. neuromuscular) disease. Take a careful history. Ask specifically about pauses in breathing signalling sleep apnoea. May lead to disrupted sleep/nocturnal enuresis/daytime somnolence/morning headaches (high CO_2)/under-achievement at school. Definitive diagnosis on polysomnography (see section 10, under *Management of Myopathies*). Treatment tailored to cause.

2.8 Tracheo-oesophageal fistula (TOF)

Failure of normal development of the primitive foregut leads to a fistula connecting the oesophagus and trachea with or without oesophageal atresia.

Oesophageal atresia presents in the immediate neonatal period with vomiting, choking (+/– an absence of gas in the abdomen, depending on the position and size of the fistula). Confirmation is obtained by attempted passage of a nasogastric tube. May exist as part of the VACTERL constellation (**V**ertebral, **A**nal, **C**ardiac, **T**OF, **E**ars, **R**enal, **L**imb).

TOF without oesophageal atresia will often present later. At its most obvious, the child may choke with feeds, but equally the history may be one of recurrent chest infections or wheeze. Diagnosis is made on a tube oesophagram (injection of radio-opaque dye into the oesophagus under pressure to force open a small fistula). It is often missed on bronchoscopy, particularly flexible bronchoscopy.

Treatment for both conditions is surgical.

3. ASTHMA

3.1 Pathophysiology

Chronic inflammatory disease of the airways with a well-recognized genetic component in which many cells are involved, including eosinophils, lymphocytes and mast cells. Airway inflammation leads to airway oedema, and hyperreactivity resulting in reversible bronchoconstriction.

If left untreated, the inflammatory changes may eventually become chronic and irreversible, a process termed 'airway remodelling'.

From both laboratory and epidemiological studies, a protective role for infection against the subsequent development of asthma has been demonstrated.

T-lymphocyte populations are biased towards a T-helper cell (T_{H2}) phenotype (interleukin (IL)-4 and IL-5 secreting, involved in IgE production), as opposed to the T_{H1} phenotype which is more commonly found in response to infection.

Symptoms:	May be classical wheeze and dyspnoea, or cough-variant. Often worst at night or in early morning.
Triggers:	Viruses
	Allergens (e.g. house dust mite, cats, dogs)
	Cold air
	Cigarette smoke
	Exercise
	Stress/emotional

675

3.2 Drug treatment

Management should include:

- Identification and avoidance of precipitating factors (e.g. house dust mite, pets, cigarette smoke)
- Education: importance of long-term prophylaxis
- Recognition and management of acute attack (written plan where appropriate)

British Thoracic Society Guidelines for asthma management

Step 1	Bronchodilators prn
Step 2	Low-dose inhaled anti-inflammatory and prn bronchodilators
Step 3	High-dose steroid or low-dose steroid plus long-acting bronchodilator and short-acting bronchodilator prn
Step 4	High-dose inhaled steroid plus regular bronchodilator
Step 5	Above plus regular oral corticosteroids

Guidelines recommend stepping down treatment when control is achieved, i.e. aim for best control on lowest dose.

Treatment options beyond step 5

- Continuous subcutaneous terbutaline
- Intravenous immunoglobulin
- Alternative immunosuppressive drugs:
  - Methotrexate
  - Azathioprine
  - Cyclosporine A
    - gum hypertrophy
    - hypertrichosis
    - leucopenia
    - renal toxicity
    - levels required

Inhaler devices (you should know how to demonstrate each device)

Very important to choose one suitable for child.

Inhaler devices	
Large volume spacers	Used with metered-dose inhalers (MDIs) Best lung deposition Used with mask in young age group, and mouthpiece when old enough to form seal Static charge reduces lung delivery: leave to dry after washing — do not dry with towel
	Single puffs best administered individually Volumatic: salbutamol, beclomethasone, fluticasone Nebuhaler: terbutaline, budesonide
Smaller spacers	(e.g. AeroChamber) more portable and versatile, although delivery not quite as good
Dry powder inhalers	Children (usually around 4–7 years) who can: • form a seal with their lips • hold their breath Includes Turbohaler, Diskhaler, Acuhaler, etc.

MDIs have poor lung deposition (most go into mouth) and are not to be recommended for use alone.

Long-acting bronchodilators useful to gain control instead of increasing steroid dose and in exercise-induced asthma.

3.3 Acute attack

Signs of severity:

- Inability to talk in sentences
- Tachypnoea/tachycardia
- Inter/subcostal recession
- Use of accessory muscles of respiration
- Quiet or silent chest (poor air entry)
- Pulsus paradoxus
- Cyanosis (very late sign — beware)

In the presence of tachypnoea, a normal CO_2 level indicates a severe attack.

Management of acute severe asthma

- Oxygen
- Bronchodilator: via spacer device has been shown to be as effective, if not more so, than via nebulizer, can be give continuously. If unsuccessful, intravenous salbutamol: cardiovascular monitoring. Watch K^+.

- Aminophylline
  - Loading dose slowly

- Systemic (usually i.v.) steroids
- If respiratory support required:
  - Lowest possible inspiratory pressures
  - Short inspiratory time; long expiratory time
  - Minimal/no PEEP to reduce air trapping

Causes of wheeze in childhood

Common

> Viral-associated recurrent wheeze
> Acute viral infection, e.g. RSV, adenovirus
> Asthma
> Gastro-oesophageal reflux (and aspiration syndromes)
> Cystic fibrosis
> Inhaled foreign body

Rare

> Distal bronchomalacia
> Obliterative bronchiolitis (see section 11.2)
> Bronchiectasis

---

4. CYSTIC FIBROSIS

4.1 Background

Cystic fibrosis is the commonest lethal recessive disease of Caucasians, with a carrier frequency of 1:25, leading to disease in 1:2,500 of the population (>6,000 patients in UK). Previously regarded as a disease of childhood, increases in survival have swelled the adult CF population. Median survival for a child born today estimated at 40 years.

The gene responsible encodes cystic fibrosis transmembrane-conductance regulator (CFTR) and is on chromosome 7. The primary function of CFTR is a chloride ion channel, but also inhibits the epithelial sodium channel, ENaC. CF respiratory epithelium therefore fails to secrete Cl^- (absorb in sweat gland, hence high sweat electrolytes), and hyperabsorbs Na^+ and thus H_2O, dehydrating the airway surface. Secretions are viscid, impairing mucociliary clearance and thus host defence.

CFTR now known to have other functions (related to transport of other substances, e.g. bicarbonate, and receptors for bacteria), but are controversial.

Other organs affected for similar reasons include gut, pancreas, liver and reproductive tract.

Diagnosis

Sweat test

- 'Gold standard'. Values of Na$^+$ or Cl$^-$ (better) >60 mEq/l diagnostic (although >40 in infants very likely to indicate CF)
- Traditionally required at least 100 mg sweat, but newer methods (e.g. macroduct) require less. Conductivity (increased in CF) also used by some labs.

Cases of CF with normal sweat electrolytes have been reported, so if high suspicion, does not rule out diagnosis.

- If values in grey area (40–60 mEq/l), fludrocortisone suppression test useful: 3 mg/m^2 b.d. for 2 days prior to sweat test: normalizes in non-CF, no effect in CF.

Possible causes of false-positive sweat test

- Technique (evaporation leads to increased concentration and decreased volume)
- Eczema/dermatitis/ectodermal dysplasia
- Malnutrition
- Flucloxacillin therapy
- Untreated hypothyroidism/panhypopituitarism
- Adrenal insufficiency
- Glycogen storage disease/mucopolysaccharidosis
- Glucose 6-phosphate dehydrogenase deficiency
- Fucosidosis
- Nephrogenic diabetes insipidus

Genetic testing (see below)

Immunoreactive trypsin (IRT)
Useful in first 6 weeks of life. Raised in CF. Often used as first test in areas with newborn screening.

Nasal potential difference (PD)
Mostly used for research purposes, but useful in grey cases. Technically challenging in children.

4.2 Genetics

Over 1,000 mutations in CFTR identified to date. Fall into five classes. Commonest is $\Delta F508$, a class II mutation which leads to defective protein folding, and thus failure to reach the apical membrane. Some relationship between pancreatic status and genotype, but poor correlations to date for lung disease. Should not be used to provide prognosis.

Most clinical laboratories test for 5–12 of commonest mutations (detects >90% of Caucasian cases). Useful for antenatal testing of subsequent pregnancies. Neonatal screening was approved by the government in 2001, although widespread implementation may take several years. It is universal in Australia and New Zealand.

4.3 Presentation and management

Neonatal

Commonest presentation with meconium ileus (MI), bowel obstruction secondary to thick inspissated gut contents. May be antenatal and lead to meconium peritonitis. Often requires surgery, although very mild cases occasionally managed with, e.g., Gastrografin.

Rarer presentations

- Pseudo-Bartter's syndrome (hypochloraemic, hypokalaemic alkalosis)
- Hypoalbuminaemia, oedema, anaemia
- Bleeding from vitamin K deficiency
- Haemolytic anaemia (vitamin E deficiency)

Pulmonary

Lungs thought to be normal at birth. Early symptoms such as cough, frequent chesty episodes and wheeze may be missed. Early infection with narrow range of organisms.

- ### *Staphlylococcus aureus*
Most children on long-term prophylaxis.

- ### *Haemophilus influenzae*

- ### *Pseudomonas aeruginosa*
Up to 80% CF patients are chronically infected by adolescence. Bacteria become mucoid and more difficult to eradicate when chronic. Treat with long-term nebulized antibiotics (colomycin +/– gentamicin or tobramycin). Intermittent courses of i.v. antibiotics (always at least two).

Allergic bronchopulmonary aspergillosis (ABPA)
Presents with dry cough, wheeze, variable infiltrates on CXR. Diagnosed with high IgE, raised RAST and precipitins. Treated with steroids +/– itraconazole.

- ### *Burkholderia cepacia*
Gram-negative, often highly resistant. Meropenem may be useful. Associated in approximately 20% with life-threatening septicaemia ('cepacia syndrome') patient-to-patient spread well-documented (segregation vital).

- ### *Stenotrophomonas maltophilia*
Emerging pathogen. Accumulating evidence that it does not lead to significant deterioration.

Atypical mycobacteria

Quite common. May be incidental finding. Treat if associated with symptomatic, persistent, or immune-suppressed, e.g. on steroids.

Airway inflammatory response excessive. May present with asthma-like symptoms (consider CF in cases of difficult/atypical asthma). End-result of infection/inflammation is (upper lobes common), chronic sputum production, clubbing (asthma DOES NOT cause clubbing), hypoxia. May have haemoptysis (high bronchial arterial flow. If severe: embolization). 90% patients die of respiratory failure.

Other treatments for lung disease

Mainstay of treatment is physiotherapy (regular even when well!). Consider bronchodilators if responsive. Many on inhaled steroids (evidence lacking).

Recombinant human DNAase (rhDNAase)

- Degrades viscous neutrophil-derived DNA
- Thins sputum
- Nebulized once daily
- Useful in approx. 30% patients with abnormal pulmonary function tests (PFTs)
- Very expensive (£7,500/patient per year)

Extrapulmonary involvement

Exocrine insufficiency

- Presents with steatorrhoea and failure to thrive
- Low stool elastase, high 3-day faecal fat
- Treat with pancreatic enzyme supplements (e.g. Creon)
- Fat-soluble vitamin supplementation
- Nutritional supplements if required
- Gastrostomy and supplemental nutrition if severe weight problems

Endocrine

- Diabetes commoner in older children (8–15%)
- Insidious, non-specific onset
- Ketoacidosis extremely rare (residual pancreatic function)
- Usually require insulin

Gastrointestinal tract (GIT)

- Distal intestinal obstruction syndrome (DIOS, previously called meconium ileus equivalent) rehydrate and Gastrografin, Golitely, etc.
- Attention to dietary fibre and enzymes
- Hepatic cirrhosis
- Ursodeoxycholic acid may be useful

Nose

- Polyps (up to 30%): topical steroid or surgery — often recur

Sinusitis

- Common
- Same organisms as lungs

Infertility

- 99% males (obstruction and abnormal development of vas deferens)
- Females subfertile, but many successful pregnancies

Arthritis

- Probably immune-complex-mediated
- Correlates with PFTs

Vasculitis

- More common in older patients

4.4 New/emerging therapies

- Ibuprofen
  - Slows reduction in lung function, but side-effects
  - Not yet in widespread use in UK
- TOBI: **tob**ramycin for **i**nhalation
  - Heavy marketing in USA where colomycin not used
  - Very expensive, not widely used in UK
- Gene therapy
  - Still at research stage
  - Liposomes or recombinant viral vectors
  - Problems with efficiency and inflammatory response
- Many others not yet in clinical arena

4.5 Transplantation

Heart–lung or bilateral lung performed. More recently living-related donors. Currently no advantage, but will possibly improve with further experience.

Psychological issues of major importance.

Possible contraindications (vary slightly with different centres)

- Long-term, high-dose steroids
- Multiresistant organisms

- Previous thoracic surgery
- Lack of family support or psychological issues

Post-transplant problems:

- Prolonged immunosuppression and infection
- Obliterative bronchiolitis common

5. OTHER CAUSES OF BRONCHIECTASIS

Symptoms/signs as for CF depending on severity. May be visible on CXR but CT more sensitive. Bronchography no longer used.

Primary ciliary dyskinesia

Previously called 'immotile cilia syndrome.'

Autosomal recessive (gene not yet identified). Rare, 1:15,000 births.

Presentation:	Neonatal respiratory distress, rhinorrhoea
	Recurrent LRTIs. May lead to bronchiectasis.
	Sinus disease. Glue ear: often does not respond well to grommets.
	50% have dextrocardia +/– abdominal situs inversus (Kartagener's)
	Male infertility (female subfertility)
Diagnosis:	Nasal brushing for ciliary beat frequency (normal >10 Hz)
	and structure (electron microscopy)
	Low exhaled/nasal nitric oxide (NO)
	Prolonged saccharin clearance time
Treatment:	Physiotherapy
	Antibiotics
	ENT and hearing assessment
	Genetic counselling

Post-infection
Classically pertussis, although may also follow measles. May occur after severe infection with any organism.

Post-airway obstruction
Highlights importance of early detection and removal of foreign bodies (see section 8)
TB — obstructive lymphadenopathy.

Recurrent infection
For example, immune-deficiency (see section 7.9).

Recurrent aspiration

Idiopathic: up to 60%. Other causes must be excluded.

Congenital: Rare.

6. BRONCHOPULMONARY DYSPLASIA (BPD)

Chronic lung disease resulting from premature delivery, surfactant deficiency and neonatal artificial ventilation.

Variable definitions all including requirement for O_2 at 28 days.

Other aetiological factors include:

- Birth asphyxia
- High-concentration O_2 administration
- Fluid overload
- Infection
- Vitamin A deficiency — antioxidant effects

Of these, barotrauma from ventilation and oxygen toxicity most important. Centres using non-invasive ventilation as first-line (e.g. nasal continuous positive-airways pressure (CPAP)), have lower incidence of BPD.

Incidence reduced greatly by both antenatal steroids (increases lung maturation and surfactant production) and exogenous surfactant. (For further details see Chapter 13, *Neonatology*.)

Treatment

- Long-term O_2
- Corticosteroids
- Diuretics and fluid restriction may be useful
- Immunization including 'flu and Pneumovax
- Consider use of palivizumab (see section 7.7)
- Aggressive treatment of infections
- Bronchodilators may be useful in wheezy cases
- Consider and treat coexisting gastro-oesophageal reflux (immature swallow, reduced muscle tone, prolonged intubation all increase risk)

Longer-term complications

- Reactive airways disease (e.g. risk of severe disease with RSV)
- Complications of intubation (e.g. subglottic stenosis, granulation tissue, tracheomalacia)
- Gastro-oesophageal reflux
- Pulmonary hypertension and cor pulmonale
- Growth and nutritional delay (neurodevelopmental disability)

7. INFECTIONS

7.1 Epiglottitis

Usually caused by *H. influenzae* type b. Rare since introduction of Hib vaccine. Presents with acute-onset stridor, fever, anxious child.

> Do not examine throat (may precipitate fatal airway obstruction)
>
> Do not X-ray (although appearances may be diagnostic, wastes time and is dangerous)
>
> Do not upset child, e.g. taking blood, lying flat

If suspected: urgent general anaesthesia (GA), visualization of upper airway and intubation. Rarely need tracheotomy. Bacterial swabs at intubation. Treat with i.v. 3rd generation cephalosporin.

7.2 Tonsillitis

Acute tonsillitis common and self-limiting in childhood. Presentation may be non-specific in small child, e.g. irritability, refusal of feeds, fever, febrile convulsion. Older child usually complains of sore throat. Bacterial and viral causes (commonly adenovirus, rhinovirus, β-haemolytic Streptococcus); exudate does not imply bacterial cause.

Indications for tonsillectomy

- Recurrent severe attacks of tonsillitis
- Tonsillar hypertrophy leading to airway obstruction/sleep disordered breathing
- Associated Eustachian tube obstruction with hearing impairment
- Recurrent OM associated with adenotonsillar infection

7.3 Croup

- Viral laryngotracheobronchitis: parainfuenza, influenza, RSV, rhinoviruses
- Common 6 months to 5 years of age
- Barking cough and stridor
- Child not usually toxic, may have low-grade fever
- Nebulized adrenaline may help **but** watch for rebound obstruction!
- Good evidence for role for steroids
  - Oral single dose seems to be as good as i.m. (dexamethasone in most studies)
  - Some evidence for high-dose nebulized steroids, e.g. budesonide
- Severe cases may require intubation and ventilation
- May be recurrent

7.4 Tracheitis

- Presentation as for croup
- Viral (same as croup) and bacterial (*S. aureus and H. influenzae*) aetiologies
- Bacterial cases often more toxic
- Severe cases may require intubation

7.5 Bacterial pneumonias

Presentation

Variable depending on severity

- Cough
- Tachypnoea +/– other signs of respiratory distress (nasal flaring, grunting, use of accessory muscles)
- Fever
- Non-specific irritability in younger infant
- Hypoxia
- CXR often patchy shadowing in infant and more commonly lobar consolidation in older child

Aetiology

- Pneumococcus commonest organism
- With increasing age, Mycoplasma more prevalent
- *S. aureus* associated with lung abscess (both Staph and Strep may follow varicella infection)
- Rarely *H. influenzae*, streptococci, Klebsiella (remember most pneumonias viral in younger child)

Management

- Mild cases can be diagnosed clinically and treated with oral antibiotics out of hospital
- More severe cases — cultures (sputum if available, upper airway secretions, blood)
  - WBC and differential and CRP useful for monitoring response to treatment (Do not differentiate well between bacterial and viral infections, i.v. antibiotics)
  - Hydration (see below)
  - O_2 therapy if required
  - Rarely, severe cases will require respiratory support

Complications

Syndrome of inappropriate secretion of antidiuretic hormone (SIADH) is common. Leads to fluid retention and thus hyponatraemia, which if severe can lead to cerebral oedema and convulsions. Monitor electrolytes and osmolality (serum and urine). Management is by fluid restriction and NOT administration of sodium. Empyema — see section 7.6.

7.6 Empyema

Collection of pus in pleural space resulting from spread of infection from lung tissue. Presents with signs of pneumonia plus decreased unilateral air entry, dull percussion note. Patient often has scoliosis toward affected side +/– mediastinal shift. Fluid demonstrated on CXR. US may confirm presence of loculation or fibrin strands.

Management

- Requires drainage (not just aspiration)
- Some recent evidence that urokinase may assist recovery by breaking down fibrinous material
- Intravenous antibiotics
- A minority may need surgery — decortication
- VATS (video-assisted thoracic surgery) gaining in popularity

Complications

- Bronchopleural fistula
- Lung abscess
- SIADH

Other causes of pleural effusion include:

- TB
- Chylothorax (especially post-surgery from thoracic duct ligation)
- Congestive heart failure
- Hypoalbuminaemia (with peripheral oedema, e.g. nephrotic syndrome)
- Malignancies (rare)
- Blood in pleural space will have similar CXR appearance, e.g. post-trauma

7.7 Bronchiolitis

Classically caused by RSV, common in autumn and winter (similar picture can be caused by 'flu, paraflu and adenovirus infections). Very common. >80% children under 4 years possess neutralizing antibodies (although not very effective, hence repeated infections). Causes a range of symptoms from URTI in older children and adults to bronchiolitis in the first 2 years of life. Commonest cause of pneumonia in the first year.

Presentation

- Respiratory distress and coryza
- Fever
- Hyperinflation
- Apnoea in very young infants
- Crackles widespread throughout lung fields +/– wheeze

Diagnosis

- Immunofluorescence on nasopharyngeal aspirate

Management

- Largely supportive
- Adequate hydration
- Humidified O_2 as required
- Evidence for use of bronchodilators (e.g. ipratropium bromide or salbutamol) not strong, but used frequently, often with apparent success

Groups at risk of severe disease

- BPD or other chronic lung disease, e.g. CF
- Congenital heart disease (especially cyanotic or associated with pulmonary congestion/hypertension)
- Immunocompromised children
- Disease in these children may lead to respiratory failure and requirement for ventilation

(Same groups of children at high risk for severe illness from influenza virus. Neuraminidase inhibitors have recently been licensed for nasal administration in high-risk patients.)

Specific treatments

Ribavirin

No longer being used to any great extent due to poor efficacy, difficulties with administration (clogs up ventilator circuits) and potential teratogenicity. Used mainly in severe immunocompromise (e.g. bone marrow recipients) sometimes in conjunction with an i.v. preparation.

Vaccination

No vaccine currently available, and early studies with attenuated virus led to increased severity in subsequent infective episode. Anti-RSV immunoglobulin useful in early studies in high-risk cases, but problems obtaining sufficient quantity and usual concerns re blood products.

Humanized monoclonal anti-RSV antibody (palivizumab, Synagis) available in Europe since 1999 (1 year earlier in USA).

- Given as monthly i.m. injections during the RSV season
- Shown in trials of BPD babies to reduce admissions, but no effect on the severe end of the disease (PICU, mortality)
- Recommendations for use vary (commonly chronically O_2-dependent in first 2 years of life)

7.8 Tuberculosis and atypical mycobacterial infection

After a fall in incidence in TB worldwide over the last two to three decades following the development of successful anti-TB chemotherapy, there is now an increase in the number of cases, both in adults and children. Largely reflects the rapid increase in numbers infected with HIV, but is also being observed in areas of extreme poverty and overcrowding in countries like the USA. Rise in cases of multi-drug resistant infection, often resulting from poor adherence to treatment in index cases.

NB. TB is a notifiable disease.

Prime example of the ability of micro-organisms either to exist within a host without causing adverse effects (TB infection) or to multiply, with or without tissue invasion and spread, and cause TB disease. Which one of these two situations evolves depends both on host (age, immune status, nutrition) and bacterial factors (numbers and virulence factors).

Pulmonary TB

The major route of infection is via the respiratory tract (more rarely via the oral route leading to gut TB — must rule out immunodeficiency).

Once organisms have been inhaled they establish themselves in the periphery of the lungs, and elicit a host inflammatory response (largely via macrophages).

Spread to regional lymph nodes may also cause hilar adenopathy.

If inflammatory response is sufficient to keep the infection in check, the lesion may calcify and form a Ghon focus, which may be identified later on CXR, and may be the only evidence of previous TB in an otherwise well subject. This is much rarer in children than in adults, and the majority of TB presenting in children results from the primary infection, resulting in the period from infection to disease often being as short as weeks.

Symptoms
Vary and may be non-specific.

- Fever
- Irritability
- Weight loss and lethargy
- Cough
- Airway obstruction from lymphadenopathy; may lead to lobar collapse or less frequently to air trapping
- Dyspnoea and respiratory distress in severe cases especially if miliary
- Erythema nodosum

Radiology

- Can vary greatly from isolated focus to hilar lymphadenopathy, lobar collapse/ consolidation to miliary (seed-like) shadowing throughout lung fields
- Large caseating lesions not common in children

Extrapulmonary

TB can infect most organs in particular the brain, kidneys, gut and bone. Children are more prone than adults to extrapulmonary infection, the details of which will not be discussed further here.

Diagnosis of TB

High index of suspicion important.

Tuberculin testing

Intradermal administration of purified tuberculin protein will lead to a T-cell-mediated reaction in sensitized individuals. Depending on the clinical situation, and whether BCG has been administered, the size of reaction considered significant may differ.

Size of reaction	Significant in:
>15 mm	Any child
10–15 mm	High risk: birth or arrival from high-risk country
	Contact with adults in high-risk group
	Young age
>5 mm	Contact with an open known case (if no BCG)
	Clinical or radiographic evidence
	HIV infection

Microbiology

- Sputum (rare in children)
- Gastric aspirates (morning)
- Bronchoalveolar lavage fluid
- Acid-fast bacilli may be visible on staining, otherwise culture requires up to 6–8 weeks

Some laboratories will test with PCR, although as very sensitive, false-positives can arise.

Treatment

Current guidelines state that all cases should receive at least three drugs. Quadruple therapy should be initiated where there is a risk of multiresistant TB, e.g. case or contact from developing country.

Drug treatment is given in an initial phase of three or four drugs, followed by a maintenance phase of two drugs.

Usual first-line treatment	Potential side-effects
Isoniazid (6 months)	Peripheral neuropathy Abnormal LFTs
Rifampicin (6 months)	Orange urine/tears Hepatic enzyme induction (drug interactions) Abnormal LFTs
Pyrazinamide (2 months)	Liver toxicity (only active against intracellular, actively dividing forms of the bacteria. Works best early in the treatment course. Good meningeal penetration if CNS disease)

Additional therapeutic agents for high-risk/drug-resistant disease

Ethambutol	Visual disturbance Perform ophthalmic examination Avoid in very young children
Streptomycin (i.m. — used rarely) Ciprofloxacin Clofazimine Kanamycin Clarithromycin	

Children are rarely open cases (i.e. smear-positive) and it is therefore unusual that they would be capable of transmitting the infection. After the first 2 weeks of treatment the child should be allowed to re-commence normal activities.

Neonatal contact

A neonate born to a mother with active TB is at serious risk of acquiring the disease. If at the time the maternal diagnosis is realized (and treatment commenced) the infant has no signs of TB, the child should receive isoniazid prophylaxis, be closely followed up, and receive a tuberculin test at approximately 3–4 months. Thereafter, the guidelines for older children should be followed.

Contact tracing is a major public health issue. Cases of paediatric TB still arise in families where a parent is known to be infected but children are not screened.

Pulmonary infection with atypical mycobacteria

Examples include *Mycobacterium avium*, *M. intracellulare*, *M. kansasii* and *M. malmoense*. Unusual except in the immunocompromised or in children with CF. Symptoms range from those seen with TB infection to much milder with fever or lethargy. In some cases, diagnosis may only be suspected after new changes are seen on CXR, or for example in CF when the organisms are identified in the sputum. In CF, difficulties may arise in determining whether such organisms are pathogens. Treatment of a CF child recommended if child unwell, or sputum persistently positive.

Treatment
Longer than for *M. tuberculosis* (up to 2 years). Choice of agents depends on organism and sensitivities. Usually a combination of:

- Rifampicin
- Clarithromycin/azithromycin
- Amikacin
- Ciprofloxacin
- Clofazimine
- Ethambutol

Notification and contact tracing are not required.

7.9 Infections in the immunocompromised host

Pneumocystis carinii pneumonia (PCP)

Presentation: Onset may be acute or insidious (especially older child)
tachypnoea, respiratory distress, fever, +/– cough
bilateral crackles, hypoxia, often normocapnic in early stages

CXR: Classically bilateral interstitial and alveolar shadowing
may be normal, unilateral, focal

Diagnosis: Occasionally found on nasopharyngeal aspirate (NPA)
Usually requires bronchoalveolar lavage (BAL)
In rare cases, lung biopsy required

Think: Severe combined immune deficiency states
HIV (common in 1st year of life)
di George syndrome
(CD40 ligand deficiency; previously called hyper-IgM syndrome)

Treatment: High-dose trimethoprim/sulfamethoxazole (pancytopenia, rash, fever)
Pentamidine or dapsone used less frequently
Steroids — role established in HIV — less certain otherwise
If ventilated, consider surfactant
Prophylaxis required after treatment

Other: Anti-PC antibodies common in healthy children

Cytomegalovirus (CMV)

Presentation: (usually insidious) radiology and likely immunodeficiencies similar to PCP
May be congenital or acquired
May coexist with extrapulmonary infection — ophthalmic examination required

Diagnosis: Antigen (DEAFF, detection of early-antigen fluorescent foci) or PCR on NPA, BAL
Detection in other body fluids, e.g. urine do not confirm CMV as cause of pneumonitis

Other: Dual infection with PCP not uncommon

Other infections

Organisms causing similar interstitial picture in immunocompromised patients:

- Measles
- Varicella
- Herpes simplex
- Adenovirus
- Fungi
- Mycobacteria

Lymphocytic interstitial pneumonitis (LIP)

Although not related to any particular pathogen, this disorder is often confused with the opportunistic infections above, and thus is included here. Seen in children with HIV or occasionally other immunodeficiency states. Less common in adults.

Tends to coexist with marked lymphadenopathy – parotid hyperplasia, and to decrease with falling CD4 count.

Presents either as chronic cough – hypoxia and clubbing if severe.
May be asymptomatic and detected radiologically only.

Treatment: Nil if well, usually responds to steroids

When to suspect immune-deficiency

Normal children may have up to 10 URTIs per year. Suspect abnormal immune function if respiratory tract infections:

- Unusually severe or prolonged
- Recurrent (although if same site suspect anatomical abnormality or foreign body)
- Any case of pneumonitis/unexplained interstitial disease
- Associated with:
  - Infections in other sites, e.g. skin, liver, gastrointestinal, bone
  - Failure to thrive
  - Persistent or generalized lymphadenopathy

693

8. INHALED FOREIGN BODY

Will not be diagnosed unless thought about. Major long-term implications if not removed: lobar collapse, bronchiectasis.

Suspect:	Sudden-onset cough/wheeze/breathlessness
	May or may not give history of aspiration
	Ask about presence of older siblings in case of infant
	Unilateral signs: wheeze, absent or diminished air entry, tracheal/mediastinal deviation if severe
CXR:	Either volume loss or hyperexpansion from air trapping on affected side
	Hyperexpansion best visualized on expiratory film
Management:	Removal under rigid bronchoscopy (flexible bronchoscopy not recommended, as removal more difficult)
	Follow-up ventilation scan should be considered, especially in cases of non-inert foreign body, e.g. food. Peanuts particular problem as nut oil very irritant and proinflammatory. If removal delayed, anti-inflammatory agents, e.g. steroids, may be useful to reduce airway narrowing
	Consider post-op antibiotics, depending on findings
	Education important, particularly avoidance of peanuts in young children

9. PNEUMOTHORAX

In children, usually associated with underlying disease.

- Gas trapping (e.g. severe asthma, CF)
- Bullae (e.g. Marfan's)
- Other: Langerhans cell histiocytosis (in association with fibrotic, honeycomb CXR changes)
- Iatrogenic (high-pressure ventilation), traumatic and post-operative

Symptoms and signs:	Dyspnoea, cough, chest pain
	Tracheal deviation, asymmetrical chest expansion and breath sounds
	Hyper-resonance
	+/– Subcutaneous emphysema
Management:	Depends on size on CXR (all patients should have one)
	If small with minimal symptoms, can be managed conservatively and observed
	If larger/significant symptoms give O_2 (aids air absorption from pleural space) and insert chest drain
Recurrent:	Consider pleurodesis
	Visceral pleura adheres to chest wall with either talc or bleomycin
	Painful. May exclude possibility of future transplantation, e.g. in CF. Consider with care
Confused with:	Neonatal cysts, diaphragmatic hernia, severe hyperinflation, e.g. inhaled foreign body

10. NEUROMUSCULAR DISORDERS

Can impair respiratory function at any of following sites: spinal cord, peripheral nerve, neuromuscular junction and muscle.

10.1 Spinal cord

Spinal muscular atrophy (SMA)

Disorder at levels of the anterior horn cells (atrophy). Autosomal recessive inheritance.

Presents as floppy infant (Werdnig–Hoffman disease; with tongue fasciculation, preservation of eye muscles giving alert facial expression) or in less severe forms, as hypotonia and delayed motor milestones.

Respiratory involvement always seen in types I and II (diaphragm spared), common in type III. Chest may be bell-shaped. Lungs small.

Previously, severe forms would have been given a grave prognosis once diagnosed and allowed to die. More and more common, particularly in the USA, parents are demanding long-term ventilation. Obvious ethical issues regarding this as currently no realistic chance of improvement or cure.

Myelomeningocele

Rarely affects respiration unless very high.

Cervical cord injury

Respiratory involvement depends on level.

10.2 Peripheral nerve

Guillain-Barré syndrome

- Post-viral inflammatory ascending polyneuropathy
- Respiratory involvement common and most serious manifestation (intercostals and diaphragm)
  - This will be underestimated, unless specifically monitored
  - Do not assess with peak flow (may be normal despite respiratory muscle compromise) — use vital capacity
- Bulbar involvement may lead to aspiration. Protective intubation may be required.
- Good prognosis, even in severe cases requiring mechanical ventilatory support. Usual course:
  - Evolution 2–4 weeks
  - Plateau variable
  - Resolution 2–4 weeks later

- Specific treatments:
  - Intravenous immunoglobulin
  - Plasmapheresis in some cases

10.3 Neuromuscular junction

Myasthenia gravis (MG)

- Autoimmune disease with antibodies directed against the acetylcholine (ACh) receptor
- Episodic muscle weakness, often mild, e.g. ptosis
- Weakness increases with exertion
- Management strategies include a trial of anticholinesterase drugs such as pyridostigmine, thymectomy or immunosuppressive treatments

Congenital MG is an autosomal recessive, non-autoimmune disease in which ACh synthesis or mobilization is defective. May respond to anticholinesterase drugs, but if not, severe cases require long-term ventilatory support (see below) and assistance with feeding.

Neonatal MG is seen in up to 15% of babies born to affected mothers and results from transplacental passage of autoantibodies.

Is transient, but affected infants may have feeding difficulties or require respiratory support. Treated with anticholinesterase drugs/exchange transfusion or plasmapheresis occasionally required.

Botulism

- Rare
- Toxins produced by *Clostridium botulinum* (usually food-borne) lead to impaired release of ACh at neuromuscular junction. Bulbar muscles involved early, with respiratory failure in most cases. Good prognosis with adequate support. (Currently being used as treatment for certain diseases with muscular spasm as major component.)

Tick paralysis

- Very rare

10.4 Muscle

Myotonic dystrophy

- Floppy infant in severe form
- Diaphragm involvement (eventration)
- Feeding problems +/– aspiration
- Maternal (when congenital) myotonia
- Later problems: learning difficulties, cardiac conduction defects, baldness
- Triplet-repeat disease (others Huntington's, Fragile X, Friedreich's ataxia) with increasing severity in subsequent generations (genetic anticipation)

Duchenne muscular dystrophy (DMD)

- X-linked
- Weakness usually noted towards end of first decade
- Death usually from respiratory failure
- Preceded by recurrent lower respiratory tract infections +/– aspiration from swallowing incoordination

Myopathies

- Respiratory involvement variable depending on type

Symptoms:	Respiratory infections
	Morning headaches (CO_2 retention)
	Daytime drowsiness
Management:	Always consider possibility of respiratory involvement
	Lung function testing
	Polysomnography (overnight O_2, CO_2, nasal airflow, chest wall movement, heart rate, resp rate +/– EEG, pH probe)
	Non-invasive ventilation increasingly used (see below). Use once evidence of respiratory failure. Some evidence against prophylactic use in DMD.

10.5 Non-invasive ventilatory support

Acute respiratory failure requiring invasive ventilation in the ITU setting will not be dealt with in this chapter, although the systems below can also be administered long-term with the aid of a tracheostomy tube in cases where this is necessary.

Children with the neuromuscular disorders above (plus those with malacic airways and very occasionally chronic lung disease) may have chronic respiratory compromise and benefit from long-term ventilatory support.

This can be administered as either positive or negative pressure:

Positive pressure
Both continuous (CPAP) or bi-level (Bi-PAP) positive airway pressure can be administered through either a nose or face mask.

Both systems can be used at home with or without oxygen depending on the pathology. The devices are in general well-tolerated, the only major problem being one of pressure sores resulting from the tight-fitting mask.

Negative pressure
Devices, including the cuirass jacket, have also been used in these settings.

The jacket is worn around the chest, with closely fitted seals at either end.

Negative pressure applied to the jacket causes inspiration.

Expiration can be passive or assisted.

The benefits of this approach include a more physiological respiratory cycle. Movement of the child is limited by the devices, which can also be very noisy.

In the UK, negative pressure is used much less frequently than positive. It is important to remember that significant weakness of the bulbar muscles, especially with any airway malacia, can lead to airway collapse and obstruction during applied negative pressure, which can lead to failure of the device.

11. RARE DISORDERS

11.1 Congenital disorders

Cystic adenomatoid malformation

Type 1: single or multiple large cysts (despite shift effects, usually good post-operative prognosis)
Type 2: multiple small cysts
Type 3: solid mass (poor prognosis)

In most cases the affected lobe needs to be removed because of infection (and possible malignant transformation) risks. May be diagnosed antenatally. Cases are reported where antenatal findings appear to have been resolved by time of birth — speculations about prognosis are therefore difficult. May be confused radiologically with congenital diaphragmatic hernia, pneumatocoeles.

Congenital lobar emphysema

Over-inflation of lobe due to intrinsic deficiency of bronchial cartilage +/– elastic tissue.

Commonest sites: LUL, RML, RUL. Rare in lower lobes.
Presentation: May be asymptomatic, detected on CXR.
Neonatal respiratory distress.
Chest asymmetry. Hyper-resonance.
CXR: Hyperlucent region. May be associated compression of other lobes.
VQ scan may show absence of ventilation/perfusion in more severe cases.
Management: In mildest cases, manage conservatively.
Most cases presenting in infancy are more severe and require surgical removal because of risks of infection and collapse of other areas.
Cardiac work-up. 1:6 have associated cardiac abnormality.

Bronchogenic cyst

- Remnant of primitive foregut derived from abnormal tracheobronchial budding
- Up to 10% of mediastinal masses in children
- Contain normal tracheal tissue, filled with clear fluid
- May exist in various sites including paraoesophageal, with symptoms varying accordingly
- Asymptomatic
- Airway compression
- Stridor
- Lobar collapse
- Obstructive emphysema
- Infection
- Haemorrhage

Barium swallow may detect filling defect. Surgical removal recommended to prevent infection, airway obstruction, malignant transformation. Pre-operatively avoid high-pressure ventilation and air travel — cysts may expand and rupture.

Lobar sequestration

Mass of non-functional lung; abnormal communication with airway and usually supplied by systemic circulation.

Intra- or extralobar (often associated with other congenital abnormalities and polyhydramnios). May have derived from accessory lung bud, although exact aetiology uncertain. Lower lobes commonest, more often left. Many asymptomatic. Present most commonly with recurrent pneumonia in same site.

CXR: Solid or cystic (if intralobar +/– air-fluid level) mass
Angiography required to demonstrate and delineate systemic blood supply

Surgical removal required even in asymptomatic cases, as infection will ensue if untreated.

Scimitar syndrome

- Hypoplastic right lung with anomalous venous drainage (usually to IVC or R atrium) +/– systemic collateral arterial supply. 'Scimitar' sign is the vertical line caused by the RUL pulmonary vein running into the RA.
- May be asymptomatic or lead to recurrent infection
- Right lung usually functions well and surgical correction of the vascular abnormalities is usually recommended

Diaphragmatic hernia

Incidence estimated at around 1:2,500–3,500 births. More common on the left. Main problems arise from the associated pulmonary hypoplasia, both on the affected side and the contralateral side when there is significant mediastinal shift. Diagnosis may be made antenatally on ultrasound.

Postnatal presentation includes respiratory distress, scaphoid abdomen and vomiting. CXR shows bowel loops inside thorax which may be confused with either cystic malformation or pneumothorax (use nasogastric tube both to confirm the diagnosis and to deflate the stomach reducing the chance of rupture).

Often associated with other malformations, in which case prognosis is worse.

Treatment: Surgery required
No clear evidence, but some suggestion that high-frequency oscillatory ventilation may help
Pulmonary hypertension quite common. May respond to NO or vasodilators

Prognosis: Even with optimal management, mortality about 50–60%
Survivors may have problems associated with underlying pulmonary hypoplasia

Alpha-1 antitrypsin deficiency

- Recessively inherited disorder
- Absence of liver-derived antiprotease leads to proteolytic destruction of pulmonary tissue and emphysema on exposure to oxidants, e.g. cigarette smoke and pollutants
- Rare for pulmonary problems to arise in children who are more likely to have the associated liver disease (eventual cirrhosis)
- PiMM refers to the homozygous normal state, PiZZ is homozygous deficient, PiSZ also causing disease

Alveolar proteinosis

Aetiology uncertain, although some cases presenting as neonates are now known to be due to deficiency of surfactant-associated protein B. Lipid-laden type II pneumocytes desquamate into the alveolar spaces leading to increasing hypoxia and respiratory distress.

CXR: Resembles interstitial proteinosis with widespread confluent airspace shadowing

Diagnosis: Made on lung biopsy

Prognosis: Poor

In older child, whole lung lavages may help, but in infants, the disease is almost universally fatal. Genetic counselling required.

Congenital pulmonary lymphangiectasia

- Rare dilatation of pulmonary lymphatics leading to severe neonatal respiratory distress and often pleural effusions
- Associated with congenital cardiac disorders such as obstructed venous drainage
- Prognosis very poor
- No specific treatment

11.2 Acquired disorders

Obliterative bronchiolitis

- Results from viral infection (usually adeno, but occasionally measles or RSV) or post lung or bone marrow transplant
- Severe, widespread small-airways obstruction
- Dyspnoea, wheeze and hypoxia with eventual pulmonary hypertension

CXR: hyperinflated lungs with patchy pruning of vascular markings
CT: patchy areas of air trapping (honeycomb) and poor perfusion

In early stages may have some response to bronchodilators or steroids, but often no treatment successful. If unilateral, may go on to Swyer-James (also called Macleod's) syndrome of unilateral hyperlucent lung with diminished vascularity.

Haemosiderosis

- Repeated episodes of pulmonary haemorrhage lead to accumulation of haemosiderin at the alveolar level
- Haemorrhage may be symptomatic with haemoptysis, or unrecognized, presenting with anaemia
- Aetiology uncertain, although a subgroup of cases are associated with cows' milk protein allergy and positive antibodies. These respond to dietary manipulation.
- Another subgroup have Goodpasture's syndrome (positive antiglomerular basement membrane antibodies)
- Similar clinical picture may occur with mitral stenosis or connective tissue diseases

Symptoms: Usually episodic
Fever, dyspnoea, wheeze +/– haemoptysis
CXR: May be normal
More commonly patchy shadowing
Diagnosis: Haemosiderin-laden macrophages in BAL
Management: Difficult
Acute: Treat hypoxia, anaemia
Longer term: Steroids
Hydroxychloroquine
Alternative immunosuppressive drugs

Sarcoid

- Extremely rare in childhood
- Multisystem granulomatous disease, may be confused with TB and chronic granulomatous disease

Symptoms: Dry cough, dyspnoea
Clinical examination often unremarkable in early stages (may lead to clubbing later)
CXR: Hilar lymphadenopathy
Patchy lung infiltrates
May be associated with extrapulmonary disease (skin, eye, kidney, gut)
Diagnosis: Usually made on biopsy (Kveim test no longer performed)
Treatment: May be self-limiting
Steroids +/– hydroxychloroquine if treatment required

Interstitial lung diseases of childhood

Group of conditions not well defined in terms of aetiology which lead to inflammation and fibrosis at the alveolar level, sometimes also termed 'cryptogenic fibrosing alveolitis' (CFA). Gradual onset dry cough, dyspnoea, hypoxia, clubbing. Widespread crackles throughout both lung fields.

CXR/CT: Ground-glass appearance
Differential diagnosis includes pneumonitis from opportunistic pathogens, e.g. PCP, extrinsic allergic alveolitis. Definitive diagnosis will require an, open lung biopsy. Histological findings vary from inflammation (more likely to respond to steroids) through to severe fibrosis (steroids less likely to succeed; antifibrotics, e.g. hydroxychloroquine may be used).
Prognosis: Highly variable ranging from subacute respiratory failure to a plateau phase with intermittent symptoms, or even recovery in some patients.

Pulmonary hypertension (PH)

Increased pulmonary pressure may be primary (rare) or more commonly occurs secondary to another disease.

These include:

- Any cause of chronic lung disease, e.g. BPD, CF. Chronic hypoxia leads to pulmonary vasoconstriction and arterial wall changes
- High pulmonary arterial flow from left to right shunt, e.g. large VSD
- Obstructed pulmonary venous drainage or left heart failure (rare in childhood)

Primary PH presents with hypoxia, dyspnoea and if severe, right heart failure. May present in the neonatal period as persistent fetal circulation (see section 1.3).

May respond to pulmonary vasodilators:

- High O$_2$
- Prostacyclin
- Nifedipine
- Nitric oxide
- Viagra

Prognosis usually poor unless transplantation an option.

12. FURTHER READING

Cystic fibrosis: Davis PB, (editor), Lung Biology in Health and Disease Series. Dekker, 1993.

Kendig's Disorders of the Respiratory Tract in Children: Chernick V and Boat TF, (editors), 6th edition. W B Saunders 1998.

Respiratory Care Anatomy and Physiology: Foundations for Clinical practice: Beachey W Mosby 1998.

Chapter 18

Rheumatology

Nathan Hasson

CONTENTS

Rheumatology

1. JUVENILE IDIOPATHIC ARTHRITIS (JIA)

This is the new classification for autoimmune arthritis in childhood and replaces 'juvenile chronic/rheumatoid arthritis'.

Definition: A chronic arthritis that persists for a minimum of 6 consecutive weeks in one or more joints, commencing before the age of 16 years and after active exclusion of other causes.

Epidemiology: 1:1,000 children under 16 years of age

Classification
- By mode of onset during the first 6 months
- 8 groups:
  - Systemic onset
  - Polyarticular rheumatoid factor-negative (RF–)
  - Polyarticular rheumatoid factor-positive (RF+)
  - Oligoarticular — persistent
  - Oligoarticular — extended
  - Enthesitis-related arthritis (enthesis = point of bony insertion of tendon)
  - Psoriatic
  - Unclassified

Systemic disease
- High remittent fever and rash with one or more of the following: hepatomegaly, splenomegaly, generalized lymphadenopathy, serositis (occasionally pericarditis)
- Arthritis may be absent at the onset, but myalgia or arthralgia are usually present

Polyarticular onset
- Five or more joints develop in the onset period, usually somewhat insidiously and symmetrically
- May be further divided by the presence of IgM rheumatoid factor

Oligoarticular onset
- The commonest mode with four or fewer joints involved, particularly knees and ankles
- Three clear subgroups have emerged, notably young children with positive antinuclear antibodies who are at risk from chronic iridocyclitis, older boys (aged 9 upwards) who

707

frequently carry the histocompatible leucocyte antigen (HLA) B27 and develop enthesitis (now classified as enthesitis related arthritis (ERA)), and those that extend past four joints (extended oligoaricular juvenile idiopathic arthritis (EOJIA))
- Others presenting in this way include juvenile psoriatic arthritis, the arthritis of inflammatory bowel disease and Reiter's syndrome, while some are as yet unclassified

1.1 Systemic onset disease

General characteristics

- Usually begins before 5 years of age, but can occur throughout childhood into adult life
- Equal in boys and girls less than 5 years old; female predominance in those over 5 years old

Clinical features

- High once-daily spikes fever for >2 weeks
- Myalgia
- Arthralgia
- Malaise
- Rash — salmon pink or red maculopapular eruption
- Lymphadenopathy — cervical, epitrochlear, axillary and inguinal
- Hepatosplenomegaly
- Serositis — occasionally pericarditis
- Hepatitis
- Progressive anaemia
- Disseminated intravascular coagulation
- Arthritis — knees, wrists and carpi, ankles and tarsi, neck, followed by other joints

Investigations

- Erythrocyte sedimentation rate (ESR) — high
- Haemoglobin — low (normochromic, normocytic)
- White blood cell count — raised (neutrophil leucocytosis)
- Platelets — raised (>400×10^6/l)
- IgM rheumatoid factor — negative
- Antinuclear antibodies (ANA) — negative

Course and prognosis

- Half will have recurrent episodes of systemic disease
- Progressive arthritis occurs in about a third, irrespective of whether there are systemic exacerbations
- The younger the age of onset, the greater the risk of poor growth, both somatic and of joints
- Amyloidosis occurs in some children with persistent disease activity, predominantly among Europeans

Management

- Physiotherapy to maintain joint mobility and muscle function
- Non-steroidal anti-inflammatory drugs (NSAIDs) to control pain, inflammation and fever
- Corticosteroids in severe disease, either as pulsed intravenous, single daily dose or given on alternate days
- Methotrexate especially for arthritis
- Cyclosporin for systemic features
- Etanercept (anti-tumour necrosis factor (TNF) receptor antibody) for disease resistant to other medical management or patients in whom there is significant drug toxicity — very little about long-term toxicity, specialist centres only

1.2 Polyarticular — RF-negative

General characteristics

- Any age, occasionally before the first birthday
- Female predominance

Clinical features

- Polyarthritis can affect any joint; the most commonly affected are the knees, wrists, ankles and proximal and distal interphalangeal joints of the hands; metacarpophalangeal joints are often spared
- Limitation of neck and temporomandibular movement is common
- Flexor tenosynovitis
- Low-grade fever, occasionally
- Mild lymphadenopathy and hepatosplenomegaly, occasionally

Investigations

- ESR — elevated
- Haemoglobin — may be reduced
- White blood count — mild neutrophil leucocytosis
- Platelets — moderate thrombocytosis
- IgM rheumatoid factor — negative
- ANA — occasionally positive

Course and prognosis

- Variable
- May be monocyclic but prolonged over several years with good functional outcome
- Recurrent episodes tend to cause progressive deformities

Management

- Physiotherapy to maintain and improve joint and muscle function
- Splinting to prevent deformity

- NSAIDs to control pain and inflammation
- Methotrexate is very effective and can be used early on to prevent deformity

1.3 Polyarticular — RF-positive

General characteristics

- Over 8 years of age at onset
- Female predominance

Clinical features

- Polyarthritis affecting any joint, but particularly the small joints of the wrists, hands, ankles, and feet; knees and hips often early, with elbows and other joints later
- Rheumatoid nodules on pressure points, particularly elbows. Vasculitis — uncommon and often late, nail-fold lesions, ulceration.

Investigations

- ESR — usually elevated
- Haemoglobin — moderate anaemia
- IgM rheumatoid factor- persistently positive and in high titre
- ANA — may be positive
- HLA DR4 — frequently present
- Radiographically — early erosive changes of affected joints, particularly of hands and feet

Course and prognosis

- Persistent activity with serious joint destruction and poor functional outcome
- Additional long-term hazards include atlantoaxial subluxation, aortic incompetence, and amyloidosis

Management

- Physiotherapy to maintain and improve joint and muscle function
- Splinting to preserve function
- NSAIDs
- Slow-acting drugs early
- Methotrexate
- Surgical intervention, such as replacement arthroplasties, often required later

1.4 Oligoarticular (persistent and extended)

General characteristics

- Under 6 years of age
- Girls more than boys

Clinical features

- Arthritis affecting four or fewer joints: commonly knee, ankle, elbow or a single finger
- Early local growth anomalies
- Risk (1:3) of chronic iridocyclitis in the first 5 years of disease, ANA associated.
- If four or fewer joints after 6 months then **persistent** oligoarticular more than four joints then **extended**

Investigations

- ESR — may be elevated or normal, initially
- Haemoglobin — normal
- While blood count — normal
- Platelets — normal
- IgM rheumatoid factor — negative
- ANA — frequently positive
- HLA A2, DR5 and DR8

Course and prognosis

- Exacerbations and remissions
- Alteration in growth of affected limb
- Long-term prognosis of joints good, except for the 1:5 who develop polyarthritis (five or more joints) over a period of years (**extended**)
- Iridocyclitis is bilateral in two-thirds, the course is independent of the joints — its prognosis depends on early detection and good management

Management

- Physiotherapy to maintain muscle and joint function
- NSAIDs
- Local corticosteroid injection — triamcinolone hexacetonide
- Frequent ophthalmological assessment (3–6-monthly)
- Methotrexate for extended oligoarticular JIA

1.5 Enthesitis related arthritis

General characteristics

- 9 years old and over
- Male predominance

Clinical features

- Peripheral arthritis predominantly affecting the joints of the lower limb
- Enthesopathies — plantar fascia, Achilles tendon, patella tendon
- Acute iritis
- Sacroiliac pain in some   } either of these can be
- Axial disease in some   } the presenting feature

Investigations

- ESR — normal to high
- Full blood count — usually normal
- IgM rheumatoid factor — negative
- HLA B27 — present 90%

Course and prognosis

- Functional outcome good in two-thirds of cases
- Some joint extension may occurs
- Over time a third can develop serious hip problems, cervical and other spinal involvement, impaired temporomandibular function, as well as other features of spondylitis

Management

- Physiotherapy, including hydrotherapy, to maintain mobility: particularly important if spinal involvement occurs
- NSAIDs
- Local corticosteroid injections, hip arthroplasty may be needed in a small proportion
- Sulfasalazine is the disease-modifying drug of choice

1.6 Juvenile psoriatic arthritis

General characteristics

- An arthritis associated, but not necessarily coincident, with a typical psoriatic rash, or arthritis, plus at least three of four minor criteria: dactylitis, nail pitting, psoriatic-like rash or family history of psoriasis
- Female predominance
- Family history of psoriasis (common) or arthritis (but less so)

Clinical features

- Asymmetrical arthritis
- Flexor tenosynovitis
- Occasionally severe destructive disease
- Systemic features rare
- Nail pitting
- Onycholysis
- Psoriasis

Investigations

- ESR — varies with number of joints, may be high
- Haemoglobin — may fall
- White blood count — may increase (neutrophils)
- IgM rheumatoid factor — negative
- ANA — can be positive

Course and prognosis

- Young onset can be associated with iridocyclitis
- Remitting and relapsing course, even into adult life
- Occasionally severely destructive
- Occasionally spondylitis (inflammation of spinal joints) develops

Management

- Physiotherapy
- NSAIDs
- Severe destructive form may require immunosuppressants such as methotrexate

1.7 Unclassified

All those that do not meet criteria for the above.

2. OTHER FORMS OF CHILDHOOD AUTOIMMUNE ARTHRITIS

2.1 Inflammatory bowel disease-related arthritis

General characteristics

- Arthritis associated with either ulcerative colitis or Crohn's disease
- Above 4 years of age
- Male and female equal

Clinical features

- Arthritis usually occurs after the onset of bowel symptoms, but occasionally begins coincident or even precedes
- Arthritis is usually oligoarticular: knees, ankles, wrists and elbows
- Two forms:
  - Benign peripheral arthritis coinciding with active bowel disease
  - In older patients, who belong to the spondylitic group, whose joint activity does not necessarily link with bowel activity

Associated features

- Erythema nodosum
- Pyoderma gangrenosum
- Mucosal ulcers
- Fever
- Weight loss
- Growth retardation
- Acute iritis — in the spondylitic group

Investigations

- Platelets — normal/elevated
- ESR — usually elevated
- Haemoglobin — usually low (normochromic, normocytic)
- White blood count — normal
- IgM rheumatoid factor — negative
- ANA — negative
- HLA B27 present in the spondylitic group

Course and prognosis

- Peripheral arthropathy involves few joints and is episodic and benign
- Prognosis for joint function is excellent
- Prognosis for the spondylitic group is similar to that of ankylosing spondylitis

Management

- Physiotherapy as appropriate
- Treatment of the underlying bowel disorder
- NSAIDs with care, because of gastrointestinal side-effects (ibuprofen may be the drug of choice and use antacids such as ranitidine, newer cyclo-oxygenase (COX)-2 inhibitors)
- Sulfasalazine may be helpful for both subgroups

Causes of erythema nodosum

- Idiopathic
- Streptococcal infection
- Tuberculosis
- Leptospirosis
- Histoplasmosis
- Epstein–Barr virus infection
- Herpes simplex virus
- Yersinia
- Sulphonamides
- Oral contraceptive pill
- SLE
- Crohn's disease
- Ulcerative colitis
- Behçet's syndrome
- Sarcoidosis
- Hodgkin's disease

2.2 Reactive arthritis, including Reiter's syndrome

Acute arthritis occurring after an intercurrent infection, without evidence of the causative organism in the joint. Any age, but particularly teenage males.

Clinical features

- Arthritis ⎫ Typical triad
- Urethritis/balanitis/cystitis ⎬ for Reiter's
- Conjunctivitis ⎭ syndrome
- Mouth ulceration
- Fever
- Rashes, including keratoderma blennorrhagica (macules — pustular on palms, soles, toes, penis)

If only two salient features occur, it is often referred to as 'incomplete Reiter's syndrome'.

Investigations

- ESR — raised
- Haemoglobin — normal
- Mild neutrophil leucocytosis
- IgM rheumatoid factor — negative
- ANA — negative
- Occasionally positive stool or urethral culture (Shigella, Salmonella, Yersinia, Campylobacter, Chlamydia)
- High incidence of HLA B27

Course and prognosis

- Usually self-limiting, but the arthritis can be severe and persistent
- Some may later develop ankylosing spondylitis

Management

- Antibiotics initially, if an organism is found
- Physiotherapy to maintain function of joints and muscles
- NSAIDs
- Sulfasalazine if joint problems persist

Conditions associated with HLA B27 positivity

- Ankylosing spondylitis — 95% of patients
- Reiter's syndrome
- Arthritis of inflammatory bowel disease and psoriasis
- Acute iridocyclitis
- Enthesitis related arthritis of older children
- Reactive arthritis following infection with Salmonella, Shigella, Yersinia Enterocolitica, Campylobacter

2.3 Rheumatic fever

General characteristics

- An inflammatory reaction in joints, skin, heart and CNS following a Group A haemolytic streptococcal infection
- Age generally over 3 years
- Both sexes, but girls more than boys

Revised Jones' criteria

Major manifestations
Carditis (severe pan-carditis can occur in first or subsequent attacks)
Polyarthritis (flitting)
Subcutaneous nodules
Chorea
Erythema marginatum

Minor manifestations
Fever
Arthralgia
Previous rheumatic fever and rheumatic heart disease
Raised acute phase (ESR, C-reactive protein
Prolonged PR interval on ECG

Plus supporting evidence of a preceding streptococcal infection

Throat swab positive for Group A Streptococcus, increased antistreptolysin 0 and anti-DNAase B titres

Investigations

- ESR — raised if not in cardiac failure
- Haemoglobin — may fall with chronic disease
- White blood count — normal or slight rise
- IgM rheumatoid factor — negative
- ANA — negative
- ECG — may be abnormal, prolonged PR
- Echocardiogram — may show valvular or myocardial dysfunction

Course and prognosis

- Average attack lasts 6 weeks
- High risk of recurrence in patients who do not receive adequate prophylaxis against streptococcal infection

Management

- Bed rest in the acute phase
- Penicillin to eradicate residual streptococcal infection
- Salicylate therapy
- Corticosteroids in patients with significant carditis
- Prophylactic oral or intramuscular penicillin after an attack required into adult life

2.4 Infectious arthritis

Viral

- Adenovirus, parvo virus, cmv, rubella, mumps, varicella

Lyme disease

- *Borrelia burgdorferi*

Bacterial

- Haemophilus (young), Staphylococcus, Streptococcus, Meningococcus, Gonococcus
- Mycobacteria — both typical and atypical

Fungal

- Blastomycosis, coccidiomycosis, cryptococcus
- *Histoplasma capsulatum*

Other

- Mycoplasma
- Guinea worm

Differential diagnosis of childhood arthritis

- Infections
- Post-infectious arthritides
- Mechanical, including hypermobility
- JIA
- Neoplasm including acute lymphoblastic leukaemia (ALL)
- Other autoimmune/vasculitic diseases
- Rheumatic fever

2.5 Notes on management of arthritis

Physiotherapy, occupational therapy (OT), podiatry, splinting

Arthritis causes contractures and the above are used to overcome this. The physiotherapist teaches active and passive joint movements aiming to maximize function and avoid contractures. Hydrotherapy is used in early disease. Splinting at night to prevent or help correct fixed flexion deformities. The podiatrist has a specific interest in foot care. The occupational therapists role is to maximize the child's functioning within as normal an environment as possible using aids/adaptations as needed.

Orthoses

- Orthoses are useful in helping to prevent contractures, in maintaining a good position if contractures have been repaired and in providing joint stability
- They are particularly useful in aiding individual children with mobility
- The type of orthoses depends on the child's individual needs

For example they may be ankle foot orthoses if there is just ankle and foot involvement, extending to the knee if the knee is involved. Should there be a scoliosis, thoracolumbar orthoses are available

Side-effects of commonly used drugs

NSAIDs — gastrointestinal (may need ranitidine, omeprazole), neurological (headaches, mood)

Steroids — bone (use calcium, vitamin D), growth, cataract, weight gain

Methotrexate — nausea (may need ondansetron). NB. Liver and bone marrow (requires monitoring of blood count and liver function)

Antinuclear antibodies

- Not diagnostic or specific for any particular disease
- React with various nuclear constituents

Causes of ANA positivity in children

- Systemic lupus erythematosus
- Juvenile idiopathic arthritis
- Chronic active hepatitis
- Scleroderma
- Mixed connective tissue disease
- Drugs, e.g. anticonvulsants, procainamide
- Epstein–Barr virus infection

---

3. CONNECTIVE TISSUE DISORDERS OF CHILDHOOD

3.1 Dermatomyositis

General characteristics

- Non-suppurative myositis with characteristic skin rash and vasculitis
- Girls more than boys
- Peak incidence 4–10 years of age

Clinical features

- Muscle pain and occasional tenderness
- Muscle weakness — limb, girdle, neck, palate, swallowing
- Oedema
- Skin rash — periorbital heliotrope eruption and oedema
- Deep red patches over extensor surface of finger joints (Gottron's patches), elbows, knees and ankle joints
- Vasculitis and skin ulceration
- Nail-fold and eyelid dilated capillaries
- Retinitis in some
- Myocarditis with arrhythmias can occur
- Arthralgia/arthritis with contractures
- Limited joint mobility
- Gastrointestinal dysfunction
- Pulmonary involvement
- Calcinosis (after 1–2 years)

Investigations

- ESR — usually normal
- Serum muscle enzymes (CK, LDH) — elevated
- EMG — shows denervation/myopathy
- Muscle biopsy shows inflammation and/or fibre necrosis and small-vessel occlusive vasculitis
- ANA — positive in some

Course and prognosis

- Variable
- Prognosis usually good with adequate treatment
- A small proportion can develop extensive muscle wasting, severe contractures and widespread calcinosis

Management

- Gentle physiotherapy and splinting, followed by more active physiotherapy as muscle inflammation subsides
- Corticosteroids in sufficient dosage to restore function and normalize enzymes
- Cytotoxic drugs cyclosporin, methotrexate, azathioprine, cyclophosphamide, if required
- Careful monitoring is essential, with particular attention to palate and respiratory function, as well as to possible gastrointestinal problems

3.2 Systemic lupus erythematosus

General characteristics

- Onset usually after 5 years of age
- Before puberty, female to male ratio is 3:1; after puberty it is 10:1
- Higher incidence in Blacks, Orientals, Asians, Native Americans and Latin Americans
- Can be associated with complement deficiencies C2 and C4
- Possible associations with HLA antigens HLA B8, DR2, and DR3

Clinical features

- General malaise
- Weight loss
- Arthralgia or arthritis
- Myalgia and/or myositis
- Fever
- Mucocutaneous lesions:
  - Malar rash
  - Papular, vesicular or purpuric lesions
  - Vasculitic skin lesions
  - Alopecia
  - Oral ulcers
  - Photosensitivity
- Renal disease common, even at onset
- Pulmonary — pleuritis, interstitial infiltrations
- Cardiac — pericarditis, myocarditis, Libman–Sacks endocarditis
- CNS involvement — seizures, headache, psychosis
- Cerebral dysfunction — blurred vision, chorea, transverse myelitis
- Gastrointestinal involvement — hepatosplenomegaly, mesenteric arteritis, inflammatory bowel disease
- Eye — retinitis, episcleritis, rarely, iritis
- Raynaud's phenomenon, occasionally

Investigations

- ESR — raised
- Haemoglobin — low: autoimmune haemolytic anaemia in some; anaemia of chronic disease
- Leucopenia — mainly lymphopenia
- Thrombocytopenia in some
- IgM rheumatoid factor — may be positive
- ANA — strongly positive
- Antibodies to double-stranded (ds) DNA usually present in 2/3
- Total haemolytic complement and its components low
- Anticardiolipin antibodies and lupus anticoagulant may be present

Course and prognosis

- Highly variable
- Relates closely to the extent and severity of systemic involvement
- Potential causes of death include infectious complications, including bacterial endocarditis
- Other problems include myocardial infarction, pulmonary fibrosis and renal failure
- Meticulous monitoring essential

Management

- Hydroxychloroquine for skin and joints
- Corticosteroids for systemically ill patients
- Cytotoxic drugs for serious intractable disease
- Antiplatelet drugs for thrombotic episodes

Revised criteria for the classification of systemic lupus erythematosus

A person shall be said to have systemic lupus erythematosus if any four or more of 11 criteria are present:

1. Malar rash
2. Discoid rash
3. Photosensitivity
4. Oral ulcers
5. Arthritis
6. Serositis:
   Pleuritis
   OR
   Pericarditis
7. Renal disorder:
   Persistent proteinuria
   > 0.5g/day
   OR
   Cellular casts

8. Neurological disorder:
   Seizures
   OR
   Psychosis
9. Haematological disorder:
   Haemolytic anaemia
   OR
   Leucopenia
   OR
   Lymphopenia
   OR
   Thrombocytopenia

10. Immunological disorder:
    (a) Positive LE cell preparation
    OR
    (b) Anti-DNA: antibody to native DNA in
    OR
    (c) Anti-Sm: presence of antibody to Sm nuclear
    OR
    (d) False-positive serological test for syphilis
11. Antinuclear antibody: An abnormal titre of ANA

3.3 Neonatal lupus

General characteristics

- Present in neonatal period, acquired transplacentally
- Associated with maternal autoantibodies (particularly Ro/La) and with maternal lupus or Sjögren's syndrome

Clinical features

- Rash — lesions of discoid lupus or subacute cutaneous lupus
- Congenital heart block — occasional endocardial fibroelastosis
- Thrombocytopenia
- Hepatic or pulmonary disease, haemolytic anaemia — uncommon

Investigations

- ANA — particularly Ro/La
- Thrombocytopenia, anaemia, leucopenia
- Platelet antibodies — positive Coombs test
- ECG

Course and prognosis

- Cutaneous and haematological manifestations transient
- Congenital heart block permanent
- Hepatic fibrosis occasional
- Some risk of systemic lupus erythematosus in teenage or adult years

Management

- Symptomatic for transient manifestations
- Heart block may require pacemaker

3.4 Behçet's syndrome

General characteristics

- A clinical triad of recurrent oral aphthous ulcers, recurrent genital ulcers and uveitis
- Male predominance
- High incidence in Japan, the Mediterranean and the Middle East

Clinical features

- Oral ulcers
- Genital ulcers
- Severe uveitis — may lead to glaucoma and blindness
- Arthritis
- Rash — skin hypersensitivity
- Bowel involvement
- Meningoencephalitis, brainstem lesions and dementia

3.5 Sjögren's syndrome

General characteristics

- Dry eyes (keratoconjunctivitis sicca)
- Dry mouth and carious teeth
- Parotitis
- May occur alone or in association with other rheumatic disease
- Occasional complication of renal disease or lymphoreticular malignancy

Scleroderma

Localized (majority of paediatric cases)

- Morphea:
  - Single patch
  - Multiple patches

- Linear:
  - Face, forehead and scalp (en coup de Sabre)
  - Limb (en bande)

Diffuse (systemic sclerosis/CREST (calcinosis cutis – Raynaud's phenomenon – [[o]esophageal hypomobility – sclerodactyly – telangiectasia))

- Rare in childhood; develop tightening of skin of hands, feet and face; systemic problems include respiratory, GI tract and renal disease

3.6 Overlap syndrome including mixed connective tissue disease

General characteristics

- Overlapping features of juvenile idiopathic arthritis, systemic lupus erythematosus, systemic sclerosis and dermatomyositis
- Affects particularly older girls

Clinical features

- Arthritis
- Tenosynovitis — both flexor and extensor tendons of fingers, causing contractures
- Raynaud's phenomenon — common
- Myositis
- Pleuropericardial involvement
- Dysphagia
- Parotid swelling

Investigations

- ESR — high
- Haemoglobin — often low

- White blood count — usually normal
- Platelets — can be low
- ANA — positive
- Anti-RNP antibodies in high titres indicate the designation of mixed connective tissue disease
- Anti-DNA antibodies — negative or in low titre
- IgM rheumatoid factor — occasionally positive

Course and prognosis

- Slowly develops over years
- May evolve into other recognizable conditions, such as sclerodactyly and, later, other features of systemic sclerosis or systemic lupus erythematosus

Management

- Mild disease managed with NSAIDs and/or antimalarials
- More severe disease may require corticosteroids, with or without a cytotoxic agent
- Careful monitoring required to detect signs of potentially serious systemic disease (e.g. nephritis)

4. CHILDHOOD VASCULITIS

Childhood vasculitis encompasses a wide range of clinical syndromes that are characterized by inflammatory changes in the blood vessels. The clinical expression of the disease and its severity depend on the type of pathological change, the site of involvement and the vessel size. The two most common forms seen in children are Henoch–Schönlein purpura and Kawasaki disease.

4.1 Henoch–Schönlein purpura

General characteristics

- Inflammation of small vessels, capillaries — pre- and post-capillary vessels
- May be precipitated by infection, particularly haemolytic streptococci
- Onset generally after the age of 3 years; there is a slight male predominance

Clinical features

- Petechiae
- Rash — urticarial lesions evolving into purpuric macules, usually on the legs, feet and buttocks
- Cutaneous nodules — particularly over the elbows and knees
- Localized areas of subcutaneous oedema that affect the forehead, spine, genitalia, hands and feet
- Arthritis — transient, involving large joints

724

- Gastrointestinal involvement — colicky abdominal pain and/or gastrointestinal bleeding
- Renal involvement — nephritis, occasionally nephrosis

Investigations

- ESR — normal or high
- Full blood count — normal
- Haematuria and/or proteinuria and/or casts
- IgA complexes in glomeruli and involved skin
- Serum IgA is often raised

Course and prognosis

- Episodes of Henoch–Schönlein purpura are self-limiting
- Recurrences occasionally occur
- Long-term morbidity related to renal involvement

Management

- Supportive care
- Corticosteroids in severe disease

4.2 Kawasaki disease (mucocutaneous lymph node syndrome)

General characteristics

- An acute febrile disease, first described in Japan after the 1940s
- Although now seen in all racial groups throughout the world, it appears to be more common in Orientals
- Occurs in young children, even before the first birthday, and has a slight male predominance

Investigations

- ESR — high
- Haemoglobin — lowered
- White blood count — raised
- Polymorph leucocytosis
- Platelets — raised
- ANA — negative
- IgM rheumatoid factor — negative
- Echocardiography — arteriograms

Diagnostic criteria

- Fever lasting 5 days or more
- Bilateral conjunctival injection
- Changes in lips and oral cavity

- Changes in extremities — reddening and oedema of palms and soles followed by desquamation
- Polymorphous erythematous rash
- Cervical lymphadenopathy

For diagnosis a fever and four features are required.

Clinical features

As in diagnostic criteria, plus:

- Irritability
- Pericarditis
- Valvular dysfunction
- Coronary artery disease
- Arthritis and/or arthralgia
- Gastrointestinal symptoms
- Urethritis
- Central nervous system problems — aseptic meningitis
- Iritis

Course and prognosis

- Acute and convalescent stage lasts up to 10 weeks
- Coronary aneurysms or widening in some 20% of cases
- Death due to coronary vasculitis causing myocardial infarction or rupture of an aneurysm occurs in about 1% of cases

Management

- Supportive care
- Careful observation to detect and manage complications
- Salicylate therapy
- Intravenous gammaglobulin

4.3 Polyarteritis nodosa

General characteristics

- A vasculitis affecting small- to medium-sized muscular arteries in either a generalized or cutaneous form
- Age range 3–16 years with equal sex distribution

Clinical features

- Fever
- Abdominal pain
- Arthralgia/myalgia

- Rash:
  - Petechial or purpuric in the generalized form, tender subcutaneous nodules and livedo reticularis in the cutaneous form
- Hypertension
- Renal involvement
- Neurological disease

Investigations

- ESR — high
- Haemoglobin — below 10 g/l
- Leucocytosis
- Urinary abnormalities
- ASOT — elevated in some
- Histology — focal necrosis in small- and medium-sized arteries

Course and prognosis

- Cutaneous form is usually benign but relapses may occur
- Prognosis is worse in the generalized form, depending on the organ involvement

Management

- Steroids — high dose (2 mg/kg per day) in the generalized form
- Steroids and immunosuppressants for severe cases
- Penicillin prophylaxis, if streptococcal aetiology is proved

4.4 Takayasu's disease (giant-cell arteritis)

General characteristics

- A panarteritis of the aorta and its large branches leading to thrombosis, stenosis or occlusion
- Primarily affects young adult women, but may occur in children
- More common in Orientals and Blacks

Clinical features

- Claudication — in the arms and also the legs, and absent pulses
- Myalgia
- Hypertension
- Malaise
- Fever

Investigations

- ESR — high
- Haemoglobin — low
- White blood count — neutrophil leucocytosis

- Using a combination of Doppler's and angiography it is possible to show occlusion, stenosis, or aneurysms

Course and prognosis

- Variable

Management

- Steroids with or without cytotoxic therapy
- Reconstructive surgery when the disease is inactive

4.5 Vasculitis with granuloma

Churg–Strauss syndrome

General characteristics

- A systemic necrotizing vasculitis of small arteries and veins, accompanying asthma and associated with eosinophilia

Clinical features

- Lung involvement — asthma, transient pulmonary infiltrates
- Rash — palpable purpuras and tender subcutaneous nodules
- Peripheral neuropathy
- Renal involvement — occasionally

Wegener's granulomatosis

General characteristics

- This also is a necrotizing granulomatous vasculitis of the upper and lower respiratory tracts, accompanied by glomerulonephritis

Clinical features

- Pulmonary granulomata
- Destructive granulomata of the ears, nose and sinuses
- Rash
- Glomerulonephritis
- Eye lesions

Special investigation

- Antineutrophil cytosolic antibodies

Management

- Combined therapy with steroids and cyclophosphamide

4.6 Differential diagnosis of childhood rheumatic disorders

- Infection
- Neoplasm
- Blood dyscrasias
- Mechanical anomalies, including injury
- Biochemical abnormalities
- Genetic and/or congenital anomalies
- Oddities do occur

5. MISCELLANEOUS ORTHOPAEDIC DISORDERS

Developmental dysplasia of the hip (DDH)

- Previously called 'congenital dislocation of the hip'
- 1:1,000 deliveries family history common, associations breech, spine abnormality, neuromuscular problem
- Varies from shallow acetabulum to full dislocation
- Commoner in females (5–10 times)
- Examination — Barlow and Ortolani's tests
- Radiology ultrasound (early), X-ray (later)
- Orthopaedic management with splinting/operation

Perthes disease

- Incidence 1:2000, males commoner (4:1), 10% of cases are bilateral
- Age at presentation 2–10 years
- Present with limp, may present with knee pain
- Pathology is of ischaemic necrosis of the femoral head involving the epiphysis and adjacent metaphysis.
- Diagnosis is by lateral X-ray of the appropriate hip joint (increased density and smaller femoral head)
- MRI shows early changes
- Differential diagnosis includes septic arthritis, osteomyelitis, transient synovitis, post fracture, neoplasia, slipped upper femoral epiphysis
- Association with congenital dislocation of the hip, mucopolysaccharidosis, achondroplasia and rickets
- Orthopaedic management

Slipped upper femoral epiphysis

- More common in boys, peak age 10–15, 20% bilateral
- Associated with obesity and microgenitalia, hypothyroidism, tall stature
- Usually presents with knee and hip pain
- Lateral X-ray of the hip diagnostic
- Orthopaedic management with pinning head/osteotomy
- Complications include premature epiphyseal fusion and avascular necrosis

Chondromalacia patellae

- Anterior knee pain after exercise
- Normal radiology
- Clark's sign — pain from patella pressure on quads contraction
- Management analgesia, physiotherapy and strapping
- Most do well

Osgood–Schlatter's disease

- Males more common
- Pain from tibial tuberosity with swelling (at the site of insertion of the patella tendon)
- Normal radiology
- Ultrasound may be useful
- Rest, then progressive mobilization
- Most do well

Reflex sympathetic dystrophy

- Autonomic nerve dysfunction in a limb results in severe immobilization due to pain
- Osteoporosis is associated
- Physiotherapy to remobilize is the best treatment

Hypermobility

- Commonest cause of musculoskeletal complaints in childhood
- Causes joint pain and swelling after exercise
- Improves with age
- Differential includes Ehlers–Danlos syndrome (skin fragility and hyperextensibility, and joint hyperextensibility), Marfan's syndrome
- Management is exercise to build up strength and reassurance

Irritable hip (transient synovitis)

- Age 2–10 years, boys more frequently than girls
- Limp or pain following viral illness
- Minimal systemic features
- Investigations include full blood count, ESR and X-ray of the hip joint (normal).
- Ultrasound may demonstrate a small effusion
- Resolves with analgesia, bed rest +/– traction within 7 to 10 days

Scoliosis (lateral curvature of the spine)

- Usually postural and easily correctable, e.g. due to leg-length discrepancy and corrected with a raised shoe
- Structural (curve plus rotation) is idiopathic or secondary, e.g. to hemivertebrae, cerebral palsy, neuromuscular, Marfan's, neurofibromatosis, tumour, TB

- Idiopathic — onset can be infantile (usually male), juvenile or adolescent (usually female)
- Diagnosis is radiological by X-ray or MRI
- Management is with exercising, bracing and occasionally surgery

Severe kyphoscoliosis (backward and lateral curvature of the spine) causes restriction of chest movement with alveolar hypoventilation, and secondary cardiorespiratory disease.

Toe walking

- Can be a normal finding up until age 3 years
- Neurological disorders include cerebral palsy, Duchenne muscular dystrophy, spinal cord problems, congenital tendo-Achilles shortening
- Leg-length discrepancy
- Habit

Foot drop

- Variety of causes
- Patient has a stepping gait and lifts the affected limb high to avoid scraping the foot on the floor
- They are unable to walk on their heel
- Possible causes
  - Lateral popliteal nerve palsy (look for signs of injury below and lateral to the affected knee)
  - Peroneal muscle atrophy
  - Poliomyelitis

6. OSTEOGENESIS IMPERFECTA

Osteogenesis imperfecta is a disorder of connective tissue characterized by bone fragility. The disease encompasses a phenotypically and genetically heterogeneous group of inherited disorders that result from mutations in the genes that encode for type 1 collagen. The disorder is manifest in the tissues in which the principal matrix is collagen, namely bone, sclerae and ligaments. The musculoskeletal manifestations vary from perinatal lethal forms, to moderate forms with deformity and a propensity to fracture to clinically silent forms with subtle osteopenia and no deformity, as discussed below

Osteogenesis imperfecta type 1

This is characterized by osteoporosis and excessive bone fragility, distinctly blue sclera and hearing loss. Autosomal dominant inheritance, 1:30,000 live births. Fractures may be obvious from birth. Hearing impairment due to otosclerosis affects most patients from the 5th decade, but is rare in the 1st decade. Some families have dentinogenesis imperfecta — with yellow transparent teeth which are fragile. There is spontaneous improvement with puberty. X-rays show generalized osteopenia, evidence of previous fractures and callus formation at the site of new bone formation. The skull X-ray shows Wormian bones.

Osteogenesis imperfecta type II

This lethal syndrome is characterized by low birth weight and typical X-ray findings of crumpled bones and beaded ribs. Autosomal recessive in a few cases, most being autosomal dominant new mutations. Affects 1:60,000 live births. 50% are stillborn, the remainder dying soon after birth from respiratory difficulty due to a defective thoracic cage. It is worth looking at a picture of the lethal form. X-rays show multiple fracture of the ribs, often beaded, and crumpled (accordion like) appearance of the long bones.

Osteogenesis imperfecta type III

This syndrome is characterized by severe bone fragility and multiple fractures in the newborn period which lead to progressive skeletal deformity. The sclera may be bluish at birth, but become less blue with age. Autosomal recessive with clinical variability suggesting genetic heterogeneity. Few patients survive into adult life. X-rays show generalized osteopenia and multiple fractures, without the beading of the ribs or crumpling of the ribs seen in type II.

Osteogenesis imperfecta type IV

This syndrome is characterized by osteoporosis leading to bone fragility without the other features of type 1. The sclera may be bluish at birth, but become less blue as the patient matures. Autosomal dominant inheritance. Variable age of onset and variable number of fractures, there is spontaneous improvement with puberty. X-rays show generalized osteopenia, and fractures, but these are generally less than the other forms of osteogenesis imperfecta.

Management

For osteogenesis imperfecta type II, no therapeutic intervention is helpful. For other forms, careful nursing of the newborn may prevent excessive fractures. Beyond the newborn period, aggressive orthopaedic treatment is the mainstay of treatment aimed at prompt splinting of fractures and correction of deformities. Genetic counselling is important. Reliable prenatal diagnosis is not available for all forms of osteogenesis imperfecta, although severely affected fetuses may be confidently recognized by X-rays, US scanning and biochemistry.

7. OSTEOPETROSIS

Osteopetrosis (marble bone disease, Albers–Schönberg disease) is characterized by a generalized increase in skeletal density. There are multiple types. The most important two are listed below:

Congenita — presents in infancy (autosomal recessive) with failure to thrive, hypocalcaemia, anaemia, thrombocytopenia and rarely fractures. Bone encroaching on the marrow cavity leads to extramedullary haemopoiesis. Optic atrophy and blindness common secondary to bone pressure. Diagnosis is by skeletal survey. Bone marrow transplant can be curative.

Tarda — presents in later childhood, usually with fractures, and manifestations are less severe and treatment is symptomatic.

8. HEMIHYPERTROPHY

This is often difficult to recognize. It may involve the whole of one side of the body, or be limited in extent, e.g. to just one leg. It may be congenital, in which case the tissues are structurally and functionally normal. It has been associated with mental retardation, ipsilateral paired internal organs and rarely with Wilms' tumours or adrenal carcinomas.

Hemihypertrophy can be confused with regional overgrowth secondary to neurofibromatosis type I, haemangiomas and lymphangiomas.

8.1 Beckwith–Wiedemann Syndrome (BWS)

A fetal overgrowth syndrome, mapped to gene locus 11p15.5. Clinically the three major features are pre- and/or postnatal overgrowth (>90th centile), macroglossia and abdominal wall defects, with minor defects of characteristic ear signs (ear lobe creases or posterior helical pits), facial naevus flammeus, hypoglycaemia, organomegaly and hemihypertrophy. The diagnosis is based on either: (1) three major features; or (2) two major plus three or more minor features.

Infants are more likely to be delivered prematurely, 35% before 35 weeks. Exomphalos occurs in 50% of cases. Hypoglycaemia, which is usually mild and transient, occurs in 50%. Deaths from BWS can occur in infancy and are mainly caused by problems related to prematurity or congenital cardiac defects (<10%). During childhood, the dysmorphic features become less apparent, although the macroglossia may cause feeding problems, problems with speech and occasionally with obstructive apnoea. Surgical tongue reduction may be required in severe cases. Overgrowth is most marked in the first few years and is associated with an advanced bone age. It tends to slow down in late childhood, and most adults are <97th centile. Hemihypertrophy occurs in 25% of cases. Visceromegaly is common and neoplasia occurs in 5%, most commonly with Wilms' tumour followed by adrenocortical carcinoma, hepatoblastoma and neuroblastoma, those children with hemihypertrophy being the most at risk. By adolescence, the majority lead a normal life. There is controversy about abdominal tumour screening which some centres advocate should be by regular abdominal palpation and others by regular ultrasound examination or both.

9. FURTHER READING

A Colour Atlas of Paediatric Rheumatology: Ansell BM, Rudge S, Schaller JG. Wolfe 1991.

Adolescent Rheumatology: Isenberg DA, Miller JJ. Martin Dunitz 1999.

Paediatric Orthopaedics: Mier RJ, Brower TJ. Kluwer Academic 1994.

Textbook of Pediatric Rheumatology: Cassidy JT, Petty RE, 4th edition. WB Saunders 2001.

Chapter 19
Statistics

Angie M Wade

CONTENTS

Statistics

1. STUDY DESIGN

1.1 Research questions

A research study should always be designed to answer a particular research question. The question usually relates to a specific population. For example:

- Does taking folic acid early in pregnancy prevent neural tube defects?
- Is a new inhaled steroid better than current treatment for improving lung function amongst cystic fibrosis patients?
- Is low birth weight associated with hypertension in later life?

Random samples of the relevant groups are taken. For example: pregnant women, cystic fibrosis patients, low and normal birth weight individuals.

Based on the outcome in the samples, inferences are made about the populations from which they were randomly sampled. Dependent on the nature of the data, averages, percentages or proportions may be calculated for the samples taken. Prevalence or incidence of a disease or occurrence may be of interest.

Prevalence is the number of cases within a defined population at a specified time, **incidence** is the number of new cases arising in a given period in a specified population. For example, diabetes has high prevalence but low incidence, whereas the common cold has low prevalence and high incidence.

For the research questions given above, the suitable summaries of the outcomes may be:

- The risk of neural tube defect (number of cases/number of women studied), compared to the offspring of those who do and don't take folic acid during pregnancy. The relative risk (risk in group taking folic acid/risk in those that take placebo treatment) would give a measure of how effective the intervention is in preventing neural tube defects.
- The difference in average lung function between those given the new steroid and those given standard therapy will provide a measure of the effectiveness of the new treatment compared to standard.
- The difference in percentages developing hypertension between those who were low and normal birth weight (sometimes known as the attributable risk reduction) would provide a useful summary measure.

Statistical analysis enables us to determine what inferences can be made. Studies are either experimental or observational.

1.2 Experimental studies

In experimental studies, individuals are assigned to groups by the investigator. For example, pregnant women will be assigned to take either folic acid or a placebo; cystic fibrosis patients will be assigned to either the new or current treatment. In both of these examples the second group is known as a control group.

Note that a control group does not necessarily consist of normal healthy individuals. In the second example the control group comprises cystic fibrosis patients on standard therapy.

Individuals should be randomized to groups to remove any potential bias. Randomization means that each patient has the same chance of being assigned to either of the groups, regardless of their personal characteristics. Note that random does not mean haphazard or systematic.

Experimental studies may be:

Double-blind: neither the patient, nor the researcher assessing the patients or the treating clinician, knows which treatment the patient has been randomized to receive

Single-blind: either the patient or the researcher/clinician does not know (usually the patient)

Unblinded (or open):   both the patient and the researcher/clinician know

Clinical trials are experimental studies.

1.3 Crossover studies

In a crossover study, each patient receives treatment and placebo in a random order. Fewer patients are needed because many between-patient confounders may be removed. For example, even though pairs of cystic fibrosis patients may be chosen and randomized to groups on the basis of their disease severity, this does not ensure that the groups will be of similar age or sex.

Crossover studies are only suitable for chronic disorders that are not cured but for which treatment may give temporary relief. There should be no carryover effect of the treatment from one treatment period to the next.

1.4 Observational studies

In observational studies the groups being compared are already defined (e.g. low and normal birth weight) and the study merely observes what happens.

Case-control, **cross-sectional** and **cohort** are particular types of observational studies that, respectively, consider features of the past, the present and the future to try and identify differences between the groups.

- If we take groups of individuals with and without hypertension with the aim of identifying different features in their past that might explain a causal route for the hypertension this is a **case-control** study.
- If we take groups of low and normal birth weight babies and follow them forward in time to see whether one group is more prone to hypertension then this is a **cohort** study.

The **relative risk** (RR) can be used as a measure of effect in a cohort study. A similar measure based on the odds (number of cases/number of non-cases) rather than risk (number of cases/number studied, i.e. cases and non-cases) in each group, known as the '**odds ratio**' (OR), is appropriate for case-control studies.

1.5 Confounding

Confounding may be an important source of error. A confounding factor is a background variable (i.e. something not of direct interest) that:

- is different between the groups being compared
and
- affects the outcome being studied

For example, in a study to compare the effect of folic acid supplementation in early pregnancy on neural tube defects, age will be a confounding factor if:

- either the folic acid or placebo group tends to consist of older women
and
- older women are more, or less, likely to have a child with a neural tube defect

When studying the effects of a new inhaled steroid against standard therapy for cystic fibrosis patients, disease severity will be a confounder if:

- one of the groups (new steroid/standard therapy) consists of more severely affected patients
and
- disease severity affects the outcome measure (lung function)

In the comparison of hypertension rates between low and not low birth weight, social class will be a confounder if:

- the low birth weight babies are more likely to have lower social class
and
- social class is associated with the risk of hypertension

If a difference is found between the groups (folic acid/placebo, new steroid/standard therapy and low/normal birth weight) we will not know whether the differences are, respectively, due to folic acid or age, to the potency of the new steroid or the severity of disease in the patient, or to birth weight or social class.

Confounding may be avoided by matching individuals in the groups according to potential confounders. For example, we could age-match folic acid and placebo pairs or deliberately recruit low and normal birth weight individuals from similar social classes. We could find pairs of cystic fibrosis patients of similar disease severity and randomly allocate one of each pair to receive the new steroid while the other receives standard therapy.

2. DISTRIBUTIONS

2.1 Types of data

Data may be either categoric (qualitative) or numeric (quantitative).

- With **categoric** variables each individual lies in one category
- **Numeric** data is measured on a number scale

Ranks give the order of increasing magnitude of numeric variables. For example:

Sample of seven readings:

| 2.3 | 5.0 | 3.9 | 1.3 | −2.1 | 1.3 | 4.2 |

In order of magnitude:

| −2.1 | 1.3 | 1.3 | 2.3 | 3.9 | 4.2 | 5.0 |

Ranks:

| 1 | 2.5 | 2.5 | 4 | 5 | 6 | 7 |

Note that there are seven values in the sample and the largest value has rank **7**. Where there are ties (for example, the two values 1.3), the ranks are averaged between the tied values.

The **mode** is the value that occurs most often. In the example above:

Mode = 1.3

The **median** is the middle value when the values are ranked. In the example above:

Median = 2.3

The **mean** is the arithmetic average. In the example above:

$$\text{Mean} = \frac{2.3 + 5.0 + 3.9 + 1.3 - 2.1 + 1.3 + 4.2}{7} = \frac{15.9}{7} = 2.27$$

2.2 Skewed distributions

The distribution of a set of values may be asymmetrical (skewed).

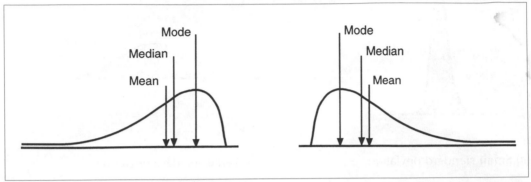

(a) Negative or downward or left skew   (b) Positive or upward or right skew

In a sample of this type the mean is 'pulled towards' the values in the outlying tail of the distribution and is unrepresentative of the bulk of the data.

Note that the skew is named according to the direction in which the tail points. In the left-hand diagram (a), the tail points to the left, to negative values and downwards.

If the distribution is skewed then the median is preferable as a summary of the data.

2.3 Normal distribution

The normal distribution is symmetrical and bell-shaped. The normal distribution is sometimes called the Gaussian distribution.

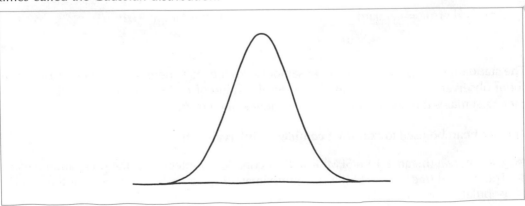

Normal distribution

2.4 Standard deviation

The standard deviation ($= \sqrt{\text{variance}}$) gives a measure of the spread of the distributor values. The smaller the standard deviation (or variance) the more tightly grouped the values.

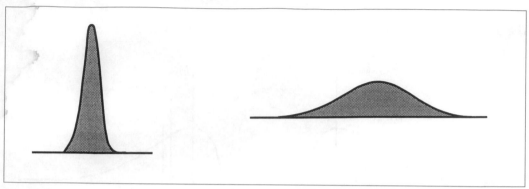

(a) Small standard deviation   (b) Large standard deviation

If the values are normally distributed, then:

- Approximately 68% of the values lie within ±1 standard deviation of the mean
- Approximately 95% of the values lie within ±2 standard deviations of the mean
- Exactly 95% of the values lie within ±1.96 standard deviations of the mean (hence 2.5% lie in each tail, total 5% outside range)

3. CONFIDENCE INTERVALS

3.1 Standard error (SE or SEM)

This is a measure of how precisely the sample mean approximates the population mean.

Standard error = $\dfrac{\text{standard deviation}}{\sqrt{n}}$ where n is the sample size

The standard error is smaller for larger sample sizes (i.e. as n increases, SEM decreases). The more observations in the sample (the bigger the value of n) the more precisely the sample mean estimates the population mean (i.e. the less the error).

The SEM can be used to construct **confidence intervals** (CI).

- The interval (mean ± 1.96 SEM) is a 95% confidence interval for the population mean.
- The interval (mean ± 2 SEM) is an approximate 95% confidence interval for the population mean.

- The interval (mean ± 1.64 SEM) is a 90% confidence interval for the population mean.

There is a 5%, or 0.05, or a 1 in 20, chance that the true mean lies outside the 95% confidence interval.

- 'We are 95% confident that the true mean lies inside the interval.'

There is a 10%, or 0.1, or 1 in 10, chance that the true mean lies outside the 90% confidence interval.

- 'We are 90% confident that the true mean lies inside the interval.'

Note the difference between the standard deviation and the standard error.

- Standard deviation (SD) gives a measure of the spread of the data values.
- Standard error (SE) is a measure of how precisely the sample mean approximates the population mean.

For example, FEV_1 is measured in 100 students. The mean value for this group is 4.5 litres with a standard deviation of 0.5 litres. If the values are normally distributed then:

approximately 95% of the values lie in the range $(4.5 \pm 2(0.5))$
$= (4.5 \pm 1)$
$= (3.5, 5.5$ litres$)$
Standard error $= \dfrac{0.5}{\sqrt{100}} = \dfrac{0.5}{10} = 0.05$

An approximate 95% confidence interval for the population mean FEV_1 is given by:

$(4.5 \pm 2(0.05)) = (4.5 \pm 0.1) = (4.4–4.6$ litres$)$

i.e. we are 95% confident that the population mean FEV_1 of students lies in the range 4.4–4.6 litres.

Confidence intervals can similarly be constructed around other summary statistics, for example the difference between two means, a single proportion or percentage, the difference between two proportions. The standard error always gives a measure of the precision of the sample estimate and is smaller for larger sample sizes.

4. SIGNIFICANCE TESTS

Statistical significance tests, or hypothesis tests, use the sample data to assess how likely some specified null hypothesis is to be correct. The measure of 'how likely' is given by a probability (p) value. Usually, the null hypothesis is that there is 'no difference' between the groups.

4.1 Null hypotheses and *p* values

To answer the research questions in section 1 we test the following null hypotheses:

- There is no difference in the incidence of fetuses with neural tube defects between the groups of pregnant women who do and do not take folic acid supplements
- Lung function is similar in cystic fibrosis patients who receive the new inhaled steroid when compared with the patients on current treatment
- Hypertension rates do not differ according to birth weight

Even if these null hypotheses were true we would not expect the averages or proportions in our sample groups to be identical. Because of random variation there will be some difference. The **p value** is the probability of observing a difference of that magnitude if the null hypothesis is true.

Since the *p* value is a probability, it takes values between 0 and 1. Values near to zero suggest that the null hypothesis is unlikely to be true. The smaller the *p* value the more significant the result:

- $p = 0.05$, the result is significant at 5%.

The sample difference had a 1 in 20 chance of occurring if the null hypothesis were true.

- $p = 0.01$, the result is significant at 1%.

The sample difference had a 1 in 100 chance of occurring if the null hypothesis were true.

Statistical significance is not the same as clinical significance. Although a study may show that the results from drug A are statistically significantly better than for drug B we have to consider the magnitude of the improvement, the costs, ease of administration and potential side-effects of the two drugs, etc. before deciding that the result is clinically significant and that drug A should be introduced in preference to drug B.

4.2 Significance, power and sample size

The study sample may or may not be compatible with the null hypothesis. On the basis of the study results, we may decide to disbelieve (or reject) the null hypothesis. In reality, the null hypothesis either is or is not true.

	Null hypothesis:	
Decision based on study results:	True	False
'Accept' null hypothesis	OK	(II)
'Reject' null hypothesis	(I)	OK

The study may lead to the wrong conclusions.

- A low (significant) *p* value may lead us to disbelieve (or reject) the null hypothesis when it is actually true — Box (I) above. This is known as a **type I error**.
- The *p* value may be high (non-significant) when the null hypothesis is false — Box (II) above. This is known as a **type II error**.

The **power** of a study is the probability (usually expressed as a percentage) of correctly rejecting the null hypothesis when it is false.

Larger differences between the groups can be detected with greater power. The power to identify correctly a difference of a certain size can be increased by increasing the sample size. Small samples often lead to type II errors (i.e. there is not sufficient power to detect differences of clinical importance).

In practice there is a grey area between accepting and rejecting the null hypothesis. The decision will be made in the light of the *p* value obtained. We should not draw different conclusions based on a *p* value of 0.051 compared with a value of 0.049. The *p* value is a probability. As it gets smaller the less likely it is that the null hypothesis is true. There is no sudden changeover from 'accept' to 'reject'.

4.3 Parametric and nonparametric tests

Statistical hypothesis tests are either parametric or nonparametric. Choosing the appropriate statistical test depends on:

- The type of data and its distribution
- Whether the data is paired or not

Parametric tests usually assume the data is normally distributed. Examples are:

- *T*-test (sometimes called 'Student's *t*-test' or 'Student's paired *t*-test')
- Pearson's coefficient of linear correlation

An unpaired (or 2-sample) *t*-test is used to compare the average values of two independent groups (e.g. patients with and without disease, treated versus placebo, etc.).

A paired (or 1-sample) *t*-test is used if the members of the groups are paired. For example, each individual with disease is matched with a healthy individual of the same age and sex; in a crossover trial the measurements made on two treatments are paired within individuals.

Nonparametric tests are usally based on ranks. Examples are:

- Wilcoxin
- Sign
- Mann–Whitney U
- Kendall's S
- Spearman's Rank Correlation
- Chi-squared (χ^2)

Chi-squared is used to compare proportions (or percentages) between two groups.

5. CORRELATION AND REGRESSION

Sometimes measurements are made on two continuous variables for each study subject, e.g. CD4 count and age, blood pressure and weight, FRC and height. The data can be displayed in a scatterplot.

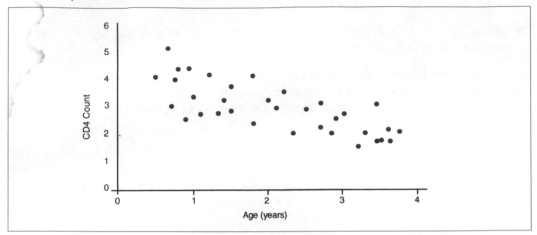

Scatterplot of CD4 count versus age

5.1 Correlation coefficients

The correlation coefficient (sometimes called Pearson's coefficient of linear correlation) is denoted by r and indicates how closely the points lie to a line.

r takes values between -1 and 1, the closer it is to zero the less the linear association between the two variables. (Note that the variables may be strongly associated but not linearly.)

Negative values of r indicate that one variable decreases as the other increases (e.g. CD4 count falls with age).

Values of -1 or $+1$ show that the variables are perfectly linearly related, i.e. the scatterplot points lie on a straight line.

Correlation coefficients:

- Show how one variable increases or decreases as the other variable increases
- Do not give information about the size of the increase or decrease
- Do not give a measure of agreement

Pearson's r is a parametric correlation coefficient. Spearman's Rank Correlation and Kendall's S are nonparametric correlation coefficients.

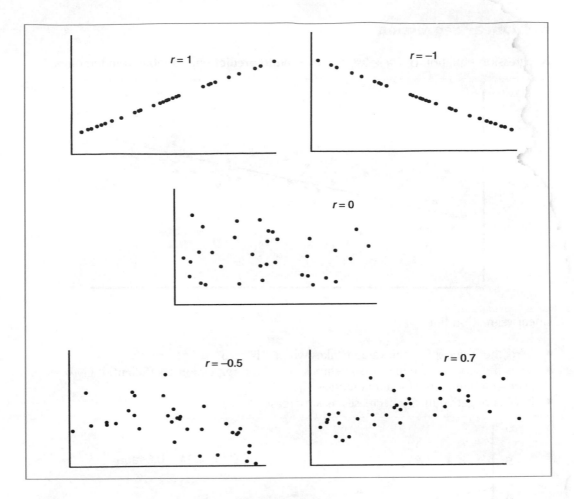

Scatterplots with different correlation coefficients

- Parametric correlation coefficients quantify the extent of any linear increase or decrease
- Nonparametric correlation coefficients quantify the extent of any tendency for one variable to increase or decrease as the other increases (for example, exponential increase or decline, increasing in steps, etc.)

A p value attached to a correlation coefficient shows how likely it is that there is no linear association between the two variables.

A significant correlation does not imply cause and effect.

5.2 Linear regression

A regression equation ($y = a + bx$) may be used to **predict** one variable from the other.

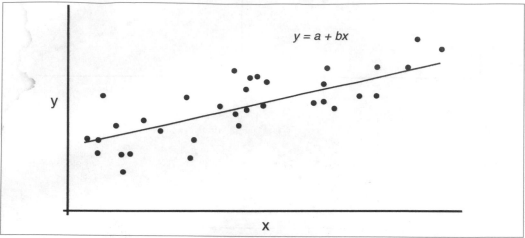

Linear regression line

- 'a' is the intercept — the value y takes when x is zero
- 'b' is the slope of the line — sometimes called the **regression coefficient**. It gives the average change in y for a unit increase in x
- If 'b' is negative then y decreases as x increases

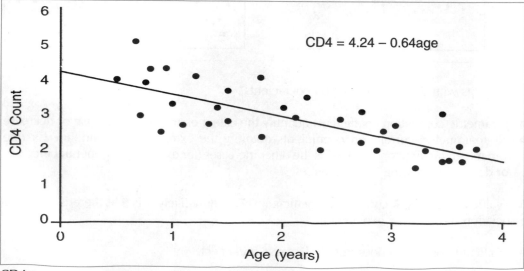

CD4 count versus age

If the units of measurement change then so will the regression equation. For example, if age is measured in months rather than years then the value of the slope (the average change in CD4 for a unit increase in age) will alter accordingly.

6. SCREENING TESTS

Screening tests are often used to identify individuals at risk of disease. Individuals who are positive on screening may be investigated further to determine whether they actually have the disease.

- Some of those who are screen-positive will not have the disease
- Some of those who have the disease may be missed by the screen (i.e. test-negative)

	Diseased	Disease-free
Screening test result:		
Positive — indicating possible disease	a	b
Negative	c	d

- **Sensitivity** is the proportion of true positives correctly identified by the test:

$$= \frac{a}{a+c}$$

- **Specificity** is the proportion of true negatives correctly identified by the test:

$$= \frac{d}{b+d}$$

- **Positive predictive value** is the proportion of those who test positive who actually have the disease:

$$= \frac{a}{a+b}$$

- **Negative predictive value** is the proportion of those who test negative who do not have the disease:

$$= \frac{d}{c+d}$$

Note that the positive and negative predictive values depend on the **prevalence** of the disease and may vary from population to population. Prevalence = proportion of diseased amongst the total ie $(a + c) = (a + b + c + d)$

Likelihood ratios

- **The likelihood ratio (LR) for a positive test result LR+** $= \dfrac{\text{sensitivity}}{1 - \text{specificity}}$

- **The likelihood ratio for a negative test result, LR–** $= \dfrac{1 - \text{sensitivity}}{\text{specificity}}$

Likelihood ratios may be multiplied by pre-test odds to give post-test odds. They are not prevalence-dependent.

Example

A screening test is applied to patients with and without disease X. Of 100 who have the disease, 60 test positive; of 200 without the disease, only 20 test positive.

The following table may be constructed:

Screening test result	Disease X	Disease-free
Positive (indicating possible disease)	60	20
Negative	40	180

Therefore, the following are true:

- Sensitivity = 60/100 = 0.6 or 60%
- Specificity = 180/200 = 0.9 or 90%
- LR+ = 0.6/(1–0.9) = 6
- LR– = (1–0.6)/0.9 = 0.44
- The positive predictive value is 60/(60 + 20) = 0.75 or 75% (i.e. 75% of those who test positive actually have the disease in this sample)
- The prevalence of the disease in this sample is ((60 + 40) (100 + 200)) = 0.33 or 33%

If a particular patient had a prior odds of 1.5 of having the disease (meaning that he or she is 1.5 times more likely to have the disease than not to have it) then 1.5/2.5 (or 60%) of patients of this type will have the disease). The **posterior odds** of the patient having the disease will thus be determined by the result of the screening test:

- If the test is positive (LR+) then the odds of having the disease will be 1.5 × 6 = 9
- If the test is negative (LR–), the odds will be 1.5 × 0.44 = 0.66

Note that, as expected, the odds of having the disease rise if the test is positive and fall if the test is negative.

A posterior odds of 9 means that the patient is nine times more likely to have the disease than not, which equates to a probability of 9/10 or 0.9 (as opposed to 0.6 before testing). A posterior odds of 0.66 equates to a probability of 0.66/1.66, or 0.4 (as opposed to 0.6 before testing).

7. FURTHER READING

An Introduction to Medical Research: Bland M, Oxford Medical Publications 1987.

Essentials of Medical Statistics: Kirkwood BR, Blackwell Scientific Publications 1988.

Practical Statistics for Medical Research: Altman DG, Chapman and Hall 1991.

Statistical Methods in Medical Research: Armitage P and Berry G, Blackwell Scientific Publications 1987.

17-OHP	17-OH progesterone
5-HT	5-hydroxytryptamine; serotonin
A–aDO_2	alveolar–arterial oxygen difference
ABPA	allergic bronchopulmonary aspergillosis
ABPM	ambulatory blood pressure monitoring
ABR	auditory brainstem response
ACE	angiotensin-converting enzyme
ACh	acetylcholine
ACTH	adrenocorticotropic hormone
AD	autosomal dominant
ADA	adenosine deaminase
ADH	antidiuretic hormone
ADHD	attention-deficit hyperactivity disorder
ADPKD	autosomal dominant polycystic kidney disease
AFI	amniotic fluid index
AFLP	acute fatty liver of pregnancy
AHG	anti-human globulin
AIDS	acquired immunodeficiency syndrome
AIHA	autoimmune haemolytic anaemia
ALA	aminolaevulinic acid
ALD	adrenoleucodystrophy
ALL	acute lymphoblastic leukaemia
ALT	alanine aminotransferase
AML	acute myelocytic leukaemia
AMN	adrenomyeloneuropathy
ANA	antinuclear antibody
ANT	alloimmune neonatal thrombocytopenia
APC	antigen-presenting cell
APLS	Advanced Paediatric Life Support [guidelines]
APTT	activated partial thromboplastin time
AR	autosomal recessive
ARF	acute renal failure
ARPKD	autosomal recessive polycystic kidney disease
ART	antiretroviral treatment
AS	aortic stenosis
ASA	American Standards Association
ASD	atrial septal defect

ASO	antistreptolysin O
ATG	anti-thymocyte globulin
ATM	ataxia-telangiectasia mutated gene
ATN	acute tubular necrosis
ATNR	asymmetrical tonic neck reflex
AV	atrioventricular
AVP	arginine vasopressin
AVSD	atrioventricular septal defect
BCAA	branch-chain amino acid
BCG	bacille Calmette–Guérin
BIE	bullous icthyosiform erythroderma
BMD	Becker muscular dystrophy
BMI	body mass index
BMT	bone marrow transplantation
BP	blood pressure
BPD	broncho-pulmonary dysplasia
BPSU	British Paediatric Surveillance Unit
BSAEP	brainstem auditory evoked potential
BSE	bovine spongiform encephalopathy
BT	Blalock–Taussig
Btk	Bruton's tyrosine kinase
BWS	Beckwith–Wiedemann syndrome
BWt	body weight
c/s	cycles per second
CA	choanal atresia
CAA	coronary artery aneurysms
CAH	congenital adrenal hypoplasia
CAL	café-au-lait
cALL	common ALL
cAMP	cyclic adenosine monophosphate
CAO	Child Assessment Order
CCAM	congenital cystic adenomatoid malformation
CD	cluster of differentiation; collecting duct
CDG	congenital disorders of glycosylation
CF	cystic fibrosis
CFA	cryptogenic fibrosing alveolitis
CFTR	cystic fibrosis transmembrane-conductance receptor
CG	Clinical Governance
CGD	chronic granulomatous disease

CHARGE	Coloboma, Heart disease, choanal Atresia, Retarded growth and development, Genital hypoplasia, and Ear abnormalities	DHEAS	dehydroepiandrosterone sulphate
		DHT	dihydrotestosterone
		DI	diabetes insipidus
		DIC	disseminated intravascular coagulation
CHD	congenital heart disease		
CHI	Commission for Health Improvement	DIOS	distal intestinal obstruction syndrome (formerly called 'MI equivalent')
CI	confidence interval		
CID	combined immunodeficiency	DKA	diabetic ketoacidosis
CJD	Creutzfeldt–Jakob disease	DLA	Disability Living Allowance
CK	creatine kinase	DMD	Duchenne muscular dystrophy
CK-MB	creatine kinase – membrane-bound	DMSA	dimercaptosuccinic acid
CLL	chronic lymphocytic leukaemia	DORV	double outlet right ventricle
CMC	chronic mucocutaneous candidiasis	DOT	directly observed therapy
CML	chronic myeloid leukaemia	DPPC	dipalmitoylphosphatidylcholine
CMT	Charcot–Marie–Tooth	DT	distal tubule
CMV	cytomegalovirus	DTPA	diethylenetriaminepenta-acetic acid
CNS	central nervous system; congenital nephrotic syndrome	DWM	Dandy–Walker malformation
CoA	coenzyme A		
COX	cyclo-oxygenase	EB	epidermolysis bullosa
CPAP	continuous positive-airways pressure	EBV	Epstein–Barr virus
CPK	creatine phosphokinase	ECF	extracellular fluid
CREST	Calcinosis cutis–Raynaud's phenomenon–[o]Esophageal hypomotility–Sclerodactyly–Telangiectasia	ECG	electrocardiogram
		ECHO	echocardiogram
		ECMO	extracorporeal membrane oxygenation
CRF	chronic renal failure	EDRF	endothelium-derived relaxing factor
CRH	corticotropin-releasing hormone	EEG	electroencephalogram
CRP	C-reactive protein	*ELA*	elastase gene
CSF	cerebrospinal fluid	ELBW	extremely low birth weight
CT	computed tomography	EM	erythema multiforme
CTFR	cystic fibrosis transmembrane regulator	EMG	electromyogram
		ENaC	epithelial sodium channel
CTG	cardio tacograph	EOG	electro-oculography
CVB	chronic villous biopsy	EPO	Emergency Protection Order; erythropoietin
CVID	common variable immunodeficiency		
CVS	chronic villous sampling	EPP	erythropoietic protoporphyria
CXR	chest X-ray	ERG	electroretinogram; electroretinography
D⁻	non-diarrhoea-associated HUS	ESM	ejection systolic murmur
D⁺	diarrhoea-associated HUS	ESR	erythrocyte sedimentation rate
DAF	decay accelerating factor	ESRF	endstage renal failure
DAMP	deficits in attention, motor control and perception	ETEC	enterotoxigenic *Escherichia. coli*
DDAVP	1-deamino-8-D-arginine vasopressin; desmopressin	FA	Freidreich's ataxia
		Fab	antigen-binding fragment of an immunoglobulin
DDH	development dysplasia of the hip		
DDT	dichlorodiphenyltrichloroethane	FACS	flow cytometric analysis
DEAFF	detection of early-antigen fluorescent foci	FAP	familial adenomatous polyposis
		FBC	full blood count

Fc	crystallizable fragment of an immunoglobulin	HA	haemolytic anaemia
FCV	forced vital capacity	HAART	highly active antiretroviral therapy
FDP	fibrin degradation factor	HACEK	*Haemophilus* spp. (*H. parainfluenzae, H. aphrophilus, H. paraphrophilus*), *Actinobacillus actinomycetemcomitans, Cardiobacterium hominis, Eikenella corrodons* and *Kingella kingae*)
FEF_{25-75}	forced expiratory fraction (25% being 75% empty)		
FENa	fractionated excretion of sodium		
FEV_1	forced expiratory volume in first second	Hb	haemoglobin
FFA	free fatty acids	HBcAg	hepatitis B core antigen
FFP	fresh-frozen plasma	HBeAg	hepatitis B e antigen
FGFR	fibroblast growth-factor receptor	HbF	fetal haemoglobin
FH	familial hypercholesterolaemia	HBsAg	hepatitis B surface antigen
FiO_2	fractional inspired oxygen	HCG	human chorionic gonadotropin
FISH	fluorescent *in situ* hybridization	HCV	hepatitis C virus
fl	femtolitre	HD	haemodialysis
FSGS	focal segmental glomerulosclerosis	HD	Hodgkin's disease
FSH	follicle-stimulating hormone	HDL	high-density lipoprotein
FVC	forced vitual capacity	HELLP	haemolysis, elevated liver enzymes, low platelets [syndrome]
		HFO	high-frequency oscillation
G 6-P	glucose 6-phosphate	HGPRT	hypoxanthine guanine phosphoribosyltransferase
G-CSF	granulocyte colony-stimulating factor		
G6PD	glucose 6-phosphate dehydrogenase	HHA	hereditary haemolytic anaemia
GA	general anaesthesia; glutaric aciduria	HHV	human herpesvirus
		Hib	*Haemophilus influenzae* b
GAG	glycosaminogen; glycosaminoglycans	HIE	hypoxic–ischaemic encephalopathy
		HIV	human immunodeficiency virus
Gal 1-PUT	galactose 1-phosphate uridyltransferase	HLHS	hypoplastic left heart syndrome
		HMSN	hereditary motor and sensory neuropathies
GBS	group B Streptococcus		
GCS	Glasgow Coma Score	HOCM	hypertrophic obstructive cardiomyopathy
GFR	glomerular filtration rate		
GH	growth hormone	HPA	human platelet alloantigen
GHRH	growth hormone-releasing hormone	HPL	human placental lactogen
G_i	inhibitory G-protein	HSCT	haematopoietic stem-cell transplantation
GIT	gastrointestinal tract		
G_M	mono-ganglioside	HSP	Henoch–Schönlein purpura
GM-CSF	granulocyte–monocyte colony-stimulating factor	HSV	herpes simplex virus
		hTLR	human Toll-like receptors
GN	glomerulonephritis	HUS	haemolytic–uraemic syndrome
GnRH	gonadotropin-releasing hormone	HVA	homovanillic acid
GnRHa	gonadotropin-releasing hormone analogues	i.m.	intramuscular
		i.v.	intravenous
G_s	stimulatory G-protein	ICF	intracellular fluid
GSD	glycogen storage disease	ICP	Integrated Care Pathway
GvHD	graft versus host defence	ICP	intracranial pressure
		IDL	intermediate-density lipoprotein
		IFN	interferon
		IGF	insulin-like growth factor

IGFBP-1	insulin-like growth factor binding protein-1		MCGN	mesangiocapillary glomerulonephritis
IL	interleukin		MCT	medium-chain triglyceride
INR	International Normalised Ratio		MCUG	micturating cystogram
Io	ionized		MCV	mean corpuscular volume
IRD	infantile Refsum disease		MDI	metered-dose inhaler
IRT	immune reactive trypsin		MELAS	mitochondrial encephalopathy, lactic acidosis, stroke-like episodes
ITP	idiopathic thrombocytopenic purpura		MEN	multiple endocrine neoplasia
IUGR	intrauterine growth retardation		Men C	meningitis C
IVA	isovaleric acidaemia		MERFF	myoclonic epilepsy, ragged red fibres
IVC	inferior vena cava		MG	myasthenia gravis
IVIG	intravenous immunoglobulin		MG-CSF	megakaryocyte colony-stimulating factor
JIA	juvenile idiopathic arthritis		MHC	major histocompatibility complex
JMML	juvenile myelomonocytic leukaemia (formerly known as juvenile chronic myeloid leukaemia, JCML)		MI	meconium ileus
			MIBG	metaiodobenzylguanidine
JVP	jugular venous pressure		MID	minimum intolerated dose
			MIF	Mullerian inhibiting factor
KD	Kawasaki's disease		MMA	methylmalonic acidaemia
kDa	kilodalton		MMF	mycophenolate mofetil
			MMR	measles, mumps, rubella
L/S	lecithin/sphingomyelin ratio		MPS	mucopolysaccharidosis
LAD	leucocyte-adhesion deficiency		MRI	magnetic resonance imaging
LBW	low birth weight		MSH	melanocyte-stimulating hormone
LCHAD	long-chain hydroxyacyl-CoA dehydrogenase		MSUD	maple-syrup urine disease
			MTD	maximum tolerated dose
LDH	lactate dehydrogenase		mtDNA	mitochondrial DNA
LDL	low-density lipoprotein		MUD	matched unrelated donor
LEA	local education authority			
LFT	liver function test		NADP	nicotinamide adenine dinucleotide phosphate
LGV	lymphogranuloma venereum		NADPH	reduced form of NADP
LH	luteinizing hormone		NAG	*N*-acetylglucosaminidase
LHRH	luteinizing hormone-releasing hormone		NAI	non-accidental injury
			NALD	neonatal adrenoleucodystrophy
LIP	lymphocytic (lymphocytic) interstitial pneumonitis		NBT	nitroblue tetrazolium
			NCL	neuronal ceroid–lipofuscinoses
LMBTS	left modified Blalock–Taussig shunt		NDI	nephrogenic diabetes insipidus
LoH	Loop of Henle		NEC	necrotizing enterocolitis
LRTI	lower respiratory tract infection		NHL	non-Hodgkin's lymphoma
LV	left ventricle		NICE	National Institute for Clinical Excellence
LYST	lysine tRNA gene			
			NK	natural killer [cell]
M-CSF	monocyte colony-stimulating factor		NKH	non-ketotic hyperglycinaemia
MAC	*M. avium complex*		NMDA	*N*-methyl-D-aspartate
MAG-3	mertiatide		NO	nitric oxide
MAS	meconium aspiration syndrome		NPPG	Neonatal and Paediatric Pharmacists Group
MCAD	medium-chain acyl-CoA dehydrogenase		NREM	non-rapid eye movement

NSAID	non-steroidal anti-inflammatory drug	PIVH	peri-intraventricular haemorrhage
NTM	non-tuberculous Mycobacteria	PKU	phenylketonuria
nv-CJD	new variant Creutzfeldt–Jakob disease	PLC	phospholipase C
		PNET	primitive neuroectodermal tumour
OA	oesophageal atresia; organic acidaemia	PNP	purine nucleoside phosphorylase
		PO_2	partial pressure of oxygen
OI	oxygenation index	PPD	purified-protein derivative
OM	otitis media	PPHN	persistent pulmonary hypertension of the newborn
OPV	oral polio vaccine	PPROM	preterm PROM
OR	odds ratio	PROM	prolonged rupture of membrane
ORS	oral rehydration solution	PS	pulmonary stenosis
ORT	oral rehydration therapy	PSM	presystolic murmur
OS	Omenn's syndrome	PT	prothrombin time; proximal tubule
OT	occupational therapist	PTH	parathyroid hormone
OTC	ornithine transcarbamylase	PTLD	post-transplantation lymphoproliferative disorder
PA	propionic acidaemia	PUJ	pelviureteric junction
PA	pulmonary artery	PUV	posterior urethral valve
PA	pulmonary atresia	PVL	periventricular leucomalacia
$PaCO_2$	arterial carbon dioxide tension		
PAF	platelet activating factor	r	correlation coefficient
PALS	Paediatric Advanced Life Support (guidelines)	RA	right aorta
		RAG	recombinase activating gene
PANDAS	psychiatric and neurological diseases associated with streptococcal infection	RAST	radioallergosorbent test
		RBP	retinol binding protein
		RCDP	rhizomelic chondrodysplasia punctata
PBG	porphobilinogenPCO polycystic ovarian syndrome	RCPCH	Royal College of Paediatrics and Child Health
PCP	*Pneumocystis carinii* prophylaxis; *Pneumocystis carinii* pneumonia	REM	rapid eye movement
		rhDNAase	recombinant human DNAase
PCR	polymerase chain reaction	RMBTS	right modified Blalock–Taussig shunt
PCT	porphyria cutanea tarda	RMS	rhabdomyosarcoma
PD	peritoneal dialysis; potential difference	ROP	retinopathy of prematurity
		RP	retinitis pigmentosa
PDA	patent ductus arteriosus; persistent ductus arteriosus; pulmonary disease anaemia	RR	relative risk
		RSV	respiratory syncytial virus
		RTA	renal tubular acidosis
PDH	pyruvate dehydrogenase	RV	residual volume; right ventricle
PEEP	positive end-expiratory pressure	RVH	right ventricular hypertrophy
PEFR	peak expiratory flow rate	RVT	renal vein thrombosis
PEG	polyethylene glycol	Rx	treatment
PET	positron-emission tomography		
PFT	pulmonary function test	s.c.	subcutaneous
PH	pulmonary hypertension	SA	surface area
PHA	phytohaemagglutinin	SaO_2	arterial oxygen saturation
PHVD	post-haemorrhagic ventricular dilat[at]ion	SAP	serum amyloid P
		SBE	suspected bacterial endocarditis
PICU	paediatric intensive-care unit	SBR	serum bilirubin
PIE	pulmonary interstitial emphysema	SCD	sickle-cell disease
PIF	peak inspiratory flow		

SCID	severe combined immunodeficiency disorder	TORCH	Toxoplasmosis, Other (congenital syphilis and viruses), Rubella, Cytomegalovirus, and Herpes simplex virus
SCBU	special care baby unit		
SD	standard deviation		
SE (SEM)	standard error of the mean	TPN	total parenteral nutrition
SEB	staphylococcal enterotoxin-B	TRH	thyrotropin-releasing hormone
SEC	staphylococcal enterotoxin-C	TRP	tubular reabsorption of PO_4
SENCO	special educational needs co-ordinator	TSE	transmissible spongiform encephalopathies
SGA	small for gestational age	TSH	thyroid-stimulating hormone
SHBG	sex-hormone binding globulin	TS	tuberous sclerosis
SIADH	syndrome of inappropriate ADH [secretion]	TSS	toxic-shock syndrome
		TT	thrombin time
SIDS	sudden infant death syndrome	TTP	thrombotic thrombocytopenic purpura
SIRS	systemic inflammatory response syndrome		
SLE	systemic lupus erythematosus	UAC	umbilical artery catheterisation
SLO	Smith–Lemli–Opitz	UCCS	uncooked cornstarch
SMA	spinal muscular atrophy	UCD	urea cycle defects
SOL	space occupying lesion	UDP	uridine diphosphate
SPA	supra pubic asparate	URTI	upper respiratory tract infection
SPEA	streptococcal pyrogenic exotoxin A	US	ultrasound
SRNS	steroid-resistant nephrotic syndrome	UTI	urinary tract infection
SSNS	steroid-sensitive nephrotic syndrome		
SSPE	subacute sclerosing panencephalitis	VACTERL	vertebral, anal, cardiac, TOF, ears, renal, limb
SSRI	serotonin-reuptake inhibitor	VATS	video-assisted thoracic surgery
STD	sexually transmitted disease	VER	visual evoked response
SVC	superior vena cava	VF	ventricular fibrillation
SVT	supraventricular tachyarrhythmia	VI	ventilation index
SWS	slow-wave sleep	VIP	vasoactive intestinal peptide
		VLBW	very low birth weight
TAPVC	total anomalous pulmonary venous connection	VLCAD	very long-chain acyl-CoA dehydrogenase
TAPVD	total anomalous pulmonary venous drainage	VLCFA	very long chain fatty acid
		VLDL	very low-density lipoprotein
TAR	thrombocytopenia and absent radius (syndrome)	VMA	vanillylmandelic acid
		VQ	ventilation–perfusion
TB	tuberculosis	VSD	ventricular septal defect
TBW	total body water	VT	ventricular tachyarrhythmia
TCR	T-cell receptor	VUR	vesicoureteric
TD	travellers' diarrhoea	vWD	von Willebrand's disease
TFT	thyroid function test	vWF	von Willebrand factor
TGA	transposition of great arteries	VZV	varicella zoster virus
T_{H1}	T-helper cell, subset 1		
THC	total haemolytic complementTMS tandem mass spectrometry	WAGR	Wilms' tumour, Aniridia, Genitourinary abnormalities, mental Retardation
TNF	tumour-necrosis factor	WAS(P)	Wiskott–Aldrich syndrome (protein)
TOBI	tobramycin for inhalation	WBC	white blood cell
TOF	tracheo-oesophageal fistula		

WCC	white [blood] cell count	XR	X-linked recessive
WPW	Wolff–Parkinson–White	XRI	X-linked recessive icthyosis
XALD	X-linked adrenoleucodystrophy		
XD	X-linked dominant	Zap	zymosan-activated plasma
XLA	X-linked agammaglobulinaemia	ZIG	zoster immunoglobulin
XLP	X-linked lymphoproliferative syndrome	ZS	Zellweger's syndrome

Index